MW00843658

The SAGES Atlas of Robotic Surgery

Yuman Fong • Yanghee Woo
Woo Jin Hyung • Clayton Lau
Vivian E. Strong
Editors

The SAGES Atlas of Robotic Surgery

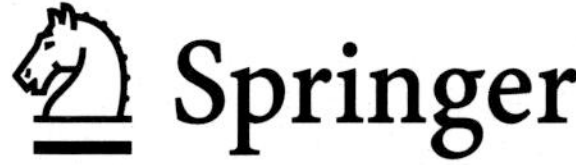

Editors
Yuman Fong
Department of Surgery
City of Hope National Medical Center
Duarte, CA
USA

Yanghee Woo
Department of Surgery
City of Hope National Medical Center
Duarte, CA
USA

Woo Jin Hyung
Robotic Surgery
Yonsei University Health System
Seoul
South Korea

Clayton Lau
Department of Surgery
Division of Urology and Urologic Oncology
City of Hope National Medical Center
Duarte, CA
USA

Vivian E. Strong
Department of Surgery
Gastric and Mixed Tumor Service
Memorial Sloan Kettering Cancer Center
New York, NY
USA

ISBN 978-3-319-91043-7 ISBN 978-3-319-91045-1 (eBook)
https://doi.org/10.1007/978-3-319-91045-1

Library of Congress Control Number: 2018948826

Printed on acid-free paper

This Springer imprint is published by the registered company Springer Nature Switzerland AG
The registered company address is: Gewerbestrasse 11, 6330 Cham, Switzerland

This book is dedicated to the memory of Jeffrey Ying (1954–2017).

I first met him on the Fourth of July 2014, at a picnic he and his wife Renee were throwing to celebrate the birth of our nation. My wife and I were new to Southern California and were invited because of who Jeffrey was: generous, welcoming of any new neighbor, and always sharing and celebrating life.

Jeffrey was an engineer and founder of the I/O Controls Corporation. In business he was known as an entrepreneur, an innovator, and a leader. He held more than 100 patents. He believed in science and engineering for the betterment of mankind. In his work and through his inventions, he has touched the lives of many.

For those who knew him, he was always the most interesting man in the room. He lived life to the fullest and was accomplished in so many areas outside of work. Whatever he did, he did the utmost. He was the first Chinese pilot from Taiwan to circumnavigate the globe in a single engine aircraft, when he and Renee performed the feat in 2010.

Jeffrey was also kind, loyal, compassionate, and generous. He and his wife Renee started the 12K Foundation to fund education for orphans in Tibet. They were also generous in support of medical research directed at engineering new cancer therapies.

We are happy to have known him and continue to be inspired by him.

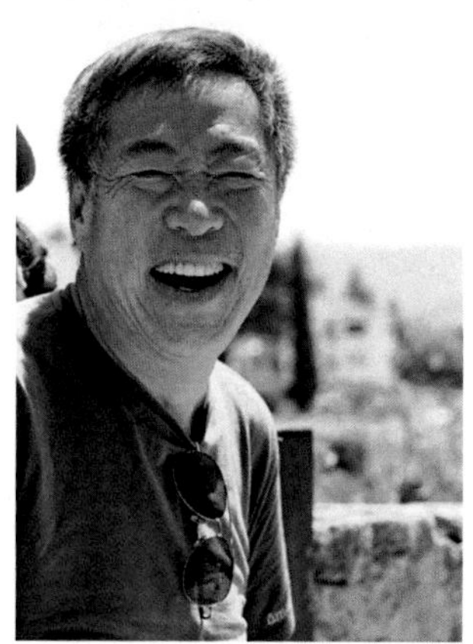

"Always be curious and adventurous; keep the heart of a child inside and fill it up with joy and peace, and be the best you can be (Jeffrey Ying)."

Preface

Robotic Surgery as the Natural Evolution of Minimally Invasive Surgery

Minimally invasive surgery (MIS) was largely restricted to diagnostic procedures until the second half of the twentieth century. Improving instrumentation, particularly in energy devices for sealing and in stapling devices for anastomosis of luminal organs, prompted rapid development of laparoscopy in the end of the last century. The first laparoscopic cholecystectomy was performed in 1985 [1] and within a decade was the standard of care [2]. The first laparoscopic colectomies were performed in 1990 and now are accepted as standard [3]. Many operations, including complex esophageal, liver, lung, and endocrine procedures, are now routinely performed using laparoscopic approaches and to the benefit of many patients. Robotic surgery, introduced to surgeons at the beginning of the twenty-first century, is the natural evolution of this MIS revolution. Using computer control of the MIS instruments, robotic surgery offers many potential advantages including improved visibility, easily controlled articulated instruments, and superb ergonomics. Complex tasks such as suturing that have challenged the laparoscopic surgeon are now easily within reach of the robotic MIS surgeon. The surgical robot has evolved from a single-purpose robot to a true surgical instrument with many potential operations. Over three million operations of many types have been performed with the assistance of the surgical robot.

The evolution of robotic surgery is reminiscent of what transpired in the evolution of industrial robots in the mid-twentieth century. Industrial robots were born as necessary safety tools for nuclear engineering. In the 1940s, mechanical teleoperators were created for handling dangerous radioactive materials. In the 1950s, computer controllers were added to the tele-manipulators to improve reliability and ergonomics. In the 1960s, General Motors deployed the first Unimation® robots in their automotive factories. In the early days, these robots were put to work just stacking boxes and unloading trucks. This is reminiscent of the first robots that arrived in the operating room. In 1992, Computer Motion Inc. brought forth the operative robot "Automated Endoscopic System for Optimal Positioning (AESOP)," which did not drive any surgical interventional instrument. AESOP was a single-purpose camera holder that reliably held and moved the laparoscopic camera, improving visualization of the MIS operation.

Industrial robots are now well advanced. Robots are now used autonomously for many of the essential steps in welding and assembling the more than 70 million vehicles produced yearly. Robots are even used to autonomously drive cars here on Earth and on Mars [4]. Most importantly, there is now general public acceptance of robotics for manufacturing and transportation.

Surgical robots are now mainly used as mechanical teleoperators in the surgical suite, allowing rapid and precise movement of the laparoscope within and between multiple operating fields. The surgical robotic tele-manipulator is also used to drive an increasingly diverse number of instruments to facilitate accessibility and performance of increasingly complex MIS tasks. We are now at a pivotal point in the field when a technology is about to transform from a tool for innovators and experts to a tool for general practitioners. To facilitate general deployment, teaching tools are necessary including comprehensive atlases such as the current volume. This book is a step-by-step guide to document the current state of the field, to increase accessibility for those venturing in the field, and to improve the safety of procedures. Ultimately, the goal is to improve outcomes for patients undergoing such procedures by providing an easy to understand, illustrated atlas of robotic surgery.

This book outlines the basics of successfully organizing, initiating, and running a robotic program. Details regarding technical, financial, and medico-legal aspects are presented, including room design and surgical team needs. This section is intended to help efficiently set up and start a robotic program. The economic cost of robot-assisted surgery is a major and consistent factor contributing to inertia against adoption [5]. Mitigating the higher cost is an essential component to the routine adoption of robotic surgery. We hope this section of the book will alert readers to the avoidable inefficiencies and wasted costs in the initial phase of launching a new program.

Safety is an important issue since extensive operations are being performed through 8 mm incisions. In cases where emergencies arise, it is critical to have meticulously rehearsed plans for urgent or emergent conversion to ensure life-saving interventions. These are described in chapters on workflow (Chap. 7) and emergencies (Chap. 9).

We then present technical steps and detailed pearls of 34 operations that are routinely performed, with room setup and instrument usage, as well as technical steps. The operations presented range from surgery in the oral pharynx to pelvic operations. Some of these, such as prostatectomy, colectomy, cholecystectomy, pulmonary resection, and gynecologic procedures, are well established and are the standard procedures for the organ involved. Some procedures described, such as radical gastrectomies, pancreatectomies, and trans-oral surgery, are emerging procedures that we anticipate will become important in the field. For some of the most complex operations, such as pancreaticoduodenectomy, we detail descriptions by more than one group to show variations in procedure.

The field of robotics is both dynamic and rapidly evolving. Many new operations are being invented and improvements in current operative technique will develop with wider deployment and increasing input from more robotic surgeons, as well as from improvements in robots and instrumentation. We hope that the reader will see our book as a living work that our robotic surgical community will shape together. If you have new variations of the current procedures or a new procedure that is becoming popularized, please let us know so we can plan to include it in the next edition.

The future for robotic MIS surgery is bright. However, for most of the operations performed by a robotic approach, there is a perception that it takes longer and costs more, especially at the initiation of a new program. Most cars in the world are created by robots because *quality is more consistent, production is faster, and it costs less*. Interventional radiologic procedures are rarely debated even when initial costs are steep because the procedures are clearly more efficient and significantly reduce morbidity. For common low-intensity robotic operations, we need to make them safer, faster, cheaper, or easier [6].

For high-end technical operations, technical enhancements including better instrumentation and workflows that enable improvements in accessibility or outcome are critical to growing this application. As physicians, we tirelessly aim to improve the learning curve for established and emerging techniques, improve outcomes for our patients, and most of all help our patients return to normal and productive lives. We hope this atlas will contribute to all of these goals.

This book is intended for anyone who plans to incorporate robotically assisted surgery into their portfolio of practice. We hope this will include surgeons, nurses, and other operating room personnel, as well as administrators and engineers. A work like this is only possible because of the contributions of many. The authorship of this work includes experienced surgical oncologists, general surgeons, thoracic surgeons, gynecologic oncologists, urologists, transplantation specialists, anesthesiologists, architects, and attorneys. We thank them for their contributions and efforts to collaborate in the creation of this comprehensive and special work.

We also thank our teachers, residents, clinical fellows, and colleagues who have shared their knowledge and experience with us. We thank our patients who inspire us to be superior clinicians, who inspire us to constantly strive to improve the field. We thank our editor at Springer Lee Klein. Finally, we thank our families, particularly Nicole, Christy, James, Jonathan, Jungwon, Boyun, and Seokwoo, for the patience and support they have given us daily for our clinical work, and then to complete a work such as this.

Duarte, CA, USA Yuman Fong
Duarte, CA, USA Yanghee Woo
Seoul, South Korea Woo Jin Hyung
Duarte, CA, USA Clayton Lau
New York, NY, USA Vivian Strong

References

1. Blum CA, Adams DB. Who did the first laparoscopic cholecystectomy? J Minim Access Surg. 2011;7(3):165–8.
2. Fong Y, Brennan MF, Turnbull A, Colt DG, Blumgart LH. Gallbladder cancer discovered during laparoscopic surgery. Potential for iatrogenic tumor dissemination. Arch Surg. 1993;128(9):1054–6.
3. Blackmore AE, Wong MT, Tang CL. Evolution of laparoscopy in colorectal surgery: an evidence-based review. World journal of gastroenterology. 2014;20(17):4926–33.
4. Baruch J. Steer driverless cars towards full automation. Nature. 2016;536(7615):127.
5. Patti JCO, Barrows C, Velanovich V, Moser AJ. Current economic analysis of robotic pancreas and liver surgery. Hepatobiliary Surg Nutr. 2017. In press.
6. Fong Y, Woo Y, Giulianotti PC. Robotic surgery: the promise and finally the progress. Hepatobiliary Surg Nutr. 2017;6(4):219–21.

Contents

Part I History and Basics of Robotic Surgery

1 **History of Robots and Robotic Surgery** ... 3
Paolo Fiorini

2 **Robotic Operating Rooms** ... 15
Jeffrey Berman, Emile Dajer, and Yuman Fong

3 **Developing a Robotic Surgery Program** ... 29
Pedro Recabal Guiraldes and Vincent P. Laudone

4 **Legal Aspects of Setting Up a Robotic Program** ... 37
Martin B. Adams and Glenn W. Dopf

5 **Financial Considerations in Robotic Surgery** ... 45
Nikhil L. Shah, Rajesh G. Laungani, and Matthew E. Kaufman

6 **Visualization in Robotic Surgery** ... 53
Mahdi Azizian, Ian McDowall, and Jonathan Sorger

7 **Workflow in Robotic Surgery** ... 67
Olivia R. Enright and Michael G. Patane

8 **Anesthetic Implications of Robotic Surgery: Positioning and Access** ... 71
John L. Raytis, Yuman Fong, and Michael W. Lew

9 **Urgent and Emergent Conversions in Robotic Surgery** ... 79
Abigail J. B. Fong and Yuman Fong

10 **Hybrid Robot-Assisted Surgery** ... 89
Aaron Lewis, Yanghee Woo, and Yuman Fong

Part II Urologic Procedures

11 **Robot-Assisted Partial Nephrectomy** ... 103
Jaspreet Singh Parihar and Clayton Lau

12 **Robot-Assisted Radical Prostatectomy** ... 113
Bertram Yuh and Greg Gin

13 **Robot-Assisted Adrenalectomy** ... 127
Jaspreet Singh Parihar and Clayton Lau

14 **Robotically-Assisted Laparoscopic Radical Cystoprostatectomy and Anterior Exenteration** . . . 131
Ali Zhumkhawala, Jonathan N. Warner, and Kevin Chan

15 **Robotic Pelvic and Retroperitoneal Lymph Node Dissection** . . . 159
Steven V. Kardos and Jonathan Yamzon

Part III Gynecologic Procedures

16 **Hysterectomy with Bilateral Salpingo-Oophorectomy** . . . 169
Ernest S. Han and Stephen J. Lee

17 **Radical Hysterectomy** . . . 181
Brooke A. Schlappe, Mario M. Leitao Jr., and Yukio Sonoda

18 **Robotically-Assisted Sacrocolpopexy** . . . 193
Steven Minaglia and Maurice K. Chung

Part IV Gastrointestinal Procedures

19 **Total Gastrectomy** . . . 209
Luke V. Selby and Vivian E. Strong

20 **Radical Distal Subtotal Gastrectomy and D2 Lymphadenectomy for Gastric Cancer** . . . 219
Yanghee Woo and Woo Jin Hyung

21 **Multiport and Single-Site Robotic Cholecystectomy** . . . 233
Eric Kubat, Dan Eisenberg, and Sherry M. Wren

22 **Colectomy** . . . 249
Kurt Melstrom

23 **Robotic Total Colectomy** . . . 263
Patricio B. Lynn, Manuel Maya, and Julio Garcia-Aguilar

24 **Robotic Low Anterior Resection** . . . 273
John V. Gahagan and Alessio Pigazzi

25 **Transanal Excision** . . . 281
Sam Atallah and Elisabeth C. McLemore

26 **Robotic Distal Pancreatectomy** . . . 295
Anusak Yiengpruksawan

27 **Robotic Pancreatoduodenectomy** . . . 311
Pier Cristoforo Giulianotti and Federico Gheza

28 **Robotic Pylorus-Preserving Pancreaticoduodenectomy** . . . 319
Sharona B. Ross, Darrell J. Downs, Iswanto Sucandy, and Alexander S. Rosemurgy

29 **Liver Resection: Right Lobectomy** . . . 335
Pier Cristoforo Giulianotti and Pablo Quadri

30 **Robotic Partial Hepatectomy** . . . 343
Susanne G. Warner and Yuman Fong

31 **Robot-Assisted Roux-en-Y Gastric Bypass** . . . 355
Vivek Bindal and Enrique E. Elli

32 **Robotic Roux-en-Y Gastric Bypass** 365
Michele L. Young and Keith Chae Kim

33 **Robotic Operations for Gastroesophageal Reflux Disease** 379
Daniel H. Dunn, Eric M. Johnson, Tor C. Aasheim, and Nilanjana Banerji

34 **Heller Myotomy** 397
Boris Zevin and Kyle A. Perry

Part V Thoracic Procedures

35 **Robotically-Assisted Minimally Invasive Esophagectomy (RAMIE): The Ivor Lewis Approach** 409
Fernando M. Safdie, Nicholas R. Hess, and Inderpal S. Sarkaria

36 **Robotic Pulmonary Resections** 425
Jae Y. Kim

37 **Robotic Mediastinal Surgery** 435
Boris D. Hristov, Prasad S. Adusumilli, and Bernard J. Park

Part VI Other Procedures

38 **Transoral Robotic Surgery** 445
Robert Kang, Thomas Gernon, and Ellie Maghami

39 **Robotically-assisted Ventral Hernia Repair** 453
Ioannis Konstantinidis and Byrne Lee

40 **Inguinal Hernia Repair** 457
Kamaljot S. Kaler, Simone L. Vernez, and Thomas E. Ahlering

41 **Robotic Transaxillary Thyroidectomy: A Modified Protocol for the Western Medical Community** 465
Sang-Wook Kang, Emad Kandil, and Woong Youn Chung

42 **Thyroidectomy: Robotic Facelift Approach** 479
Jonathan H. Dell, William S. Duke, and David J. Terris

43 **Transaxillary Robotic Modified Radical Neck Dissection** 489
Eun Jeong Ban and Woong Youn Chung

Index 501

Contributors

Tor C. Aasheim, MD Department of Surgery, Abbott Northwestern Hospital, Minneapolis, MN, USA

Martin B. Adams, JD Dopf, P.C., New York, NY, USA

Prasad S. Adusumilli, MD Thoracic Service, Department of Surgery, Memorial Sloan Kettering Cancer Center, New York, NY, USA

Thomas E. Ahlering, MD Department of Urology, University of California, Irvine School of Medicine, Urologic Oncology & Robotic Surgery, Irvine, Orange, CA, USA

Sam Atallah, MD Professor of Surgery, University of Central Florida—College of Medicine, Orlando, FL, USA

Chair, Department of Colorectal Surgery, Florida Hospital, Orlando, FL, USA

Director, Colorectal Surgery, Oviedo Medical Center, Orlando, FL, USA

Mahdi Azizian, PhD Image-Guided Robotics, Intuitive Surgical, Sunnyvale, CA, USA

Nilanjana Banerji, MS, PhD Neuroscience and Rehabilitation Research, Abbott Northwestern Hospital, Minneapolis, MN, USA

Eun Jeong Ban, MD Department of Surgery, Yonsei University College of Medicine, Seoul, South Korea

Jeffrey Berman, AIA, ACHA Jeffrey Berman Architect, New York, NY, USA

Vivek Bindal, MS, FNB Institute of Minimal Access, Metabolic and Bariatric Surgery, Sir Ganga Ram Hospital, New Delhi, India

Kevin Chan Division of Urology and Urologic Oncology, Department of Surgery, City of Hope Comprehensive Cancer Center, Duarte, CA, USA

Maurice K. Chung, MD, RPh Midwest Regional Center of Excellence for Endometriosis, Pelvic Pain and Bladder Control, Lima, OH, USA

Woong Youn Chung, MD, PhD Department of Surgery, Yonsei University College of Medicine, Seoul, South Korea

Emile Dajer Jeffrey Berman Architect, New York, NY, USA

Jonathan H. Dell, DO Department of Otolaryngology-Head and Neck Surgery, Augusta University, Augusta, GA, USA

Glenn W. Dopf, JD, LLM Dopf, P.C., New York, NY, USA

Darrell J. Downs, BS Department of Surgery, Florida Hospital Tampa, Tampa, FL, USA

William S. Duke, MD Department of Otolaryngology, MultiCare Health System, Tacoma, WA, USA

Daniel H. Dunn, MD Department of Surgery, Abbott Northwestern Hospital, Minneapolis, MN, USA

Dan Eisenberg, MD Department of Surgery (General Surgery), Stanford University School of Medicine, Palo Alto Veterans Administration Health Care Center, Palo Alto, CA, USA

Enrique E. Elli, MD Department of Surgery, Mayo Clinic, Jacksonville, FL, USA

Olivia R. Enright, MSPA-C Memorial Sloan Kettering Cancer Center, New York, NY, USA

Paolo Fiorini, PhD Department of Computer Science, University of Verona, Verona, Italy

Abigail J. B. Fong, MD, MBA Department of Surgery, University of Washington Medical Center, Seattle, WA, USA

Yuman Fong, MD Department of Surgery, City of Hope National Medical Center, Duarte, CA, USA

John V. Gahagan, MD Division of Colon and Rectal Surgery, Department of Surgery, University of California, Irvine, Orange, CA, USA

Julio Garcia-Aguilar, MD, PhD Colorectal Service, Department of Surgery, Memorial Sloan Kettering Cancer Center, New York, NY, USA

Thomas Gernon, MD Department of Surgery, City of Hope National Medical Center, Duarte, CA, USA

Federico Gheza, MD Division of General, Minimally Invasive and Robotic Surgery, Department of Surgery, University of Illinois at Chicago, Chicago, IL, USA

Greg Gin, MD VA Long Beach Healthcare System, Long Beach, CA, USA

Pier Cristoforo Giulianotti, MD Division of General, Minimally Invasive and Robotic Surgery, Department of Surgery, University of Illinois at Chicago, Chicago, IL, USA

Pedro Recabal Guiraldes, MD Department of Surgery, Urology Service, Memorial Sloan Kettering Cancer Center, New York, NY, USA

Ernest S. Han, MD, PhD Division of Gynecologic Oncology, City of Hope National Medical Center, Duarte, CA, USA

Nicholas R. Hess, BS University of Pittsburgh School of Medicine, Pittsburgh, PA, USA

Boris D. Hristov, MD Thoracic Service, Department of Surgery, Memorial Sloan Kettering Cancer Center, New York, NY, USA

Eric M. Johnson, MD Department of Surgery, Abbott Northwestern Hospital, Minneapolis, MN, USA

Kamaljot S. Kaler, MD Department of Urology, University of California, Irvine, Orange, CA, USA

Emad Kandil, MD Department of Endocrine Surgery, Tulane University School of Medicine, New Orleans, LA, USA

Robert Kang, MD Division of Otolaryngology/Head & Neck Surgery, Department of Surgery, City of Hope National Medical Center, Duarte, CA, USA

Sang-Wook Kang, MD Department of Surgery, Yonsei University College of Medicine, Seoul, South Korea

Steven V. Kardos, MD Urology and Urologic Oncology, Northeast Medical Group, Yale New Haven Health, Fairfield, CT, USA

Matthew E. Kaufman, MHA Piedmont Atlanta Hospital, Atlanta, GA, USA

Jae Y. Kim, MD Division of Thoracic Surgery, Department of Surgery, City of Hope National Medical Center, Duarte, CA, USA

Keith Chae Kim, MD Center for Metabolic and Obesity Surgery, Florida Hospital Celebration Health, Celebration, FL, USA

Ioannis Konstantinidis, MD Department of Surgery, City of Hope National Medical Center, Duarte, CA, USA

Eric Kubat, MD Department of General Surgery, Stanford University School of Medicine, VA Palo Alto Health Care System, Palo Alto, CA, USA

Clayton Lau, MD Department of Surgery, City of Hope National Medical Center, Duarte, CA, USA

Vincent P. Laudone, MD Department of Surgery, Urology Service, Memorial Sloan Kettering Cancer Center, New York, NY, USA

Rajesh G. Laungani, MD Robotic Service Line, Piedmont Atlanta Hospital, Atlanta, GA, USA

Byrne Lee, MD Department of Surgery, City of Hope National Medical Center, Duarte, CA, USA

Stephen J. Lee, MD Division of Gynecologic Oncology, City of Hope National Medical Center, Duarte, CA, USA

Mario M. Leitao Jr, MD Department of Surgery, Memorial Sloan Kettering Cancer Center, New York, NY, USA

Aaron Lewis, MD Division of Surgical Oncology, Department of Surgery, City of Hope National Medical Center, Duarte, CA, USA

Michael W. Lew, MD Department of Anesthesiology, City of Hope National Medical Center, Duarte, CA, USA

Patricio B. Lynn, MD Department of Surgery, New York University School of Medicine, New York, NY, USA

Colorectal Service, Department of Surgery, Memorial Sloan Kettering Cancer Center, New York, NY, USA

Ellie Maghami, MD Department of Surgery, City of Hope National Medical Center, Duarte, CA, USA

Manuel Maya, MD Instituto de Investigaciones Médicas Alfredo Lanari, Universidad de Buenos Aires, Buenos Aires, Argentina

Hospital Alemán de Buenos Aires, Buenos Aires, Argentina

Ian McDowall, BaSc Hon Vision Engineering, Intuitive Surgical, Sunnyvale, CA, USA

Elisabeth C. McLemore, MD Department of Surgery, Southern California Permanente Medical Group, Los Angeles, CA, USA

Kurt Melstrom, MD City of Hope National Medical Center, Duarte, CA, USA

Steven Minaglia, MD, MBA Division of Urogynecology and Pelvic Reconstructive Surgery, Department of Obstetrics and Gynecology, John A. Burns School of Medicine, University of Hawaii, Kapi'olani Medical Center for Women and Children, Honolulu, HI, USA

Michael G. Patane, MS, PA-C Department of Surgery, Memorial Sloan Kettering Cancer Center, New York, NY, USA

Jaspreet Singh Parihar, MD Division of Urology and Urologic Oncology, City of Hope National Medical Center, Duarte, CA, USA

Bernard J. Park, MD Thoracic Service, Department of Surgery, Memorial Sloan Kettering Cancer Center, New York, NY, USA

Kyle A. Perry, MD Division of General & Gastrointestinal Surgery, Center for Minimally Invasive Surgery, The Ohio State University, Columbus, OH, USA

Alessio Pigazzi, MD, PhD Division of Colon and Rectal Surgery, Department of Surgery, University of California, Irvine, Orange, CA, USA

Pablo Quadri, MD Division of General, Minimally Invasive and Robotic Surgery, Department of Surgery, University of Illinois at Chicago, Chicago, IL, USA

John L. Raytis, MD Department of Anesthesiology, City of Hope National Medical Center, Duarte, CA, USA

Alexander S. Rosemurgy, MD Department of Surgery, Florida Hospital Tampa, Tampa, FL, USA

Sharona B. Ross, MD Department of Surgery, Florida Hospital Tampa, Tampa, FL, USA

Fernando M. Safdie, MD Department of Cardiothoracic Surgery, University of Pittsburgh Medical Center, Pittsburgh, PA, USA

Inderpal S. Sarkaria, MD Department of Cardiothoracic Surgery, University of Pittsburgh Medical Center, Pittsburgh, PA, USA

Brooke A. Schlappe, MD Department of Surgery, Memorial Sloan Kettering Cancer Center, New York, NY, USA

Luke V. Selby, MD, MS Department of Surgery, University of Colorado Health Sciences Center, Aurora, CO, USA

Nikhil L. Shah, DO, MPH Minimal Access & Robotic Surgery, Piedmont Health Care, Atlanta, GA, USA

Yukio Sonoda, MD Department of Surgery, Memorial Sloan Kettering Cancer Center, New York, NY, USA

Jonathan Sorger, PhD, MBA Research, Intuitive Surgical, Sunnyvale, CA, USA

Vivian E. Strong, MD Department of Surgery, Memorial Sloan Kettering Cancer Center, New York, NY, USA

Iswanto Sucandy, MD Department of Surgery, Florida Hospital Tampa, Tampa, FL, USA

David J. Terris, MD Department of Otolaryngology-Head and Neck Surgery, Augusta University Thyroid and Parathyroid Center, Augusta University, Augusta, GA, USA

Simone L. Vernez, BA Department of Urology, University of California, Irvine, Orange, CA, USA

Jonathan N. Warner, MD Division of Urology and Urologic Oncology, Department of Surgery, City of Hope Comprehensive Cancer Center, Duarte, CA, USA

Susanne G. Warner, MD Department of Surgery, City of Hope National Medical Center, Duarte, CA, USA

Yanghee Woo, MD International Surgery, Department of Surgery, City of Hope National Medical Center, Duarte, CA, USA

Sherry M. Wren, MD Department of General Surgery, Stanford University School of Medicine, VA Palo Alto Health Care System, Palo Alto, CA, USA

Jonathan Yamzon, MD Department of Surgery, City of Hope National Medical Center, Duarte, CA, USA

Anusak Yiengpruksawan, MD Department of Surgery, Faculty of Medicine, Siriraj Hospital, Mahidol University, Bangkok, Thailand

Michele L. Young, PA-C Center for Metabolic and Obesity Surgery, Florida Hospital Celebration, Celebration, FL, USA

Bertram Yuh, MD, MSHCPM, MISM Division of Urology and Urologic Oncology, City of Hope Comprehensive Cancer Center, Duarte, CA, USA

Boris Zevin, MD, PhD Department of Surgery, Queen's University, Kingston General Hospital, Kingston, ON, Canada

Ali Zhumkhawala, MD Division of Urology and Urologic Oncology, Department of Surgery, City of Hope Comprehensive Cancer Center, Duarte, CA, USA

Part I

History and Basics of Robotic Surgery

History of Robots and Robotic Surgery

1

Paolo Fiorini

Introduction

This chapter presents a brief history of robotics and one of its most successful applications, surgical robotics. The first section describes the beginning of this technology, from 1950 to 1980, when the basic concepts and technologies were developed. The second section addresses the development of robotic surgery, which has established itself as a necessary complement to standard surgical practice. The third section briefly summarizes some of the current research efforts in robotic surgery, and the fourth section introduces the main commercial surgical robots available on the market. The final section describes the most important robotic concepts that are necessary to understand the main features of any surgical robot.

The Beginnings

Robots are among the good byproducts of the Second World War. Their technology derived from the early teleoperation systems developed in 1948 by Raymond Goertz at the Argonne National Laboratory in the United States, to handle radioactive material [1]. The word "robot" and the concept of a mechanical entity able to carry out tasks that a person cannot do or does not want to do pre-date this technology development. The word "robot" started to be used in the 1920s following a play by the Czech author Karel Capek, called R.U.R. (Rossum's Universal Robots), in which artificial biological organisms in human form obey their master's orders [2]. These organisms were called "robots," a word derived from the Czech "robota," meaning "forced labor." They were more similar to androids than to current humanoid robots, as they could also think for themselves, which eventually led to a rebellion that destroyed the human race. The word "robot" then came to identify all devices developed to display an animate behavior.

In ancient times, many mythological figures and brilliant devices have been described that mimic human or animal functions. It is worth remembering the clay golems of Jewish legend [3], the clay giants of Norse legend, and the Greek myth of Talos [4], in which a bronze warrior guarded the island of Crete in 400 BC. The quest to develop mechanical humans is present in most cultures. In early China, about 900 BC, the inventor Yan Shi developed for King Mu of Zhou a life-sized, human-shaped figure made of leather and wood [5]. In 1066, the Chinese inventor Su Song built a water clock shaped as a tower with mechanical figures indicating the hours [6]. About 1495 in Italy, Leonardo da Vinci drew in his notebooks the plans for a mechanical knight able to sit up, wave its arms, and move its head and jaw [7]. In Japan, complex animal and human automata were built in the seventeenth to nineteenth centuries [8], such as the "karakuri ningyō," a type of mechanical device used to recreate different events, such as the tea ceremony. In France, between 1738 and 1739, Jacques de Vaucanson developed several life-sized automatons, including his famous mechanical duck, which could flap its wings, move its neck, swallow food, and give the illusion of digesting it by excreting matter stored in its body [9]. To impress the Empress Maria Theresa of Austria, in 1770 the Hungarian inventor Kempelen Farkas developed a mechanism that was unbeatable at chess. The machine was called the "Mechanical Turk"; only in 1820 was it exposed as a hoax, with a person hidden inside the structure [10].

The word "robotics" has also a nontechnical origin. It was created in the 1940s by the Russian writer Isaac Asimov to represent the study of mechanical robots of human appearance. The robots' behavior was programmed in a "positronic" brain and satisfied certain rules of ethical conduct, which came to be known as the Three Laws of Robotics [11].

The first teleoperation system credited to Raymond Goertz consisted of a master device, held by the operator,

P. Fiorini, PhD
Department of Computer Science, University of Verona, Verona, Italy
e-mail: paolo.fiorini@univr.it

Y. Fong et al. (eds.), *The SAGES Atlas of Robotic Surgery*, https://doi.org/10.1007/978-3-319-91045-1_1

and by a slave mechanical arm, in contact with the environment, in the so-called master-slave configuration. The slave was coupled to the master through a series of mechanical linkages, and it duplicated the motions of the operator's hands and fingers. These linkages were eventually replaced by electric or hydraulic coupling; the operator could then control the position of the slave arms but lost the perception of contacts provided by the mechanical linkages. Force feedback was then added to the teleoperation system to prevent crushing glass containers, and the operator could again feel the interaction forces of the slave with the environment. This solution was called "teleoperator" to represent a teleoperation system that was not mechanically linked with the operator. The term "telepresence" was also introduced to describe the added sensory feedback, from the remote environment to the operator, who thus has increased sensory and decision-making abilities.

In 1949, the US Air Force sponsored the development of numerically controlled milling machines [12] that combined servo systems with the newly developed numerical computers. In 1953, the MIT Radiation Laboratory demonstrated the prototype of a computer numerically controlled (CNC) machine. In 1954, George Devol replaced the master device of the teleoperator with the computer control of a CNC machine and called this device a "programmed articulated transfer device" for which he filed a patent [13]. The patent rights were bought by a Columbia University student, Joseph Engelberger, who founded a company called Unimation in 1956. In 1960, the first Unimation robot was demonstrated, and the first installation was done the following year at a General Motors plant. This industrial robot could be reprogrammed to perform different pick-and-place tasks, but all parts needed to be accurately positioned in the working cell, as the robot could not adapt to any position error [14]. The first applications were for material handling in steel plants. To overcome the need for precise part positioning, in 1961 a robot with force sensing was developed at MIT [15], which enabled the robot to stack blocks in an unstructured environment without explicitly programming the robot motions. Other sensors were added to robots to increase the perception of their environment. In the 1960s, binary and halftone vision systems were also developed for obstacle detection [16], followed later by a camera vision system [17]. One of the most influential early designs was the Stanford arm designed in 1969 by Victor Scheinman at the Stanford Artificial Intelligence Lab (SAIL) (Fig. 1.1). It was a six-joint, all-electric mechanical manipulator designed exclusively for computer control [18].

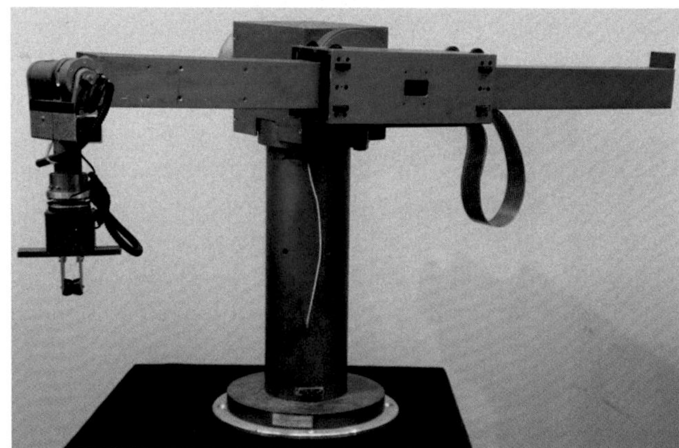

Fig. 1.1 The Stanford Arm (courtesy of Prof. Oussama Khatib, Stanford University)

This robot was enhanced with artificial intelligence algorithms that enabled it to solve puzzles [19]. These sensor-equipped robots were able to perform tasks requiring the control of the interaction forces with the environment. Japanese researchers developed the automatic selection of force and position control, and this led to the development of a mechanical manipulator with compliance control [20]. Roughly at the same time, in 1973, Stanford researchers developed the first language for programming a robot [21]. The first anthropomorphic industrial robot was developed in 1976 by Cincinnati Milacron Inc. The Tomorrow Tool (T3) could lift 50 kg and track objects on a moving conveyor belt [22]. In 1973, Victor Scheinman developed the Vicarm, which was sold in 1977 to Unimation. Figure 1.2 shows the brochure of the robots produced by Scheinman company. The following year, with support from General Motors,

VICARM
MANIPULATOR SYSTEMS
• ROBOTS
• SENSORS
• SERVOS
• COMPUTERS
• MICROPROCESSORS
• SOFTWARE
Vicarm currently offers two different six degree of freedom, computer controlled electromechanical manipulators designed for research and development in the robotics and automation areas. These manipulators are available with interfaces for the user's computer or as part of a complete computer based system, including terminal devices and software.
VICARM, INC. • 154 EAST DANA STREET • MOUNTAIN VIEW, CA 94041 • (415) 965-0557

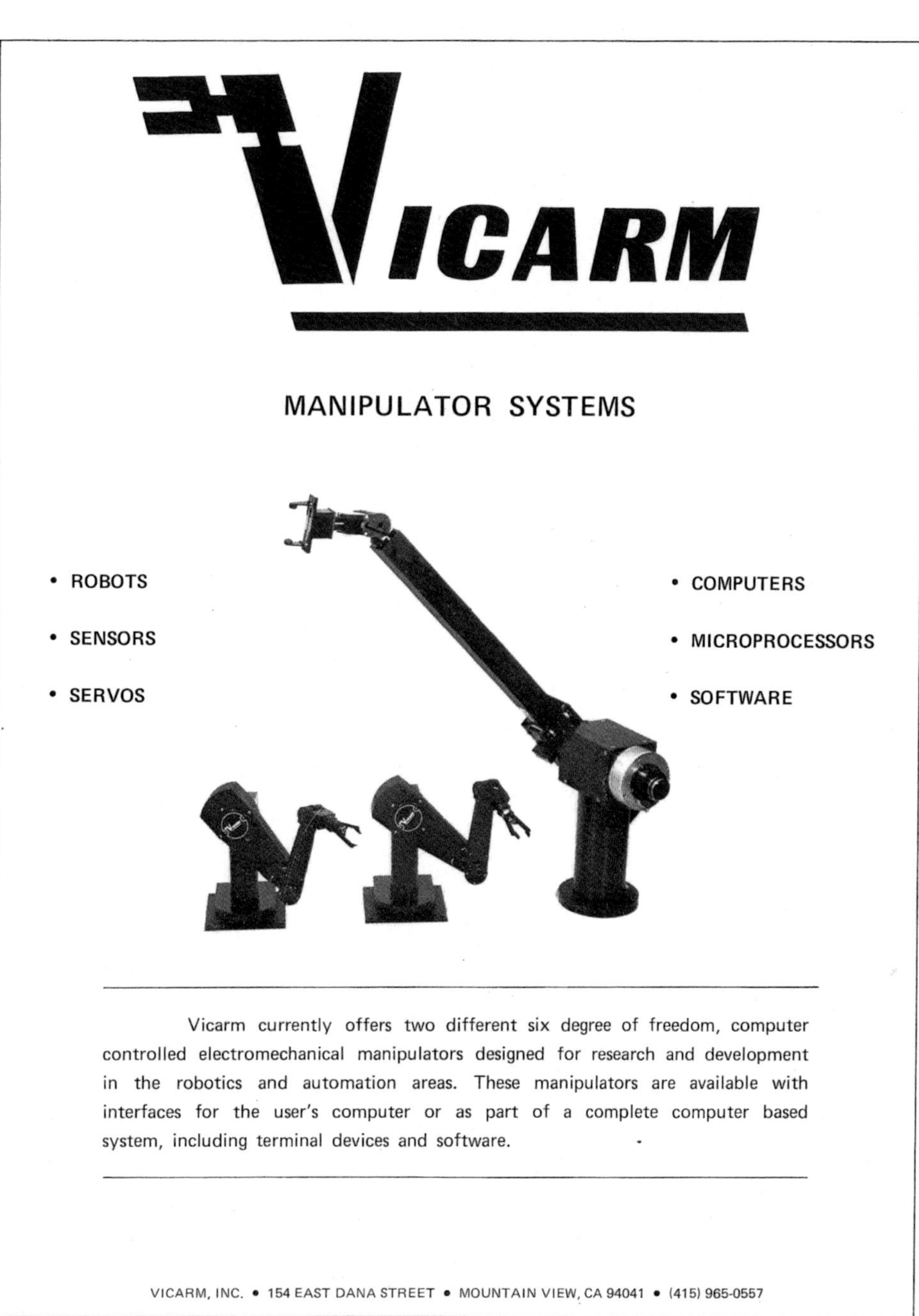

Fig. 1.2 Brochure of Vicarm, the first manufacturer of commercial robots (courtesy of Prof. Paolo Fiorini, University of Verona)

Unimation developed the Vicarm into the PUMA (Programmable Universal Machine for Assembly) family of robots, which would become the workhorse of robotics research (Figs. 1.3 and 1.4). In the mid-1970s, Antal Bejczy at Caltech NASA-Jet Propulsion Laboratory (JPL) developed the first dynamic model of a robotic arm and later began the teleoperation program for space-based manipulators, which led to robotic surgery. In 1979, the SCARA (Selective Compliant Articulated Robot for Assembly) was developed. Based on these results, the group of Antal Bejczy developed the Advanced Teleoperation Laboratory to demonstrate the feasibility of space repair from Earth and developed some of the technologies for bilateral teleoperation used in later telesurgical systems (Figs. 1.5 and 1.6).

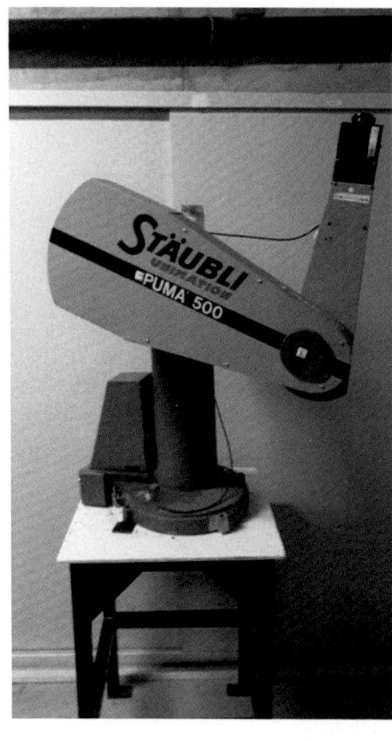

Fig. 1.3 The Puma 500 robotic arm (courtesy of Prof. Paolo Fiorini, University of Verona)

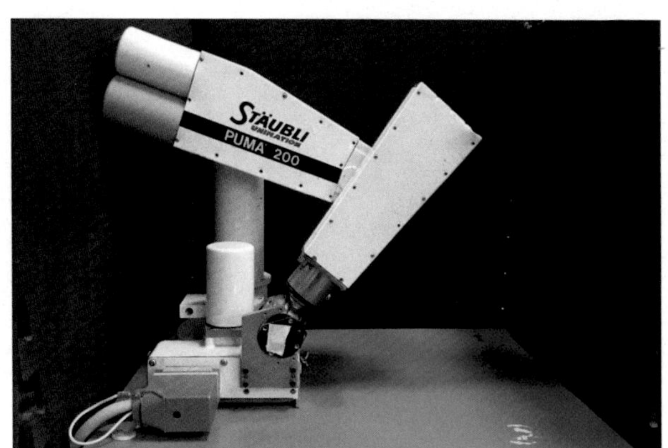

Fig. 1.4 The Puma 200 robotic arm (courtesy of Prof. Paolo Fiorini, University of Verona)

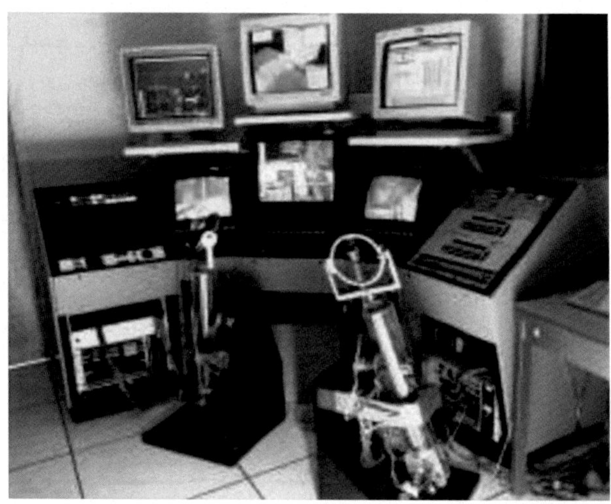

Fig. 1.5 The master station of the Advanced Teleoperation Laboratory at NASA-JPL (courtesy of NASA/JPL-Caltech)

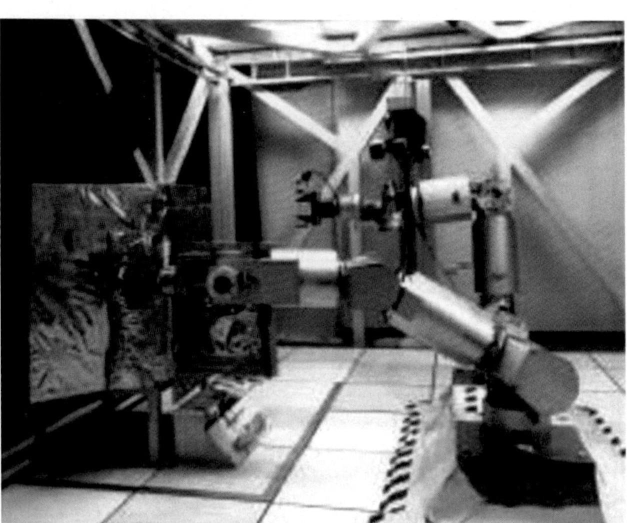

Fig. 1.6 The slave station of the Advanced Teleoperation Laboratory at NASA-JPL (courtesy of NASA/JPL-Caltech)

The introduction of force and touch sensing raised the attention of the medical community, and in 1963 researchers at the Institute Mihajlo Pupin in Belgrade developed the first robotic prosthetic device capable of programmed grasping patterns, later known as the Belgrade hand [23]. Shortly afterward, in 1972, the same Institute developed a powered exoskeleton, one of the first assistive devices for walking disabilities. Papers on robotic research carried out by scientists at the Institute Mihajlo Pupin started to appear in the western press in 1973 [24], together with the results of Russian scientists [25]. English editions of books summarizing the results achieved by the Russian robotics community [26] and books reporting on the activities of the Pupin Institute [27] were published shortly afterward.

The other important player in the early days of robotics and teleoperation research was the Paris laboratory of CEA (the French "Commissariat à l'énergie atomique et aux énergies alternatives"), where Jean Vertut established his laboratory in 1962. The other leading French laboratory in robotics was the Laboratory for Automation and Microprocessing, Monipellier (LAMM), led by Philippe Coiffet. Both laboratories are still very active in teleoperation and robotic research. These early developments and the results achieved by the French robotics community are well documented in several books [28].

In the 1920s, robots began appearing in department stores in Japan under the shape of a humanoid robot named Gakutensoku. Later, the robotic idea was carried on by the cartoon character Astro Boy, a manga series running from 1952 to 1968 [29]. Industrial robots made their appearance in Japan through Kawasaki's acquisition of a license from Unimation in 1968. In 1972, researchers were able to program a robot to build a block structure after examining the drawings of a final configuration [30]. The following year, researchers at the Waseda University in Tokyo developed the "WABOT-1," a full-scale humanoid robot with two arms, capable of walking on two legs and seeing with stereo cameras [31]. The introduction of new force sensors prompted the development of efficient algorithms for the control of dynamic interactions between the robot and its environment, such as the automatic turning of a crank [32].

The 1980s saw the development of many robotic products for industrial automation, and of new algorithms to improve robot speed and position accuracy, leading to an in-depth understanding of the capabilities and limitations of robotic systems, identifying promising applications. During this period, robotics became a recognized field of research with regular conferences and scientific publications. Research results were initially reported by two international organizations, the American Nuclear Society and the International Federation for Theory of Machines and Mechanisms (IFToMM), which started organizing at the Centre International des Sciences Mecaniques (CISM, Udine, Italy) the Robot and Manipulator Symposiums (RO.MAN.SY), still an important forum for today's robotics community. Later, also other major robotics conferences began to be organized: the International Conference on Advanced Robotics (ICAR), the IEEE International Conference on Automation and Robotics (ICRA), and the International Conference on Intelligent Robotic Systems (IROS).

The Development of Surgical Robotics

Together with the development of basic robotic technologies, researchers started considering the use of robots in areas in which human performance could be improved [33, 34]. The idea of robotic surgery was probably born in the early 1970s, proposed in a study for the National Aeronautics and Space Administration (NASA) to provide surgical care for astronauts with remote-controlled robots [35].

The first robot that was designed for patient treatment was the Arthrobot in 1983, for arthroscopic procedures. The development was led by J. McEwen, G. Auchinlec, and B. Day at the University of British Columbia, Canada [36]; the first procedures were carried out in 1984. At the same time, experiments were carried out in California of robot-assisted stereotaxic brain surgery. A joint team from Memorial Medical Center in Long Beach and NASA-JPL led by Y. S. Kwoh and Samad Hayati used a Puma 200 to hold and manipulate a biopsy cannula, navigated by a stereotactic frame mounted on the base of the robot [37]. In the same period, similar interventions were also performed in China.

In the late 1980s, the idea of robot-assisted minimally invasive telesurgery was primarily developed under the leadership of Richard Satava within the US Army, which funded SRI International's development of a prototype telesurgical system [38]. The prototype was demonstrated in animal experiments, described by Bowersox et al. [39]. Contemporary to the US development, at the University of Karlsruhe (Germany), the team led by Gerhard Buess, already a pioneer of endoscopic surgery, developed (together with the Nuclear Research Center in Karlsruhe) the surgical robot prototype ARTEMIS, with seven degrees of freedom (DoF) [40, 41], shown in Fig. 1.7.

In the mid-1980s, Brian Davies and his team at Imperial College (London, UK) started to work on prostate surgery and developed the system called PROBOT for transurethral resection of the prostate (TURP) procedures in 1991 [42]. In Milano, the team lead by Alberto Rovetta also developed a robot for TURP, which was used in a clinical trial [43].

The first robotic system for orthopedic surgery was developed in 1986 by a team formed by two surgeons, Dr. Howard Paul and Dr. William Bargar, and researchers at IBM Watson Research Center (Yorktown Heights, NY) led by Russell Taylor. This system was further developed by Integrated Surgical Systems (ISS, Santa Monica, CA), which in 1992 created the first orthopedic surgical system, in collaboration with the University of California–Davis. This system was called ROBODOC and was used for robot-assisted human hip replacement [44]. The team at Imperial College also addressed orthopedic surgery and developed the Acrobot® system for total knee replacement procedures [45]. Other robots developed for orthopedic surgery were CRIGOS [46] and Orto Maquet CASPAR [47].

In 1989, Yulan Wang founded Computer Motion Inc. (Goleta, CA), and, with a NASA-JPL grant, in 1992 he developed a robotic system able to move an endoscope during laparoscopic surgeries. He then commercialized this device as the Automated Endoscopic System for Optimal Positioning (AESOP), the first commercial robot to be routinely used in the operating room [48]. The AESOP system was later extended with the addition of more arms and different surgical instruments, and it became the Zeus Robotic Surgical System (Fig. 1.8), which included three arms [49].

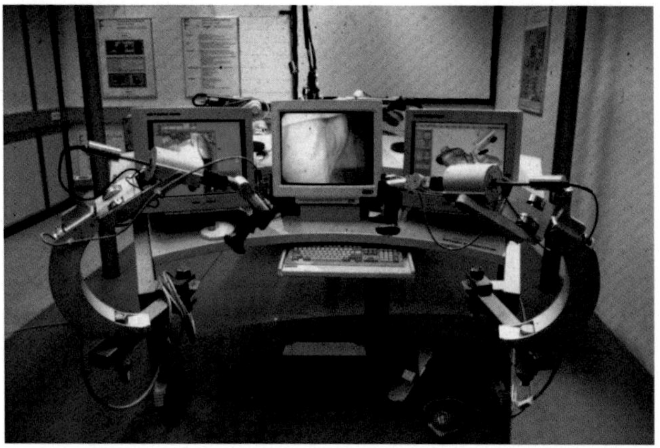

Fig. 1.7 The master station of the ARTEMIS surgical robot (courtesy of Prof. Alberto Arezzo, University of Torino)

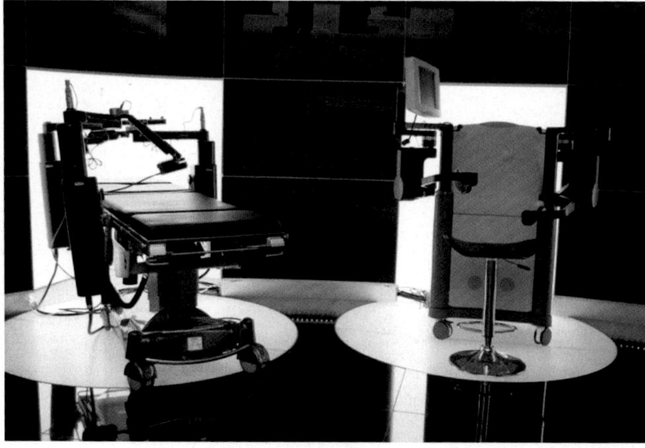

Fig. 1.8 The Zeus surgical robotic system (courtesy of Prof. Guang-Zhong Yang, The Hamlyn Center, Imperial College)

A collaboration between the ophthalmic surgeon Steve Charles and the NASA-JPL team of Antal Bejczy led to the development by Hari Nayar of the Advanced Teleoperation (ATOP) Lab of the robot-assisted microsurgery (RAMS) system in 1994, a robotic system for microsurgery with force feedback (Fig. 1.9) [50]. The RAMS capabilities were later demonstrated in coronary artery anastomoses on animals [51].

Intuitive Surgical Inc. (Mountain View, CA) was founded in 1995 by Frederic Moll. After acquiring some of the patents of SRI for their surgical robotic system, Intuitive Surgical created a first prototype of the da Vinci surgical system in 1997 to carry out clinical trials, which led to the first closed-chest, multivessel cardiac bypass procedure in 1999. The da Vinci system was cleared by the US Food and Drug Administration (FDA) for human use in 2000 and commercialized as shown in Fig. 1.10. After several attempts to create a market for beating-heart procedures, the da Vinci system found its niche in urology and gynecology, where it is now the gold standard for intervention. After a long patent dispute, Intuitive Surgical acquired Computer Motion, its only competitor, in 2003, and shortly afterward it discontinued the production of the Zeus system [52].

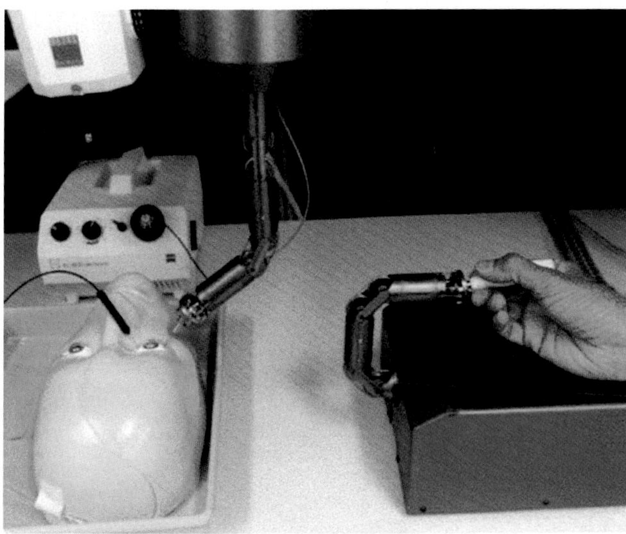

Fig. 1.9 The robot-assisted microsurgery system (courtesy of NASA/JPL-Caltech)

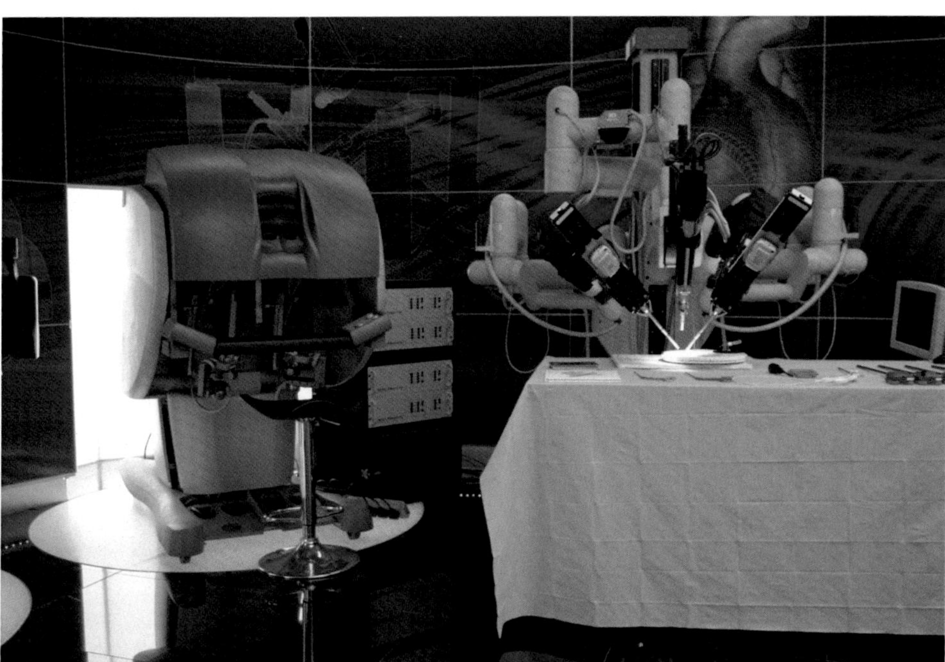

Fig. 1.10 The first generation of the da Vinci Surgical System (courtesy of Prof. Guang-Zhong Yang, The Hamlyn Center, Imperial College)

There have also been a few attempts at long-distance telesurgery. The first experiment was performed in 1993 between NASA-JPL (Pasadena, CA) and Milan, Italy, by the teams of Antal Bejczy and Alberto Rovetta [53]. A few years later, Jacques Marescaux performed a cholecystectomy on a patient in Strasbourg (France) from New York, controlling a Zeus robot in France [54]. The Zeus robot was also involved in the 2004 NEEMO experiments of undersea simulated surgery controlled remotely from the Centre for Minimal Access Surgery, London, UK. In 2005, the US Department of Defense launched its long-distance medical assistance project, the Trauma Pod [55], to demonstrate the feasibility of the original idea of Richard Satava, an emergency surgical unit in combat areas [56]. Although all these experiments were successful, long-distance telesurgery has not yet entered clinical practice because of safety and certification issues.

Several robots were also developed for neurosurgery. In 1997, the team of Alim Louis Benabid in Grenoble developed the NeuroMate system [57], a stereotaxic targeting device for neurosurgery, which was the first neurosurgical robot to receive FDA clearance. This robot was initially marketed by Innovative Medical Machines International (Lyon, France) and now is a Renishaw product [58]. Minerva [59] was designed for stereotactic brain biopsy to meet specifications incorporating safety and geometry, to perform single-dimensional incursions into the brain while the patient is within a CT system that continuously provides real-time imaging data to the robot. The PathFinder was an image-guided, frameless, six-axes robot to accurately position a tool for neurosurgery [60].

Development Directions in Surgical Robotics

Robotic surgery is a very active area of research, and it is worth mentioning some of the most successful prototypes. The German Space Agency DLR has developed the MIRO surgical system [61], whose fast dynamics could allow beating-heart interventions. It has been designed to achieve the requirements of a broad range of surgical applications in endoscopic and open surgery. Integrated multimodal sensors and different control modes allow system configurations for telepresence (Fig. 1.11).

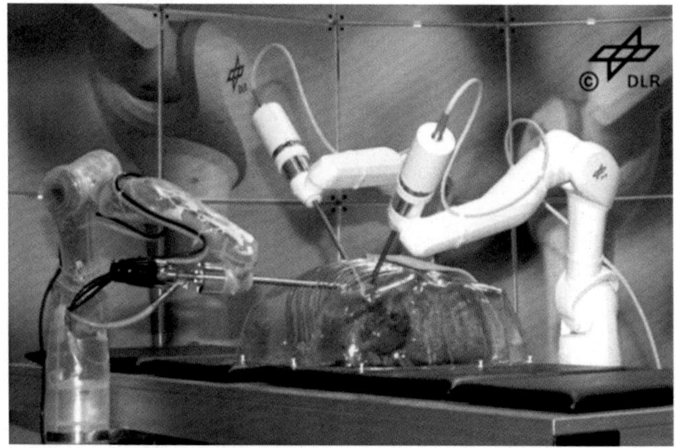

Fig. 1.11 The MIRO surgical system (courtesy of Deutschen Zentrums für Luft- und Raumfahrt [*DLR*])

Force feedback is implemented in the Surgeon's Operating Force-feedback Interface Eindhoven (SOFIE) robotic system, developed at the Eindhoven University of Technology. The arms are mounted on a single frame, which is attached to the patient table [62].

The RAVEN robot (Fig. 1.12) is a surgical system developed specifically for laboratory research. It was developed in the BioRobotics Laboratory at the University of Washington as a cable-driven arm that duplicates the kinematics of the da Vinci robot and can use the da Vinci instruments. With the support of the National Institutes of Health (NIH), eight robots have been built and distributed. To support development and distribution of the RAVEN robot, Applied Dexterity (Seattle, WA) was founded in 2013 [63].

The Surgenius robot (Fig. 1.13) was developed by the company Surgica Robotica (Verona, Italy) in 2010 under license from JPL-NASA of the RAMS system. The robot addressed some of the shortcomings of the da Vinci system, such as its monolithic structure, high cost, and lack of force feedback. The robot received European CE certification in 2013 [64].

Automation-aided surgery was demonstrated by Davies [42] and Rovetta [43] during TURP interventions and in automatic needle placement [65], and the interest in automation is increasing because it could implement the concept of "solo surgery" in which the functions of the assistant surgeon are replaced during surgery by a robot, so that the main surgeon can operate on his or her own [66].

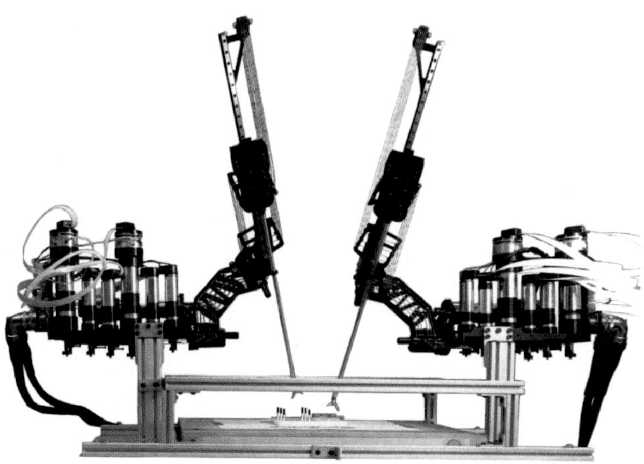

Fig. 1.12 The Raven II surgical robot (courtesy of Applied Dexterity)

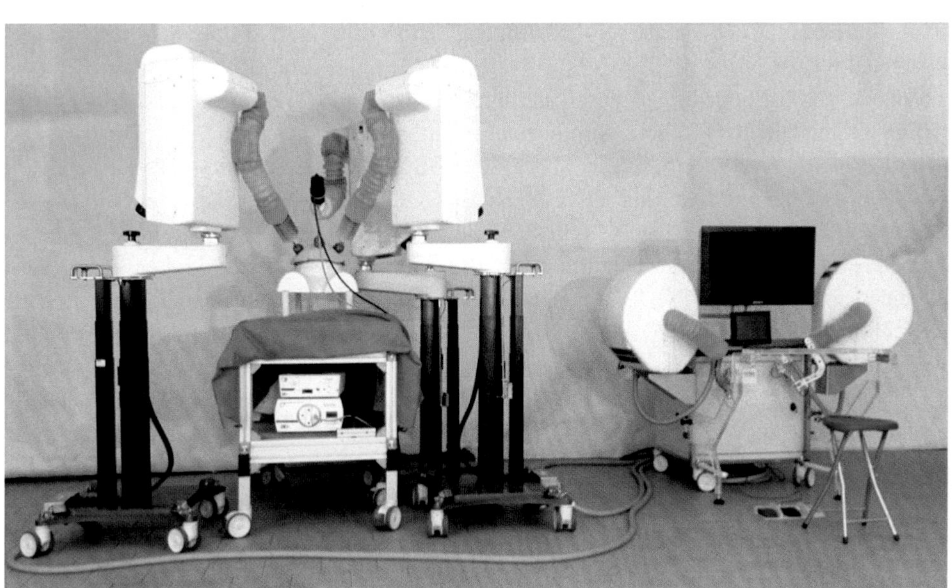

Fig. 1.13 The Surgenius surgical robot (courtesy of Prof. Paolo Fiorini, University of Verona)

Some Commercial Surgical Robots

Besides the best-known da Vinci robotic system, other commercial robots are available on the market for a number of surgical applications. Minimally invasive surgery is targeted by Titan Medical Single Port Orifice Robotic Technology (SPORT), which relies on a single incision and expendable flexible tools [67]. The Advanced Laparoscopy through Force refleCT(X)ion (ALF-X) robot is an advanced laparoscopic system that uses a modular configuration of several mobile robots positioned around the operating bed [68]. Of a completely different scale is the Renaissance system for spine screw positioning, by Mazor Robotics. The system mounts directly on the patient's spine, thus automatically compensating for respiratory motion and ensuring very high position accuracy [69]. Medrobotics Corp. is using the concept of a snake robot to develop its robotics product Flex, targeting interventions in the oral cavity. They achieved approval for Europe in 2014 and aim for a first limited commercial launch on selected European markets [70].

There are several commercial robots for radiation treatment. The CyberKnife is composed of an industrial KUKA robot carrying a linear accelerator as the radiation source. The patient is placed on a bed that can move to compensate for breathing, and the target is tracked by markers placed on the patient's body. The system can target the tumor with 0.2 mm accuracy, and the overall treatment precision is better than 0.95 mm [71]. In the Novalis system, the radiation source is constructed in an L shape and can rotate around the patient along a horizontal axis [72]. The Gamma Knife system consists of a half sphere, which houses the fixed radiation source and moveable focusing mechanism. The patient's head is fixed to a stereotactic frame and placed on a moveable bed in the center of the sphere. Through the movement of the bed and the focal adjustment, tumors can be targeted very precisely [71].

Robots for orthopedic surgery are represented by ROBODOC and the RIO Robotic Arm Interactive Orthopedic system. Since 1994, ISS has sold about 80 ROBODOC systems across Europe and Asia. In 2008, ROBODOC was acquired by Curexo Technology Corporation and was FDA-approved for automated bone milling. ROBODOC was rebranded to Curexo ROBODOC in 2007 and to THINK Surgical in 2014 [73]. The RIO system by MAKO Corp. consists of a moveable base and a robotic arm on which a milling tool is mounted. It uses image guidance to control the milling tool mounted at the end of a robotic arm, but it leaves the actual milling to the surgeon, creating resistance on predefined boundaries. MAKO was acquired by Stryker in 2015 [74].

The ARTAS is a robotic system for hair follicle harvesting. A robotic arm carries the harvesting tool, containing a camera and the extraction needles [75]. The camera captures the hair positions, and the control program computes the harvesting pattern for evenly thinning out the hair. The system can adapt to patient movements during the procedure, but the harvested hairs must be implanted by the surgeon by hand.

Some Basic Concepts and Terminology

The official definitions of robot come from the Robot Institute of America (RIA) and the ISO standard (ISO 8373:2013 Robots and robotic devices—Vocabulary): "A robot is an actuated mechanism programmable in two or more axes with a degree of autonomy, moving within its environment, to perform intended tasks." The key elements here are the "axes" of motion, also called "degree of freedom (dof)" of the robotic structure and "degree of autonomy." This last term is not defined in the standard, and it is left to the developer to define how much autonomy a robotic device has. In the case of robotic surgery, the level of autonomy is very low, and the surgeon is always in charge of the motions of the robot. Autonomy in robotic surgery is used in a protective way—for example, to force the surgeon to follow the right cutting path, as in the RIO orthopedic robot, or to keep the joystick masters aligned with the instrument tools, as in the da Vinci system. The capability of limiting the surgical tool motions to avoid delicate areas or to enforce a prescribed path is called a "virtual fixture," and it has been proved very useful also in robotic surgery training. Surgical robots consist of a "slave" station, located at the bedside, and a "master" station, where the surgeon inputs the motion commands to the robot.

Many books describe the mathematical and physical foundations of robotics [76]. Here we give a very brief summary of the main concepts. The key element in a surgical robot is the surgical instrument, which allows an intervention to be performed under the surgeon's guidance. The most sophisticated robotic instruments are those for robot-assisted minimally invasive surgery (RAMIS) procedures, which are endowed with several dofs in position (they can move linearly in the X, Y, and Z directions) and in rotation (the distal end of the instrument can rotate around one or more axes). The linear dofs determine the position of the instrument's distal end, and the rotation dof determines its orientation. Furthermore, the distal end carries the surgical tool (gripper, scissor, hook, etc.) to interact with the tissues, and the tool has its own dof (such as opening and closing of the gripper). A dof of a robot is also called a "joint"; the part connecting two adjacent dofs is called "link." The distal end of the surgical instrument is called the "wrist" of the instrument, as its articulation is similar to a human wrist.

The number and the configuration of the robot axes determine the kinematic structure of the robot. For example, the instruments of the da Vinci robot have seven dofs, three of which refer to the linear motion of the instrument tip, three to the rotation dofs, and one to the opening and closing of the instrument tool. This number of dofs is computed by adding the number of dofs of the instrument, typically three, with the number of dofs of the supporting arm, typically six, and by subtracting the number of constraints imposed by the fixed pivot point, typically two. The number of dofs of the robot and their range of motion determine the "work space" of the robot—that is, the volume that the robot or the robotic instrument can reach. The position and orientation of the instrument tool are measured with reference to a "coordinate system" that permits the instrument position and orientation to be related to the position and orientation of the master joysticks. The robotic system measures the motion of its arms, both master and slave, by using sensors located in the robot joints, and moves the joints with actuators (typically electrical motors), which are coupled to the joints by a transmission system, cables, or gears, to reduce the motor speed and to transfer the motion to links far away from the motor, as in the case of the surgical instruments.

Surgical robots for minimally invasive surgery are "teleoperated" systems, in which the robot follows the motions of the master joysticks handled by the surgeon's hands. This control paradigm is different from how industrial robots are controlled; they are programmed in advance, and all their motions are repeated over and over. This type of control is called "position" or kinematic control, in which the robot reaches the commanded position in spite of obstacles on its motions. This can be a potential safety risk because the robot can damage its surrounding environment if it is given a wrong command. An alternative control method is "force" control, in which the robot is commanded to exert a given force to the environment. If the robot is not in contact with an object, this command makes the robot move in the direction of the desired force. When a contact is detected, the contact force is limited by the force commanded to the robot. This control mode is more complex than position control because it requires the use of contact sensors. In the case of surgical robots, there are no instruments yet equipped with contact sensors, and the master station is not capable of "force feedback." That is, the interaction force between the instrument and the environment is not transmitted to the surgeon commanding the robot. The interaction between the surgeon and the master station that uses forces is called "haptics." A different control approach is when the surgeon holds the surgical tool directly, as in the RIO orthopedic system. This control method is called "hand-on compliant control," and the robot prevents the human from making wrong motions. In this case, the "master" and the "slave" stations are the same, as the surgeon commands the robot by directly moving the robot instrument. Instability can happen in certain situations, for example, when there is a delay between the master commands and the slave motions, and is obviously a dangerous situation that must be avoided. Suitable control algorithms have been designed to avoid these forms of instability but they are not used yet in clinical practice.

To analyze the motions of the robot, to train surgical students, and to plan difficult interventions, surgical simulators can be used. The simulator can represent a general anatomy or a "patient-specific" anatomy derived from preoperative images of the patient. The simulator can be physical or virtual, meaning that the anatomy is represented by a physical object or by a computer program visualizing anatomical images on a display. These computer simulators are often called "virtual reality" simulators and may give the user a three-dimensional perception of the anatomy using a stereo display. However, most virtual reality simulators lack the ability to reproduce contact forces, because the biomechanical properties of the tissues are hard to estimate. Furthermore, a simulation that computes the contact forces and the deformations of the simulated organs is very computation-intensive, so it may not display images and render forces in real time. Force feedback and accurate biomechanical simulations are the next frontiers of surgical robotics.

References

1. Goertz RC. Fundamentals of general-purpose remote manipulators. Nucleonics. 1952;10:36–42.
2. https://en.wikipedia.org/wiki/R.U.R.
3. https://en.wikipedia.org/wiki/Golem
4. https://en.wikipedia.org/wiki/Talos
5. Needham J. Science and civilisation in China: volume 2, history of scientific thought. Cambridge: Cambridge University Press; 1991.
6. Fowler CB. The museum of music: a history of mechanical instruments. Music Educ J. 1967;54:45–9.
7. https://en.wikipedia.org/wiki/Leonardo%27s_robot
8. Law JM. Puppets of nostalgia—the life, death and rebirth of the Japanese Awaji Ningyo tradition. Princeton, NJ: Princeton University Press; 1997.
9. Wood G. Living dolls: a magical history of the quest for mechanical life. London: Faber & Faber; 2003.
10. https://en.wikipedia.org/wiki/The_Turk
11. https://en.wikipedia.org/wiki/Three_Laws_of_Robotics
12. Rosenberg J. A history of numerical control 1949–1972: the technical development, transfer to the industry, and assimilation. University of Southern California Information Science Institute, Marina del Rey, CA. Report No. ISI-RR-72-3; 1972.
13. Malone B. George Devol: a life devoted to invention, and robots. IEEE Spectrum; 2011. http://spectrum.ieee.org/automaton/robotics/industrial-robots/george-devol-a-life-devoted-to-invention-and-robots
14. Engelberger JF. Robotics in practice. Kempston: IFS Publications; 1980.
15. Ernst HA. A computer-operated mechanical hand. ScD Thesis, Massachusetts Institute of Technology; 1961.
16. Roberts LG. Homogeneous matrix representation and manipulation of N-dimensional constructs. Massachusetts Institute of Technology Lincoln Laboratory: Lexington, MA; 1966.
17. Wishman MW. The use of optical feedback in computer control of an arm. Stanford AI Laboratory, AIM56; 1967.
18. http://infolab.stanford.edu/pub/voy/museum/pictures/display/1-Robot.htm
19. Feldman J. The use of vision and manipulation to solve the instant insanity puzzle. Proceedings of the Second International Conference on Artificial Intelligence. London, UK; 1971. p. 359–64.
20. Paul RP. Modeling, trajectory calculation and servoing of a computer controlled arm. AIM 177. Stanford: Stanford AI Laboratory; 1972.
21. Paul RP. WAVE, a model-based language for manipulator control. Ind Robot. 1977;4:10–7.
22. Hon RE. Application flexibility of a computer controlled industrial robot. SME Technical Paper, MR 76-603; 1976.
23. https://en.wikipedia.org/wiki/Rajko_Tomović
24. Vokobrovitch M, Potkonjak V. Scientific fundamentals of robotics 1: dynamics of manipulation robots. Heidelberg: Springer Verlag; 1982.
25. Popov EP, Yurevich EI. Robotics. Moscow: Imported Pubn; 1989.

26. Kuleshov VS, Lakota NA. Remotely controlled robots and manipulators. Moscow: MIR Publishers; 1988.
27. Vokobrovitch M, Stokic D. Control of manipulation robots: theory and application. Scientific fundamentals of robotics series 2. Heidelberg: Springer-Verlag; 1982.
28. Coiffet P, Chirouze M. An introduction to robot technology. Paris: Hermes Publishing; 1982.
29. Profile: Tezuka Osamu. Anime Academy. 6 November 2007.
30. Ejiri M, Uno T, Yoda H. A prototype intelligent robot that assembles objects from plane drawings. IEEE Trans Comp. 1972;21: 199–207.
31. http://www.humanoid.waseda.ac.jp/booklet/kato_2-j.html
32. Inue H. Computer controlled bilateral manipulators. Bull Japanese Soc Mech Eng. 1971;14:199–207.
33. Hoeckelmann M, Rudas IJ, Fiorini P, Kirchner F, Haidegger T. Current capabilities and development potential in surgical robotics. Int J Advanced Robotic Syst. 2015;12:1–39.
34. Siciliano B, Khatib O, editors. Springer handbook of robotics, vol. LXXVI. 2nd ed. Berlin: Springer; 2017. 2227 p. 1375 illus. isbn:978-3-540-30301-5.
35. Alexander AD. Impacts of telemation on modern society. Proceedings of the 1st CISM–ITOMM Symposium. 1972. p. 121–136.
36. https://en.wikipedia.org/wiki/Robot-assisted_surgery
37. Kwoh YS, Hou J, Jonckheere EA, Hayati S. A robot with improved absolute positioning accuracy for CT guided stereotactic brain surgery. IEEE Trans Biomed Eng. 1988;35:153–60.
38. https://www.youtube.com/watch?v=3YpidnNUID4
39. Bowersox JC, Shah A, Jensen J, Hill J, Cordts PR, Green PS. Vascular applications of telepresence surgery: initial feasibility studies in swine. J Vasc Surg. 1996;23:281–7.
40. Schurr MO, Arezzo A, Buess GF. Robotics and systems technology for advanced endoscopic procedures: experiences in general surgery. Eur J Cardiothorac Surg. 1999;16(Suppl 2):S97–105.
41. Rininsland H. ARTEMIS. A telemanipulator for cardiac surgery. Eur J Cardiothorac Surg. 1999;16(Suppl 2):S106–11.
42. Harris SJ, Arambula-Cosio F, Mei Q, Hibberd RD, Davies BL, Wickham JE, et al. The Probot—an active robot for prostate resection. Proc Inst Mech Eng H. 1997;211:317–25.
43. Rovetta A, Sala R, Molinari Tosatti L. A robotized system for the execution of a transurethral laser prostatectomy. ISIR, International Symposium on Industrial Robots, Milano, October 1996.
44. Rassweilera J, Binderc J, Frede T. Robotic and telesurgery: will they change our future? Curr Opin Urol. 2001;11:309–20.
45. Jakopec M, Harris SJ, Rodriguez y Baena F, Gomes P, Davies BL. The Acrobot® system for total knee replacement. Ind Robot. 2003;30:61–6.
46. Brandt G, Radermacher K, Lavallée S, Staudte HW, Rau G. A compact robot for image guided orthopedic surgery: concept and preliminary results. In: 4th International Symposium on Medical Robotics and Computer Assisted Surgery (CVRMed-MRCAS'97), Grenoble, France; 1997. p. 767–776.
47. Debandi A, Maeyama A, Lu S, Hume C, Asai S, Goto B, et al. Biomechanical comparison of three anatomic ACL reconstructions in a porcine model. Knee Surg Sports Traumatol Arthrosc. 2011;19:728–35.
48. Kraft BM, Jäger C, Kraft K, Leibl BJ, Bittner R. The AESOP robot system in laparoscopic surgery: increased risk or advantage for surgeon and patient? Surg Endosc. 2004;18:1216–23.
49. https://en.wikipedia.org/wiki/ZEUS_robotic_surgical_system
50. Das H, Ohm T, Boswell C, Steele R, Rodriguez G. Robot-assisted microsurgery development at JPL. In: Akay M, Marsh A, editors. Information technologies in medicine. New York: John Wiley & Sons; 2001. p. 85–99.
51. Stephenson ER Jr, Sankholkar S, Ducko CT, Damiano RJ Jr. Robotically assisted microsurgery for endoscopic coronary artery bypass grafting. Ann Thorac Surg. 1998;66:1064–7.
52. http://surgrob.blogspot.com/2010/03/vintage-report-on-intuitive-vs-computer.html
53. Rovetta A, Sala R, Cosmi F, Wen X, Milanesi S, Sabbadini D, et al. A new telerobotic application: remote laparoscopic surgery using satellites and optical fiber networks for data exchange. Int J Robot Res. 1996;15:267–79.
54. https://en.wikipedia.org/wiki/Lindbergh_operation
55. https://www.sri.com/newsroom/press-releases/darpa-selects-sri-international-lead-trauma-pod-battlefield-medical-treatmen
56. Garcia P, Rosen J, Kapoor C, Noakes M, Elbert G, Treat M, et al. Trauma pod: a semi-automated telerobotic surgical system. Int J Med Robot. 2009;5:136–46.
57. Benabid AL, Hoffman D, Ashraff A, Koudsie A, Le Bas JF. Robotic guidance in advanced imaging environments. In: Alexander III E, Maciunas RJ, editors. Advanced neurosurgical navigation. New York: Thieme Medical Publishers; 1999. p. 571–83.
58. http://www.renishaw.com/en/neuromate-stereotactic-robot--10712
59. Glauser D, Fankhauser H, Epitaux M, Hefti JL, Jaccottet A. Neurosurgical robot Minerva: first results and current developments. J Image Guid Surg. 1995;1:266–72.
60. Morgan PS, Carter T, Davis S, Sepehri A, Punt J, Byrne P, *et al.* The application accuracy of the PathFinder neurosurgical robot. In: Lemke HU, Inamura K, Vannier MW, Farman AG, Doi K, Reiber JHC, editors. CARS 2003—computer assisted radiology and surgery: proceedings of the 17th international congress and exhibition, London, 25–28 June 2003 London: Elsevier; 2003.
61. Hagn U, Nickl M, Jörg S, Passig G, Bahls T, Nothhelfer A, et al. The DLR MIRO: a versatile lightweight robot for surgical applications. Ind Robot. 2008;35:324–6.
62. https://en.wikipedia.org/wiki/Sofie_(surgical_robot).
63. http://applieddexterity.com
64. Monticello G, Morselli M, Fiorini P. The development of the surgical robot Surgenius. In: International Federation of Robotics. World robotics 2011: service robots. New York: United Nations; 2011. p. 144–148. ISBN 978-3-8163-0616-0.
65. Bauer J, Lee BR, Stoianovici D, Bishoff JT, Micali S, Micali F, Kavoussi LR. Remote percutaneous renal access using a new automated telesurgical robotic system. Telemed J E Health. 2001;7:341–6.
66. Muradore R, Fiorini P, Akgun G, Barkana DE, Bonfe M, Boriero F, et al. Development of a cognitive robotic system for simple surgical tasks. Int J Adv Robot Syst. 2015;12:37. https://doi.org/10.5772/60137.
67. http://www.titanmedicalinc.com
68. http://www.alf-x.com/en
69. http://www.spine-health.com/video/spine-surgery-mazor-robotics-renaissance-guidance-system-sponsored
70. http://medrobotics.com
71. Coste-Manière E, Olender D, Kilby W, Schulz RA. Robotic whole body stereotactic radiosurgery: clinical advantages of the Cyberknife integrated system. Int J Med Robot. 2005;1:28–39.
72. Teh BS, Paulino AC, Lu HH, Chiu JK, Richardson S, Chiang S, et al. Versatility of the Novalis system to deliver image-guided stereotactic body radiation therapy (SBRT) for various anatomical sites. Technol Cancer Res Treat. 2007;6:347–54.
73. http://thinksurgical.com
74. http://www.makosurgical.com/physicians/products/rio
75. http://restorationrobotics.com
76. Siciliano B, Sciavicco L, Villani L, Oriolo G. Robotics modelling, planning and control. London: Springer-Verlag; 2009.

Robotic Operating Rooms

2

Jeffrey Berman, Emile Dajer, and Yuman Fong

Operating rooms (ORs) have been developed to provide a sterile environment in which to perform invasive procedures on patients. ORs are contained in suites that provide sterile support instruments and supplies necessary to perform the sterile procedures in a restricted environment, limiting access by the public and others not trained in or not involved with the procedures. Over the years, many new technologies to assist or augment surgeons have been added to ORs. The recent popularity and ubiquitous presence of robots in this environment raises complex design and planning issues worthy of consideration.

The Development of Robotic Systems

After the development of manually operated laparoscopic tools and instruments, machines that could operate these instruments with different physical abilities from the human hand (i.e., robots) were developed. These robots can be organized into several categories, including guidance systems, high-accuracy manipulators and scaled motion devices that incorporate enhanced vision, and other guidance systems such as magnification with stereo depth of field viewing, image guidance using X-rays and other devices, or navigation based on anatomical landmarks or fiducial markers. These robots seek to perform work not easily accomplished by hand and not accessible to manually operated or manipulated instruments or to assist with work in a difficult or hazardous environment.

Early in the adoption of robot-assisted surgery, robots were generally mobile, stand-alone instruments and systems, which were wheeled into general ORs to assist with parts of various specialized surgeries. These robots finally became the principal operating tool in many complex surgeries. As both ORs and robots have become more sophisticated, it has become functionally critical for these rooms to be designed specifically for the integration of the robotic system with the other video and integration systems incorporated within a modern surgical/interventional environment.

J. Berman, AIA, ACHA (✉) · E. Dajer, AIA
Jeffrey Berman Architect, New York, NY, USA
e-mail: jberman@jbarch.com

Y. Fong, MD
Department of Surgery, City of Hope National Medical Center,
Duarte, CA, USA

Y. Fong et al. (eds.), *The SAGES Atlas of Robotic Surgery*, https://doi.org/10.1007/978-3-319-91045-1_2

Space Requirements

As defined by the Facility Guidelines Institute (FGI; 2010, 2018), an *operating room (OR)* is a room in the Surgical Suite, designated and equipped for performing invasive procedures that require a restricted environment [1]. A *restricted environment* is a designated space with limited access eligibility. Such space has one or more of the following attributes: specific signage, physical barriers, security controls, and protocols that delineate requirements for monitoring, maintenance, attire, and use. The term is generally applied to operating rooms and the suites within which they are contained.

A *surgical suite* is defined as a space that includes operating rooms and support areas [1].

Our robotic surgical OR would be part of this suite, and we would expect these procedures to be performed under anesthesia in a Class C OR [1].

The design of an OR to support robotic procedures must first start with a basic OR to support any type of general or specialized surgery. The size of these rooms now starts at the code-prescribed minimum of 400 square feet, with dedicated space within the room for sterile surgical instruments, circulating nurses, doctors, desk and charting, and space for anesthesiology, including the anesthesia machine supplies and medicines [2]. These basic functions, as well as circulation around the sterile field and space for instrument and supply carts and bins for trash and other used materials, reside in the 400 square feet [2]. To add a robot or another large piece of equipment to this room while maintaining proper circulation, sterile field, and functionality requires the addition of a substantial amount of square footage, not less than 200–300 addtional square feet. Figure 2.1 shows the physical footprint of a typical OR and the footprints of a typical robotic system and other support systems equipment. Often more than one of these machines is used in the same case, requiring even more room for logistics, movement, and equipment during the procedure and staging prior to and after the use of each system. Figure 2.2 shows the actual sizes of these machines when parked and the additional space required to operate with the equipment in and around the surgical fields. Note the operator space required and the additional circulation space required to maintain the sterile fields.

Critical dimensions and clearances are similar to those required in a general OR. These have to do with circulation around the table, maintenance of the sterile field, sterile zones to lay out and prepare instruments, and circulation patterns to, from, and around the field. In robotic surgery, space is also required for the consoles that operate the robots and other equipment related to the controls in the video distribution of the robot images. The size of the expanded surgical workspace at the table pushes the circulation space further from the field and increases it substantially (Figs. 2.3 and 2.4).

Typically, a substantial amount of time is required for the robot to be set up and draped and have the necessary instruments installed on its arms. This procedure should take place while the patient is being brought into the room and prepared for the procedure. These two operations need to be separated, as the instruments must be handled in a sterile environment with no through traffic, both to protect the arms of instruments from mechanical damage due to impact and to maintain the sterile field when the instruments are placed and the arms are draped prior to the case. The zone for preparation of a robot should be specifically related to the way it will dock to the patient and the OR table once the case starts. The less movement required to bring the robot into position, the better: The robots are hard to drive when unfolded, and the extension of their large and delicate arms for surgery makes complex movement difficult.

Fig. 2.1 Plan of a typical operating room (OR) layout for open or minimally invasive surgery (MIS), with three staff work desks with computer and a picture archiving and communication system (PACS) station and dedicated space for anesthesia and medicines. When all personnel along with fixed and movable equipment is included. An area of 550 square feet is reasonable—slightly larger than the 400 square feet minimum space required by the Facility Guidelines Institute

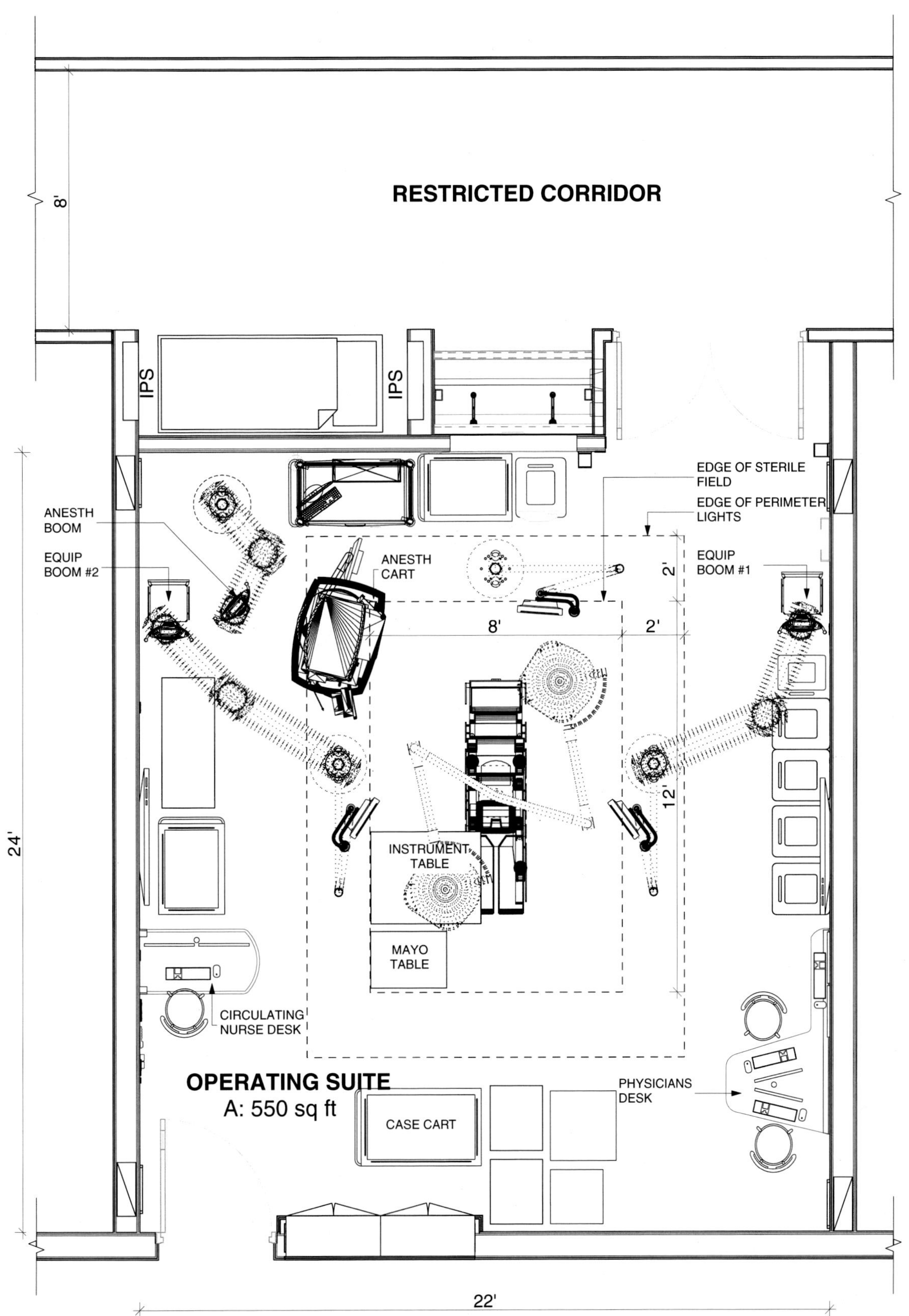
RESTRICTED CORRIDOR
8'
IPS
IPS
ANESTH
BOOM
EQUIP
BOOM #2
ANESTH
CART
EDGE OF STERILE
FIELD
EDGE OF PERIMETER
LIGHTS
EQUIP
BOOM #1
2'
8'
2'
12'
24'
INSTRUMENT
TABLE
MAYO
TABLE
CIRCULATING
NURSE DESK
OPERATING SUITE
A: 550 sq ft
CASE CART
PHYSICIANS
DESK
22'
STERILE CORE

RESTRICTED CORRIDOR
8'
IPS
IPS
ANESTH
BOOM
EQUIP
BOOM #2
ANESTH
CART
EDGE OF STERILE
FIELD
EDGEOFPERIMETER
LIGHTS
EQUIP
BOOM #1
24'
CIRCULATING
NURSE DESK
PHYSICIANS
DESK
OPERATING SUITE
A: 550 sq ft
22'
STERILE CORE
ROBOTIC SURGERY EQUIPMENT WILL REQUIRE SPATIAL ACCOMMODATIONS WITHIN THE SURGICAL SUITE. THIS APPROXIMATELY EQUATES TO 140 SQUARE FEET FOR THE EQUIPMENT FOOT PRINT AND ADDITIONAL CIRCULATION NEEDS.
140 sq ft
VC
VISION
CART
PATIENT
ROBOT
SURGEON
CONSLE (X2)

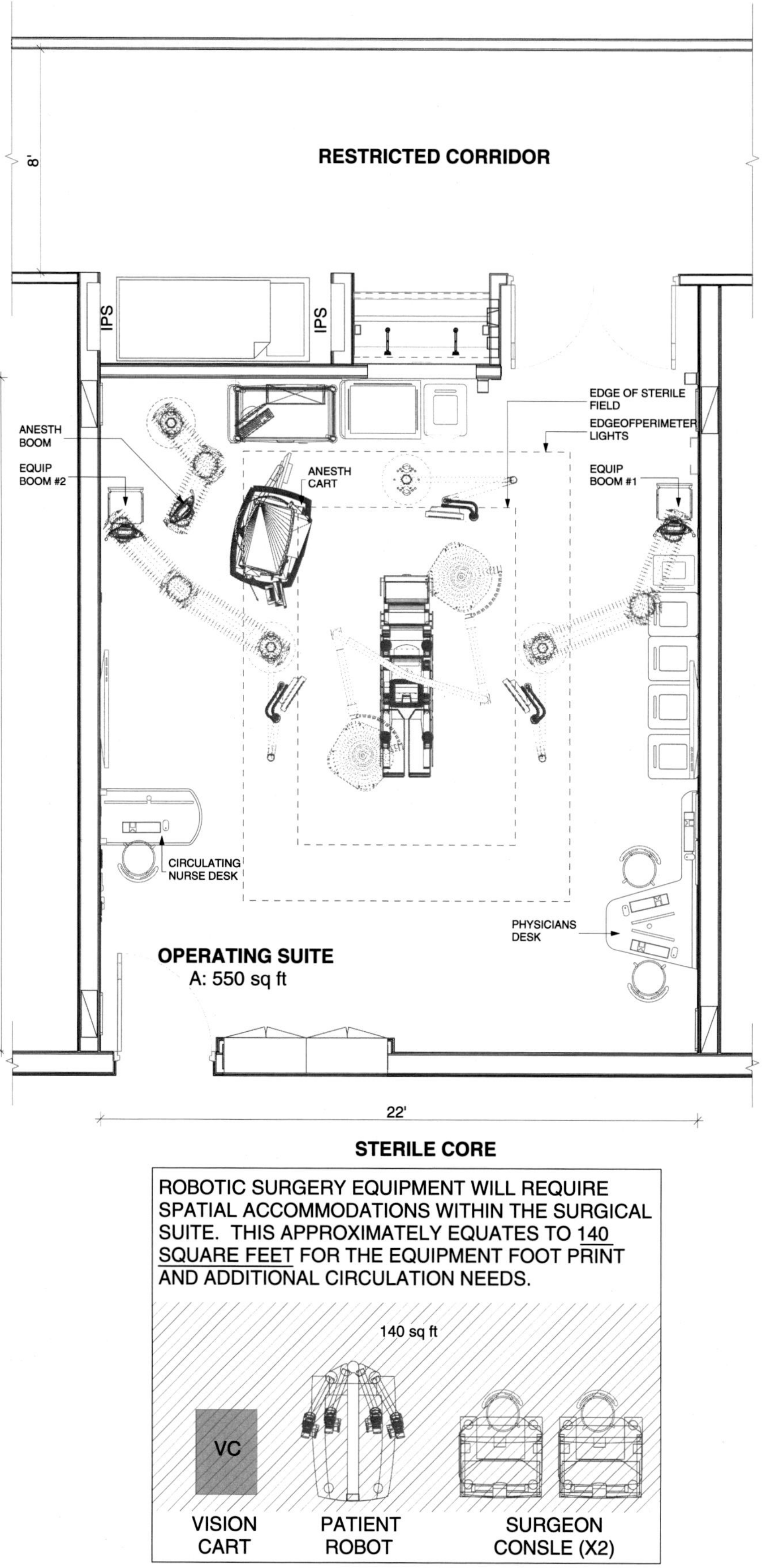

Fig. 2.2 A Da Vinci® robot (Intuitive Surgical; Sunnyvale, CA) with two consoles, circulation, setup, and operation requires a minimum area of 140 square feet, increasing the size of the OR by approximately one third

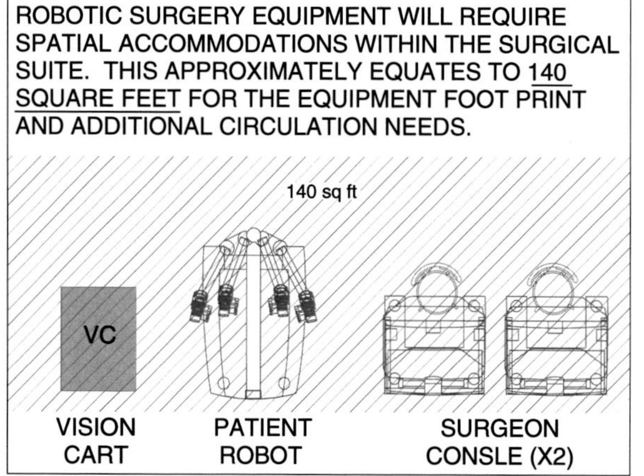

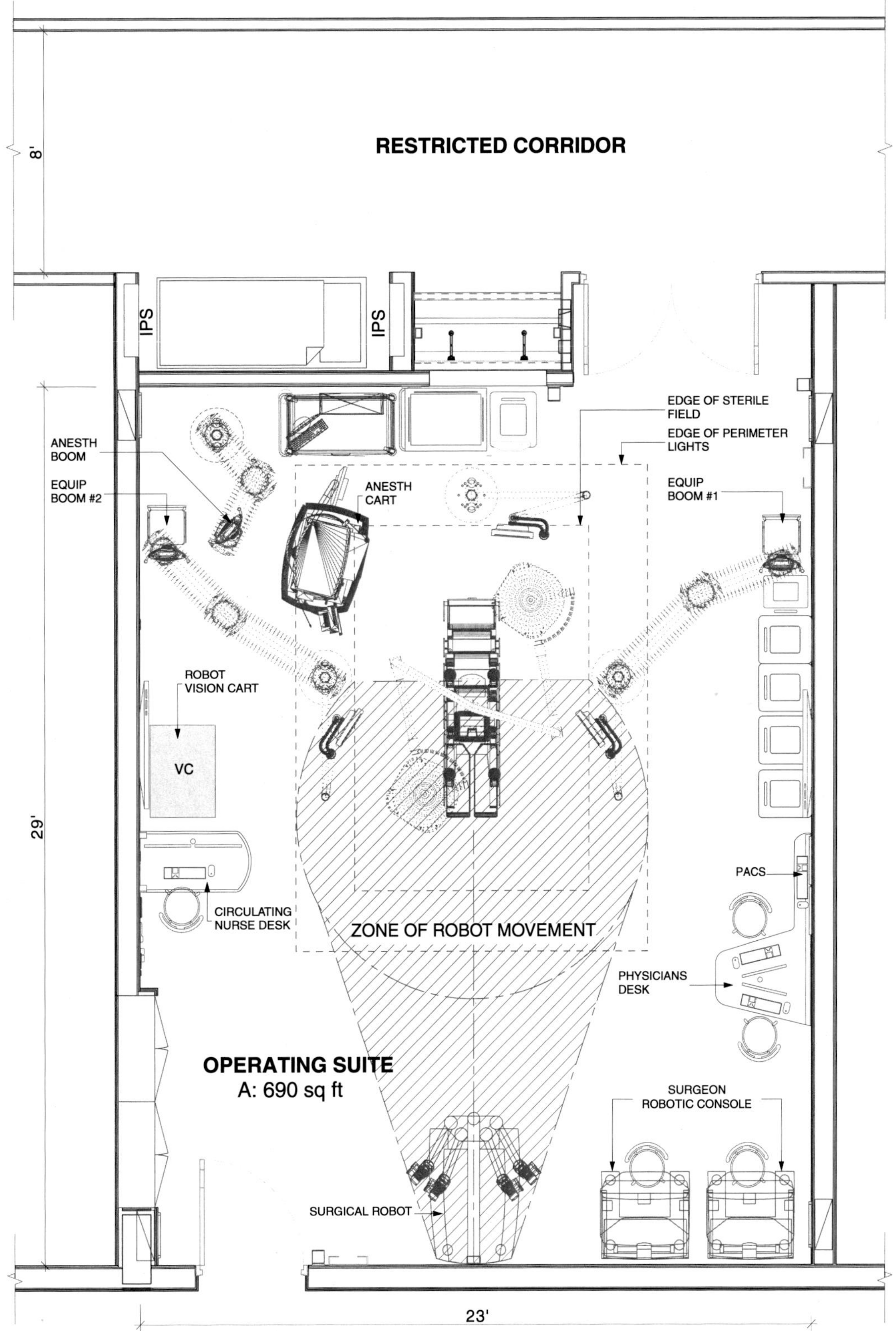

Fig. 2.3 This arrangement is designed to leave the consoles permanently parked near the surgeons' desks in the corner and to minimize the travel of the robot within the room during setup. The robot is shown parked when not in use. Additional space in the room allows the OR to be used for other procedures when the robot is parked

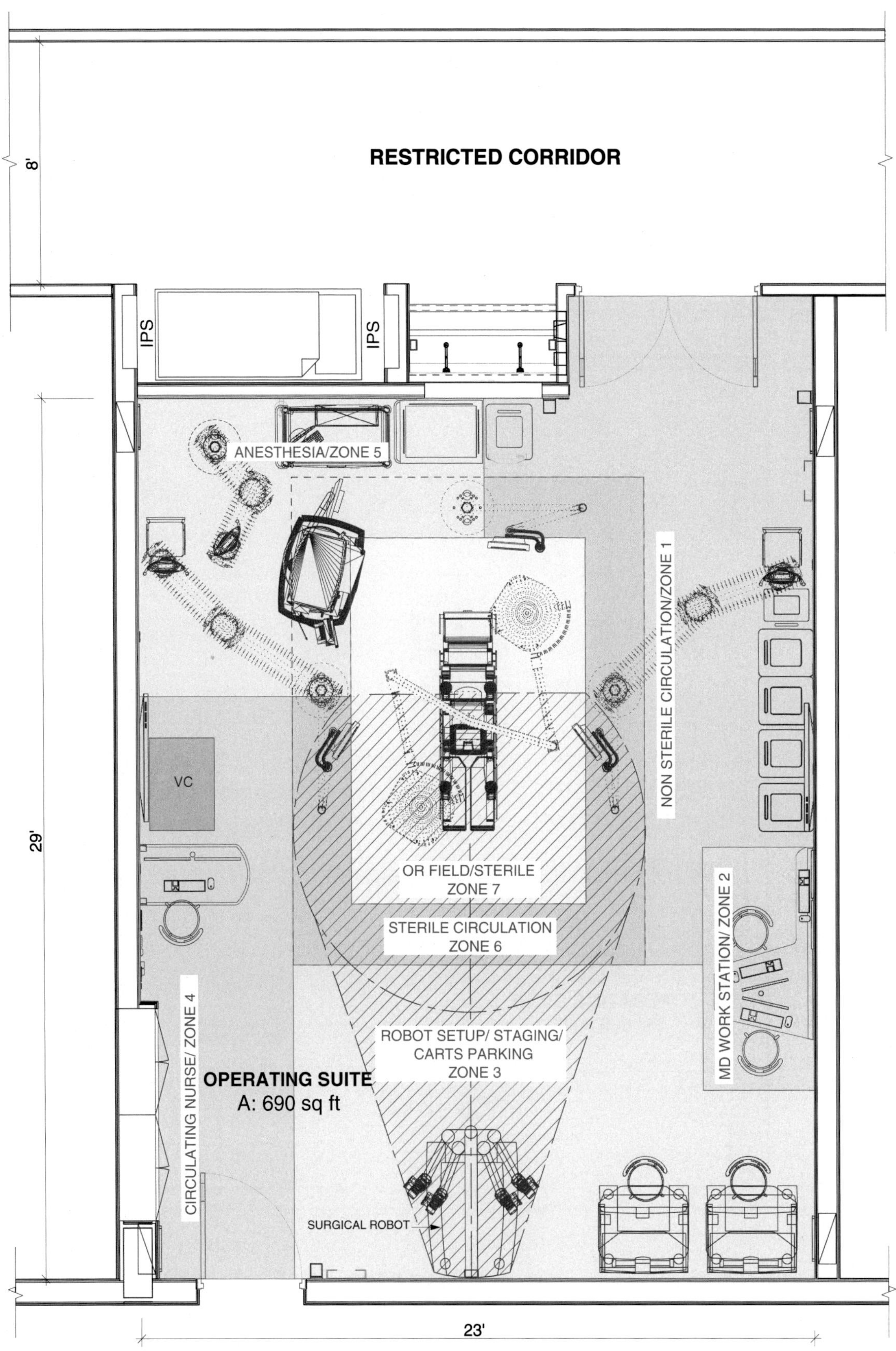

Fig. 2.4 This diagram of a robotic OR shows work zones for different functions during setup and during surgery

Support and Infrastructure Beyond the OR

Spaces for program support, training rooms, and operational support areas have a major impact on the design of new ORs. These areas must be provided for when planning a new OR suite, or identified and implemented within the building when retrofitting existing ORs for robotics or adding a robotic surgery program to an existing facility, even where the changes within the ORs are minimal.

Ancillary support space is significant in terms of space and resources required to support a functional robotics program. The spaces fall into two major categories: support/repair and training.

Support and Repair Spaces

These areas include repair and working space to house additional parts of the system, including consoles, video carts, and robots when not in use in a specific room, if the facility cannot dedicate ORs to robotic surgery or expand rooms with robots sufficiently to provide adequate parking spaces. A repair space is needed outside of the operating rooms, but preferably on the same floor as the ORs and in the restricted corridor. In this space, systems can be set up for testing and taken apart over time to be repaired and serviced without leaving the area. Hallways and doorways between service areas, storage areas, and ORs should be carefully planned to facilitate movement of these large, heavy instruments without damage to the building or the robot.

The additional instruments and specialty tools required to support the robot will require special processing in a sterile environment, generally a central sterile processing department. Additional storage space for this inventory, instruments, case carts, and supplies must be available in a sterile core adjacent to the robotic operating rooms. These resources are specific to the robot; a full complement of general surgical instruments and supplies will always be required to manually support the procedure and to assist and supplement the robot's capabilities.

Training Spaces

The training requirements for staff require space to develop skills and test new procedures using simulators, dry lab and wet lab training and experimentation. This training can be performed as part of a comprehensive surgical skills center, or it can be located in another simulation and training center. Facilities can be developed with the ORs and be proprietary to the hospital, but often training is provided on a contract basis in schools or at other dedicated surgical training and simulation facilities that are available to rent on a class or project basis. Workflow and support between these training and education functions and the actual support of surgery need to be carefully coordinated because of the great expense and difficulty of moving robots between distant facilities and the scheduling conflicts that arise between surgery schedules and training classes. The actual robots used for surgery must be available for training and testing in the OR suite at prearranged times.

Case Study: Modification of ORs for Robotics

An interesting case study that illustrates many of the issues involved with integration of a robot into a surgical environment is a project we completed in 2016 at the Josie Robertson Surgery Center in New York City. The hospital had extensive experience with robotic surgery on its inpatient platform and was building a new ambulatory surgery facility. The initial goal for design was to build three dedicated special OR suites over three floors: 1 for robotics, 1 for general surgery and laparoscopic work, and 1 for breast and plastic surgery, for a total of 12 operating rooms, four suites per specialty per floor. The rooms were all constrained to the same size by the footprint area of the new building, and the initial design developed three unique room layouts to support each specialty. What we learned was that there were many common, even identical, elements across the surgical platforms and specialties. These included the staff support spaces such as desks, computer workstations, charting, anesthesia, medicines, supplies, instruments, and communication systems. The patients and all the other elements remain the same size. What changed was the circulation in the room, the logistics and workflow around the surgical field to provide instruments and to service the robot. Space for the robot and all of its ancillary and support equipment is substantial when compared with the overall footprint of a general surgery OR (Figs. 2.5 and 2.6).

The major change or difference between a more traditional OR and a robotics room is the additional space needed for the setup of the robot and multiple sterile fields and the more restrictive requirements for circulation and flow of the room. The additional space is not just for the robot. The size of the sterile field also expands significantly, both during room setup and during the case, because the robot will occupy the space normally taken by the instrument table during surgery. A separate area for the instrument table away from the field and a sterile setup prior to the case away from the table are required. The space between the instrument table and the setup area for the robot is significant and falls in a critical area immediately adjacent to the table at the foot and to one side of the patient (Fig. 2.7).

When the robot is not in use, it can be parked out of the way of other procedures. The surgical staff appreciated the extra space for supplies and case carts when the robot was not in the room (Fig. 2.8).

Cabling between the parts of the robot needs to be managed carefully. These cables are heavy and delicate and interfere with both staff walking and cart and supply traffic into the room and to the sterile field, the work area, and the robot. The options for managing and routing these cables are currently limited, and it is important in planning and equipping these rooms to protect them from damage and to prevent the staff from tripping.

Lighting design for these rooms is very similar to that of a traditional or laparoscopic operating room: the general lighting needs to be bright enough for the setup and cleaning of the room as well as the repair and maintenance of the equipment. This lighting also needs to be dimmed so as to not produce intereference with the main surgical light which is designed to provide accurate color rendering of organic tissues and eliminate shadows caused by physical interference between light and patient. The surgeons at the robotic consoles have separately controlled and dimmed lighting overhead in order to control any glare preferentially. All the lighting must be dimmable, and controls must allow the room to be minimally lit to allow circulation between work areas around the robot and the surgical field without glare on the screens. The surgical lights often can be used as task lighting when they are not needed for surgery, but detailed consideration of task lighting requirements for the instruments, the circulating nurse, and the anesthesia work area is critical to the ability of staff to operate equipment and chart the case [3].

The fact that the surgeons are not working in the sterile field but instead are at remote consoles provides opportunities and challenges and raises a series of questions that need to be answered early in the planning and design of the rooms. The major question is whether the consoles should be in the OR or separated from the OR to provide isolation and concentration for the surgeons. The general consensus is to provide console space within the ORs and adjacent to workspace for the surgeons, including the medical record computer and picture archiving and communication system (PACS) terminals used in reviewing the case and preparing for the surgery. This workspace and the consoles should be located away from the surgical field and away from the sterile work zone between and including the circulating nurse desk access to the sterile core and the sterile setup zone between the instrument table, the surgical table, and the front of the robot where instruments are put on and the arms draped before beginning the case.

The expansion of the sterile field poses some interesting opportunities as well as challenges in the layout of the organization of the room and the workflow. Sterile work areas can be consolidated with their circulation and access to the instruments and supplies; the less sterile traffic of trash, in and out room cleaning, traffic from surgeons and others prior to the case, and the arrival, preparation, and departure of the patient can be segregated in a separate area (Figs. 2.9, 2.10, and 2.11). These layouts can yield a more efficient workflow with reduced setup and turnaround times between cases, as well as better infection control and less damage to instruments and parts of the robot. Another part of the basic plan should be dedicated robot rooms with parking space and permanent space for the non-moving parts. Better outcomes result when moving of equipment is minimized between cases and in the setup of cases.

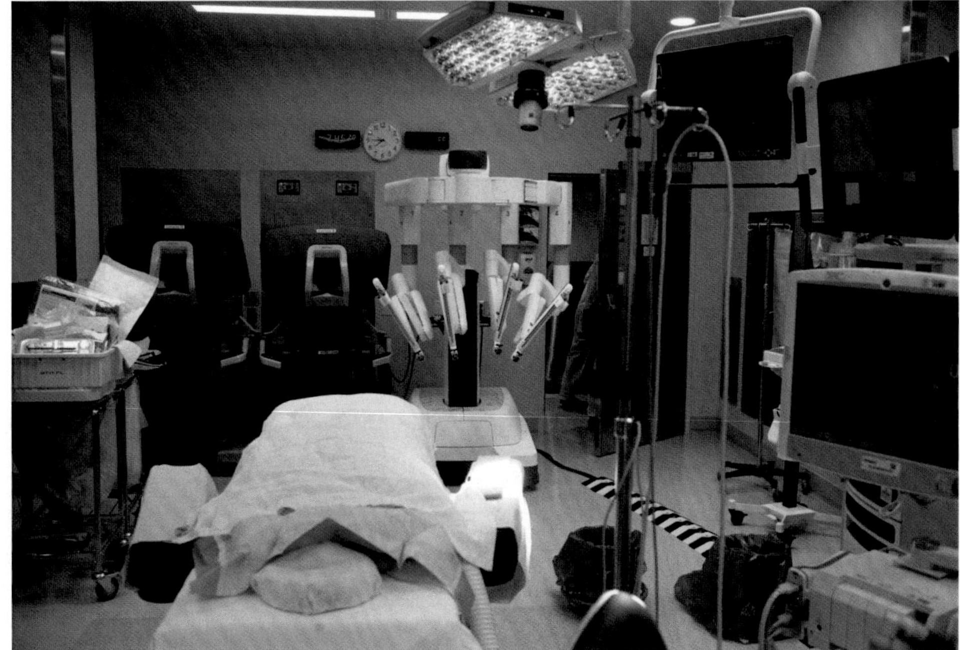

Fig. 2.5 A view from the restricted corridor door, looking at the robot parked against the wall with the consoles

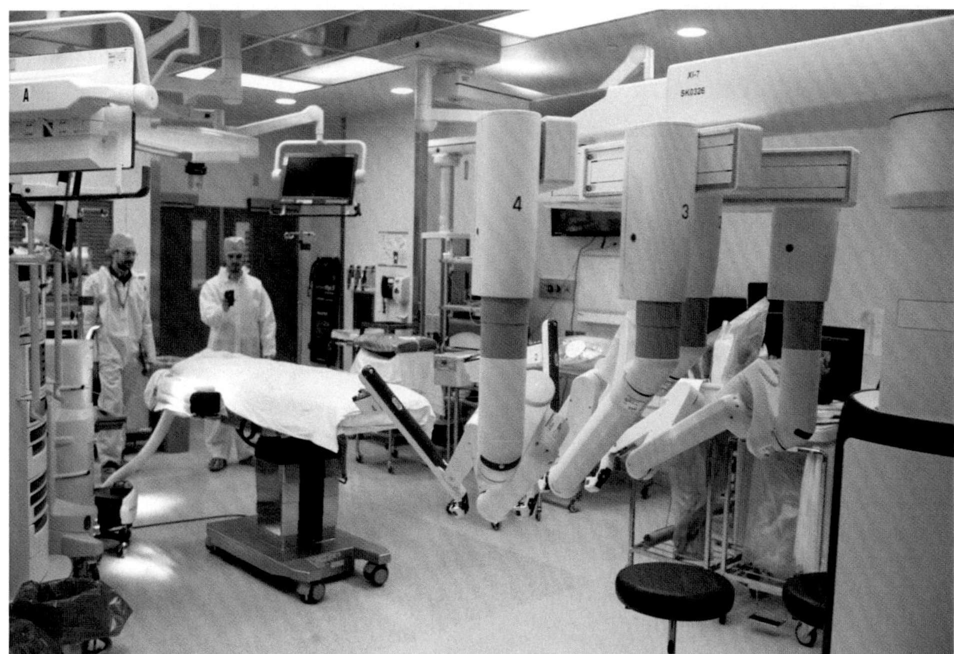

Fig. 2.6 A robot ready to be prepared for a case. The view is from the position of the anesthesiologist. The door to the sterile core is visible on the right. The consoles are on the left

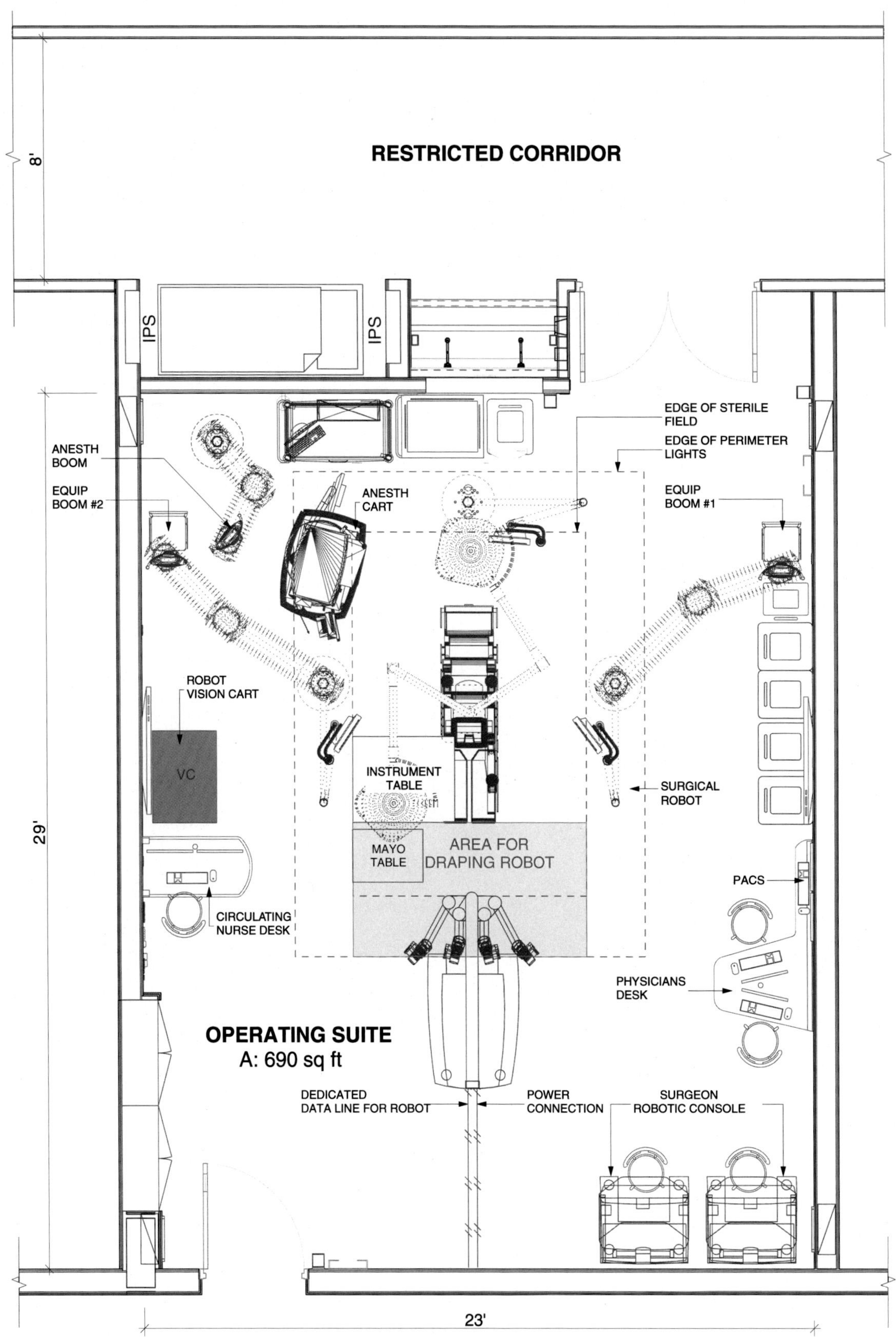

Fig. 2.7 A robot ready to be draped and have instruments installed on its arms. This occurs at the foot of the table so that the patient can be prepped at the same time. Circulation is around the back of the robot during this period to protect the arms of the robot, the sterile field, and the instruments

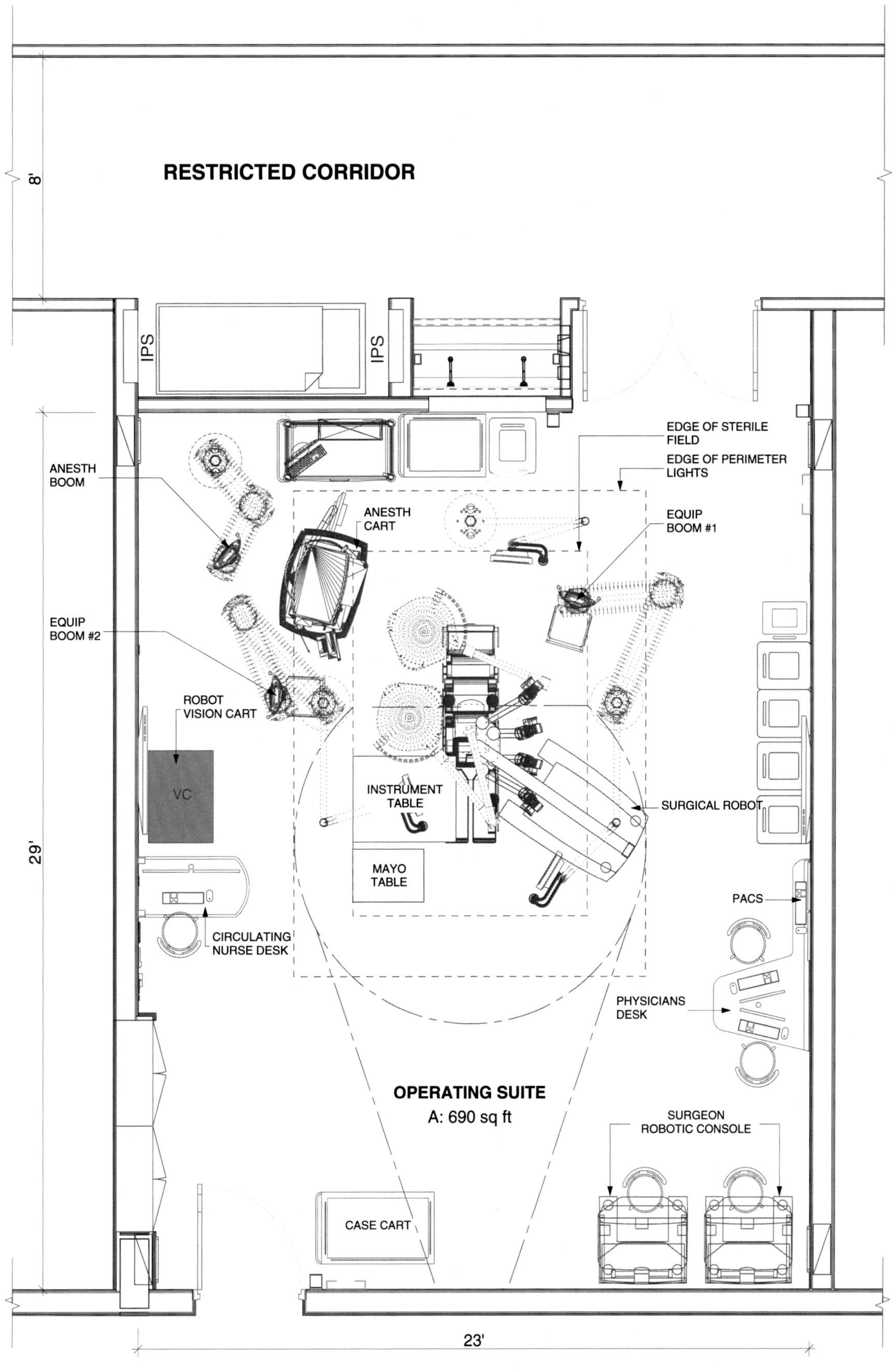

Fig. 2.8 An optional position of the robot in relation to the table for certain procedures that require the table to be shifted laterally to leave clear the aisles along the sides of the field, with adequate space behind the robot

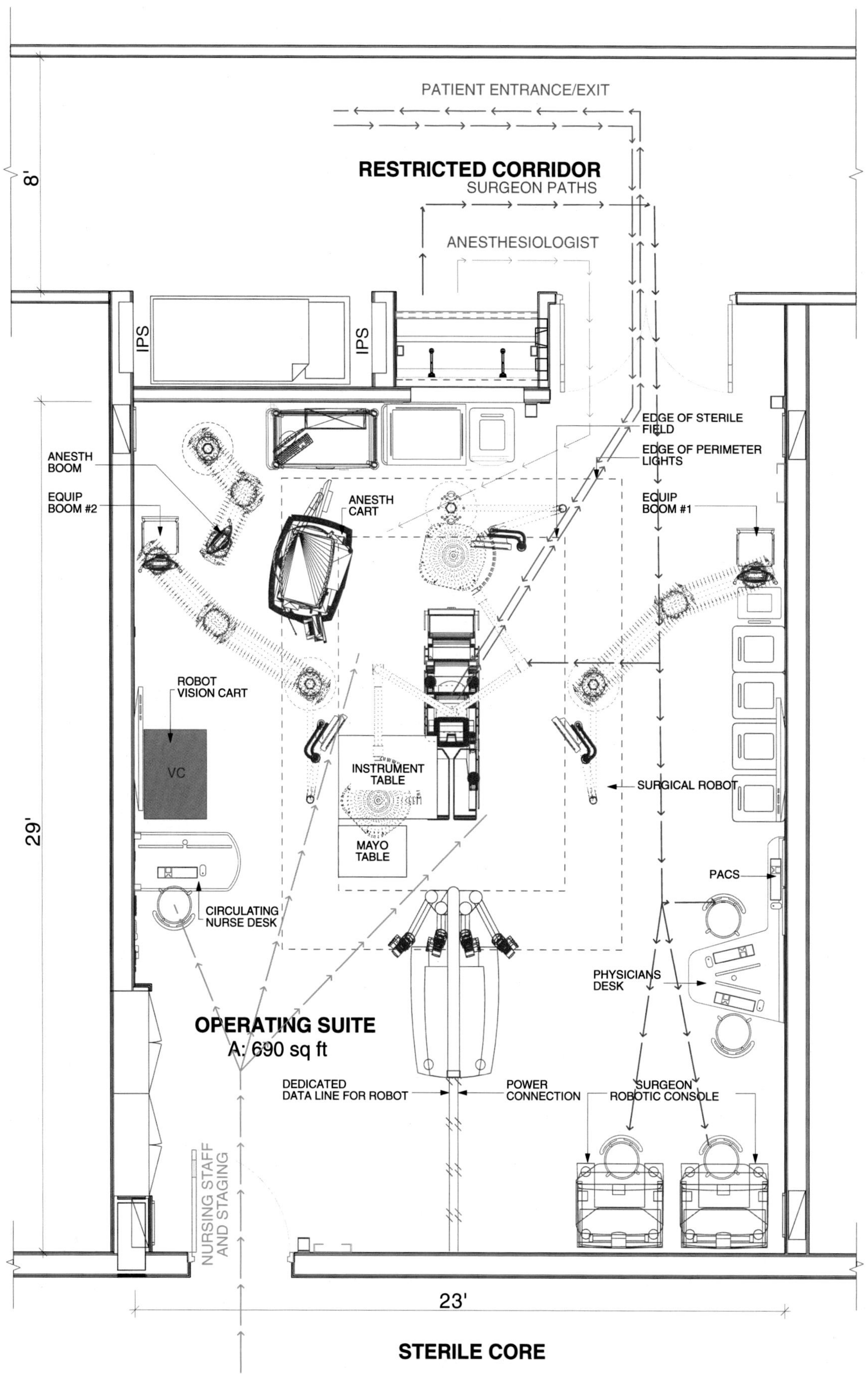

Fig. 2.9 During setup, preparation, and between cases, work areas are distributed around the room and separated to minimize disruption of independent tasks necessary to begin the surgery. There is more traffic in and out of the OR, and the sterile areas and paths are extended to prepare multiple functions

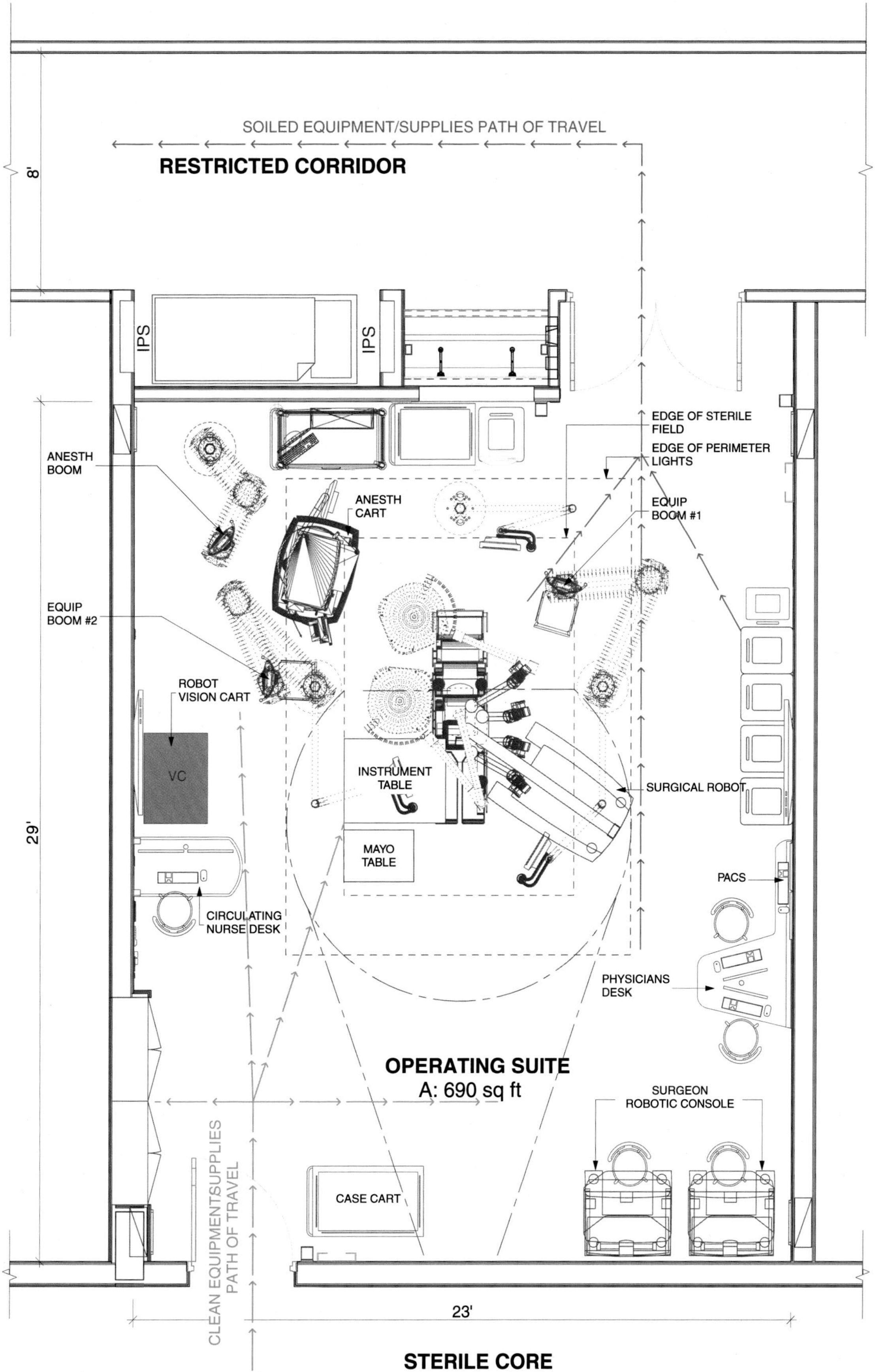

Fig. 2.10 Once the procedure begins, all instruments, supplies, and equipment are staged within the OR or in the sterile core just outside the room. The workflow and traffic are defined and limited to protect the sterile operating field from contamination and disturbance

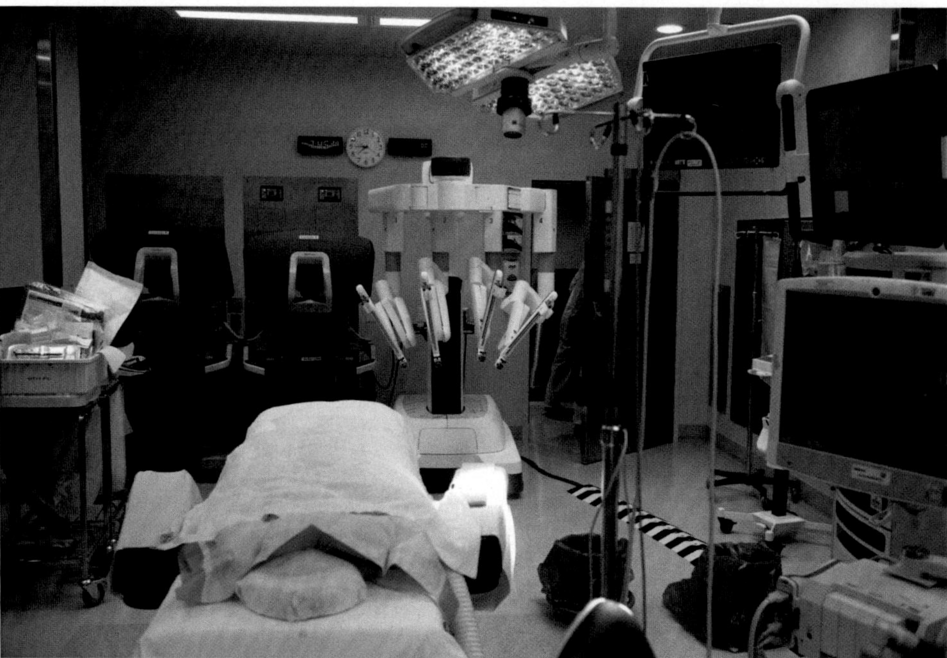
Fig. 2.11 A robotic OR viewed from the sterile core/circulating nurse position just before the start of setup. The equipment is in the room, the OR table is ready for patients, and the robot is on and ready to be draped and set up

The robot can function as a stand-alone device, but the efficiency of the OR staff will be improved by integrating the robotic video images into a routing system and making them available to the staff working within the room and the surgical field. As the case progresses, the ability to monitor progress and to see what is happening has proven to be an asset to the fellows, assistants, and surgical nurses assisting with the case. The anesthetist also benefits, and the surgeons, although focused on the display in the console, will need at times to see vital signs, general information displayed on the patient PACS, and other imaging that may be produced in the field, such as ultrasound or fluorescence imaging. Many robots have stereo imaging that can be displayed for viewing with and without special glasses on capable displays that can also be viewed without special devices. In general, however, stereo views are necessary only for the surgeons operating at the console, and the provision of only one channel or eye view simplifies the viewing in the room and the development of the video system in the routing of signals. Provisions should be made for routing of signals to outside classrooms or conference rooms, and for a viewing position in the room for visitors, which will allow them to see the general workflow and the room overall on wall-mounted or boom-mounted displays; they can then be kept clear of the immediate vicinity of the table, the surgical field instruments, and the robot where staff is working. The current signals most often used in operating rooms are 1080p, but displays are quickly evolving to the 4K and 8K standards. Even though all the signals are not produced at this resolution, the room should be prepared for these high-resolution and high-frame rate signals. The laparoscopic instruments and PACS images are already at these high resolutions, and we should expect all video to eventually migrate to this standard. The higher frame rates on the displays will allow support of 3-D visualization with glasses like those in theaters and for home video.

Conclusions

The addition of a robot or robotic surgery system to an OR adds significant space requirements to the room and technical complexity to the systems in the room. Special consideration must be given to the room layout and the space required to operate the system efficiently. When proper planning and design are implemented and the workflow and process in the room are properly understood, the impact on other cases performed in the room, the movement required to set up and put away the robot between cases, and wear and tear on the equipment can be minimized and staff functionality can be optimized.

References

1. Facilities Guideline Institute. Guidelines for design and construction of Hospitals. Dallas: FGI; 2018.
2. Berman J, Fong Y. Designing interventional environments in the treatment of cancer. In: Dupuy DE, Fong Y, WN MM, editors. Image-guided cancer therapy: a multidisciplinary approach. New York: Springer Science+Business Media; 2013. p. 201–12.
3. Berman J, Leiter RB, Fong Y. Lighting in the operating room: current technologies and considerations. In: Fong Y, Giulianotti PC, Lewis J, Koerkamp BG, Reiner T, editors. Imaging and visualization in the modern operating room: a comprehensive guide for physicians. New York: Springer Science+Business Media; 2015. p. 3–15.

3 Developing a Robotic Surgery Program

Pedro Recabal Guiraldes and Vincent P. Laudone

Successful implementation of a robotic surgery platform can result in increased value for patients, surgeons, and the institution, but building a robotic surgery program is a challenging endeavor that requires a multidisciplinary team. A steering committee is essential because coordinated efforts are required at different levels. Some of the committee's duties include defining goals, writing institutional guidelines, credentialing and privileging surgeons, coordinating the multidisciplinary robotic team, and educating the community. Robotic surgery is expanding and sooner or later will be available at most surgical institutions. The success of these programs will depend mainly on the commitment of the team and strong leadership from the steering committee.

Introduction

Initially devised to perform telesurgery, the first robotic platform based on an immersive interface (da Vinci® surgical system, Intuitive Surgical, Sunnyvale, CA) received US Food and Drug Administration (FDA) clearance to be used in human surgery in 2000. In the ensuing decade, the world witnessed a major transformation in minimal access surgery. Robotically-assisted surgery was disseminated across many different specialties, including urologic, gynecologic, general, colorectal, thoracic, cardiac, and head and neck surgery, often replacing laparoscopy in the process. Over 2000 da Vinci units are currently in use in the United States, where

P. Recabal Guiraldes, MD · V. P. Laudone, MD (✉)
Department of Surgery, Urology Service,
Fundacion Arturo Lopez Perez Center, Santiago, Chile

Y. Fong et al. (eds.), *The SAGES Atlas of Robotic Surgery*, https://doi.org/10.1007/978-3-319-91045-1_3

robotic surgery programs have been implemented in different settings ranging from small community hospitals to high-volume tertiary care centers. According to Intuitive Surgical's most recent annual report [1], the number of robotically-assisted surgeries continues to rise. In 2014, approximately 449,000 procedures were performed in the United States and an additional 121,000 elsewhere in the world (Fig. 3.1).

In the early 2000s, urology and gynecology were the primary uses of the robotic platform, but over the past 5 years, continued market expansion in the United States has been driven mainly by general surgery procedures, including cholecystectomy, hernia repair, and colorectal surgeries. The fourth generation of da Vinci surgical systems (Xi model) was launched in 2014. Currently, 65 different da Vinci surgical instruments are available, as well as a fluorescence imaging system (Firefly®, Intuitive Surgical), which allows real-time visualization of the vasculature, lymph nodes, or bile ducts, using specialized imaging hardware in combination with an injectable fluorescent dye. Because this chapter deals with establishing a new robotic surgery program and currently the most commonly used platform is da Vinci, this chapter will primarily refer to da Vinci systems. The authors' experience is greatest with these systems, so we can give specific details that should be helpful to surgeons contemplating such a program, no matter which system they may eventually choose.

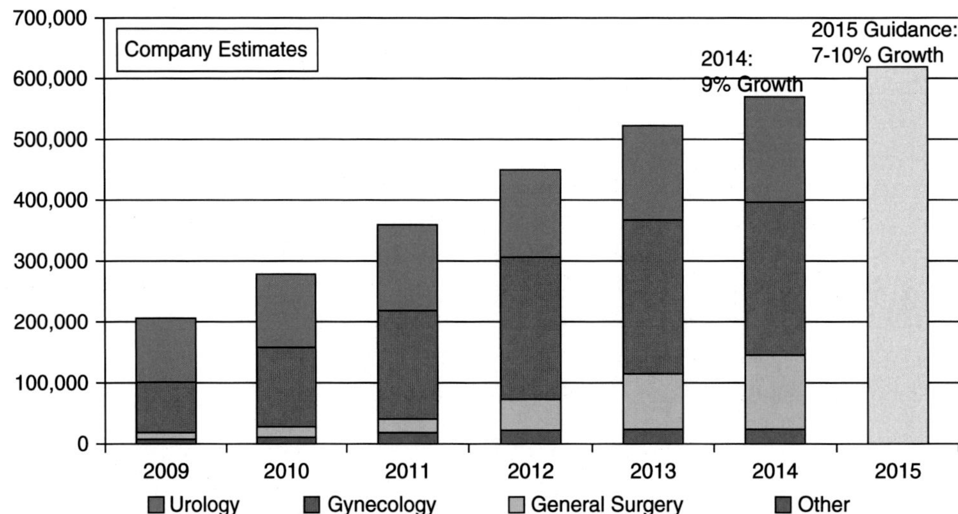

Fig. 3.1 Number and type of annual worldwide procedures using da Vinci surgical system, 2009–2014 [1]

Evidence-Based Medicine: Is the Robotic Surgical System Justified?

The emergence of robotic surgery programs across the United States was highly market-driven, as clinical studies investigating outcomes of robotically assisted surgery were lacking. This sophisticated surgical tool became a marketing strategy on its own, attracting both patients and surgeons to institutions that possessed this cutting-edge technology. In recent years, a body of evidence demonstrating benefits of robotically assisted surgery has been built, albeit some of it has come from sources with risk of bias. Over 400 peer-reviewed journal articles comparing robotically assisted surgery and alternative treatments were published in 2014. A number of meta-analyses have compared outcomes of robotic procedures in several specialties versus those performed using an open or conventional laparoscopy approach (Table 3.1) [2–16]. Robotic surgery has been associated with a lower rate of conversion to open surgery [3, 11, 12], reduced intraoperative blood loss [4, 5, 12–14], and a shorter length of hospitalization [5–7, 9, 12–15]. With few exceptions [12], most meta-analyses have also reported similar or lower complication rates. The information in these meta-analyses must be considered carefully, however, as most have included studies with significant risk of bias.

Procedure-specific meta-analyses have reported a reduced incidence of postoperative erectile dysfunction following robotically assisted rectal resections [2] and total mesorectal excision [3], reduced time to recovery of bowel function following robotically-assisted colectomy for benign and malignant disease [4–6], reduced positive surgical margin rate and anastomotic stricture rate following robotically-assisted radical prostatectomy [10], and reduced warm ischemia time and estimated glomerular filtration rate decline following robotically-assisted partial nephrectomy [11]. These benefits must be weighed against a consistent increase in cost and operative time.

There is still a lack of high-level evidence to support the superiority of the robotic approach for long-term and oncologic outcomes, however. Another caveat is that most studies showing the superiority of robotically-assisted surgery have evaluated outcomes of oncologic procedures; the evidence favoring the use of the robotic system for benign diseases is less robust. As such, institutions considering acquiring a robotic surgical system should carefully scrutinize their own procedure mix, and this investment should be in line with the institution's vision and mission.

Financial Considerations

The implementation of a robotic surgery platform poses a significant financial challenge to any institution. The substantial capital investment needed to make this technology available for patient treatment calls for a careful examination of several factors. As of 2016, the da Vinci Surgical System generally sells for between $0.6 million and $2.5 million depending upon configuration and geography, and the annual rate for a service contract is between $100,000 and $170,000. Disposable supplies can run more than $1000 per case. Before an institution decides to acquire a robotic surgical system, a thorough analysis is crucial to gauge feasibility, let alone profitability. This analysis should consider the impact of a robotic surgery program on current and projected case volume; payor mix and reimbursement; expected benefits (e.g., decrease in complications and length of hospitalization); direct and indirect expenses such as the cost and depreciation of the da Vinci unit, the service contract, supplies, and possible renovation to the operating room (OR) facility to suit the robotic surgical system; marketing; and training, proctoring, and credentialing of the robotic surgery staff.

In a market crowded with robots, for most programs length-of-stay savings are not enough to offset the increased cost derived from the unit, the service fee, and the supplies. A few years ago (but much less so today), a robotic surgical system was perceived as a strategic advantage that would attract out-of-area patients to the institution, resulting in increased surgical volume. From a purely procedural cost accounting perspective, the investment is rarely justified, and this should not be the driving motivation. Nonetheless, institutions can still derive value from making robotically assisted surgery available to their patients. Advantages for the institution include a possible increase in surgical volume, availability of latest technology that will attract younger and insured patients, and creating a culture of excellence that allows recruiting and retaining of top surgical talent. Many fellowship-trained surgeons feel more comfortable operating with the robotic platform than using conventional laparoscopic or open approaches and simply won't consider working at institutions that don't have robotics available.

Concrete evidence of the cost-effectiveness of robotic surgery compared with the alternatives is limited. Several studies confirm that the procedural cost of robotic surgery is higher than the cost for open or conventional laparoscopic cases [9, 17], but very few have used economic models that are representative of the disease pathway—that is, that are sufficiently detailed and include longer-term costs of care, extending beyond the perioperative period. Decisionmakers are in need of studies that capture relevant differences in outcome across strategies within their own systems, by accounting not only for procedural cost but also for quality-adjusted life-years (QALYs) and incremental cost-effectiveness ratio [17].

Table 3.1 Summary of comparative results in 15 recent (2013–2015) meta-analyses

	Broholm [2]	Xiong [3]	Rondelli [4]	Trastulli [5]	Chang [6]	Chuan [7]	Montalti [8]	Liu [9]	Robertson [10]	Choi [11]	Ran [12]	Shazly [13]	Fonseka [14]	Marano [15]	Cao [16]
Technique compared with robotic	Lap	Lap	Lap	Lap	Lap	Lap	Lap	Lap	Lap	Lap	Lap; open	Lap; open	Lap; open	Open	Open
Procedure	Rectal CA surgery	TME	Right col	Col	Col	Gastr	Hepat	Gyn surgery	Prost	Partial nephr	Endometrial CA resection	Hyst	Cyst	Gastr	Mitral valve surg
Meta-analysis showed advantage for following outcomes[a]															
Conversion to open surgery		+robot	NCSD	NCSD	NCSD		NCSD	NCSD	NCSD	+robot	+robot; —				
Operative time		NCSD	+lap	+lap	+lap	+lap	+lap	+lap		NCSD	NCSD; +open		+lap; +open	+open	
Estimated blood loss		NCSD	+robot	+robot	NCSD	NCSD	+lap			NCSD	+robot; +robot	NCSD; +robot	NCSD; +robot	NCSD	
Length of stay		NCSD	NCSD	+robot	+robot	+robot	NCSD	+robot			NCSD; +robot	NCSD; +robot	NCSD; +robot	+robot	NCSD
Complications		NCSD	NCSD	+robot	+robot	NCSD	NCSD	NCSD	+robot	NCSD	+lap; +robot	NCSD; +robot	—; +robot	NCSD	
Lymph node yield		NCSD	NCSD	NCSD	NCSD	+robot					NCSD; NCSD	NCSD; NCSD	—; NCSD	NCSD	
Surgical margins		+robot					NCSD		+robot	NCSD			—; NCSD		
Anastomotic leak			NCSD	NCSD		NCSD			+robot						
Time to recovery of bowel function			+robot	+robot	+robot				NCSD						
Postoperative ED	+robot	+robot													

\+ indicates the approach with the most favorable given outcome; NCSD indicates no clinically significant difference

The following outcomes were reported in only one meta-analysis: for the International Prostate Symptom Score (IPSS), Broholm [2] favored robotic; for local recurrence, Xiong [3] observed NCSD; and for urinary continence, Robertson [10] observed NCSD. Choi results [11] favored robotic for conversion to radical surgery, warm ischemia time, and change in eGFR and observed NCSD for change in creatinine. Cao results [16] favored robotic for perioperative mortality and open for cross-clamp time and cardiopulmonary bypass time, with NCSD for reoperation and stroke

CA cancer, *col* colectomy, *ED* erectile dysfunction, *eGFR* estimated glomerular filtration rate, *gastr* gastrectomy, *gyn* gynecologic, *hepat* hepatectomy, *hyst* hysterectomy, *lap* conventional nonrobotic laparoscopic surgery, *NCSD* no clinically significant difference, *nephr* nephrectomy, *prost* prostatectomy, *robot* robotic, *surg* surgery, *TME* total mesorectal excision

The Robotic Surgery Steering Committee

Institutions that have successfully implemented robotic surgery have recognized the importance of a dedicated robotic taskforce. Early engagement of and collaboration between the hospital's board, medical staff, and administration are critical to ensure operational success, as all parties must join efforts toward the same objectives. Creating a robotic surgery steering committee is necessary to ensure patient safety and the highest standards when integrating robotic technology, considering the significant operational challenges associated with establishing robotically-assisted surgery at any institution. The composition of the committee should include, on the clinical side, a robotics coordinator (usually a registered nurse with OR coordination experience) and representatives from all surgical specialties performing robotically-assisted surgery, anesthesia, OR nursing, surgical physician assistants, equipment techs, and supply personnel. On the administrative side, a marketing specialist, a financial advisor, and a senior executive should be included.

The committee's duties include defining goals and a timeline, writing institutional guidelines, overseeing training and credentialing of the robotic surgery staff, coordinating scheduling of robotic procedures, supervising patient outcomes, coordinating the multidisciplinary robotic team, and educating the community. The committee must determine which procedures should be performed and who is privileged to use the robotic system. Although maximizing the number of robotic cases might make economic sense, the misuse of the robotic system for "inappropriate" procedures or having many surgeons performing only a few cases each is simply not a good medical practice.

Credentialing and Privileging Surgeons

In the early 2000s, completion of Intuitive Surgical's preparatory training was the only requirement for surgeons to be cleared to perform robotic surgery on the da Vinci system. The program—consisting of 1 day of hands-on training and completion of two cases proctored by an expert—became the base of credentialing requirements at many institutions. However, a recent ruling in the trial of *Taylor v Intuitive Surgical, Inc.* [18] has challenged the responsibility of the manufacturer in the credentialing process, implying that the medicolegal risks related to the use of the robotic platform are jointly shared by physicians and hospitals, in addition to the manufacturer. As such, institutions are responsible for certifying the competence of surgeons (credentialing) and granting permission for them to perform specific procedures (privileging).

As of 2016, there is no universal credentialing process. Scientific societies have created guidelines recommending structured robotic training [19, 20], but each robotic steering committee is responsible for defining the institutional credentialing requirements. Credentialing within an institution may vary according to the surgeon's prior training. (Table 3.2 shows an example from the authors' institution.) This process should be clearly specified and stringently held; it is better to have fewer surgeons who are truly committed than to privilege many surgeons who will get little console time and therefore never gain the necessary competency.

Training requirements should be tailored according to the surgeon's previous exposure to minimal access and robotic surgery. Naïve surgeons should complete a formal didactic course providing the basic knowledge to understand the mechanics of the technology. Surgeons need to be familiar with device function and malfunction, including basic troubleshooting and how to safely remove the device in an emergency. This curriculum should also include review of recorded specialty-specific cases, observation of specialty-

Table 3.2 Faculty credentialing and privileging to perform robotic surgery at Memorial Sloan Kettering Cancer Center (MSKCC)

Current faculty
• Documentation of completion of the Web-based training modules for the platforms that are available at MSKCC
• Completion of an animal-based training module. This is available off-site, and there are costs associated with this training
• Completion of at least one dry-lab training session held at MSKCC prior to a live surgical procedure
• Simulation training on the currently available system
• Ten surgical cases proctored by an experienced robotic surgeon. Although highly preferable, this need not be by a surgeon of the same specialty, nor must all ten cases be proctored by the same surgeon. The proctor(s) must complete a form attesting to completion of the proctored cases. If the proctor(s) identify any concerns during the proctoring of cases, more than ten cases may need to be proctored
New faculty
• New faculty who have received robotic training in their residency/fellowship will be credentialed to independently perform robotic procedures if they can provide an adequate list of cases, describing the nature of the cases as well as their role (assistant and/or console surgeon) in each case. A letter from their training program documenting completion of adequate robotic training and competency in robotic surgery is required. Documentation of completion of the most current Web-based training modules is also required. An animal-based training module is not required
• New faculty who have performed robotic procedures since completing their training program will be credentialed to perform robotic procedures independently if they can provide an adequate list of cases that they have performed as the surgeon. Documentation of completion of the most current Web-based training modules is also required. An animal-based training module is not required
• New faculty who do not meet one of the above two sets of criteria must meet all the other criteria for current faculty above

specific live cases, dry-lab practice and/or practice on a robotic simulator, and a procedure dry run. The first cases performed by a surgeon transitioning to robotically assisted surgery should be proctored to decrease stress in the OR and minimize risks for the patient. After completion of the prespecified curriculum and proctored cases, surgeons are credentialed by the steering committee and privileged to perform that particular procedure. The steering committee is responsible for monitoring the outcome of procedures performed by the newly trained surgeons. Proficiency should be reassessed for maintenance of surgical privileges. This process is aimed at ensuring patient safety when introducing new technology in the OR.

The Robotic Surgery OR Team

Knowledge and commitment are essential characteristics of a team that successfully performs robotically assisted surgery. The adoption of novel technology requires training of all the OR staff to ensure patient safety and operational success. This team faces unique logistical challenges in the OR, and collaboration is critical.

Dedicated robotic surgeons in each specialty performing robotically assisted surgery must champion this team. Institutions should strive to have their higher-volume, most efficient surgeons on the console, to reduce operative time and improve patient outcomes. Studies comparing the learning curve of robotically-assisted surgery to that of conventional laparoscopy for complex procedures suggest that mastering robotically-assisted surgery may require fewer cases [21–23]. Most surgeons recognize the learning advantage of concentrating cases over a short period of time, and the institution should encourage and facilitate this concentration.

A bedside assistant with laparoscopic experience and comprehensive understanding of the procedure is essential. The operating surgeon—who is at the console and not scrubbed in—may not perform several tasks, including changing the robotic instruments, cleaning the laparoscope, passing sutures, using suction and irrigation, and removing needles and specimens. Studies have shown that formal laparoscopic training and an organized robotic training course consisting of hands-on training, video review, and simulation increased the assistants' level of satisfaction at work, could improve trocar placement and the insertion of laparoscopic instruments and hemostatic maneuvers, and could reduce docking and undocking times [24, 25]. A skilled laparoscopic assistant can significantly reduce operative times—particularly in complex operations—by predicting the surgeon's following moves and providing better exposure when retracting tissue and using suction to remove blood and smoke. The use of a fourth robotic arm cannot replace the role of the bedside assistant. Every robotic surgeon should make an effort to establish partnership with the bedside assistant in order to increase the assistant's predictive ability and streamline the operations.

The OR staff, including the scrubbed and circulating nurse, must also be trained and knowledgeable about the robotic instruments, the docking and undocking process, and basic troubleshooting. The anesthesiology team should be familiar with specific issues of robotic surgery, such as patient setup and the ventilatory and hemodynamic changes induced by the pneumoperitoneum and the Trendelenburg positioning utilized in many procedures.

Careful surgical planning is important to reduce the costs associated with instrument use, as robotic instruments can be used a certain number of times before expiring. Each instrument has a limited number of "lives," so surgeons should only use the instruments that are truly required to perform the procedure, to avoid incurring extra costs. Training and careful manipulation and reprocessing of instruments help ensure these will be in good condition until they expire. For example, inappropriate use of the robotic scissors causes them to lose sharpness, but replacing them during the case increases the overall cost.

Every member of the robotic team must be aware of his or her own responsibilities in the unlikely scenario of an emergency conversion to open surgery. It is advisable to review this plan before every case, as some of the steps may be counterintuitive (e.g., it is recommended *not* to undock the robot until everything is ready to perform the incision, because the robotic arms may be tamponading the hemorrhage). A formal checklist approach is highly recommended (Table 3.3).

Table 3.3 Checklist for emergent conversion from robotic to open procedure

Who	What
Attending surgeon	1. Call for emergent conversion to open procedure, *designate person in charge of maintaining tamponade*
Circulating RN	2. Push code "blue" button and/or call central desk. Turn on OR lights
Circulating RN	3. Open robotic emergency tray
Anesthesia team	4. Notify anesthesia attending via Vocera
Anesthesia team	5. Initiate IV fluid resuscitation. Confirm adequacy of IV access
Anesthesia team	6. Request blood products. *Request confirmation when sent*
Bedside assistant	7. Maintain tamponade; may initiate removal of some robotic instruments at the direction of attending surgeon
Attending surgeon	8. Direct one of the staff to undock robot
Attending surgeon	9. Proceed to open procedure
Circulating RN	10. Notify all available service attendings for additional help

IV intravenous, *OR* operating room, *RN* registered nurse

Marketing and Community Education

After the training and credentialing process is complete, a marketing strategy should be developed to raise awareness about the da Vinci surgery program. A recent study of a Web-based survey, in which half of participants worked in the healthcare industry, confirmed that the public still has significant misperceptions about robotic surgery. For example, the main concern for two thirds of respondents was that the robot would malfunction, causing internal damage during the surgery; 21% thought the robot had some autonomous function during surgery; and 14% had never heard of robotic surgery. Less than half of respondents would prefer a robotically assisted surgery over conventional minimal access surgery, indicating an ongoing need for patient education [26].

The marketing goals include making patients and referring physicians aware of the availability of robotic surgery; educating patients, referring physicians, and internal staff about potential benefits of the robotic system; promoting the expertise of specific surgeons; and positioning the institution as a leader in state-of-the-art medical technology. Diverse marketing initiatives have contributed to the success of robotic surgery programs across the United States, with tactics that include press releases, physician presentations, traditional media, social networks, newsletters, open houses, direct mail, brochures, and even robot test drives. Launching the marketing strategy after the first cases have been successfully completed is advisable, so that local outcomes can be included as part of the campaign.

Mistakes to Avoid

- Marketing as the focus for program development. Building a robotic surgery program is a resource-consuming endeavor. The objective must be to increase value for the patients, the surgeons, and the institution. After the program is established, procedures are standardized, and the learning curves have been overcome, it is appropriate to use a marketing strategy to raise awareness about the availability of the platform and the outcomes from the institution. Marketing should never be the initial or the final objective for acquiring the device.
- Marketing the robot by referencing outcomes from other institutions. The robotic platform is a surgical tool, and the outcomes of robotic surgery depend on the surgeon who is using the tool. Outcomes cannot be extrapolated across institutions just because the procedures are performed with the same tool.
- Privileging too many surgeons at once. Privileging too many surgeons prolongs the learning curves and standardization of the procedures, creates confusion within the OR team, and frustrates the committed surgeons who can't get enough console time. Key personnel should be identified in advance and allowed to standardize the procedure before other naïve surgeons begin their training.
- Buying the robot for a single surgeon or specialty. A robotic surgery program is unlikely to succeed if only one surgeon or one specialty is using the robot. Most successful programs are multidisciplinary.
- Forcing open surgeons who are not interested in robotic surgery to use the robot. If a surgeon is not interested, encouraging him or her to use the device is a recipe for disaster.
- Failing to foresee the need for additional platforms. Some programs are very successful, and volumes can grow quickly. Institutions should not wait until the robotic scheduling reaches full capacity to acquire a second platform; doing so causes scheduling delays, frustrates surgeons and patients, and prolongs the learning curve for recently incorporated surgeons.

Conclusions

Building a robotic surgery program is challenging in many ways and requires a dedicated, multidisciplinary team. In an economic environment where healthcare cost is under intense scrutiny and the system often rewards quantity rather than quality, the current controversy surrounding the value of robotic surgery is basically driven by its high cost and by the paucity of evidence showing an improvement on "hard" outcomes such as survival and recurrence. Nevertheless, the current robotic platform increases value to various stakeholders by decreasing invasiveness; improving dexterity, visualization, and ergonomics; providing motion scaling; and eliminating tremor. In addition, most studies have shown similar or better short-term outcomes for most complex procedures, with very few reporting higher incidence of complications in specific settings. The robotic surgery field is expanding, and there is still much room for improvement in areas such as tactile feedback, single-site surgery, telepresence surgery, and augmented reality. As technology evolves and cost decreases, robotic surgery will be available sooner or later at most surgical institutions. The success of these programs will depend mainly on the commitment of the team and strong leadership from the steering committee.

Acknowledgment We thank Amy Plofker, Memorial Sloan Kettering Cancer Center editor, for the editorial input.

References

1. Intuitive Surgical, Inc. Annual Report 2014. Sunnyvale, CA: Intuitive Surgical; 2015. http://investor.intuitivesurgical.com/phoenix.zhtml?c=122359&p=irol-irhome. Accessed 10 Sept 2015.
2. Broholm M, Pommergaard HC, Gögenür I. Possible benefits of robot-assisted rectal cancer surgery regarding urological and sexual dysfunction: a systematic review and meta-analysis. Color Dis. 2015;17:375–81.
3. Xiong B, Ma L, Huang W, Zhao Q, Cheng Y, Liu J. Robotic versus laparoscopic total mesorectal excision for rectal cancer: a meta-analysis of eight studies. J Gastrointest Surg. 2015;19:516–26.
4. Rondelli F, Balzarotti R, Villa F, Guerra A, Avenia N, Mariani E, Bugiantella W. Is robot-assisted laparoscopic right colectomy more effective than the conventional laparoscopic procedure? A meta-analysis of short-term outcomes. Int J Surg. 2015;18:75–82.
5. Trastulli S, Cirocchi R, Desiderio J, Coratti A, Guarino S, Renzi C, et al. Robotic versus laparoscopic approach in colonic resections for cancer and benign diseases: systematic review and meta-analysis. PLoS One. 2015;10:e0134062.
6. Chang YS, Wang JX, Chang DW. A meta-analysis of robotic versus laparoscopic colectomy. J Surg Res. 2015;195:465–74.
7. Chuan L, Yan S, Pei-Wu Y. Meta-analysis of the short-term outcomes of robotic-assisted compared to laparoscopic gastrectomy. Minim Invasive Ther Allied Technol. 2015;24:127–34.
8. Montalti R, Berardi G, Patriti A, Vivarelli M, Troisi RI. Outcomes of robotic vs laparoscopic hepatectomy: a systematic review and meta-analysis. World J Gastroenterol. 2015;21:8441–51.
9. Liu H, Lawrie TA, Lu D, Song H, Wang L, Shi G. Robot-assisted surgery in gynaecology. Cochrane Database Syst Rev. 2014;12:CD011422.
10. Robertson C, Close A, Fraser C, Gurung T, Jia X, Sharma P, et al. Relative effectiveness of robot-assisted and standard laparoscopic prostatectomy as alternatives to open radical prostatectomy for treatment of localised prostate cancer: a systematic review and mixed treatment comparison meta-analysis. BJU Int. 2013;112:798–812.
11. Choi JE, You JH, Kim DK, Rha KH, Lee SH. Comparison of perioperative outcomes between robotic and laparoscopic partial nephrectomy: a systematic review and meta-analysis. Eur Urol. 2015;67:891–901.
12. Ran L, Jin J, Xu Y, Bu Y, Song F. Comparison of robotic surgery with laparoscopy and laparotomy for treatment of endometrial cancer: a meta-analysis. PLoS One. 2014;9:e108361.
13. Shazly SA, Murad MH, Dowdy SC, Gostout BS, Famuyide AO. Robotic radical hysterectomy in early stage cervical cancer: a systematic review and meta-analysis. Gynecol Oncol. 2015;138:457–71.
14. Fonseka T, Ahmed K, Froghi S, Khan SA, Dasgupta P, Shamim Khan M. Comparing robotic, laparoscopic and open cystectomy: a systematic review and meta-analysis. Arch Ital Urol Androl. 2015;87:41–8.
15. Marano A, Choi YY, Hyung WJ, Kim YM, Kim J, Noh SH. Robotic versus laparoscopic versus open gastrectomy: a meta-analysis. J Gastric Cancer. 2013;13:136–48.
16. Cao C, Wolfenden H, Liou K, Pathan F, Gupta S, Nienaber TA, et al. A meta-analysis of robotic vs. conventional mitral valve surgery. Ann Cardiothorac Surg. 2015;4:305–14.
17. Tandogdu Z, Vale L, Fraser C, Ramsay C. A systematic review of economic evaluations of the use of robotic assisted laparoscopy in surgery compared with open or laparoscopic surgery. Appl Health Econ Health Policy. 2015;13:457–67.
18. *Taylor v Intuitive Surgical, Inc.*, No. 09-2-03136-5 (Wash Super Ct, Kitsap County, March 25, 2013). http://www.citronresearch.com/wp-content/uploads/2013/02/Taylor-vs-Intuitive-Surgical-Suit.pdf [published 5 February 2013; Accessed 20 Oct 2015]. http://www.law360.com/articles/444699/intuitive-not-negligent-in-surgery-death-jury-rules [published 24 May 2013; Accessed 20 Oct 2015]. http://www.bloomberg.com/news/articles/2013-05-23/intuitive-wins-trial-defeats-negligent-training-claims [published/corrected 10 June 2014; Accessed 20 Oct 2015].
19. Herron DM, Marohn M, SAGES-MIRA Robotic Surgery Consensus Group. A consensus document on robotic surgery. Surg Endosc. 2008;22:313–25. discussion 311–2
20. Ahmed K, Khan R, Mottrie A, Lovegrove C, Abaza R, Ahlawat R, et al. Development of a standardised training curriculum for robotic surgery: a consensus statement from an international multidisciplinary group of experts. BJU Int. 2015;116:93–101.
21. Melich G, Hong YK, Kim J, Hur H, Baik SH, Kim NK, et al. Simultaneous development of laparoscopy and robotics provides acceptable perioperative outcomes and shows robotics to have a faster learning curve and to be overall faster in rectal cancer surgery: analysis of novice MIS surgeon learning curves. Surg Endosc. 2015;29:558–68.
22. Pierorazio PM, Patel HD, Feng T, Yohannan J, Hyams ES, Allaf ME. Robotic-assisted versus traditional laparoscopic partial nephrectomy: comparison of outcomes and evaluation of learning curve. Urology. 2011;78:813–9.
23. Passerotti CC, Franco F, Bissoli JC, Tiseo B, Oliveira CM, Buchalla CA, et al. Comparison of the learning curves and frustration level in performing laparoscopic and robotic training skills by experts and novices. Int Urol Nephrol. 2015;47:1075–84.
24. Sgarbura O, Vasilescu C. The decisive role of the patient-side surgeon in robotic surgery. Surg Endosc. 2010;24:3149–55.
25. Thiel DD, Lannen A, Riche E, Dove J, Gajarawala NM, Igel TC. Simulation-based training for bedside assistants can benefit experienced robotic prostatectomy teams. J Endourol. 2013;27:230–7.
26. Boys JA, Alicuben ET, DeMeester MJ, Worrell SG, Oh DS, Hagen JA, DeMeester SR. Public perceptions on robotic surgery, hospitals with robots, and surgeons that use them. Surg Endosc. 2015 (Epub ahead of print). https://doi.org/10.1007/s00464-015-4368-6.

Legal Aspects of Setting Up a Robotic Program

4

Martin B. Adams and Glenn W. Dopf

Robotic surgery presents challenges to surgeons and hospitals in the defense of medical and hospital malpractice lawsuits. The practitioner's awareness of potential legal pitfalls is essential for establishing a practice in which robotic surgery plays a central role. This chapter explores the various legal theories that may be asserted by patients against surgeons and hospitals and provides advice for confronting and avoiding legal liability.

Elements of a Robotic Surgical Malpractice Action

A surgical robotic platform is claimed by manufacturers to be "safe and safer than other comparative surgery methods" [1].

"Serious complications may occur in any surgery, including da Vinci® [robotic] Surgery, up to and including death" [2]. Manufacturers warn that "patients who are not candidates for non-robotic minimally invasive surgery are also not candidates for" robotic surgery [3]. So, for example, if multiple prior pelvic surgeries are a contraindication for laparoscopic surgery, then they are also a contraindication for robotic surgery. To proceed otherwise would expose the surgeon to potential liability should an injury occur.

A patient's negative experiences following surgery using a robotic platform can result in a lawsuit involving claims of, inter alia, surgeon malpractice, hospital malpractice, lack of informed consent, strict product liability, and negligent credentialing of the surgeon who utilized the surgical robotic product.

A patient ["plaintiff"] who sues a defendant, such as a hospital or a surgeon, for malpractice "must establish four elements to prevail on a negligence cause of action: (1) A duty by a defendant to act according to an applicable standard of care; (2) A breach of the applicable standard of care; (3) An injury; and (4) A causal connection between the breach of care and the injury" [4].

Courts define "negligence" as the "lack of ordinary care." A physician or hospital is negligent upon the physician's or hospital's "failure to use that degree of care that a reasonably prudent person would have used under the same circumstances" [5]. "Malpractice is professional negligence and medical malpractice is the negligence of a doctor" [6]. A medical act or a health-care provider's failure to act is a "proximate cause" of a patient's injury if the act or omission "was a substantial factor in bringing about the injury" [7].

In a lawsuit involving surgical malpractice, plaintiff must produce expert testimony as to a departure from good and accepted practice in the surgeon's treatment of the patient. Plaintiff must also demonstrate a causal connection between the surgeon's alleged departures from good and accepted practice and the injuries claimed to have been suffered on account of the surgical malpractice [8].

The patient must prove that his or her robot-assisted surgical care "fell below the standard of care [and] that any negligence proximately caused his injury" [9]. "Expert testimony is generally required" to determine whether a physician or a hospital has breached a duty [10].

A jury "would need expert medical testimony to explain whether [a surgeon] breached the standard of care by proceeding with the surgery and choosing to convert it to the traditional procedure" after a robotic platform malfunctions during the surgery [11]. "Where… medical personnel make on-the-spot decisions, requiring sophisticated medical insights, a jury cannot be expected to evaluate those judgment calls without the aid of expert opinion" [12].

Plaintiff may allege that a hospital used a defective surgical robot. A surgical robot may have a known history of defective performance of a particular surgical task. The hospital and the surgeon then would have a duty to ensure against the possibility of the robot misperforming that surgical task [13]. A surgeon who is aware of a defect in surgical equipment prior to plaintiff's surgery may not "allow that

M. B. Adams, JD · G. W. Dopf, JD, LLM (✉)
Dopf, P.C., New York, NY, USA
e-mail: bbenjamin@dopfnyc.com

Y. Fong et al. (eds.), *The SAGES Atlas of Robotic Surgery*, https://doi.org/10.1007/978-3-319-91045-1_4

type of [equipment] to be used in surgical procedures performed in the hospital..." [14].

A patient can allege against a hospital that the facility failed to, inter alia, procure the patient's informed consent, properly maintain a surgical robot, have on staff properly trained personnel, and have an agreement with the manufacturer of the surgical robot that would require the availability of the manufacturer's technician to respond to a surgical emergency involving the robot [15]. An issue of fact may exist for the jury as to whether a surgeon committed malpractice by taking an unduly long period of time to perform a robot-assisted procedure [16].

A hospital may breach its duty of care to a surgical patient by allowing a health-care provider less qualified than the attending surgeon to perform or supervise a surgical procedure [17]. The presence in the operating room of a manufacturer's representative does not relieve the surgeon from liability arising from the use of a surgical robot. The reason is that the surgeon exercises his own medical judgment and discretion [18].

"Medical ethics and practice dictate that the doctor must be an intervening and independent party between patient and... manufacturer" [19]. A surgeon has a "duty to the patient, as dictated by medical ethics and practice, to act independently and intervene between the patient and device manufacturer...." Should a conflict of interest arise "affect[ing] the physician's duty to exercise 'independent professional judgment' on the patient's behalf, it is the physician who would be held liable to the patient for any violation of that duty - not the device manufacturer" [20].

In a case involving a surgeon's use in a spinal fusion operation of an internal fixation device manufactured by defendant, plaintiff's complaint against the manufacturer, alleging breach of warranty, negligence, fraud, negligent design, and inadequate warning, was dismissed. The court found that the manufacturer provided appropriate and adequate warnings. The surgeon had a consulting agreement with the manufacturer, but plaintiff failed to show that the agreement "improperly influenced [the surgeon's] decision" to use the manufacturer's device. The surgeon also "use[d] other internal fixation systems in spinal fusion surgeries - the choice of which depend[ed] on the particular patient." The court noted that if the surgeon was "influenced to use [defendant's] device because of his financial arrangement with [defendant], the more appropriate course would be to pursue a claim against" the surgeon [21].

Proximate Cause in Surgical Robot Litigation

A patient's injuries can be "the direct result of selecting the robot-aided surgical procedure and the repercussions suffered when that procedure could not be completed." A court may find that a patient's "injuries would not have occurred if she had not selected the robot-aided procedure" [15].

A medical expert may opine that a surgical robot is the competent producing cause of the patient's injury and that the injury would not occur in the absence of deviation from accepted surgical care [22].

Plaintiff must provide an "explanation of how the malfunction" of a surgical robot "caused his injuries." A malfunction of a surgical robot may "directly cause a bodily rupture or injury of some sort." The malfunction may alternatively "cause a delay in the surgery's completion" with the delay resulting in the patient's injuries [23].

Plaintiff's ability to establish that a surgeon's conduct is the proximate cause of plaintiff's injuries can be problematic in surgery involving a robotic platform. Plaintiff's medical expert must be able to testify that, had the patient undergone a procedure other than the robotic procedure at issue, the patient would not have sustained his injury. Plaintiff's lawsuit may be defeated if the testimony of plaintiff's expert "indicates the injury could have occurred absent defendants' allegedly negligent conduct" [24].

A physician may argue that even if injury occurred when a surgeon utilized a particular surgical device, there may be no causal connection to the robotic platform, because the device is "routinely used" in the surgery "regardless of whether robotic equipment is involved." Still, a jury may need to determine whether the degree and quality of difference between a surgical device used in robot-assisted surgery and the device when used in surgical procedures without robotic assistance are significant enough to make the robotic device and its use "unique to robot-assisted procedures" [25].

Informed Consent for Surgery Involving a Robotic Platform

The law of informed consent, at its simplest, involves the practitioner disclosing to the patient the risks, benefits, and alternatives of the proposed medical procedure or treatment. A jury may decide whether there is a greater "risk" for a surgical misadventure when the procedure represents the first time that the surgeon has undertaken a robotically performed procedure.

"Surgeons should counsel their patients that serious complications may occur with any surgery, including *da Vinci* Surgery, up to and including death," warns a manufacturer of robotic surgical systems [26].

"Careful preoperative assessment of patient risk is critical for preventing perioperative complications" arising from robotic surgery.... "Risks for robot-assisted surgery should be thoroughly explained in the context of the patient's clinical condition, surgical options, pathology and anatomy. Patients should be advised on the experience of the surgeon in performing the recommended robotic procedure," advises the Massachusetts Board of Registration in Medicine [27].

Of course, the patient is entitled to know the alternatives to the robotic procedure. Once again, this should be documented. Keep in mind that it is quite customary for there to be a multiple-year hiatus between the surgery and a trial. That is all the more reason to maintain proper documentation.

Dr. Lee Char and his team have argued that, "[t]o promote informed decision-making and autonomy among patients considering innovative surgery, surgeons should disclose the novel nature of the procedure, potentially unknown risks and benefits, and whether the surgeon would be performing the procedure for the first time. When accurate volumes and outcomes data are available, surgeons should also discuss these with patients" [28].

If a decision is made to advise the patient that the patient will be, for example, the "third patient" on which the physician has ever performed robotic surgery, then that decision should be documented in the medical chart. Otherwise, should a trial ensue, the patient may allege that he or she was never told that she was the "third patient."

In some states, a physician's raw success rate for a procedure does not constitute risk information that is reasonably related to a patient's medical procedure for the purpose of informed consent. In other states, a physician's prior experience with a procedure may have a direct bearing on the risks to the patient from the procedure, and provider-specific information related to the risks posed by the circumstances under which the physician will perform a procedure may need to be disclosed as part of the patient's informed consent.

Corporate Negligence and Surgical Robotic Liability

Under the doctrine of corporate negligence, "a hospital owes its patients the duty to furnish to the patient supplies and equipment free of defects, among others" [29]. "Hospitals have a duty to supply the required equipment and instrumentalities for the care of their patients" [30].

"The standard of care to which the hospital will be held is that of an average, competent health-care facility acting in the same or similar circumstances. This standard is generally defined by the Joint Commission on Accreditation of Hospitals (JCAH) standards and the hospital's bylaws" [31].

Credentialing and Proctoring of a Surgeon

A hospital has a "duty of care in granting physicians privileges to use the hospital's facilities generally or for certain procedures…" [32]. A hospital "has a direct duty to grant and continue staff privileges only to competent doctors." A hospital also "has a duty to remove 'a known incompetent'…" physician on the hospital's staff [33].

A hospital can be liable to a patient for failing to exercise due care in the selection and retention of a physician on the hospital staff [34]. A "failure of a hospital to develop and adhere to reasonable procedures for reviewing a physician's qualifications creates a foreseeable risk of harm thus establishing an independent duty to such patients…" [35].

A surgeon may receive training from the manufacturer of a surgical robot. The hospital where the surgeon performs surgery can credential the surgeon in the operation of a robotic surgical system [36].

A robotic surgical device manufacturer has warned that a surgeon "considering using computer-assisted surgery… shall only do so after successfully completing required medical training and certification as well as the relevant training mandated in the professional guidelines of their own hospital, institution, or society – including training on the use of" the particular robotic surgical system under consideration [3].

"Guidelines set forth by [professional medical organizations]… may be helpful in establishing robotic surgery credentialing protocols" [27]. Professional organizations have issued criteria for the "credentialing and privileging for robotic procedures" [37]. Professional societies have prepared formal guidelines for credentialing of surgeons in the use of surgical robots and guidelines for robotic surgery training [38].

The American Urological Association has promulgated requirements for granting of urologic robotic privileges and maintenance of privileges [39]. The Massachusetts Board of Registration in Medicine has recommended that credentialing for robot-assisted surgery "should be based on proven competency and proficiency, rather than the completion of a set number of cases" [27].

A patient may claim that a hospital "was negligent for failing to ensure that [a surgeon] was properly credentialed to use the robotic equipment…" [40].

A hospital must "undertake due diligence in determining whether [a] surgeon had the requisite training and experience to utilize" a surgical robot in a particular type of surgery. A jury may need to determine whether a hospital negligently permitted a surgeon to utilize a robot in performance of the surgery [41].

A hospital may or may not "have a distinct delineation of privilege (DOP or proctoring requirement) for the use of [a] robotic system." The hospital may decide that, instead of a proctoring requirement, surgeons with advanced experience and evidence of training with a robotic system may use the device. A plaintiff may introduce evidence concerning the applicable standard of care required proctoring with respect to a robotic procedure and whether a hospital should have had such a proctoring requirement [42].

The American Urological Association has issued standard operating practices for proctors during robotic surgery [39]. A hospital's failure to proctor a surgeon may constitute a breach of the applicable standard of care. In that situation, a hospital may be independently liable to a patient injured during a robotically assisted surgery. The failure of a hospital to proctor a surgeon in robotic surgery can create liability, provided plaintiff presents "evidence showing that the applicable standard of care required proctoring" [43].

The patient must "show a causal connection between credentialing to use the robotic equipment" and the patient's injury [44].

Strict Product Liability and Robotic Surgery

Strict liability, simply stated, is the legal responsibility for an injury without the need for the injured party to prove carelessness or fault.

Surgeons and surgical equipment "may combine in the performance of a medical procedure culminating in an unexpected, mysterious and disastrous result." Plaintiffs' lawyers will sometimes sue the company that manufactured the surgical equipment and the hospital that supplied the equipment to the surgeon. Negligence on the part of the hospital or the manufacturer may be "just as possible as some unspecified and indeterminate lack of care on the surgeon's part" [45].

Plaintiffs can sue under a doctrine called "strict product liability." Under that doctrine, a manufacturer or others involved in the distribution of a surgical robot can be liable for injury caused by a "defect" in the product. This type of liability is imposed so long as the surgical robot "is used for its intended or reasonably foreseeable purpose." A surgical robot is "defective if it is not reasonably safe – that is, if the product is so likely to be harmful" to the patient that "a reasonable person who had actual knowledge of its potential for producing injury would conclude that it should not have been marketed in that condition" [46].

Strict product liability issues may arise in a robotic surgical malpractice action against a hospital and a surgeon. The medical defendants may want to allocate and shift responsibility onto the manufacturer of the surgical robot by impleading the manufacturer as a third-party defendant—that is, adding a third party into the underlying lawsuit.

A plaintiff may not maintain a valid cause of action sounding in either breach of warranty or product liability with respect to a medical device whose use "was only a procedure incidental to medical treatment" [47] "…[I]t has been widely held that strict liability may not be invoked by a patient against a hospital or physician in the use of a defective medical implement" [47]. Courts have held that a "health-care provider cannot be held strictly liable for a latent defect in a medical device manufactured by a third party" [48].

"Generally, hospitals are not engaged in the business of selling the products or equipment used in the course of providing medical services…. Consequently, the products used are intimately and inseparably connected with the provision of medical services" [49]. However, despite the difficulty in "establishing an isolated sale as opposed to a whole transaction for services," a patient may be able to plead against a hospital a cause of action for breach of an implied warranty arising out of a defective surgical device implanted into the patient [30].

A state statute relating to product liability actions may be found by a court to preclude any product liability actions against health-care providers [50]. A hospital's charging of a patient for the use of surgical equipment is not a "sale" within the meaning of the Uniform Commercial Code [51].

A hospital can reasonably argue that use of a surgical robot in the course of surgery does not constitute a "sale" of the robot. Such a sale would be required for plaintiff to maintain a cause of action sounding in product liability and breach of warranty [52]. A hospital may "properly" be "regarded as itself a consumer" of a surgical robot, which the hospital "merely employs… in performing its actual function of providing medical services" [53].

A hospital is not in the business of independently selling surgical robots to the public. A hospital is not "in the business of providing them outside of its primary purpose of providing medical facilities." Under those circumstances, a court may conclude that a defective surgical robot is "inseparable from the services rendered by the hospital." The hospital in that case may avoid being held liable under a strict liability claim [54].

Malfunction of a Surgical Robot

A product may fail to "perform the function that it is designed and intended to perform…." The product may cause "harm when the product is being used for its intended purpose." In at least one jurisdiction (Pennsylvania), plaintiff is not required to provide more specific proof of the specific defect in order to recover damages [30].

A patient may argue that a surgical robot malfunctioned. To succeed, plaintiff must not only show a malfunction but also that the malfunction caused his injury [55].

In one case, a patient suffering from prostate cancer underwent a prostatectomy. The patient alleged that a "da Vinci robot" used by his surgeon "malfunctioned during the surgery and displayed 'error' messages." The surgical team tried unsuccessfully to make the robot operational. A da Vinci representative in the operating room was unable to render the robot functional. The surgeon decided to complete the surgery using laparoscopic equipment instead of the robot. The patient later complained of erectile dysfunction and severe groin pain [56]. The patient sued the hospital and the manufacturer of the robot. The patient claimed strict product liability, negligence, and breach of warranty. The court granted summary judgment to the manufacturer and dismissed all claims. The patient failed to adduce "evidence that would permit a jury to infer [the patient's] erectile dysfunction and groin pain were caused by the robot's alleged malfunction…" [57].

Learned Intermediary Doctrine

"Product warnings are intended for the physician, 'whose duty it is to balance the risks against the benefits' of various treatments and to prescribe the treatments he or she thinks best" [57]. A "physician acts as an 'informed intermediary'… between the manufacturer and the patient; and, thus, the manufacturer's duty to caution against a [product's] side effects is fulfilled by giving adequate warning through the prescribing physician, not directly to the patient…" [58].

"Under the learned intermediary doctrine, a defendant manufacturer has an obligation to inform the treating physician of the risks of a medical device" [59]. "When a manufacturer gives a warning regarding its product, the issue is whether the warning provided to the physician is adequate" [60].

A warning issued by a manufacturer to a surgeon, who is a learned intermediary, may be sufficient for the manufacturer to meet the requisite standard of care and may defeat plaintiffs' claim of negligent failure to warn [61].

A surgeon may have been "aware of a potential dangers in using" a surgical device and may have "chose[n] to use [the device] despite those risks." Under that circumstance, "the adequacy of the [manufacturer's] warning is not a producing cause of the injury," and the plaintiff may not recover against the manufacturer of the surgical device under a theory of failure to warn [62].

A "manufacturer of a medical device does not have a duty to directly warn a patient of risks associated with the device, but instead discharges its duty by providing the physician with sufficient information concerning the risks of the device" [63]. A "manufacturer has no duty directly to a patient to warn of risks associated with the product when the manufacturer has provided accurate, clear and unambiguous information about the risks associated with a product to the patient's physician…. It is then incumbent upon the now-learned physician to evaluate those risks and the use of the product in treating a particular patient" [64].

A manufacturer of a surgical robot owes to the surgeon a duty to warn. That duty to warn does not necessarily also run to the hospital where the robotic surgery is performed [65]. A hospital, though, may escape liability for inadequate warnings under the learned intermediary doctrine where the patient's claim against the hospital arises from an alleged lack of proper warnings as to a medical product used during surgery [66].

In a recent surgical case, a surgeon had performed a prostatectomy upon a patient who, because of the patient's morbid obesity, "was not an optimal candidate." The surgeon "understood that he should only operate on thin patients while he was still new to the da Vinci System." During the surgery, the surgeon switched from use of a da Vinci System to an open prostatectomy. The patient sustained a tear of the rectal wall at some point in the surgery and suffered anesthesia complications [67]. The court held that even if the learned intermediary doctrine applied, the hospital did not "act[ ] as a second learned intermediary," and the manufacturer had no duty to provide warnings to the hospital. A hospital "that facilitates the distribution of a medical product, yet does not exercise its own individualized medical judgment, is not a learned intermediary," explained the court. The hospital "did not take [the patient's] individualized circumstances or medical history into account… [the hospital did not] play[ ] any role in deciding whether [the patient] should receive a da Vinci System surgery" [66].

Collateral Estoppel in Surgical Robot Litigation

Collateral estoppel, also known as issue preclusion, precludes a party from litigating in a later lawsuit an issue that was clearly raised in an earlier lawsuit and decided against that party, even if the courts or the theories of liability in the two lawsuits are not the same. For example, in medical malpractice action, if a court dismisses some physicians on the ground that those physicians correctly diagnosed a condition in a timely fashion, then the patient who is suing other physicians still in the lawsuit can no longer argue that the condition was not correctly or timely diagnosed.

During the course of litigation, manufacturers of surgical robots frequently file written applications in court for "summary judgment," that is, for a court order dismissing plaintiff's claims. The manufacturer's application, which is called a "motion," will also seek a court order dismissing any claim [a "cross-claim"] that another defendant, such as a physician or hospital, has asserted against the manufacturer. The cross-claim is designed to force the manufacturer to share in any liability that a jury may assess at trial in favor of the injured plaintiff.

The court may deny the manufacturer's application on the ground that an issue exists for the jury's determination as to whether a surgical robot was defective or contributed to the patient's claimed injuries. In that situation, the manufacturer has a substantially increased incentive to settle. The reason is that a finding by the jury against the manufacturer may prevent the manufacturer from defending on the merits identical allegations brought in the future by other plaintiffs.

Once a jury decides a particular issue against the manufacturer, the manufacturer is "collaterally estopped" from defending on the merits against that same issue in future litigation. This "collateral estoppel" can be of great benefit to future plaintiffs. To prevent that from happening, a manufacturer who has been unsuccessful in its effort to dismiss a lawsuit before trial will redouble its efforts to settle the case before trial, before a jury decides an issue against the manufacturer and collateral estoppel sets in.

References

1. *Darringer v Intuitive Surgical, Inc.*, 2015 WL 4623935 (N.D. Cal.). (Products liability and negligence action against the manufacturer of a da Vinci robotic platform; plaintiff sustained injuries after undergoing a laparoscopic left pyeloplasty using a da Vinci robot.)
2. Intuitive Surgical: Welcome to Intuitive Surgical. intuitivesurgical.com/company/. Clinical Evidence, Accessed 11 Aug 2015.
3. Intuitivesurgical.com, Medical Advice Disclaimer. Accessed 20 Aug 2015.
4. *Cobb v Dallas Fort Worth Medical Center-Grand Prairie*, 48 S.W.3d 820 (Ct. App., Waco, Tex. 2001). (Pedicular hardware was inserted into plaintiff for treatment of an internal disc disruption in her lower back; several days after the surgery, the surgeon discovered that the screws used to install the pedicular hardware were made for a child patient and were not safe for use in a patient of plaintiff's weight and size; plaintiffs alleged that the transpedicular hardware and screws were the wrong size and non-FDA-approved; hospital's motion for summary judgment was denied as to the negligence claim and granted as to the strict liability claim.)
5. New York Pattern Jury Instruction 2:10 (2015).
6. New York Pattern Jury Instruction 2:150 (2015).
7. New York Pattern Jury Instruction 2:70 (2015).
8. *Rivera v Kleinman*, 16 N.Y.3d 757, 944 N.E.2d 1119, 919 N.Y.S.2d 480 (2011). (A surgeon operated on an infant's dislocated right and left hips; the surgeries were performed 2 weeks apart and entailed cutting and repositioning the bones that join at the hip and fixing them with a plate with side screws and a hip screw; plaintiff claimed that the surgeon improperly positioned the screw implanted in the infant's left hip; that screw broke through the infant's skin and was taken out during emergency surgery; the surgeon's motion and the hospital's cross motion seeking summary judgment were granted.)
9. *Rex v Univ of Cincinnati College of Medicine*, 2013 WL 6095889 (Ct. App., 10th Dist., Franklin Co., Ohio). (A surgeon performed a robotic wide excision radical prostatectomy; such surgery typically lasts for about 2 to 3 hours and the patient normally returns home the next day and can return to work in a little over 1 week; plaintiff's surgery lasted for approximately 7 hours and plaintiff unexpectedly lost a massive amount of blood, About 2.3 liters; plaintiff was subsequently diagnosed with ischemic optic neuropathy; plaintiff failed to prove the surgeon's preoperative and surgical treatment fell below the standard of care or that any alleged negligence proximately caused plaintiff's eye injury.)
10. *Espalin v Children's Medical Center of Dallas*, 27 S.W.3d 675 (Ct. App., Dallas, Tex. 2000). (After undergoing surgery to repair a coarctation of the aorta and a patent ductus arteriosus, an infant sustained paraplegia of her lower extremities; plaintiffs claimed that a cooling blanket supplied by the hospital did not work.)
11. *Silvestrini v Intuitive Surgical, Inc.*, 2012 WL 380283 (ED La 2012). (During performance of a robotic transaxillary total thyroidectomy, the robot malfunctioned; neither the surgeon nor any other hospital staff member was able to repair it; the patient was under general anesthesia with the robot "inserted" in her neck when the malfunction occurred; the patient's thyroid was removed using a traditional, non-robot-aided procedure; that technique required opening the patient's neck with a long surgical cut; plaintiff claimed she now had an "extensive, unattractive scar" on her neck that would require significant plastic surgery, and that remaining remnants of her thyroid would need to be surgically removed.)
12. *Rolon-Alvarado v Municipality of San Juan*, 1 F.3d 74 (1st Cir. 1993). (An endotracheal tube, reinserted in the immediate aftermath of surgery, snapped; when a physician attempted to replace the broken tube, the patient went into cardiorespiratory arrest and died; defendant's motion for judgment as a matter of law was granted after plaintiff rested at trial.)
13. See, *e.g.*, *Mirabella v Mount Sinai Hosp.*, 43 A.D.3d 751, 842 N.Y.S.2d 17 (1st Dep't 2007). (Plaintiff suffered a leak of bowel contents into her abdomen during bariatric surgery; during the operation, the surgeon did not seem to have any problems with the disposable surgical staplers he used; he visually observed that staples were in place, and he performed a leak test using saline irrigation with blue dye that confirmed no leaking; the surgeon observed that the staples were "closed and firm" on the anti-mesenteric side of the bowel, but there were no staples on the mesenteric side, as there should have been; the surgeon concluded that there was a "misfiring of the stapler"; the surgeon testified that such misfirings, while not common, were known to occur and were a matter of concern.)
14. *Goldfarb v St. Charles Hosp. & Rehabilitation Cent*er, 2 A.D.3d 579, 769 N.Y.S.2d 575 (2d Dep't 2003). (While conducting a laparoscopy, a surgeon inserted into plaintiff's abdomen a trocar; the surgeon then noticed heavy internal bleeding, converted the procedure to a laparotomy, and stopped the bleeding, using sutures and clips; a general surgeon, who was brought into the operating room, inspected the operative site, identified a punctured artery as the source of the bleeding, and recommended consulting a vascular surgeon, was granted summary judgment; plaintiffs' theory, that the general surgeon was aware of a defect in the trocar prior to plaintiff's surgery and nonetheless allowed that type of trocar to be used in surgical procedures performed in the hospital, was speculative.)
15. *Silvestrini v Intuitive Surgical, Inc.*, *supra*, at note 11.
16. See, *e.g.*, *Morrison v Altman*, 278 A.D.2d 135, 718 N.Y.S.2d 319 (1st Dep't 2000). (Defendants doctor's and hospital's motions for summary judgment were denied; issues of fact existed as to how and when an infectious agent was introduced, whether defendant doctor committed malpractice in administering a lumbar epidural steroid injection by taking 17 minutes to perform the procedure and using the same needle in more than one location, and whether defendant hospital's nurse committed malpractice by failing to prepare proper records, obtain a full history, properly examine plaintiff, and properly evaluate the injection site.)
17. *Siebe v University of Cincinnati*, 117 Ohio Misc.2d 46, 766 N.E.2d 1070 (Court of Claims, Ohio 2001). (Defendant violated its own policy because a central venous line was not installed under the direction of an anesthesiologist; it was the standard of care at defendant hospital to have an attending anesthesiologist perform or supervise installation of a central venous line; it was against defendant's hospital policy to have a resident supervise placement of a central venous line by a trainee nurse anesthetist; misplacement of the central venous line and the lack of follow-up care by defendant proximately caused a hydrothorax to develop in the patient's chest cavity.)
18. *Wolicki-Gables v Arrow Intern., Inc.*, 641 F.Supp.2d 1270 (M.D. Fla. 2009), *aff'd*, 634 F.3d 1296 (11th Cir. 2011). (A surgeon implanted into a patient with back pain and physical limitations an Arrow pump system; summary judgment was granted to defendant sales representative, who was present at the initial implantation procedure; the sales representative's role was limited to carrying "back up" products in their sterile packages to have available for

the surgeon's use, if necessary, and to observing preparation of the products; the sales representative did not "scrub in" for the procedure and did not enter the sterile field; he did not come into contact with the pump, which never left the sterile field.)
19. *Hill v Searle Laboratories, a Div of Searle Pharmaceuticals, Inc.*, 884 F.2d 1064 (8th Cir. 1989). (A copper intrauterine device perforated plaintiff's uterus and was partially embedded in her small bowel.)
20. *Talley v Danek Medical, Inc.*, 7 F.Supp.2d 725 (E.D. Va. 1998), *aff'd*, 179 F.3d 154 (4th Cir. 1999).
21. *Talley v Danek Medical, Inc.*, *supra*, at note 20.
22. See, *e.g.*, *Svoboda v Our Lady of Lourdes Memorial Hosp., Inc.*, 31 A.D.3d 877, 817 N.Y.S.2d 772 (3rd Dep't 2006). (Plaintiff underwent right knee replacement surgery; a continuous passive motion machine was used as part of his postoperative care at the hospital; after being discharged, plaintiff discovered an ulcer on his right calf; hospital's motion for summary judgment was denied.)
23. *O'Brien v Intuitive Surgical, Inc.*, 2011 WL 3040479 (N.D. Ill.). (Plaintiff alleged that a da Vinci surgical robot manufactured by defendant was defectively designed and malfunctioned during plaintiff's pancreatectomy and islet cell transplant surgery; the complaint was dismissed; plaintiff did not allege that the malfunction directly caused a bodily rupture or injury or that the malfunction caused a delay in the surgery's completion and that the delay led to plaintiff's injuries.)
24. Balding v Tarter, 2013 WL 4711723 (4th Dist., Ill.). (A urologist performed a laparoscopic robot-assisted radical prostatectomy; the complaint against the urologist was dismissed; plaintiff's expert urologist was unable to say that had plaintiff undergone an open procedure, as opposed to the robotic procedure, he would not have sustained his median nerve injury; to the extent that a longer surgery may increase the risk of that complication, the expert stated it was "hard to say how much increase" there would be if the operation had lasted only 90 minutes; plaintiff's treating plastic surgeon stated that compression injuries to the median nerve could occur at any point in time after 2 hours, and if plaintiff's surgery had taken 2 hours, "he could have" had the same result.)
25. *Mohler v St. Luke's Medical Center, LP*, 2008 WL 5384214 (Ct. App., Div 1, Dep't B, Ariz.). (A patient's small intestine was perforated during a laparoscopic robotically-assisted surgery to remove the patient's gallbladder; the procedure was the first robotically-assisted surgery of any kind that the surgeon performed; an issue of fact on proximate causation existed as to whether the perforation occurred at the start of the procedure or through use of robotic equipment; there was evidence that trocars used with the robotic equipment were different from regular trocars used in laparoscopic procedures and that the trocars were an integral part of robotically-assisted procedures.)
26. Intuitivesurgical.com, Important Surgical Risks. Accessed 1 Sep 2015.
27. Commonwealth of Massachusetts Board of Registration in Medicine, Quality and Patient Safety Division, Advisory on Robot-Assisted Surgery, March 2013.
28. Lee Char SJ, Hills NK, Lo B, Kirkwood KS. Informed consent for innovative surgery: a survey of patients and surgeons. Surgery. 2013;153:473–80.
29. *Ripley v Lanzer*, 152 Wash.App. 296, 215 P.3d 1020 (2009). (Medical malpractice action; during an arthroscopic medical meniscectomy surgery, a scalpel blade detached from its handle and lodged in the patient's knee joint; plaintiff's corporate negligence claim against defendant hospital was dismissed because plaintiff failed to adduce expert medical evidence to establish the standard of care.)
30. *Cobb v Dallas Fort Worth Medical Center-Grand Prairie*, *supra*, at note 4.
31. *Ripley v Lanzer*, *supra*, at note 29.
32. *Kenneson v Johnson & Johnson, Inc.*, 2015 WL 1867768 (D. Conn.). (Action against a hospital alleging negligence and violation of the Connecticut Unfair Trade Practices Act, arising out of surgery involving implantation of a "Prolene Mesh.")
33. *Schelling v Humphrey*, 123 Ohio St.3d 387, 916 N.E.2d 1029 (2009).
34. *Newbold-Ferguson v AMISUB (North Ridge Hospital), Inc.*, 85 So.3d 502 (4th Dist., Fla. 2012).
35. *Raschel v Rish*, 110 A.D.2d 1067, 488 N.Y.S.2d 923 (4th Dep't 1985). (Plaintiff raised issues of fact relating to the hospital's breach of its duty to investigate the competency of defendant plastic surgeon before renewing his staff privileges; defendant physician had been sued at least three times for malpractice for surgery and for silicone injections.)
36. *Taylor v Intuitive Surgical, Inc.*, 188 Wash.App. 776, 355 P.3d 309 (Wash. 2015), *review granted*, 9 Feb 2016.
37. See, *e.g.*, American College of Obstetricians and Gynecologists, Society of Gynecologic Surgeons, Committee Opinion, Robotic Surgery in Gynecology, Number 628, March 2015.
38. *See, e.g.*, The Society of American Gastrointestinal and Endoscopic Surgeons and the Minimally Invasive Robotic Association, A Consensus Document on Robotic Surgery, November, 2007.
39. American Urological Association, Standard Operating Practices (SOPs) for Urologic Robotic Surgery.
40. *Mohler v St. Luke's Medical Center*, supra, at note 25.
41. *Vaccaro v St. Vincent's Medical Center*, 71 A.D.3d 1000, 898 N.Y.S.2d 163 (2d Dep't 2010). (Plaintiffs claimed that a hospital negligently permitted a surgeon to utilize a Met–RX procedure in performance of a posterior foraminotomy decompression; the hospital's neurosurgery expert noted that the Met–RX procedure was FDA-approved and the decision to use it was "within the sole province of the operating surgeon"; plaintiffs raised a triable issue of fact through the surgeon's deposition testimony that the hospital permitted him to use the system, but never inquired into his background and training with the procedure, and that he had used the system in cervical spine surgery only once or twice before; plaintiffs' neurosurgery and anesthesiology experts opined that the hospital failed to undertake due diligence in determining whether the surgeon had the requisite training and experience to utilize the procedure in cervical spinal surgery.)
42. *Pedraza v Silverman*, 2013 WL 2633596 (4th Dist., Div 1, Cal. 2013). (Medical malpractice action by a patient who underwent a robotically assisted laparoscopic surgery.)
43. *Pedraza v Silverman*, *supra*, at note 42.
44. *Mohler v St. Luke's Medical Center, LP*, *supra*, at note 25.
45. *Inouye v Black*, 238 Cal.App.2d 31, 47 Cal.Rptr. 313 (3rd Dist., 1965). (Plaintiff underwent surgery performed by defendant neurosurgeon; defendant wired vertebrae together using two pieces of stainless steel wire; two years later, plaintiff learned that the wire had broken into relatively small fragments, an event not expected by defendant; at the close of plaintiff's case, defendant's counsel made a nonsuit motion which the trial court granted.)
46. New York Pattern Jury Instruction 2:120 (2015).
47. *Goldfarb v Teitelbaum*, 149 A.D.2d 566, 540 N.Y.S.2d 263 (2d Dep't 1989). (Plaintiff claimed that defendant dentist inserted an allegedly defective mandibular prosthesis into her mouth; complaint dismissed.)
48. *North Miami General Hosp., Inc. v Goldberg*, 520 So.2d 650 (3rd Dist., Fla. 1988). (When plaintiff awoke from a routine operation, she had sustained burns at the places on her body where an electrosurgical grounding pad had been used during the surgery; the trial court erroneously submitted a strict liability issue to the jury.)
49. *Rolon-Alvarado v Municipality of San Juan*, *supra*, at note 12.
50. *Cheshire v Southampton Hospital Assoc.*, 53 Misc.2d 355, 278 N.Y.S.2d 531 (Sup. Suffolk 1967). (Plaintiff alleged that surgical insertion of an intramedullary pin was warranted as properly manu-

factured and free of defects; the pin broke despite the surgeon's alleged statement that the pin would not break and was as strong as, if not stronger than, the original bone; surgeon's motion to dismiss the complaint was denied.)

51. *Budding v SSM Healthcare System*, 19 S.W.3d 678 (Sup. Mo. 2000). (Action for strict product liability arising from allegedly defectively designed Vitek Proplast Teflon temporomandibular joint implants; jury verdict for hospital affirmed.)
52. *Von Downum v Synthes*, 908 F.Supp.2d 1179 (N.D. Okla. 2012). (Plaintiff underwent a lumbar interbody fusion with the placement of medical devices; plaintiff alleged that the medical device implants were defective and had to be replaced; plaintiff was unable to state a cognizable claim for strict liability against the hospital.)
53. *Goldfarb v Teitelbaum, supra*, at note 47.
54. *North Miami General Hosp., Inc. v Goldberg, supra*, at note 48.
55. *Liberty Mut. Fire Ins. Co. v Sharp Electronics Corp.*, 2011 WL 2632986 (M.D. Pa.), *adopted in part and rejected in part*, 2011 WL 2632880. (Plaintiffs claimed that a restaurant fire began in a cash register because of an electrical defect.)
56. *Mracek v Bryn Mawr Hosp.*, 363 Fed.Appx. 925 (3rd Cir. 2010).
57. *Mracek v Bryn Mawr Hosp., supra*, at note 56.
58. *Sita v Danek Medical, Inc.*, 43 F.Supp.2d 245 (E.D.N.Y. 1999). (Action against the maker of a surgical screw system used by an orthopedic surgeon in spinal surgery performed upon plaintiff; plaintiff's "failure to warn" claim, whether sounding in negligence or strict liability, was barred under the informed intermediary doctrine.).
59. *Martin v Hacker*, 83 N.Y.2d 1, 628 N.E.2d 1308, 607 N.Y.S.2d 598 (1993). (A patient became severely depressed after ingesting medications manufactured by defendant and prescribed by a physician to treat the patient's hypertension; the depression allegedly led to the patient's suicide; the manufacturer's warning regarding the adverse reaction of drug-induced depression resulting in suicide was adequate as a matter of law.)
60. *Henson v Wright Medical Technology, Inc.*, 2013 WL 1296388 (N.D.N.Y. 2013). (During hip replacement surgery, the surgical team implanted defendants' Wright ProFemur Total Hip System; about 8 years later, the system broke, requiring emergency surgery for a total hip replacement; the court could not determine the adequacy of the warnings on defendants' motion to dismiss; defendants failed to prove that the learned intermediary doctrine bars plaintiff's claim of failure to warn.)
61. *Rounds v Genzyme Corp.*, 440 Fed.Appx. 753 (11th Cir. 2011). (Plaintiff underwent an autologous chrondrocyte implantation involving defendant manufacturer's Carticel, which was a biologic product comprised of autologous cultured chondrocytes used to repair articular cartilage injuries; plaintiff's negligence claim against the manufacturer was dismissed; the manufacturer's package insert expressly and clearly warned the surgeon about how to identify Carticel patients and about the risk of the exact injury of which plaintiff complained.)
62. *Parkinson v Guidant Corp.*, 315 F.Supp.2d 741 (W.D. Pa. 2004). (A guidewire manufactured by defendant fractured during the course of an angioplasty procedure; defendant provided physicians who utilize its guidewire with a list of instructions and a warning relating to the use of the guidewire; the physician who performed plaintiff's procedure testified that he was familiar with those warnings prior to performing the procedure on plaintiff and that, as an interventional cardiologist, he was familiar with the concept of tip separation; defendants were entitled to summary judgment on plaintiffs' negligent failure to warn claim.)
63. *Smith v Johnson & Johnson, Inc.*, 483 Fed.Appx. 909 (5th Cir. 2012). (Plaintiffs' product liability claims arose from manufacturers' alleged failure to warn of risks associated with the use of Mersilene mesh as part of an abdominal sarcoplexy; the surgeon was aware of the potential dangers in using Mersilene mesh and chose to use the mesh in plaintiff's surgery despite those risks; defendants were granted summary judgment.)
64. *Sita v Danek Medical, Inc., supra*, at note 58.
65. *Rounds v Genzyme Corp., supra*, at note 61.
66. *Taylor v Intuitive Surgical, Inc., supra*, at note 36.
67. *Tortorelli v Mercy Health Center, Inc.*, 242 P.3d 549 (Court of Civil Appeals, Okla. 2010). (A surgeon removed a bone tumor from plaintiff's tibia; during the surgery, an allograft bone putty was used; defendant hospital's motion for summary judgment was granted.)

Financial Considerations in Robotic Surgery

5

Nikhil L. Shah, Rajesh G. Laungani, and Matthew E. Kaufman

Introduction

The adoption of any new technology in surgery or any other field of medicine brings new challenges. There will always be advocates on the cutting edge of innovation, while others will be slower to change. The greatest factors inhibiting the adoption of new technology are the often-higher costs associated with product acquisition and the absence of a formal pathway to best practice and surgical excellence. When robotic surgery was first clinically introduced in late 2000, only about 1000 robotic surgeries were being performed worldwide, and the cost for each procedure was largely prohibitive [1–3]. Among these costs were the cost of the system, instruments, training, and prolonged operative times. Between 2000 and 2012, the number of robotic procedures performed increased from approximately 1000–2000 per year to nearly 450,000 [4]. It is evident that robotic surgery has established itself as a standard of care for certain disease states, yet challenges still arise as the new healthcare environment balances both cost and quality [5–9].

There is no question in our minds that robotic surgery has found a place in surgery; one can expect to continue to receive questions from peer physicians, patients, and hospital administration about the value of the technique, defined as the relationship between cost and quality [9–12]. In today's complex healthcare environment, the feasibility of new technology must balance both clinical outcomes and cost factors. Although many complexities in American healthcare contribute to the changing landscape in surgical practice, nothing causes such dramatic change as the introduction of a revolutionary, and perhaps disruptive, technology. As this technique continues to grow from predominantly pelvic uses, the possibilities of the technology will continue to expand and inspire continued scrutiny.

In a recent evaluation completed by Blue Cross Blue Shield Association in regard to "Critical Issues in Robotic Surgery," cost and economics were evaluated [3–5, 9, 10]. Review of the CADTH (Canadian Agency for Drugs and Technologies in Health) database revealed data regarding robotic prostatectomy. Results of a CADTH analysis comparing robotic and open prostatectomy were based on an average case load of 130 cases per year and equipment life of approximately 7 years. Incremental costs for robotic surgery were higher in terms of capital costs for equipment, consumables and disposables, and maintenance. A major cost offset was a decrease in hospitalization associated with a shortened length of stay. The aggregate cost difference, including surgical fees, anesthesia costs, and training costs, was also higher for robotic surgery [3–5, 13].

Financial justification of the cost for a hospital or a hospital system is a major challenge when it comes to implementation of a single or multiple robotic surgical systems. In this chapter, we explore the key elements of financially and operationally evaluating the feasibility of the purchase of a surgical robot and outline the key elements that we have found in building and sustaining a high-quality, physician-governed, and financially sustainable robotic surgical program.

N. L. Shah, DO, MPH (✉)
Minimal Access & Robotic Surgery, Piedmont Health Care, Atlanta, GA, USA
e-mail: Nikhil.shah@piedmont.org

R. G. Laungani, MD
Robotic Service Line, Piedmont Atlanta Hospital, Atlanta, GA, USA
e-mail: Rajesh.laungani@piedmont.org

M. E. Kaufman, MHA
Piedmont Atlanta Hospital, Atlanta, GA, USA

Y. Fong et al. (eds.), *The SAGES Atlas of Robotic Surgery*, https://doi.org/10.1007/978-3-319-91045-1_5

Operational Concerns

Three critical operational concerns must be considered prior to the purchase of a robotic surgical system:

- Operating room (OR) logistics
- Surgeon factors and training
- Governance and oversight

These factors must be considered as a part of the entire investment in a robotic surgical system. Compromising on any of them can leave a program vulnerable to quality and efficiency gaps.

Operating Room Space

Space considerations in the operating room are very important, but with each new generation of robotic surgical system, the newer models have become more facile, ergonomic, and often increasingly compact, making space demands less of an issue. Each room that houses a robotic surgical system must have space to allow for appropriate positioning and manipulation of the robotic system over the patient, ample room for the console and video tower, and enough space to house the disposables for the robot with easy access if the need for an instrument or scope replacement arises during a case. Furthermore, movement of team members such as anesthesia, circulating nurse, scrub technician, and the first assistant must be taken into consideration when assessing operating room square footage. The OR team's access to the patient, a line of sight and communication between the surgeon and the team, and the comfort of the surgeon and OR team while maintaining a sterile environment are also important setup considerations.

Robotic Surgery Coordinator

Beyond the surgeon in the OR, the robotic surgery coordinator is key to an efficiently run and maintained program. This coordinator, who is typically a registered nurse, must help in the selection and training of dedicated robotic teams. The robotic surgery coordinator in the OR must also be well versed in maintenance and troubleshooting with the robotic surgical system. Though technical issues with the robots occur infrequently, the ability of the robotic surgery coordinator to problem-solve quickly and understand how to troubleshoot the issues quickly is a core competency of this role. Not all hospitals have staffing models in the OR that allow for the development of designated teams to assist with specific programs and service lines, but it is our experience that the technical expertise required to help with the robotic procedure makes this a worthwhile investment. We have found that assignment of dedicated teams with specialized training in a particular robotic subspecialty has led to decreased cost, more efficient room turnover, a decrease in "technical mistakes," and greater surgeon satisfaction. Our teams are split into pelvic-based, general, bariatric and colorectal, and cardiothoracic groups. In our metrics, time in the OR is a major driver of procedural expense, so OR efficiency is a key driver in the overall contribution margin.

Robotic First Assistant

Technical knowledge and skill in robotic surgery by dedicated robotic first assistants (RFAs) at the bedside will only serve to ensure the success of a robotic program. The skill set required for an assistant participating in a robotic case must be based in both laparoscopy and robotic surgery. Laparoscopic assistance translates into port placement, understanding of spatial relationships of instruments within the body, and general principles of traction, countertraction, and suctioning. Robotic assistance by an RFA includes understanding docking, handling, changing, and loading of instruments, as well as troubleshooting. An assistant lacking in any of these areas may negatively impact the case from a clinical outcome standpoint, a time standpoint, and a financial standpoint. Laparoscopic skill sets are an absolute requirement for those persons assigned as surgical assistants on robotic cases.

Training and Surgeon Factors

Surgeon expertise on robotic surgical techniques directly correlates with both cost and quality. In general, a robotic surgeon, defined as an individual that builds a surgical practice around procedures that are performed using a robotic surgical system, has higher value (less cost and better outcomes) than an individual that simply offers the technology in his or her suite of services. This is especially true when all of the aforementioned operating room environmental and personnel factors are included. Not every surgeon needs to go through a formal fellowship training program, but in lieu of this education, the surgeon must complete a large volume of procedures to achieve proficiency. Currently, at the hospital level, no formal national training standards exist for physicians to use the robot. And because the responsibility for quality and safety falls upon the hospital, it falls to the robotic surgical physician governing body, which is discussed later in this chapter, to establish and enforce standards for surgical practice and training on the robot.

A successful training curriculum may include the time using the robotic simulator to achieve understanding and skill development in regard to the technical aspects of robotic surgery—camera movement, use of clutch, positioning of arms at the console, and basic skill building. An established proctoring program is also important, whether the proctoring surgeon is on site for training purposes or the surgeon who is performing robotic surgery travels to an outside facility to acquire the necessary skills.

Governance and Oversight

Establishment of a Governance Committee, which is peer-review enabled and protected, to oversee a robotic surgery program is absolutely critical. This group must consist of surgeon champions from each of the subspecialties performing robotic surgery, a leader from anesthesiology (included in order to address anesthetic concerns with robotic surgery), a nurse champion (which could be the robotic surgery coordinator), and relevant administrative and/or hospital quality department analytic support. This committee must put into place quality controls to evaluate performance, including but not limited to individual surgeon robotic volume, department volume, hospital time, and individual robot utilization. This committee must also take responsibility for the credentialing, mentoring, and proctoring of new surgeons. We hold surgeons accountable by flagging those with consistently low volumes of robotic surgery, high complication rates, frequent intraoperative consultations, and any patient readmissions within 30 days of discharge.

Establishment of quality and safety standards for robotic surgery is important to keep complication rates low for those surgeons that are adjusting to the new technology. The governance and oversight committee must also serve as a platform for peer review, so that the performance of robotic surgeons is overseen by other robotic surgeons, keeping the evaluation fair. The development and distribution of a regular physician scorecard will allow for continuous discussion around practice variation and individual practice performance (Fig. 5.1).

These data should be transparent and individually reviewed by surgeons or sections practicing within the same institution. The goal of the scorecard is also to bring to light the cost associated with each procedure, as well as the profit margin for a particular procedure. The ultimate goal of the surgeon scorecard is not meant to be critical or to expose flaws. It is simply a tool for optimization and continued development of a robotic surgical program.

Analytic Profle of Piedmont

# of hysterectomies performed in (Sep/1/2016–Apr/30/2016 : 548

# of qualified hysterectomies for benchmark analysis : 401

# of surgeons performed at least 12 hysterectomies in the study period : 8

ECONOMICAL OUTCOME	Piedmont	South Atlantic	National
Avg. Hyst. Cost	$5,520	$4,019	$4,224
Inpatient Cost	$5,458	$4,203	$4,556
Outpatient Cost	$5,578	$3,918	$3,980
Surgical Cost*	$4,020	$2,817	$3,018
OPEN Cost	$5,112	$3,918	$4,336
LAP Cost	$5,564	$3,692	$3,967
Robotic Cost	$6,532	$5,044	$4,883
VAH Cost	$4,179	$2,899	$3,242

*include OR, supplies, and Observation Room

ANALYTICAL SYNTHESIS

Major Cost Categories

- Surgery Cost (Avg.): $4,020
- Room & Board Cost (Avg.): $686
- LAB Cost (Avg.): $296

Primary Cost Driver

- Surgery Cost: 1.33 times higher than national avg.
- LAB Cost: 2 times higher than national avg.
- High cost in robotic surgery

OPERATIONAL & CLINICAL OUTCOME	Piedmont	South Atlantic	National
Inpatient Volume (%)	194 (48.4%)	35.4%	42.3%
Avg. LOS (days)	2.60	2.27	57.7%
Avg. OR Time (mins)	172.3	148.2	150.7
OPEN Volume (%)	145 (36.2%)	23.0%	23.0%
LAP Volume (%)	102 (25.4%)	35.6%	32.3%
Robotic Volume (%)	111 (27.7%)	28.1%	30.2%
VAG Volume (%)	43 (10.7%)	13.3%	14.4%
# of Readmission (%)	6 (1.50%)	2.18%	2.48%
# of Complications (%)	61 (15.2%)	9.13%	9.55%

HIGH VOLUME SURGEON	ANALYZED VOLUME	AVG. COST	ADJ, AVG COST
	40	$5,908	$4,656
	39	$5,300	$3,844
	36	$6,954	$4,643
	26	$6,014	$4,187
	20	$5,768	$4,129
	17	$6,430	$4,157
	14	$4,910	$3,739
	12	$6,023	$4,630
	12	$4,875	$4,035

Fig. 5.1 Example of a scorecard for a robotic surgery program. This scorecard provides cost, complication, and key operational (average length of stay, surgical time and volume) information for the same surgery performed using different techniques and compares regional performance. This is likely to be more information than the hospital has access to for any single specialty, but it provides a comprehensive snapshot of cost and quality for the program

Credentialing, Training, Proctoring, and Mentoring

Credentialing

Because of the advanced technology used, robotic surgery requires specific training and proctoring. The procedure may be the same as when using a traditional laparoscopic technique, but an element of technical complexity is added that requires appropriate and adequate training, peer proctoring and mentoring, and eventual credentialing by the hospital. Safety and quality standards are established developing credentialing and re-credentialing criteria. There are no nationally set guidelines or standards for robotic credentialing, but many programs, including ours, use a minimum annual procedure requirement as a condition for credentialing. Review of performance metrics leads to case-specific operative and quality outcome benchmarking (even if it is only internal), with the goal of reaching the highest standard of quality among all surgeons performing robotic surgery.

Development and Implementation of Video Game-Based Simulation

Historically, surgeons learn new surgical procedures through observing, practicing skills and techniques, and then performing the procedure on patients under the supervision of an experienced surgeon. Today, training continues to be a serious safety issue for surgeons, hospitals, credentialing departments, surgical associations, and perhaps most importantly, the patients. If a surgeon expresses interest in robotic surgery, training is often conducted by a 1-day basic training course involving simple tasks but no emphasis on technique or in-depth knowledge of the individual steps required. Although this course is sufficient to gain familiarity with the controls of the robotic system, it is inadequate to perform complex and technically demanding techniques in operations such as radical prostatectomy with any degree of precision and expertise. In order for a fighter pilot to fly a jet, he or she must complete technique- and task-oriented flight simulation to gain sufficient skills captured through metrics. Simulators for open surgery have never really been practical, and surgical residencies are a graded and structured environment where surgeons develop their skills under constant supervision and guidance, but the advent of laparoscopic and robotic surgery, which depends on imaging using video scopes inserted into the body, allows for the very real possibility of simulation [14]. Inadequate or suboptimal training is a serious safety concern that has yet to be adequately addressed via current simulators. In addition, current robotic training lacks any objective metrics with which to gauge a surgeon's skills [15]. Development of metric-based task- and technique-driven simulated and interactive training programs will address serious safety concerns in the operating theater.

Robotic Program Acquisition Cost and Operational Expense Analysis

Completely identifying and transparently stating all of the start-up and ongoing operational expenses associated with a robotic surgical program will help build trust and minimize long-term disagreement with the hospital's finance department. The two major cost considerations that must be taken into account are the start-up fixed capital costs associated with a robot—capital, annual service contracts, and robot-specific supplies—and the costs associated with operational excellence, including the robotic surgery coordinator, OR team, and robotic first assistant (RFA).

Robot-Specific Expenses

The primary cost commitments associated with the acquisition of the robot are the cost of the robotic system itself, the accompanying annual service contract, the incremental disposables specific to the robotic system (arms, drape kit, etc.), and the incremental time associated with using a new technology. The inevitable learning curve for the OR staff and physicians will increase near-term costs (Table 5.1).

A new robotic surgical system (da Vinci Xi, Intuitive Surgical, Sunnyvale, CA) will cost a hospital $1.5 million USD. Add to this $150,000 to $200,000 USD for service contracts associated with annual maintenance. An average instrument will cost approximately $2500 USD for ten uses per instrument. On average, a case will require the use of five or six instruments, resulting in a minimum instrument cost of about $1250 USD per case. When starting a program, it is also prudent to factor in expenses associated with instrument misuse as surgeons are forced to adapt to the new technology.

Table 5.1 Robot-specific costs associated with a single robotic surgery system at a hospital or ambulatory surgical center[a]

Cost	Expense
Robotic system	$1,500,000
Robotic system depreciation (7 year)	$214,286
Service contract (annual)	$150,000
Robot disposables (per case)	$1300
Operating room time (hours)[b]	2.5

[a]All costs depicted are estimates and not reflective of actual facility direct costs

[b]Time estimate (from start to end of procedure) is based on an average time calculated across multiple specialties. This is the suggested time to be used when comparing the efficiency of completing a procedure using a laparoscopic, open, or robotic technique

Table 5.2 Cost distribution by major cost category by specialty[a]

Expense type	General surgery	GYN	Thoracic	Transplant	Urology	Colorectal
OR time (1st hours)	28%	34%	22%	22%	28%	20%
OR time (15 min)	6%	8%	20%	12%	13%	15%
OR supplies (da Vinci)	16%	20%	13%	13%	16%	12%
All other OR supplies	31%	26%	13%	28%	22%	23%
% of Total expenses	**81%**	**88%**	**68%**	**75%**	**70%**	**70%**
Average OR time	1.85	1.87	4.41	3.05	2.67	3.69
Length of stay (inpatient only)	1.89	1.83	2.62	1.72	1.77	3.90
Room and board (inpatient only)	13%	–[b]	17%	10%	13%	20%
All other expenses (inpatient only)	6%	12%	15%	14%	8%	10%
Total direct cost	**$8,000**	**$6,500**	**$10,000**	**$10,000**	**$8,000**	**$11,000**

[a]The various cost components of a robotic surgical procedure, showing the relative magnitude of each cost component in the total cost of the robotic procedure. All costs depicted are estimates and not reflective of actual facility direct costs

[b]A room and board percentage is not shown because more than 90% of the total patient mix is outpatient

Operational Cost Categories

The major cost drivers for robotic surgery are within the operating room. Based on our study of the costs across the different procedure groups and service lines, we consistently see the operating room expenses drive overall financial performance of the program. Because of the documented wide cost variations for healthcare across the United States, these expenses will vary based on each hospital's cost accounting methodology and local dynamics such as employee salaries, but the expenses shown on Table 5.2 give the relative magnitude of the costs per specialty.

Operating Costs

The overall robotic costs are relatively fixed, but cost variation between surgeons and specialties does exist, based on type of procedure performed, length of stay, physician preference items, and the duration of the procedure. The advancement in the technology has driven down the length of stay to a point where the largest operating expense risk is in the operating room. The greatest expenses in the OR—the first-hour charge and robot-specific supplies—are fixed, so the opportunity for cost containment exists through improving the procedure time and physician surgical preference items. Working within the governance structure and facilitated by the robotic surgery coordinator, it is recommended that as many instruments and supplies as possible are standardized. The operating room is also where the largest overall cost and quality risk exist. Less proficient surgeons can take longer in completing the procedure, which is inherently costly (time is cost in the OR), and can lead to complications, which can add avoidable costs. Constructing a robotic program designed around highly trained OR staff, dedicated physicians, and tightly managed preference supplies will lead to a higher-quality, financially sustainable program.

Accounting for Depreciation and Service Contracts

Volume in a robotic program not only is important for a simple contribution margin equation but also helps to spread the high fixed costs associated with the capital outlay and associated annual service contract. Opinions differ as to whether to include the full burden of the depreciation and service contracts (which amount to upwards of $250,000 to $350,000 per year) when assessing the program. At our institution, we allocate the depreciation and service contract expenses when financially evaluating the performance of our various programs because the capital asset was specifically purchased for programmatic support. This becomes the second largest hurdle for financial success in the program.

Growth, Development, and Optimization of a Robotic Surgery Program

The Robotic Strategy

The theory of "if you build it, they will come" is the premise that many hospitals use to attract patients and surgeons to use their facility, but using the robot as an enticement does not make sense. Many hospitals make the mistake of believing that success is based solely on attracting volume; they minimize the risks associated with training, governance, and specialty diversification, which will help with the financial performance of the robot. A program rooted in physician expertise and built on principles of governance and specialty diversification are the keys to success.

Benefits of a Multidisciplinary Program

Surgical case diversification within a robotic program also can contribute to increased profits with minimized costs and overhead. Diversity with multiple surgeons using a single system or multiple systems results usually in larger volume and less reliance on a specific specialty or procedure, a problem if the surgeon or group departs or the procedure falls out of popular favor (e.g., single-site laparoscopic cholecystectomy). Based on analysis completed by Intuitive Surgical and by our health system and others, the average number of cases that needs to be completed per robotic surgical system is 250–300 cases per year, which translates to 21–25 cases per month. This is a challenging load for an individual surgeon, but it may be more easily achieved by a group of surgeons.

A number of specialties have embraced robotic surgery:

- Urology
- Gynecology
- General surgery (including bariatric surgery)
- Colorectal surgery
- Cardiothoracic surgery
- Ear, nose, and throat surgery
- Transplant surgery

If a program exhibits diversity in regard to its case load, the result is typically increased use of a surgical system by a greater number of surgeons, which ultimately may result in a higher volume of cases. A case load per robotic system of 200–250 typically warrants purchase of an additional system so as to accommodate the needs of each surgeon, but it is possible to support more, depending on the proficiency of the surgeons. In the year leading up to acquiring an additional robot, we reached an average volume of about 500 cases per robot.

As a national trend, among the procedures most frequently performed on the robot is robot-assisted hysterectomy, which is associated with lower reimbursement, but even with lower or minimal comparative reimbursement, an efficient surgeon can produce a positive contribution margin (net patient revenue minus direct costs) that can help to absorb the costs of depreciation and the service contract. The other specialty that often uses robotic technology is urology. Urological cases completed with robotic assistance continue to show profitability, but as with all robotic surgery, this can be influenced by the level of efficiency by which cases are completed in the operating room. Both urology and gynecology are typically associated with larger oncology strategies, however, which can have lucrative downstream revenue opportunities (i.e., imaging, radiation therapy, chemotherapy, etc.), so it is important to assess these specialties in the context of a larger strategy. Nevertheless, this chapter specifically refers to the benefit directly associated with robot-assisted procedures.

Conclusions

Rapid innovations in surgical technique are occurring at a faster pace than the hospital's ability to develop standards that ensure quality and safety of services. It is therefore the responsibility of the physician leaders to partner with hospital administration to develop standards to help protect our patients and communities. A program that is built on the fundamentals of physician leadership, dedicated operating room teams and leadership, and an overall governance system to monitor physician performance will ensure long-term programmatic viability. Though several major societal drivers, such as affordability, quality, and personalized care, can be addressed by emerging robotic technology, overall advancement will only occur if the development revolves around responsible investment in the key elements that drive performance.

References

1. Herron DM, Marohn M, SAGES-MIRA Robotic Surgery Consensus Group. A consensus document on robotic surgery. Surg Endosc. 2008;22:313–25. discussion 311–2
2. Zorn KC, Gautam G, Shalhav AL, Clayman RV, Ahlering TE, Albala DM, et al.; Members of the Society of Urologic Robotic Surgeons. Training, credentialing, proctoring and medicolegal risks of robotic urological surgery: recommendations of the society of urologic robotic surgeons. J Urol. 2009;182:1126–1132.
3. Tandogdu Z, Vale L, Fraser C, Ramsay C. A systematic review of economic evaluations of the use of robotic assisted laparoscopy in surgery compared with open or laparoscopic surgery. Appl Health Econ Health Policy. 2015;13:457–67.
4. Mehr SR, Zimmerman MP. Robotic-assisted surgery: a question of value. Am J Manag Care. 2014;20:E13.
5. Wright JD, Tergas AI, Hou JY, Burke WM, Chen L, Hu JC, et al. Effect of regional hospital competition and hospital financial status on the use of robotic-assisted surgery. JAMA Surg. 2016;151:612–20.
6. Chan JK, Gardner AB, Taylor K, Blansit K, Thompson CA, Brooks R, et al. The centralization of robotic surgery in high-volume centers for endometrial cancer patients--a study of 6560 cases in the U.S. Gynecol Oncol. 2015;138:128–32.
7. Tabib CH, Bahler CD, Hardacker TJ, Ball KM, Sundaram CP. Reducing operating room costs through real-time cost information feedback: a pilot study. J Endourol. 2015;29(8):963.
8. Szold A, Bergamaschi R, Broeders I, Dankelman J, Forgione A, Langø T, et al.; European Association of Endoscopic Surgeons.

European Association of Endoscopic Surgeons (EAES) consensus statement on the use of robotics in general surgery. Surg Endosc. 2015;29:253–288.

9. Williams SB, Prado K, Hu JC. Economics of robotic surgery: does it make sense and for whom? Urol Clin North Am. 2014;41:591–6.
10. Barbash GI, Friedman B, Glied SA, Steiner CA. Factors associated with adoption of robotic surgical technology in US hospitals and relationship to radical prostatectomy procedure volume. Ann Surg. 2014;259:1–6.
11. Salman M, Bell T, Martin J, Bhuva K, Grim R, Ahuja V. Use, cost, complications, and mortality of robotic versus nonrobotic general surgery procedures based on a nationwide database. Am Surg. 2013;79:553–60.
12. Geller EJ, Matthews CA. Impact of robotic operative efficiency on profitability. Am J Obstet Gynecol. 2013;209:20.e1–5. Erratum in: Am J Obstet Gynecol. 2014;211:546
13. Turchetti G, Palla I, Pierotti F, Cuschieri A. Economic evaluation of da Vinci-assisted robotic surgery: a systematic review. Surg Endosc. 2012;26:598–606.
14. Kranzfelder M, Staub C, Fiolka A, Schneider A, Gillen S, Wilhelm D, et al. Toward increased autonomy in the surgical OR: needs, requests, and expectations. Surg Endosc. 2013;27:1681–8.
15. Abboudi H, Khan MS, Aboumarzouk O, Guru KA, Challacombe B, Dasgupta P, Ahmed K. Current status of validation for robotic surgery simulators - a systematic review. BJU Int. 2013;111:194–205.

Visualization in Robotic Surgery

6

Mahdi Azizian, Ian McDowall, and Jonathan Sorger

Visualization can be defined as "a technique for creating images, diagrams, or animations to communicate a message" [1]. Visualization in surgical robotics involves displaying images of patient anatomy to the surgeon. Such images can be provided by optical or tomographic imaging techniques.

The first application of robotics in surgery relied heavily on tomographic imaging, utilizing the PUMA 200 robot for CT-guided stereotactic neurosurgical procedures [2]. Since then, volumetric imaging has been a critical component of subsequent surgical robots, from the PROBOT (Imperial College, London), which used transrectal ultrasound to guide prostate resection, to the ROBODOC® system (Think Surgical, Fremont, CA), which uses CT scans combined with fiducial markers to guide joint replacement. Years later, Computer Motion (Goleta, CA) realized the importance of stable endoscopic visualization during surgery, as evidenced by the development of the Automated Endoscopic System for Optimal Positioning (AESOP®), a robotic endoscope positioning device that responded to voice commands. The da Vinci® Surgical System (Intuitive Surgical, Sunnyvale, CA) was the first to use a stereoscopic endoscope to guide soft tissue resection, further highlighting the importance of an improved visual experience for the robotic surgeon.

It is helpful to briefly review what the past, present, and future hold for each of these areas.

M. Azizian, PhD
Image-Guided Robotics, Intuitive Surgical, Sunnyvale, CA, USA
e-mail: mahdi.azizian@intusurg.com

I. McDowall, BaSc Hon
Vision Engineering, Intuitive Surgical, Sunnyvale, CA, USA
e-mail: ian.mcdowall@intusurg.com

J. Sorger, PhD, MBA (✉)
Research, Intuitive Surgical, Sunnyvale, CA, USA
e-mail: jonathan.sorger@intusurg.com

Optical Endoscopy

Robotic surgery has employed several generations of technology to provide the surgeon with a clear view of patient anatomy. These systems were created in the context of expanding laparoscopic techniques. Laparoscopic surgery is a relatively young field, with the first cholecystectomy having been performed in 1985, and robotic surgery has borrowed a number of design ideas from laparoscopy in the way that it provides visualization to the operating surgeon.

The earliest robotic surgery systems emerged in the early 1990s, including the development of systems using stereo microscopes as the viewing apparatus, exemplified by NASA Jet Propulsion Laboratory's Robot Assisted MicroSurgery workstation (RAMS) [3]. This system afforded six degrees of freedom manipulation but was primarily a research tool. Stereoscopic camera-based implementations were demonstrated as part of research work at Stanford Research International, with the system put together by the team led by Dr. Philip Green [4]. This system used a pair of cameras interfaced to a field sequential stereoscopic display viewed with stereo glasses to achieve the desired 3D visual effect. This early work was researched at various academic institutions and supported with funding from the National Institutes of Health and Defense Advanced Research Projects Agency. Robotic surgery was championed in the US government by Dr. Richard Satava and others, and this government investment in new technology exploration formed the basis for the technology commercialized by Intuitive Surgical and its da Vinci® systems.

At the present time, two main technologies are employed to capture endoscopic imagery in robotic surgery. Recent systems use optical endoscopes that contain a number of small relay lenses to enable a camera outside the cannula to image inside the patient. Optical endoscopes contain imaging optics comprised of an objective lens group and a series of relay lenses, as shown in Fig. 6.1; illumination is typically delivered through incoherent fiber optic bundles. The image formed may be captured by a camera integrated into the

Y. Fong et al. (eds.), *The SAGES Atlas of Robotic Surgery*, https://doi.org/10.1007/978-3-319-91045-1_6

endoscope or a camera attached to the endoscope. Stereo endoscopes contain two sets of imaging optics, and these two imaging optical trains are identical between the right and left eyes to provide a carefully matched stereo pair of images [5]. Designs may incorporate the camera and the optics into one unit, as shown in Fig. 6.1.

Alternatively, if the camera is draped, then a sterile drape interface may be employed between the cleaned and sterilized endoscope and the camera assembly [6]. The Intuitive Surgical Si systems take this approach. One side effect of having the camera and endoscope paired in the OR is that the stereo calibration for appropriate image alignment may need to be performed each time the system is used, as the endoscopes and cameras are not necessarily known pairs that were calibrated a priori by the manufacturer. The calibrations required would typically include white balance and left-right eye alignment. The alignment in the vertical direction is particularly important, as vertical offsets and cyclorotations in stereo displays are visually objectionable; correct horizontal alignment is also important for long-term visual comfort [7].

The latest systems employ cameras that are small enough and of sufficient performance to be placed in the distal tip of the shaft of the endoscope, as shown in Fig. 6.2. These cameras have been miniaturized so that they may be placed at the tip of an articulated tool. Flexible endoscopes of this design afford the surgeon the ability to realize much better image quality than an endoscope employing a flexible coherent image fiber bundle. This design approach also minimizes the number of optical elements before the image is formed, enabling the creation of complete cameras that can be used in vivo. Examples of these articulated stereo endoscopic systems include the Olympus Endoeye® Flex 3D, shown in Fig. 6.3, and the Intuitive Surgical da Vinci® Sp system, shown in Fig. 6.4. There are fewer optical components in these endoscopic cameras, so the alignment may be performed at the time of manufacture and stored with the camera device, simplifying the device setup time in the OR. This design approach enables the creation of endoscopes with long, thin shafts, which would not be possible with a rod lens approach. Monoscopic endoscopes can have long, very thin shafts, as image misalignment can be tolerated. In a stereo system, however, the two images must be matched and must stay well aligned; maintaining optical alignment in a device with a long, thin shaft in a hospital environment is generally impractical.

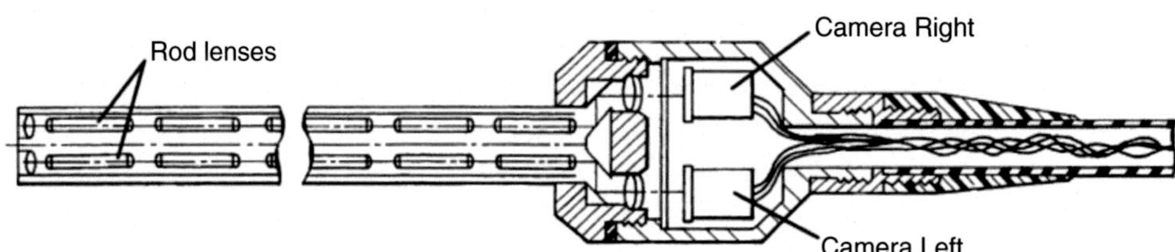

Fig. 6.1 An example, from US patent 5,588,948 [5], of a stereo endoscope designed with the camera elements outside the body. Note the trains of relay lenses, which deliver the image from inside the patient to the cameras

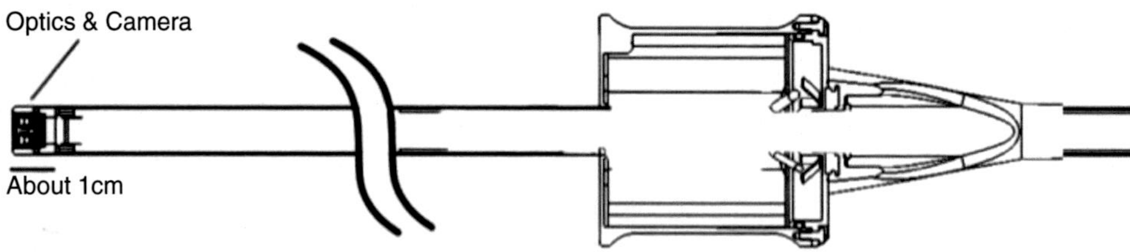

Fig. 6.2 An example of the latest generation of stereo endoscope with the camera and optics in the tip of the device, reducing the number of lens elements that can become misaligned and reducing the mass of the endoscope. (Image provided by Intuitive Surgical)

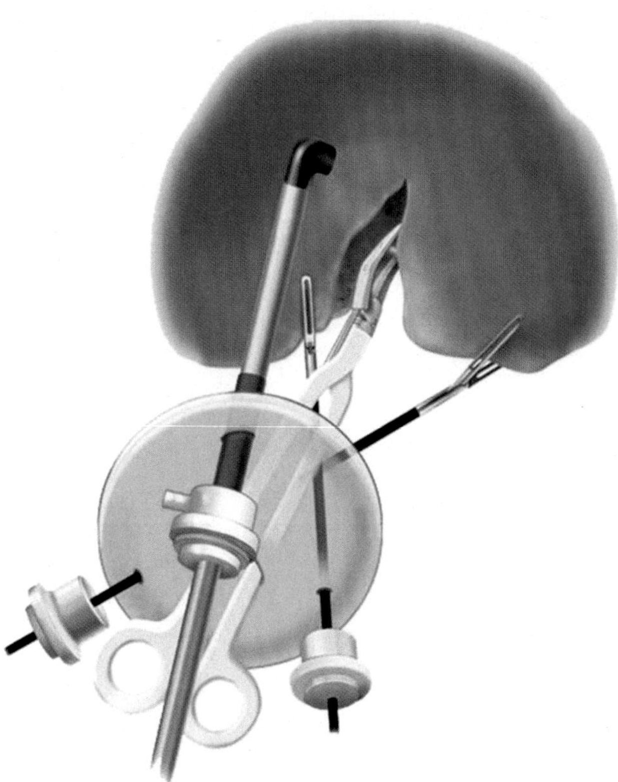

Fig. 6.3 The Olympus Endoeye® Flex 3D. In this case, the endoscope is employed for single gel port liver resection. (*Courtesy of* Dr. Yuman Fong)

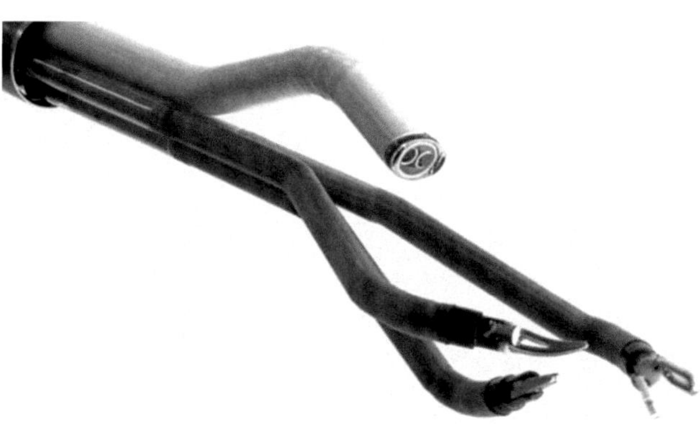

Fig. 6.4 Intuitive Surgical's Sp system with a small, articulated camera tip. (Image provided by Intuitive Surgical)

Fluorescence Imaging

Further innovation in visualization during robotic surgical procedures is exemplified by near-infrared fluorescence imaging. Fluorescence imaging is accomplished by administering a fluorescent agent, a corresponding light source, and a detector. In microscopy, a wide range of agents are available, with a variety of excitation and emission wavelengths. The surgical application of fluorescence imaging requires agents with demonstrated clinical utility that are approved by the US Food and Drug Administration (FDA). The first of these to be widely used in robotic surgical procedures is indocyanine green (ICG). Upon systemic administration, ICG rapidly binds to plasma proteins in the blood and thus offers surgeons the ability to see vasculature and tissue perfusion. The ICG is removed from the blood by hepatic parenchymal cells and is secreted into bile. This pathway for ICG excretion accounts for the rapid decrease in apparent brightness of fluorescence in vasculature after administration in patients with healthy hepatic systems. The ICG concentration in bile enables surgeons to image the bile duct structures, as illustrated in Fig. 6.5 [8]. In general, the bile duct structures become visible about 45 min after systemic administration of the agent. The excitation and emission wavelengths of ICG are in the near-infrared region, and as adipose tissue and fascia are somewhat transparent at these wavelengths, it is possible to see the ICG fluorescence through a modest thickness of intervening tissue. Researchers continue to explore other applications of ICG and its application to conditions suited to robotic surgery. There is ongoing research and exploration in the field regarding the use of ICG to image lymphatic system drainage (Fig. 6.6) and localize lymph nodes [9] in order to reduce surgical morbidity. It is important to note that a host of other fluorescent imaging agents also are being developed for intraoperative use, many of which will be suitable for use in robotic systems [10], as shown in Fig. 6.7.

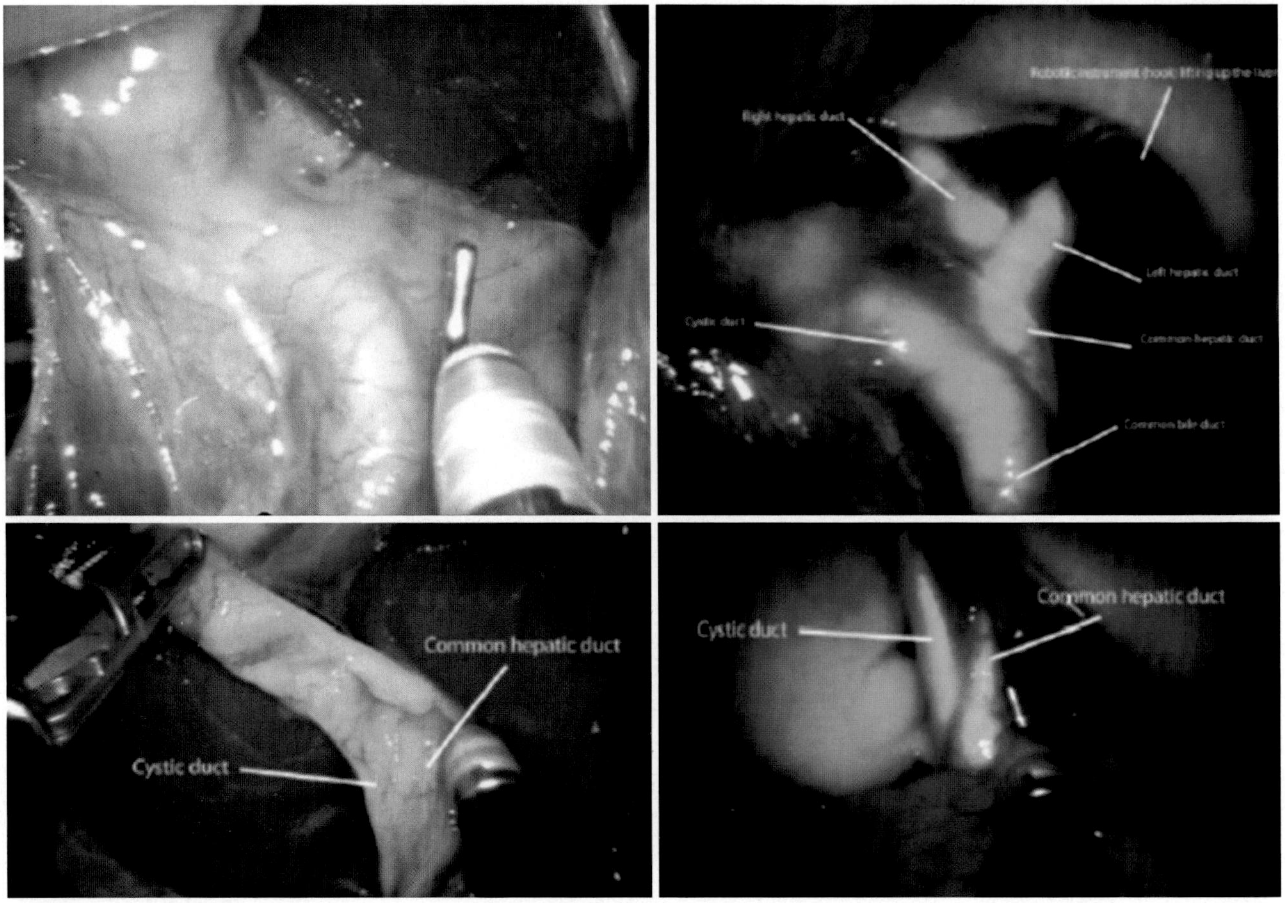

Fig. 6.5 Indocyanine green (ICG) used to visualize the hepatic ducts (*Reproduced from* Spinoglio et al. [8]; *with permission*)

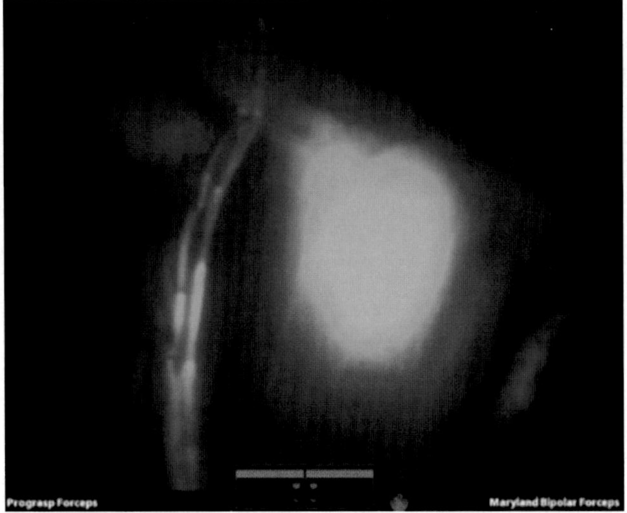

Fig. 6.6 An example of lymph node imaging using ICG. Lymphatic channels (*left*) can be seen leading to a lymph node (*right*)

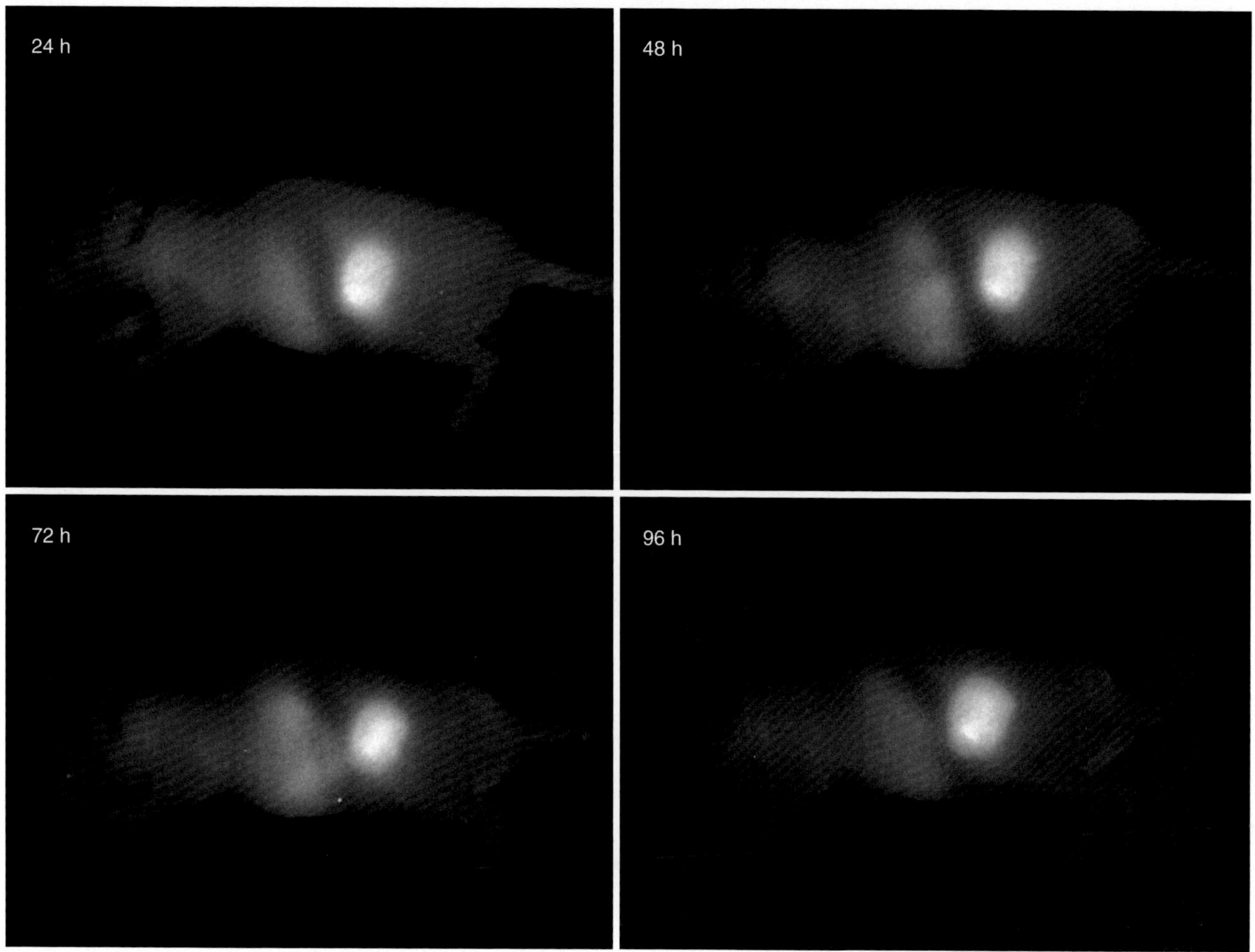

Fig. 6.7 Fluorescent near-infrared imaging of mouse bearing human colorectal cancer HT29 xenograft, 24, 48, 72, 96 h after injection of anti-CEA M5A-IRDye800. These images show long-lasting imaging of tumor suitable for operative use. (*Courtesy of* Dr. Paul Yazaki)

Other Optical Imaging Techniques

Even though surgical robotics has been successful in increasing the percentage of procedures performed in a minimally invasive manner, the opportunity to use endogenous optical signals to reduce positive margins and adverse event rates promises further benefits for patients and healthcare systems. Many of these techniques can be combined with white light endoscopy, described in the previous section. Though some of these technologies are not necessarily specific to robotics, the inherent stability of robotic vision systems will enable easier integration and implementation. Despite some limitations, it is possible that these vision-based techniques will lead to improved surgical outcomes in the future [11].

Vicini and colleagues [12] applied narrowband imaging (NBI), which uses selective bands of red, blue, and green illumination to better visualize topical tissue features, in an attempt to bring the positive margin rates in head and neck surgery down from as high as 20%. As an inherently surface-based technology, NBI shows promise in helping to evaluate suspicious superficial lesions in the head and neck (Fig. 6.8), as well as bladder cancers [13].

Many spectral-based technologies cannot easily be applied to current robotic surgical procedures because of a limited field of view. Robotics can make the acquisition of image mosaics easier, as acquisition speed and instrument travel over tissue can be specifically controlled. Mosaicking has been applied to Mauna Kea's Cellvizio® microendoscope, which traditionally offers a field of view in the hundreds of micron range, as shown in Fig. 6.9. Though individual images are only large enough to display a single gland or crypt of the colon, reconstructed mosaics can show a larger region. This specific modality may require extensive training on the part of the surgeon, or corroboration by a pathologist for definitive diagnosis.

The use of polarized light may help to visualize nuances in tissue microstructure that affect how a surgeon performs a procedure. By taking advantage of the fact that tissue scattering and absorption changes a a function of wavelength, microvessels and ultrastructure can be presented simply by exploiting white light endoscopy, as shown in Fig. 6.10.

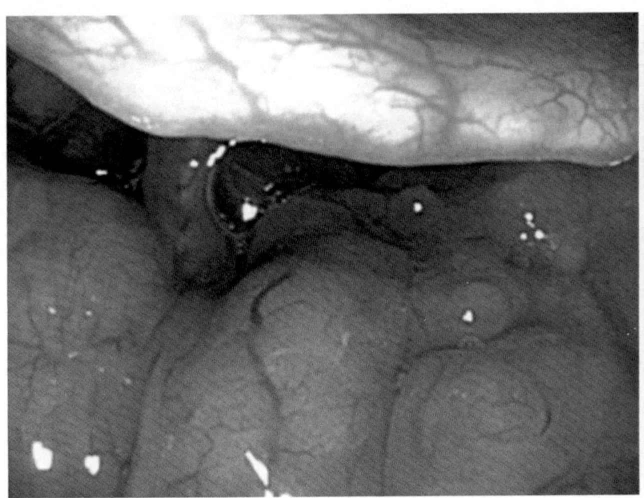

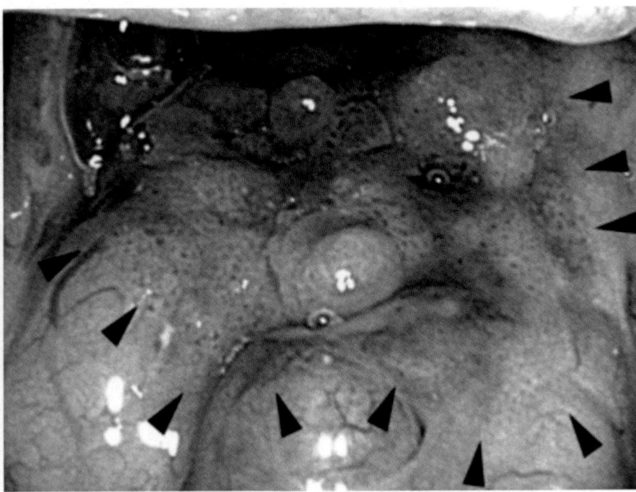

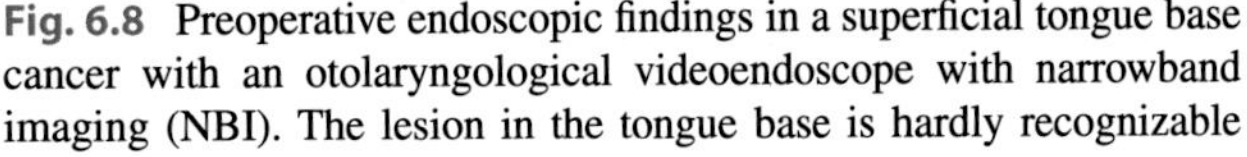

Fig. 6.8 Preoperative endoscopic findings in a superficial tongue base cancer with an otolaryngological videoendoscope with narrowband imaging (NBI). The lesion in the tongue base is hardly recognizable under white light (*left*). NBI visualizes the lesion as a brownish area with scattered brownish dots (*right*, *arrowheads*). (*Reproduced from* Tateya et al. [14]; *with permission*)

Fig. 6.9 Examples of mosaics of microscopic colorectal structures created using freehand and endoscope scanning. (*Reproduced from* Hughes and Yang [15]; *with permission from* The Optical Society)

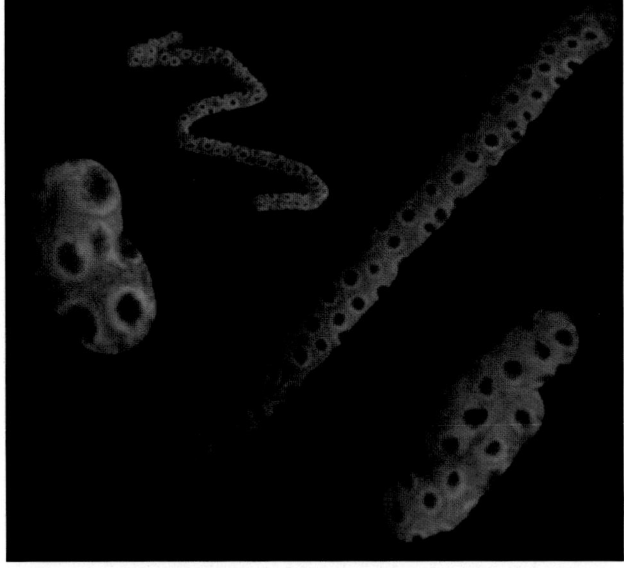

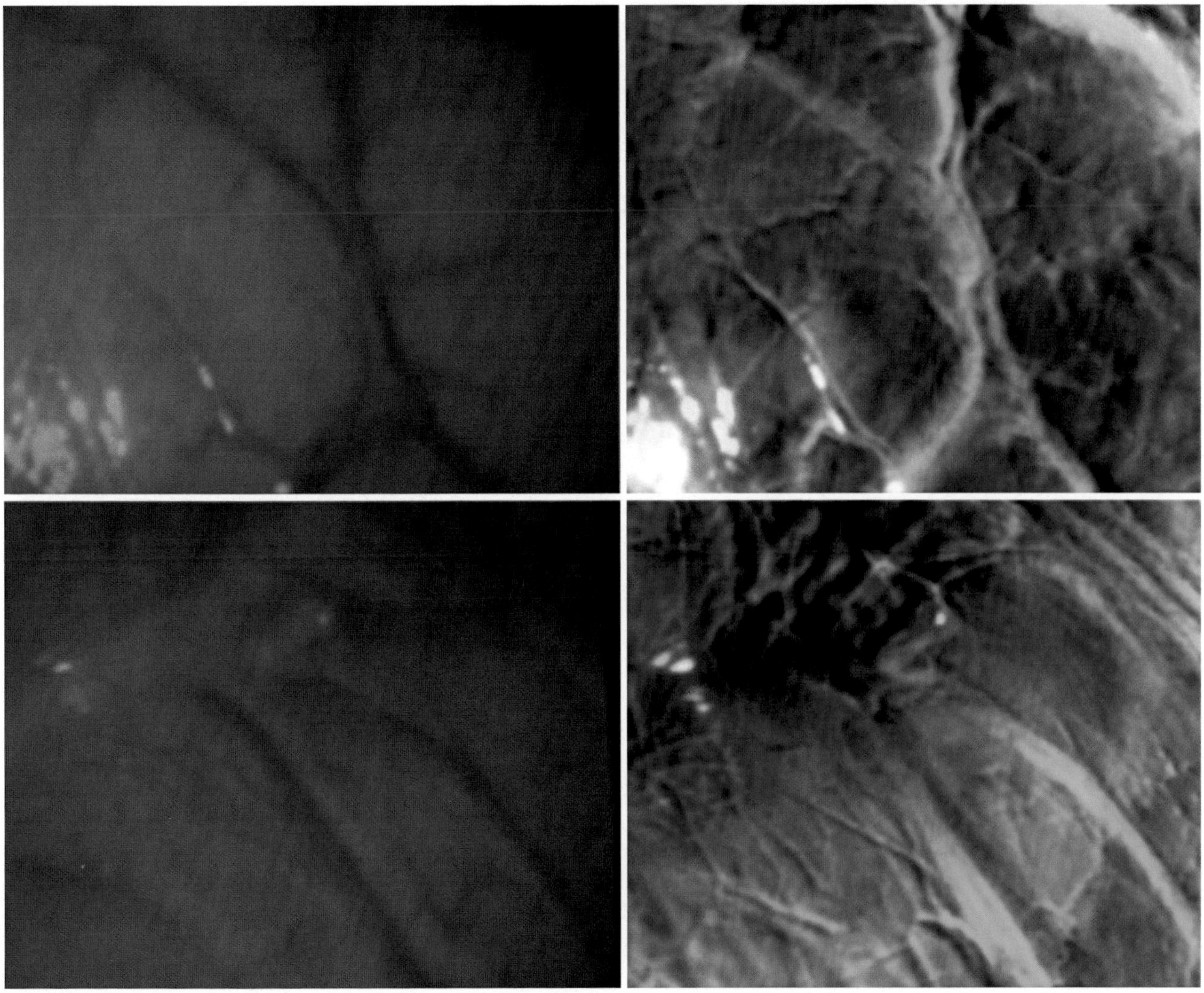

Fig. 6.10 Standard color (*left*) and polarized (*right*) images encoded in color, with *red* representing the signal from deep structures and *blue/green* corresponding to more superficial tissue. (*Reproduced from* Clancy et al. [16]; *with permission from* The Optical Society)

Tomographic Imaging

The endoscopic imaging techniques described above provide superficial projective images of tissue with a few millimeters of penetration. Tomography is another class of imaging techniques, which provides images of sections of an object using penetrating waves such as x-rays (e.g., computed tomography [CT]), gamma rays (e.g., single-photon emission computed tomography [SPECT]), radiofrequency waves (e.g., magnetic resonance imaging [MRI]), or mechanical waves (e.g., ultrasound). Tomographic imaging provides sectional images, which can provide information beyond the surface of tissue, as opposed to projective images captured by endoscopes or traditional vision.

Robotic surgery for soft tissue has been mostly focused on projective endoscope images, which show only the visible surface of organs. More recently, fluorescence imaging has also been used to provide subsurface information as an integrated solution, as described in the previous section, and has been applied to colorectal surgery [17]. Although tomographic imaging is not currently an integral part of soft tissue surgical robotic systems, it is often used to provide insight into deep tissue structures such as solid tumors and vasculature.

The use of tomographic images during robot-assisted surgery can increase accuracy and speed [18] in addition to reducing the number of complications and the chance of recurrence. On the other hand, it can disrupt the typical surgical workflow, so it is important to consider changes required. The main causes of change to the surgical workflow are the steps required for image acquisition, segmentation, registration, and visualization. These steps not only require changes in the workflow but also may require new staff to perform tasks such as image segmentation.

Workflow for Robotic Surgery

Figure 6.11 illustrates a workflow to accommodate the use of tomographic images during robotic surgery. Preoperative images are captured for diagnostic or therapeutic purposes prior to the intervention. After these images go through some preprocessing and segmentation, they also may be used for surgical planning. After operating room setup, patient preparation, and placement of the surgical robot, preoperative images must be registered to the intraoperative coordinates, which are dependent on the positions of the patient and robot. After registration is performed, the surgery can begin. Patient or robot motion can necessitate re-registration during the operation, depending on the required accuracy. If an intraoperative imaging modality is used, it also must be registered to the patient and/or robot coordinate frames. Visualization methods and parameters may need to be adjusted repeatedly. As shown in Fig. 6.11, multiple new steps are added to the workflow for robotic surgery. The following sections provide more details and examples regarding the registration, segmentation, and visualization steps.

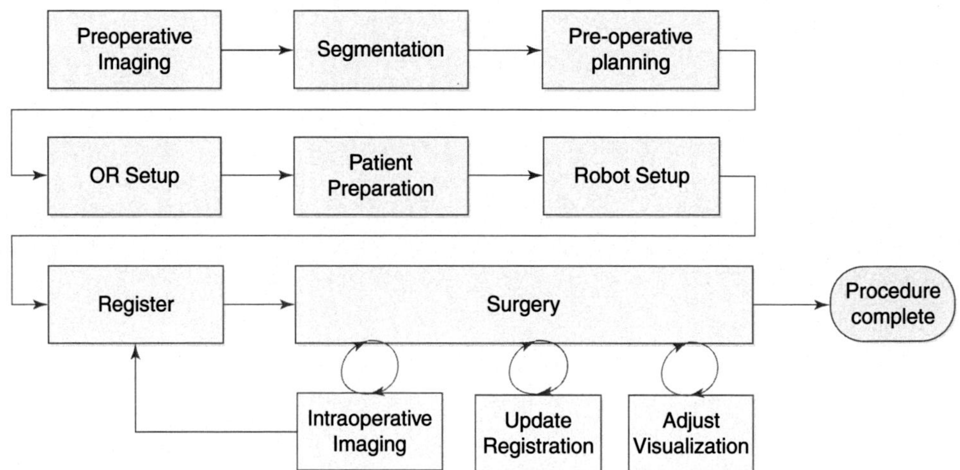

Fig. 6.11 A workflow for an image-guided, robot-assisted surgery

Registration

Endoscopic images provide the primary frame of reference during robot-assisted laparoscopic surgery. To make use of any other information during the procedure (including information provided by tomographic images), mapping of the coordinate frames should be performed. Sometimes the surgeon does this mapping using his or her perception of patient anatomy, how the robot and endoscope are set up, and the contents of the endoscopic images. This rather difficult task may require frequent switching between viewing of the preoperative images, endoscopic images, relative position of the patient and the endoscope. Finding a corresponding object within the endoscopic and tomographic image is usually a good confirmation; for example, a pulsating blood vessel may be matched to a blood vessel that was observed in a CT angiogram or a Doppler ultrasound image. Figure 6.12 shows an example in which printed renderings of a patient's CT scan were attached to a da Vinci® surgeon console.

As one could imagine, although it is possible to mentally map tomographic images to endoscopic images, it is often an extremely difficult and nonintuitive process. Several research efforts have focused on using computer-assisted techniques to facilitate this registration process. There are also commercial products offering semiautomated registration techniques, mainly for bony anatomy or for brain tissue where deformations are not large.

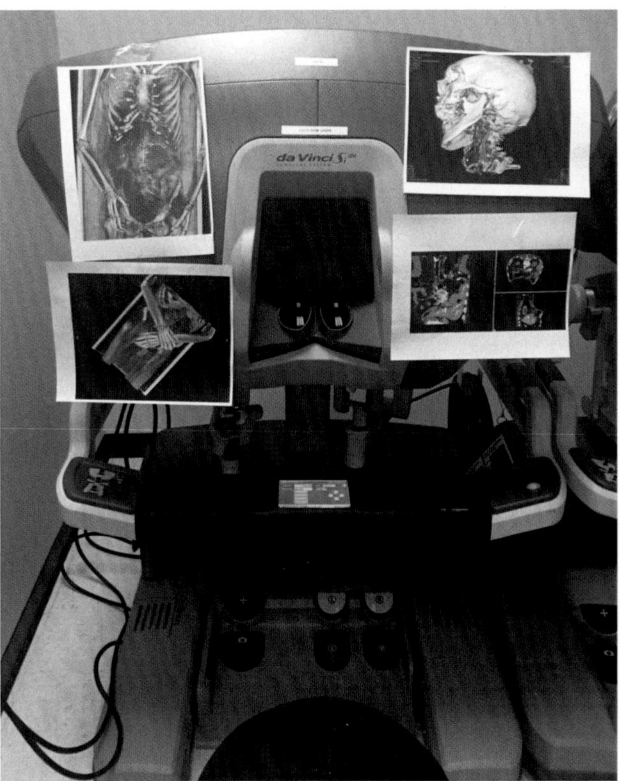

Fig. 6.12 Preoperative imaging used as a reference during da Vinci® surgery

Registration for Bony Anatomy

Registration of tomographic images for soft tissue surgery is challenging and often requires intraoperative updates because of the deformation of soft tissue. In orthopedic surgery, the organ of interest is usually some bony anatomy or regions close to bones. In these cases, nonrigid deformations can often be neglected, and bones can be fixed to prevent motion during surgery. Tracking systems such as optical or electromagnetic tracking can be used to find the rigid transformation between bony anatomy and the surgical tools operated by robots.

ROBODOC® (now TSolution One®) provides a robot-assisted solution for total hip replacement. Preoperative CT images are used for planning the surgery. A surface-based registration technique is then used by touching multiple points on the femoral surface using a tracked probe [19]. The same process is utilized for verification, and the registration is then applied to map the preoperative plan to the current patient coordinate system. This process is illustrated in Fig. 6.13.

Registration Using Intraoperative Imaging

Registration of preoperative images to intraoperative coordinates can also be performed using another imaging device. Mountney et al. [20] used a cone beam CT (CBCT) device to acquire an image of the patient in the intraoperative pose and then registered the CBCT images to the preoperative images for a minimally invasive liver surgery. This process is shown in Fig. 6.14.

As a commercially available example, the Renaissance system (Mazor Robotics Ltd., Caesarea, Israel) uses two X-ray snapshots for registration in spine surgery [21].

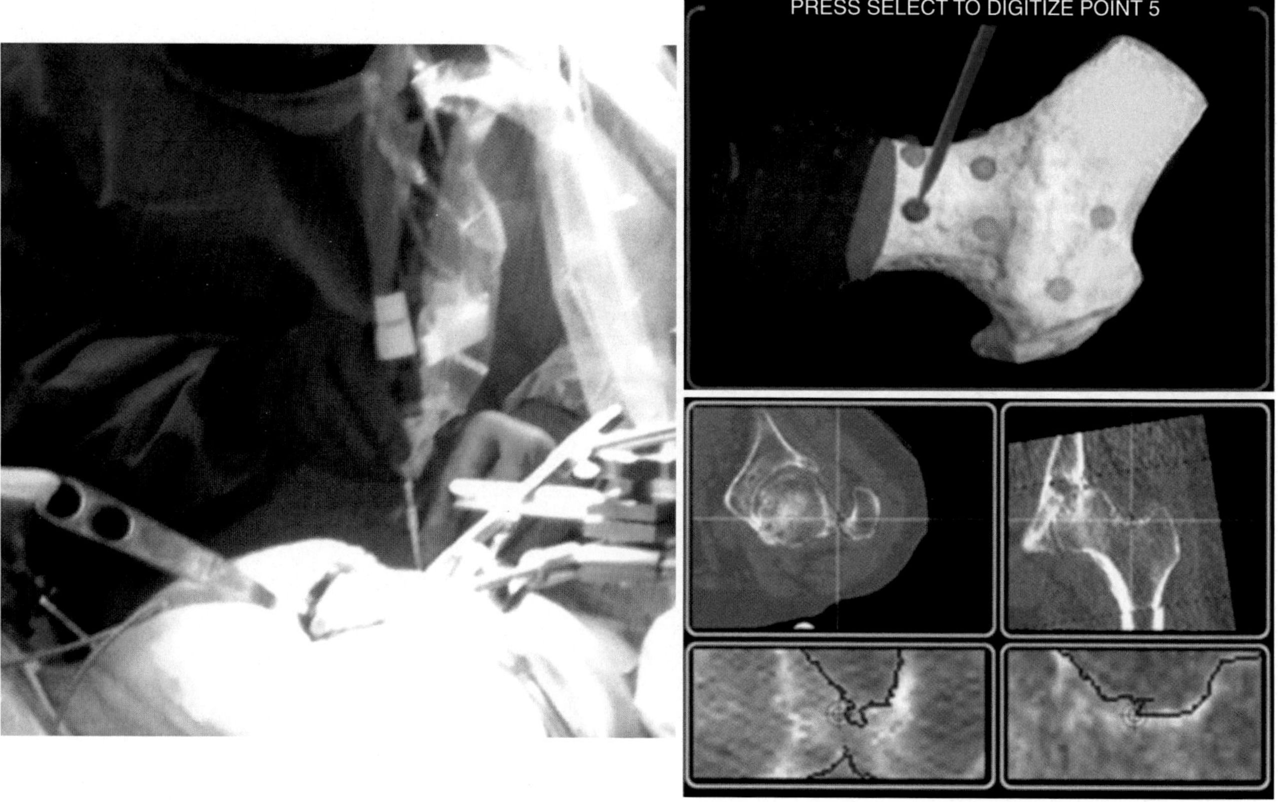

Fig. 6.13 The ROBODOC® registration is performed by touching multiple points on the femoral surface using a tracked probe. (*Modified from* Nakamura et al. [19]; *with permission*)

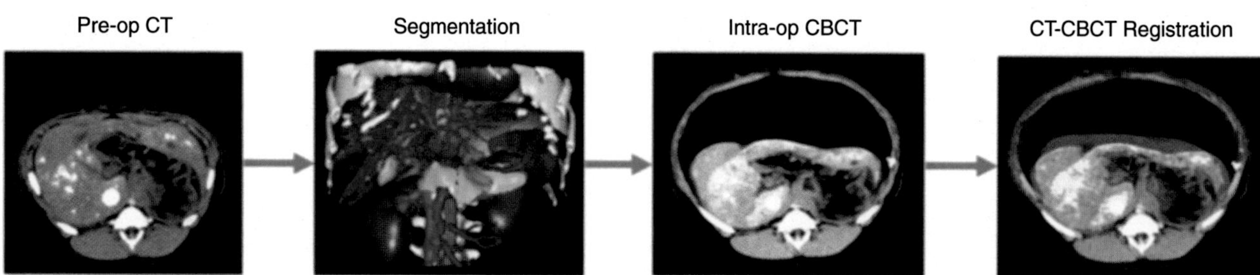

Fig. 6.14 Cone beam CT images used for registration of preoperative CT images. (Reproduced from Mountney et al. [20])

Segmentation

Visualization of the information in tomographic images is not as straightforward as visualization of endoscopic images. Three-dimensional images provided by modalities such as CT and MRI are usually displayed as orthogonal slices after multiplanar reconstruction or are rendered as volumetric images. Volumetric rendering of three-dimensional data without processing often does not provide useful visualization because of obstructed views, a cluttered environment, and lack of proper depth perception. Segmentation is the process of partitioning an image into various parts (or segments) in order to simplify visualization of the image. Segmentation of volumetric images can provide valuable information that cannot be easily captured by looking at nonsegmented images; it naturally involves modifying the raw image data.

Segmentation of volumetric images can be challenging, depending on the modality, the anatomy of interest, and the quality of the images. In some cases, segmentation can be done automatically using computer-assisted techniques such as automatic segmentation of bones based on Hounsfield units in CT images, as in Fig. 6.15. This figure shows examples of segmentation on a cadaver skull. The segmented images of the bones and carotid arteries provide completely different information that is not directly visible in the simple volume-rendered image. In some cases, algorithms are initialized manually as image processing software is used to perform the segmentation. The results are then refined by manual input from an expert user. A wide range of algorithms, from those used in conventional computer vision to advanced machine learning techniques, can be utilized to perform image segmentation.

Commercial medical image segmentation services are also available, in which a preoperative image set is uploaded and segmented by a group of experts using computer-assisted techniques; the results are provided in formats that can be used for visualization and planning purposes [22]. Small studies have demonstrated the potential of volumetric data to speed up surgical procedures [23], but caution must be taken when relying on these images for guidance, as other studies have shown the quality of the rendered volumes to be highly dependent on the person performing the segmentation [24].

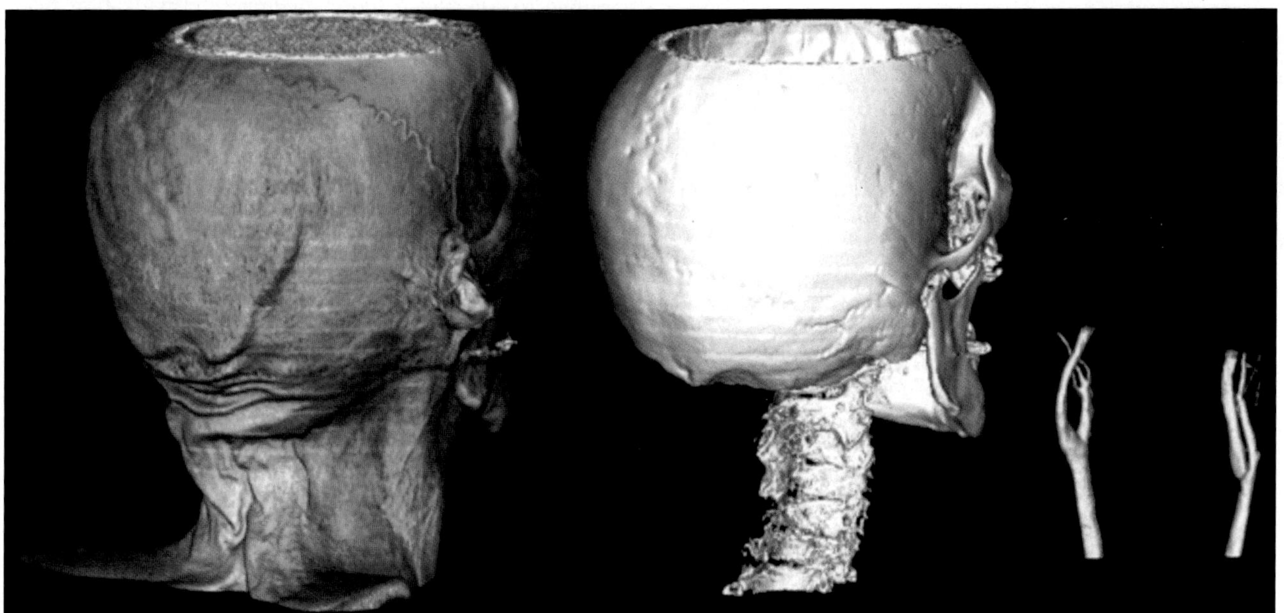

Fig. 6.15 Volume rendering of a CT image of a cadaver skull (*left*); segmented images of bones (*middle*) and carotid arteries (*right*). (Image provided by Intuitive Surgical)

Visualization

When a relatively accurate registration between tomographic and endoscopic images is possible, it might be helpful to use augmented reality techniques to provide a more integrated display of the information. Figure 6.16 shows an overlay of a rendered segmented CT angiogram over a gray-scale endoscopic image. The overlay is used as a guide to identify the correct renal artery, in order to clamp it before performing a partial nephrectomy.

Another example of visualization is shown in Fig. 6.17, in which intraoperative ultrasound images are blended with endoscopic images. This technique provides an easier interpretation of the ultrasound images and their geometric correlation with the current endoscopic view and solves the hand-eye coordination issue when looking at images.

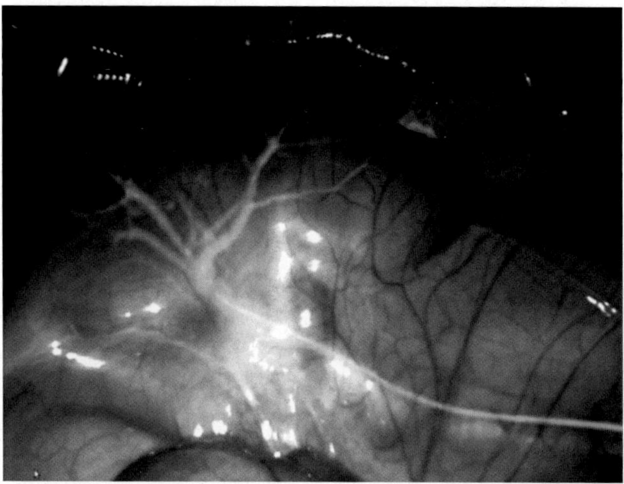

Fig. 6.16 Overlay of a segmented CT angiogram of the kidney on the endoscopic images of a da Vinci® Xi system in a partial nephrectomy case. (Image provided by Intuitive Surgical)

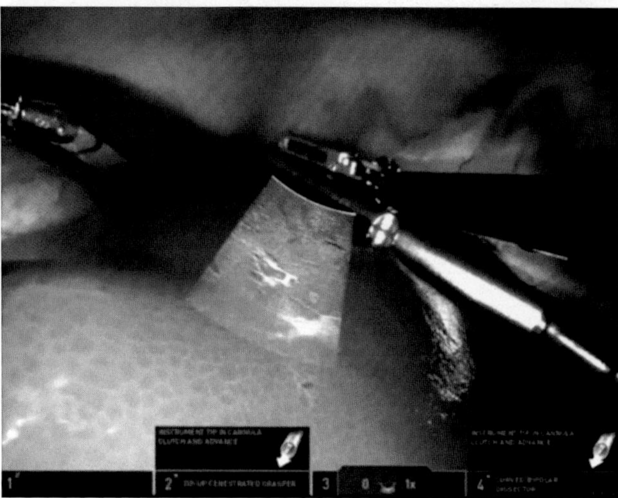

Fig. 6.17 Live ultrasound overlay on endoscopic images during liver surgery. Doppler ultrasound is used to highlight blood flow, as can be seen in this image

Conclusion

Optical endoscopy techniques used in robotic surgery are usually real-time and often benefit from an inherent co-registration with the surgeon's field of view. An example is the da Vinci® Firefly® system, which provides fluorescence information overlaid on top of endoscopic images. This technique typically is made possible by using collocated detectors for capturing white light and other optical images. On the other hand, limited penetration depth is the major drawback with optical endoscopic images.

The use of tomographic images during surgery is similar to using a map while navigating through the wilderness. Although it is possible to navigate without a map, it is often more convenient to use one. Proper registration provides GPS functionality to this map, and segmentation provides highlighted areas of interest while hiding the clutter. Tomographic images have been used for image-guided surgery by a number of research groups and also have been used in a number of commercial products [25]. Robotic surgery makes the integration of tomographic imaging more streamlined, because robotic arms often act as digitizers; their position and orientation can be tracked at high rates, which can facilitate the registration process. In addition, robotic surgical systems often provide more stable vision and a more integrated visualization platform, making it more convenient to use more advanced visualization techniques, including those in virtual reality systems. Despite all the benefits provided by tomographic imaging modalities, registration to the surgeon's field of view remains the major drawback for using tomographic imaging in robotic surgery.

References

1. Visualization (graphics). Wikipedia, The Free Encyclopedia. https://en.wikipedia.org/w/index.php?title=Visualization_(graphics)&oldid=739661476. Accessed 16 Sept 2016.
2. Kwoh YS, Hou J, Jonckheere EA, Hayati S. A robot with improved absolute positioning accuracy for CT guided stereotactic brain surgery. IEEE Trans Biomed Eng. 1988;35:153–60.
3. RAMS: Robot assisted microsurgery. NASA JPL, NASA Office of Aeronautics and Space Technology (Code R); Project completed 1997.
4. Saraf S. Robotic assisted microsurgery (RAMS): application in plastic surgery. In: Bozovic V, editor. Medical robotics. Rijeka: InTech; 2008. ISBN: 978-3-902613-18-9.
5. Takahashi S, Uehara M, Kato S, Kidawara A, Saito K, Goto M, et al., Inventors; Olympus Optical, assignee. Stereoscopic endoscope. US Patent 5 588 948, 24 Feb 1998.
6. Hopf NJ, Kurucz P, Reisch R. Three-dimensional HD endoscopy—first experiences with the Einstein Vision system in neurosurgery. Innovative Neurosurg. 2013;1:125–31.
7. Banks MS, Read JC, Allison RS, Watt SJ. Stereoscopy and the human visual system. SMPTE Motion Imaging J. 2012;121:24–43.
8. Spinoglio G, Priora F, Bianchi PP, Lucido FS, Licciardello A, Maglione V, et al. Real-time near-infrared fluorescent cholangiography in single-site robotic cholecystectomy: a single-institutional prospective study. Surg Endosc. 2013;27:2156–62.

9. Rossi EC, Ivanova A, Boggess JF. Robotically assisted fluorescence-guided lymph node mapping with ICG for gynecologic malignancies: a feasibility study. Gynecol Oncol. 2012;124:78–82.
10. Sorger J. Clinical milestones in optical imaging. In: Fong Y, Giulianotti PC, Lewis J, Koerkamp BG, Reiner T, editors. Imaging and visualization in the modern operating room: a comprehensive guide for physicians. New York: Springer; 2015. p. 133–43.
11. Rosenthal EL, Warram JM, de Boer E, Chung TK, Korb ML, Brandwein-Gensler M, et al. Safety and tumor specificity of cetuximab-IRDye800 for surgical navigation in head and neck cancer. Clin Cancer Res. 2015;21:3658–66.
12. Vicini C, Montevecchi F, D'Agostino G, De Vito A, Meccariello G. A novel approach emphasising intra-operative superficial margin enhancement of head-neck tumours with narrow-band imaging in transoral robotic surgery. Acta Otorhinolaryngol Ital. 2015;35:157–61.
13. Zheng C, Lu Y, Zhong Q, Wang R, Jiang Q. Narrow band imaging diagnosis of bladder cancer: systematic review and meta-analysis. BJU Int. 2012;110:E680–7.
14. Tateya I, Ishikawa S, Morita S, Ito H, Sakamoto T, Murayama T, et al. Magnifying endoscopy with narrow band imaging to determine the extent of resection in transoral robotic surgery of oropharyngeal cancer. Case Rep Otolaryngol. 2014;2014:604737.
15. Hughes M, Yang GZ. High speed, line-scanning, fiber bundle fluorescence confocal endomicroscopy for improved mosaicking. Biomed Opt Express. 2015;6:1241–52.
16. Clancy NT, Arya S, Qi J, Stoyanov D, Hanna GB, Elson DS. Polarised stereo endoscope and narrowband detection for minimal access surgery. Biomed Opt Express. 2014;5:4108–17.
17. Hellan M, Spinoglio G, Pigazzi A, Lagares-Garcia JA. The influence of fluorescence imaging on the location of bowel transection during robotic left-sided colorectal surgery. Surg Endosc. 2014;28:1695–702.
18. Herrell SD, Kwartowitz DM, Milhoua PM, Galloway RL. Toward image guided robotic surgery: system validation. J Urol. 2009;181:783–9. discussion 789–90
19. Nakamura N, Sugano N, Nishii T, Miki H, Kakimoto A, Yamamura M. Robot-assisted primary cementless total hip arthroplasty using surface registration techniques: a short-term clinical report. Int J Comput Assist Radiol Surg. 2009;4:157–62.
20. Mountney P, Fallert J, Nicolau S, Soler L, Mewes PW. An augmented reality framework for soft tissue surgery. Med Image Comput Comput Assist Interv. 2014;17:423–31.
21. Hu X, Scharschmidt TJ, Ohnmeiss DD, Lieberman IH. Robotic assisted surgeries for the treatment of spine tumors. Int J Spine Surg. 2015;9. https://doi.org/10.14444/2001.
22. Visible patient. https://www.visiblepatient.com/en/service. Accessed 11 Oct 2015.
23. Velayutham V, Fuks D, Nomi T, Kawaguchi Y, Gayet B. 3D visualization reduces operating time when compared to high-definition 2D in laparoscopic liver resection: a case-matched study. Surg Endosc. 2016;30(1):147–53.
24. Hughes-Hallett A, Pratt P, Mayer E, Clark M, Vale J, Darzi A. Using preoperative imaging for intraoperative guidance: a case of mistaken identity. Int J Med Robot. 2016;12(2):262–7.
25. Peters T, Cleary K, editors. Image-guided interventions: technology and applications. New York: Springer; 2008.

7 Workflow in Robotic Surgery

Olivia R. Enright and Michael G. Patane

The introduction of a robotic system into the operating room (OR) creates the need for an organized workflow. This chapter discusses the workflow in robotic surgery, including room setup, positioning, room flow, staffing, and instrumentation. A case workflow checklist (Table 7.1) outlines all the major steps to promote a seamless operation.

Room Setup

Workflow in robotic surgery begins with the initial preparations in the OR even before the patient is brought to the room. The nursing staff will prepare the sterile table with all the necessary equipment for each specialized case. When beginning robotic cases, it is very important to have all of the correct equipment ready and in the correct place so that the least amount of time is wasted in the operating room. To ensure that the case is able to begin promptly and continue through its various steps in a timely manner, the setup of the room is very important. Before the patient enters the room, the OR bed must be placed in the position that is best suited for the anesthesia team to be able to intubate safely and efficiently.

Positioning

To lessen downtime, the operating room team should place various padding and/or instrumentation on the bed before the patient enters. Efficacy requires communicating the decision about patient positioning during the case, which will determine what is placed on the bed. A preoperative huddle of the entire team allows these informations to be communicated. Antislip devices can be placed on the bed at this time, and any needed bed add-ons can be procured, such as stirrups, spreader bars, bed extensions, arm sleds, gel rolls/pads, tape, and gauze bandage rolls. The goal at this time is to have all equipment either in place or available for immediate use. Also at this time, any needed specific medications for the robotic procedure should be obtained or ordered, such as

Table 7.1 Case workflow checklist

- Room setup
  - OR table set up with padding if necessary, or other padding and tape available
  - Stirrups, spreader bars, bumps, pillows, arm extenders set up as necessary
  - Draping robot and having OR table set up with necessary robotic instruments as well as laparoscopic instruments
- Port placement
  - The surgeon discusses with the surgical team the best possible port placement for initial access and insufflation
  - The surgical team inserts remaining ports to best access the target anatomy
- Docking
  - Communication from the bedside to the circulating nurse to direct the robot/patient cart next to the operating table to avoid injury to the patient
  - Bedside assistant will guide the robotic arms and dock them to avoid collisions externally and internally and to provide clearance from the patient while also allowing significant range of motion
- Procedure
  - Communication between the surgeon in the console and the bedside assistant is critical
  - Instruments can be changed, the camera inserted and removed to be cleaned; retraction as directed by the surgeon; and irrigation and suctioning
- Undocking
  - The surgeon announces the end of the robotic portion of the operation
  - Instruments can be removed, but it is critical to make sure that all the instruments are in clear view and not holding any tissues prior to removing them
  - Once the instruments are removed and the robotic arms are undocked from the ports, the robot/patient cart can be safely guided away from the OR table

O. R. Enright, MSPA-C
Memorial Sloan Kettering Cancer Center, New York, NY, USA
e-mail: enrighto@mskcc.org

M. G. Patane, MSPA-C (✉)
Department of Surgery, Memorial Sloan Kettering Cancer Center, New York, NY, USA
e-mail: patanem@mskcc.org

Y. Fong et al. (eds.), *The SAGES Atlas of Robotic Surgery*, https://doi.org/10.1007/978-3-319-91045-1_7

indocyanine green (ICG) for any fluorescence imaging during the robotic case.

Room Flow

Once the patient is positioned safely and securely on the OR bed and has been intubated, the OR bed should be moved and positioned to provide optimal spacing. This spacing should take into consideration the position and angle of the robot as it relates to the patient, the bed, and the target anatomy. In addition, the position of the OR bed should also allow space for both the instrument table and the bedside assistant.

After the OR bed is positioned correctly, the patient may then be prepped and draped. At this time, attention should focus on securing and positioning of the various cords, tubes, and cables to be used during the case. These include, but are not limited to, insufflation tubing, smoke evacuation tubing, suction/irrigation tubing, cautery cords, and any laparoscopic or robotic instruments with cords. These should all be secured in a way that does not limit the ability of the bedside assistant to adequately access the patient. It is important to ensure that not too much or too little cord is kept on the sterile field. Too much cord can lead to tangling, but too little cord can prevent instruments from being used, as not enough length is available to reach target anatomy.

Staffing

In general, a robotic team will be assigned to the room designated for robotic cases. This team will consist of a circulating nurse, a scrub nurse or scrub tech, an anesthesiologist, a physician assistant, a surgical fellow and/or resident, and the attending surgeon. Obviously there will be some variations in staffing, but ideally there should be staff that is already trained in robotic surgery to facilitate the best outcomes. It is also recommended to have specialized technical support present during robotic cases to make sure the system is working smoothly and to troubleshoot should there be any system errors or instrument malfunctions.

Communication is one of the most important and critical tools in robotic surgery. The operating surgeon is no longer at the bedside and now relies on the assistant at the bedside to clearly communicate and guide the surgeon to protect the patient. The anesthesia team also must clearly communicate with the surgical team to ensure that the robot is not hitting the patient, or the insufflation is not poorly affecting the patient. The nursing staff will make sure that all necessary equipment is available. The physician assistant helps set up the room to facilitate a seamless operation. The entire team can use the checklist (see Table 7.1) to confirm that all necessary steps are completed to ensure patient safety and a successful operation.

Instrumentation

This section focuses on instrumentation as a whole, fully acknowledging that most surgeons will prefer specific equipment and tools that are required for specific procedures. Some instruments should not be opened until the surgeon confirms the need for them, as they are costly—especially the single-use instruments like the vessel sealer. When starting a robotic case, the first instruments used are for entering the target anatomic cavity to provide insufflation or access; the technique can vary among needle insufflation, cutdown entry, or other various modes. The next step is to have the camera ready, with the availability of either hot water or another warming method to ensure that once the camera is placed in the target anatomic cavity, fogging of the lens is kept to a minimum.

Once ports are placed, traditional laparoscopic equipment is also needed, usually on a per-case basis. Adhesions, for instance, would require a form of grasper and an instrument for cutting and cautery. During the robotic portion of the case itself, each surgeon and procedure will require specific instrumentation. There should be special attention to any extra equipment needed in addition to robotic instrumentation. Ultrasound, stapling, handheld cautery, and other ancillary tools should be easily accessible to ensure availability for the entirety of the case.

In all cases, an open conversion tray should be available. This should be confirmed during the "robotic emergency conversion time-out," a time during the "time-out" for the case when the OR team should go over what each member is responsible for in the event of an emergency conversion due to either hemorrhage or airway emergency (in transoral robotic surgery). Each member of the team should be aware of his or her role and what is required to be able to fulfill that role. An emergency conversion tray should always be available, containing the necessary equipment and tools to convert to an open procedure in a timely manner, should the situation warrant it (Tables 7.2 and 7.3).

Table 7.2 Emergent conversion from robotic to open procedure

Who	What
Attending surgeon	1. Call for emergent conversion to open procedure, *designate person in charge of maintaining tamponade*.
Circulating RN	2. Push code "blue" button or call central desk. Turn on OR lights. 3. Open robotic emergency tray. 4. Notify all available service attendings for additional help.
Anesthesia team	5. Notify anesthesia attending via Vocera/paging. 6. Initiate IV fluid resuscitation. Confirm adequacy of IV access. 7. Request blood products. *Request confirmation when sent*.
Bedside assistant	8. Maintain tamponade; may initiate removal of some robotic instruments at the direction of attending surgeon. 9. Undock robot at the direction of the attending surgeon.
Attending surgeon	10. Direct bedside assist to undock robot when appropriate. 11. Proceed to open.

Table 7.3 Head and neck robotic emergency

Who	What
Attending surgeon	*Airway*—Call for emergent tracheostomy *Bleeding*—Designate person in charge of maintaining tamponade Call for assistance from another attending surgeon if indicated
Circulating RN	*Airway*—Open tracheostomy tray *Bleeding*—Open Head and Neck dissecting tray (if necessary)
Anesthesia team	Notify Anesthesia attending via Vocera/paging *Airway*—Communicate with surgeon to maintain secure airway and decide on tracheostomy if indicated *Bleeding*—Initiate IV fluid resuscitation. Confirm adequacy of IV access. Request blood products
Bedside assistant	*Airway*—Ensure correct position of endotracheal tube at all times *Bleeding*—Local tamponade with packing under direction of operating surgeon May initiate removal of robotic instruments at the direction of the attending surgeon
Attending surgeon	Direct Bedside assist to remove robot arms when appropriate and proceed to open if necessary

Suggested Reading

Ahmad N, Hussein AA, Cavuoto L, Sharif M, Allers JC, Hinata N, et al. Ambulatory movements, team dynamics and interactions during robot-assisted surgery. BJU Int. 2016;118(1):132–9.

Ballantyne GH. Robotic surgery, telerobotic surgery, telepresence, and telementoring. Review of early clinical results Surg Endosc. 2002;16(10):1389–402.

Catchpole K, Perkins C, Bresee C, Solnik MJ, Sherman B, Fritch J, et al. Safety, efficiency and learning curves in robotic surgery: a human factors analysis. Surg Endosc. 2016;30(9):3749–61.

Fong Y, Woo Y, Giulianotti PC. Robotic surgery: the promise and finally the progress. Hepatobiliary Surg Nutr. 2017;6(4):219–21.

Kassahun Y, Yu B, Tibebu AT, Stoyanov D, Giannarou S, Metzen JH, et al. Surgical robotics beyond enhanced dexterity instrumentation: a survey of machine learning techniques and their role in intelligent and autonomous surgical actions. Int J Comput Assist Radiol Surg. 2016;11(4):553–68.

Leung U, Fong Y. Robotic liver surgery. Hepatobiliary Surg Nutr. 2014;3(5):288–94.

Mantoo S, Rigaud J, Naulet S, Lehur PA, Meurette G. Standardized surgical technique and dedicated operating room environment can reduce the operative time during robotic-assisted surgery for pelvic floor disorders. J Robot Surg. 2014;8(1):7–12.

Nota CL, Rinkes IHB, Hagendoorn J. Setting up a robotic hepatectomy program: a Western-European experience and perspective. Hepatobiliary Surg Nutr. 2017;6(4):239–45.

Patti JC, Ore AS, Barrows C, Velanovich V, Moser AJ. Value-based assessment of robotic pancreas and liver surgery. Hepatobiliary Surg Nutr. 2017;6(4):246–57.

Randell R, Greenhalgh J, Hindmarsh J, Dowding D, Jayne D, Pearman A, et al. Integration of robotic surgery into routine practice and impacts on communication, collaboration, and decision making: a realist process evaluation protocol. Implement Sci. 2014;9:52.

Yuh B. The bedside assistant in robotic surgery—keys to success. Urol Nurs. 2013;33(1):29–32.

Anesthetic Implications of Robotic Surgery: Positioning and Access

8

John L. Raytis, Yuman Fong, and Michael W. Lew

Introduction

Robot-assisted surgery has many implications for the anesthesiologist. In addition to well-described implications—such as the changes in patient hemodynamics and ventilation seen with the combination of pneumoperitoneum and Trendelenburg (or reverse Trendelenburg) position used in robotic surgery—the size, the shape, and orientation of robotic surgical equipment also have implications for the anesthesiologist. For example, in order to dock the robotic surgical system, the head of the patient is often rotated away from proximity to the anesthesiologist. This affects the position of other equipment in the operating room, reduces access to the patient's airway, and affects the use of monitoring cables and arterial, central, and intravenous lines. There is an added layer of complexity when converting from a robotic to an open procedure, in which case the orientation of the operating room table must be turned from the robotic positioning to the standard position in order to make optimal use of fixed lighting designed for open surgery. Also, an emergency plan must be in place, and all operating personnel need to be aware of how to quickly undock the robot and turn the patient should conversion to open surgery become urgent or should the administration of emergency therapy such as electronic pacing or defibrillation become necessary. In this chapter, we will summarize the most important anesthetic issues seen with robotic surgery (Table 8.1) and offer some recommendations for operating room practice in order to prevent possible complications associated with robotic surgery (Table 8.2) [1–3].

Table 8.1 Issues for the anesthesiologist for various procedures

	Category	Description	Issues	Prevention/management
Pelvic procedures (prostatectomy, gynecologic oncology, rectal surgery)	Positioning	Steep Trendelenburg	• Compromised blood return • Compromised ventilation • Slippage and nerve injury • Corneal abrasion	• Hydration • Increased inspired O_2 • Padding of pressure points • Nonslip pads • Checking position • Eye protection
Upper oral/GI/thoracic surgery (gastrectomy, esophagectomy, pneumonectomy, TORS)	Restricted access	Difficulty in emergency	• Access to airway • Access for defibrillation • Difficulty converting	• Preparation with placement of all necessary access • Short access line for emergency medications • Rehearse undocking and converting
All	Hypothermia	Long procedures	• Use of cold fluids • Use of cold gases	• Temperature monitoring • Warmers • Use warmed fluids and gases
All	Pneumoperitoneum	Prolonged insufflation	• Atelectasis • Gas embolism • Ventilator difficulties	• Monitoring • Pressure control mode of ventilation • CPAP or BiPAP post-op

J. L. Raytis, MD · M. W. Lew, MD
Department of Anesthesiology, City of Hope National Medical Center, Duarte, CA, USA
e-mail: jraytis@coh.org; mlew@coh.org

Y. Fong, MD (✉)
Department of Surgery, City of Hope National Medical Center, Duarte, CA, USA
e-mail: yfong@coh.org

Y. Fong et al. (eds.), *The SAGES Atlas of Robotic Surgery*, https://doi.org/10.1007/978-3-319-91045-1_8

Table 8.2 Some complications specifically associated with robotic surgery

1.	Upper body edema
2.	Postoperative visual loss
3.	Nerve injury
4.	Soft tissue injury
5.	Compartment syndrome
6.	Pneumothorax
7.	Pneumomediastinum
8.	Air embolism
9.	Deep venous thrombosis
10.	Hypothermia
11.	Renal failure

Anesthesia Issues for Robotic Surgery in General

Risks of Prolonged CO_2 Insufflation

- Respiratory compromise particularly in patients with COPD
- Decreased lung compliance
- Respiratory acidosis

Cardiopulmonary Risks

- Atelectasis
- Ventilation/Perfusion Mismatch

Hyperventilation and use of positive end-expiratory pressure (PEEP) is often combined to prevent the above cardiopulmonary issues. Vigilance for these complications and making sure both end-tidal CO_2 and CO_2 in blood gas have returned to normal prior to extubation are additional means of ensuring smooth recovery.

There is no data suggesting superiority of total intravenous anesthesia over inhalational anesthesia [4].

Anesthetic Issues Arising from Robotic Positioning

A wide variety of surgical procedures—urologic, gynecologic, hepatobiliary, colorectal, otolaryngologic, thoracic, and cardiothoracic—can be performed robotically. It is important to recognize the positioning requirements of different surgical procedures and of varying robotic systems.

da Vinci Si System

An important characteristic of the da Vinci Si system is that the robotic arms on the patient side unit do not rotate relative to the base of the unit. This fact leads to the requirement of turning the patient relative to the anesthesiologist in order to orient the robotic arms in the correct position above the patient.

Position for Pelvic Procedures (Including Prostatectomy and Rectal and Gynecological Procedures)

For robotic prostatectomy with the da Vinci Si system, the patient is typically turned 45 degrees from the standard position and placed in steep Trendelenburg position (Fig. 8.1). Typically, the anesthesia machine does not need to be moved. As the patient's face and airway are rotated away from the anesthesiologist, care must be taken to ensure that the face and eyes are protected and that the airway tubing is not kinked or stretched. Intravenous and arterial lines as well as monitoring cables must be long enough to accommodate this turn. The patient also must be monitored for unintended contact with the robotic surgical arms (Table 8.3).

The steep Trendelenburg position can restrict respiration. In addition, prolonged procedures in this position can produce facial, pharyngeal, or laryngeal edema. These changes can, in turn, compromise respiration after extubation. Many would thus recommend minimizing fluids during the procedure [5]. Resuscitation after surgery is imperative to prevent compromise of renal function.

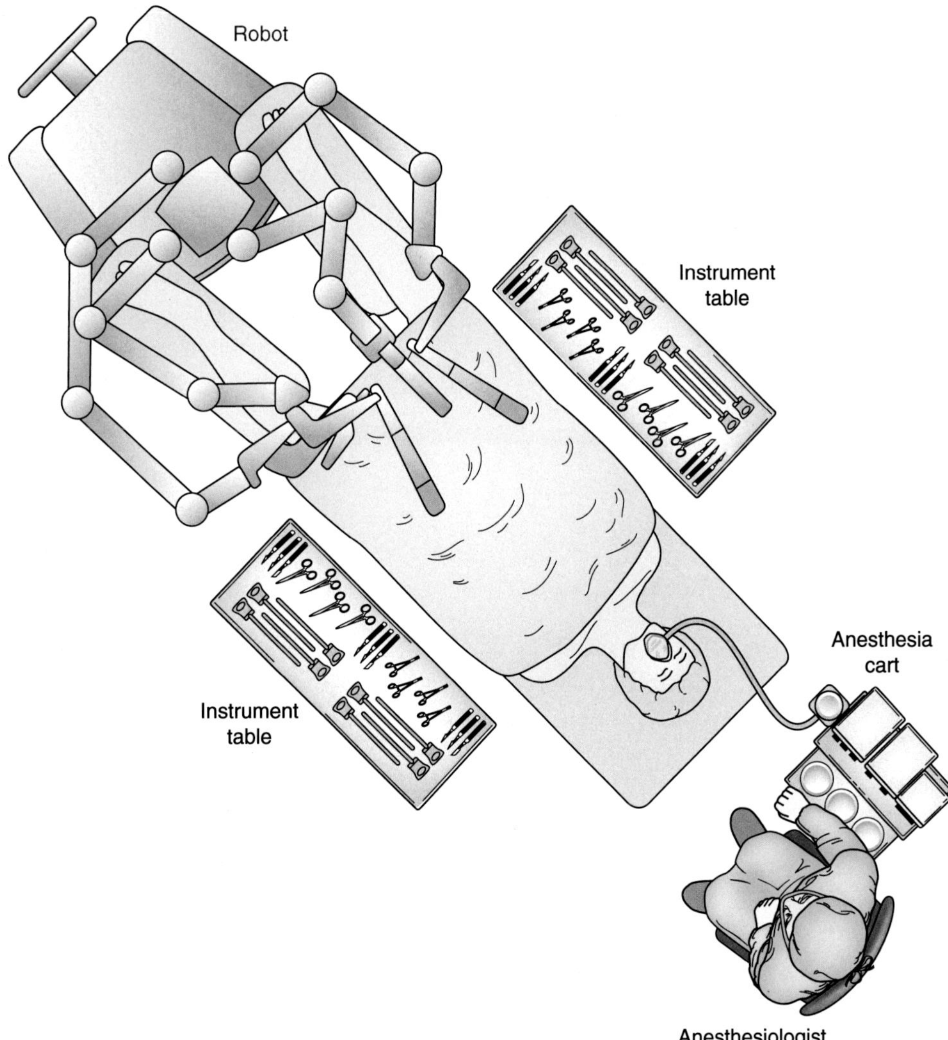

Fig. 8.1 Typical position for using Si robot for pelvic procedures such as for prostatectomy. Patient is in steep Trendelenburg

Table 8.3 Important steps to ensure favorable outcome

1. Check anesthesia tubing to ensure no kinking
2. Make sure there is adequate vascular access prior to docking
3. Protect eyes
4. Make sure all stress points are padded
5. Make sure patient is secured to prevent slippage
6. Check for clearance of all arms from patient
7. Minimize fluids during procedures in steep Trendelenburg position
8. Resuscitate as soon as possible to prevent renal injury

Monitoring urine output may be difficult due to the position compromising flow into a Foley, as well as spillage of urine when the bladder, or urethra, is open.

The steep position can also lead to slippage of the patient and stress placed on nerves or vessels. Prolonged stress on these can cause postoperative motor or sensory nerve dysfunction. Pressure on the vessels can cause muscle necrosis, swelling, and compartment syndrome [6].

Alternative Position for Robotic Gynecological Surgery

Implications for robotic gynecological surgery with the da Vinci Si are similar to those of the prostatectomy. Often, the patient is not turned relative to the anesthesiologist, and the patient side unit of the robot is brought in at an angle to the operating room table (Fig. 8.2) [7]. This allows the gynecologic surgeon to maintain access to the perineum.

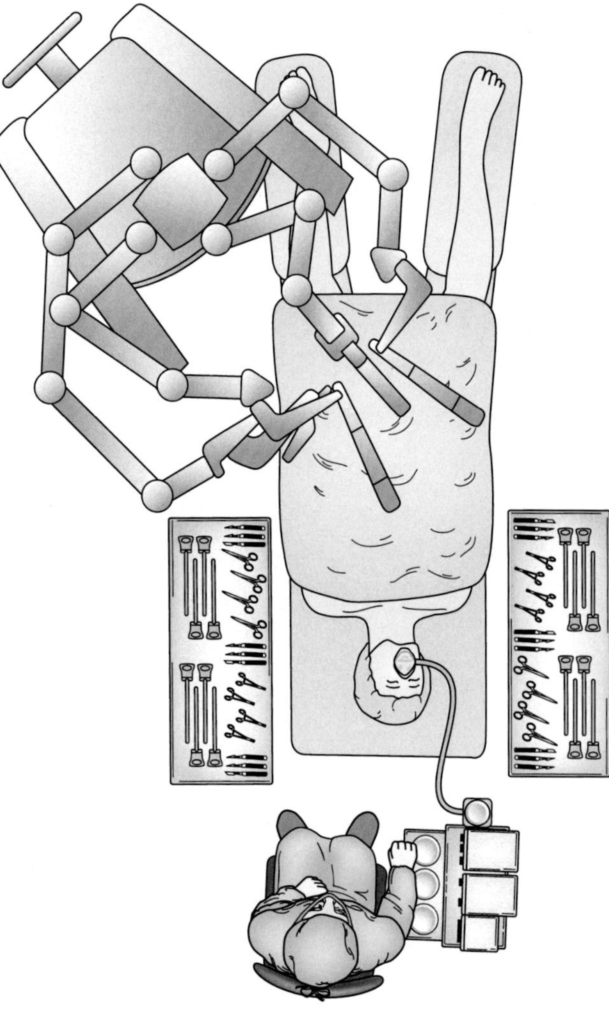

Fig. 8.2 Alternative position for gynecologic or rectal procedure. Angled docking of the robot allows vaginal and anal access

Lateral Positions for Robotic Surgery (Including Nephrectomy, Pulmonary Resections, Lateral Liver Procedures, and Distal Pancreatic Procedures)

The anesthetic implications for robotic nephrectomy or pulmonary resections using the da Vinci Si system are similar to those for the prostatectomy. There are several exceptions. Airway access is further reduced as the patient is farther from the anesthesiologist, and there are often surgical equipment and personnel between the anesthesiologist and the patient. In addition, the operating table is flexed rather than placed into Trendelenburg position (Fig. 8.3). Also, all lines, monitoring cables, and the airway circuit need to run to the patient together to allow for access of surgical personnel between the anesthesiologist and patient.

The positioning places nerves in the axilla at risk, as well as the arms. An axillary roll is helpful in preventing pressure injury to the axillary nerves. The arms will have to be positioned to allow no stress on the shoulder and to prevent inadvertent collision of the robotic arms with the patient's arms.

A foot board will help prevent the patient from accidentally slipping when placed in reverse Trendelenburg. This lateral position with the robotic arms directly over the chest greatly restricts access for chest compressions or cardioversion. Thus, rehearsals to ensure the team is capable of rapid undocking, rotation of patient, and conversion to open procedure are important (see Chap. 9).

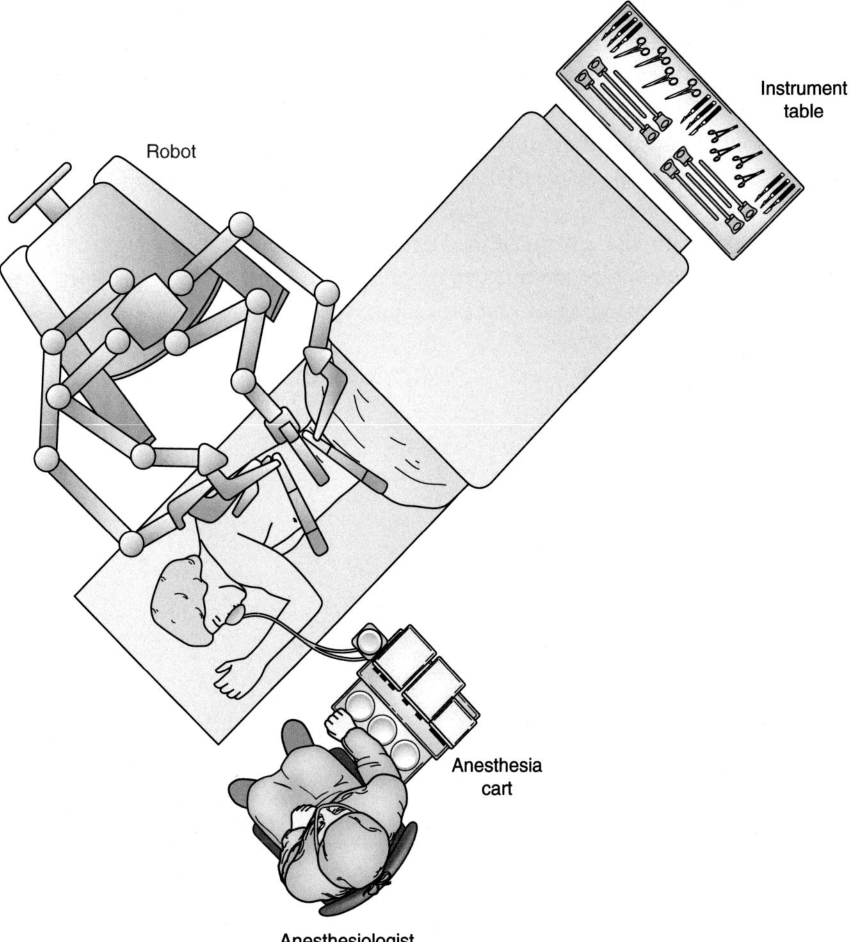

Fig. 8.3 Lateral position for nephrectomy, for thoracic procedures, for lateral liver procedures, or for distal pancreatic procedures

Position for Upper Abdominal Robotic Surgery (Hepatobiliary, Gastric, or Anterior Thoracic Surgery)

The position for hepatobiliary and thoracic surgery using the da Vinci Si includes the patient's head being rotated 135° away from the anesthesiologist (Fig. 8.4). As the patient's head is underneath the robotic arms, airway access and access to the patient's face are reduced more than for other procedures. Also, depending on the procedure, the patient may be placed in the Trendelenburg or reverse Trendelenburg positions. The anesthesia machine often needs to be moved to ensure that the airway circuit and monitoring cables reach the patient, and extensions to intravenous lines and central lines are usually needed.

The most important difference for this position is that the head and airway of the patient is completely removed from control of the anesthesiologist. Protecting the face and eyes is essential. Making sure the airway is secure is imperative.

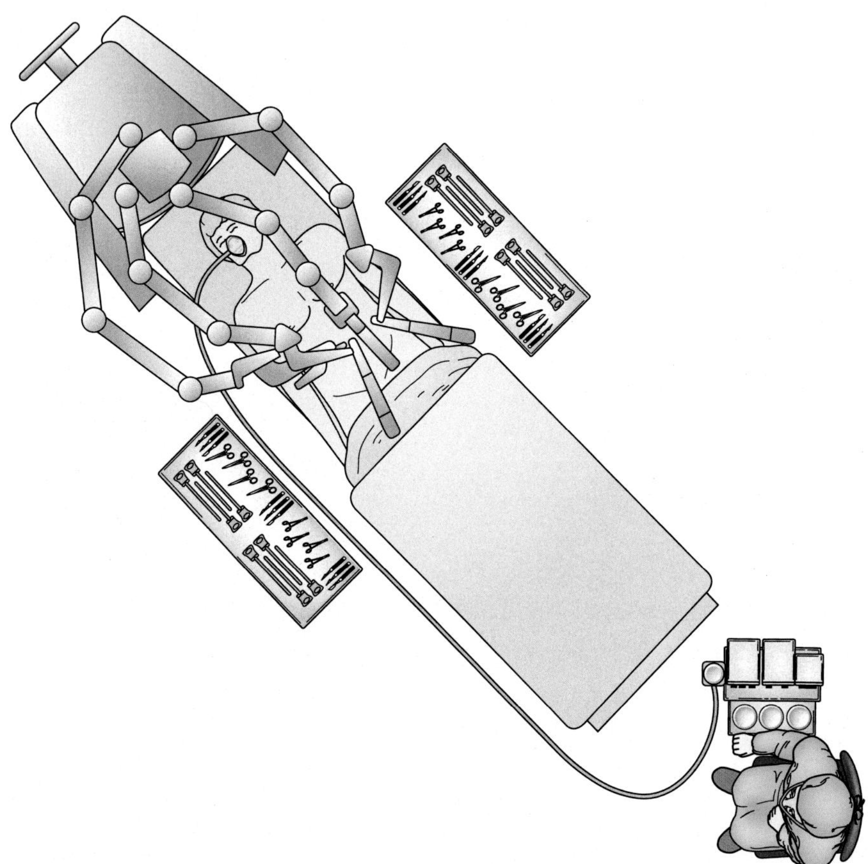

Fig. 8.4 Typical position for upper abdominal procedures. Note that access to the head or the airway is compromised

Position for Procedures with the da Vinci Xi Surgical System

One notable difference between the da Vinci Si and Xi surgical systems is that the robotic arms on the patient's side of the Xi system rotate relative to the base of the unit [8]. As a result, most of the above procedures can be performed without turning the patient relative to the anesthesiologist (Fig. 8.5). Airway access is similar to a standard laparoscopic procedure, and extensions to monitoring cables, the airway circuit, and intravenous and arterial lines are generally not required. Depending on the procedure, the patient may be in the supine or lateral positions, and the operating room table may be flexed or placed into the Trendelenburg or reverse Trendelenburg orientations. Due to the larger footprint size of the patient-side unit of the Xi robot (1.46 m^2) compared to the S and Si robots (1.15 m^2), and due to the physical position of the Xi robot relative to the patient, access to the patient's arm and to any line or monitor placed on the arm ipsilateral to the patient-side unit of the Xi robot is reduced relative to such access with da Vinci S and Si systems.

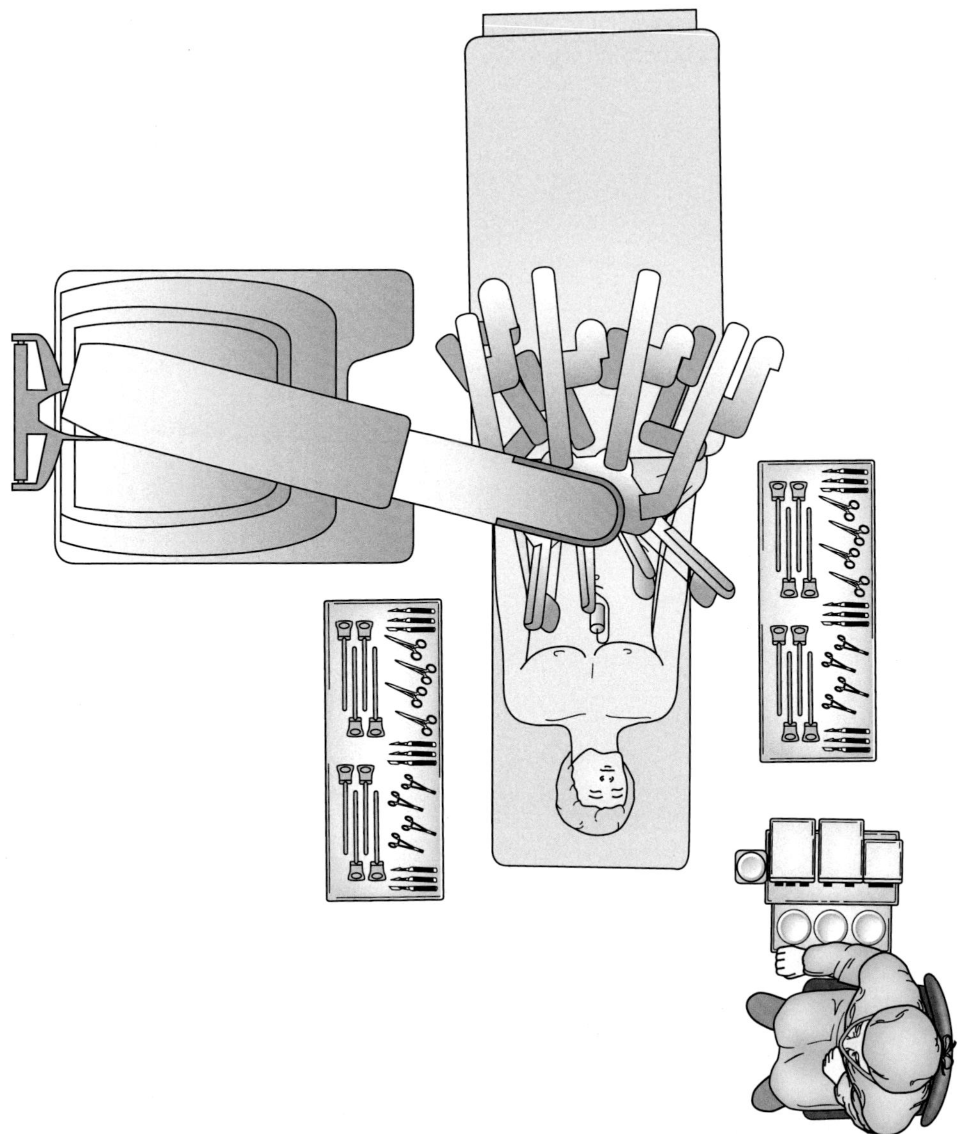

Fig. 8.5 Most procedures with the Xi can have the head and airway of the patient under complete control of the anesthesiologist

Communications and Patient Access for Robotic Surgery

As described above, access to the patient's airway and intravenous and arterial line sites are affected by the use of a robotic surgical system. In addition, it is important to recognize that access to the surgical site itself and sites for emergency therapy such as cardioversion or defibrillation are affected as well. It is essential that communication occur between the anesthesiologist, surgeon, and operating room personnel and that prior to incision, a plan is in place for undocking the robot and turning the operating room table, should urgent conversion to an open procedure or administration of emergency therapy become necessary.

References

1. Awad H, Walker CM, Shaikh M, Dimitrova GT, Abaza R, O'Hara J. Anesthetic considerations for robotic prostatectomy: a review of the literature. J Clin Anesth. 2012;24(6):494–504.
2. Arunkumar R, Rebello E, Owusu-Agyemang P. Anaesthetic techniques for unique cancer surgery procedures. Best Pract Res Clin Anaesthesiol. 2013;27(4):513–26.
3. Campos J, Ueda K. Update on anesthetic complications of robotic thoracic surgery. Minerva Anestesiol. 2014;80(1):83–8.
4. Herling SF, Dreijer B, Wrist Lam G, Thomsen T, Moller AM. Total intravenous anaesthesia versus inhalational anaesthesia for adults undergoing transabdominal robotic assisted laparoscopic surgery. Cochrane Database Syst Rev. 2017;4:CD011387.
5. Hsu RL, Kaye AD, Urman RD. Anesthetic challenges in robotic-assisted urologic surgery. Rev Urol. 2013;15(4):178–84.
6. Lee JR. Anesthetic considerations for robotic surgery. Korean J Anesthesiol. 2014;66(1):3–11.
7. Kaye AD, Vadivelu N, Ahuja N, Mitra S, Silasi D, Urman RD. Anesthetic considerations in robotic-assisted gynecologic surgery. Ochsner J. 2013;13(4):517–24.
8. Yuh B, Yu X, Raytis J, Lew M, Fong Y, Lau C. Use of a mobile tower-based robot—the initial Xi robot experience in surgical oncology. J Surg Oncol. 2016;113(1):5–7.

Urgent and Emergent Conversions in Robotic Surgery

9

Abigail J. B. Fong and Yuman Fong

Introduction

Robotically-assisted operations are now commonplace at many hospitals. Recent development of new instrumentation for robotic surgery and increasing expertise at many centers now allow the most intricate of operations to be accomplished by robotically assisted techniques. Esophagectomies, low anterior resections, hepatectomies, pancreaticoduodenectomies, and pneumonectomies are just some of the major operations routinely performed at specialty centers by robotically assisted techniques [1].

The dexterity of the fine-controlled, wristed instruments and the superior visibility afforded by binocular vision offer the possibility of a facile minimally invasive surgery approach for advanced procedures as never before, but the large robot that towers over the patient and the lack of a large incision produce obstacles to the control and repair of major injuries. Consequently, reports are mounting of rare but catastrophic results in some emergency situations. The limited access to the patient could delay the start of effective treatment of a life-threatening emergency, with possible fatal outcome [2]. As the use of robotic systems has increased, the number of patients undergoing robotically assisted surgery with severe comorbidities and the risk of critical incidents during surgery have increased as well [3–5].

This chapter presents examples of some of the urgent and emergent situations that require undocking of the robot and/or conversion from robotically assisted to open operation. We offer a plan to prepare, rehearse, simulate, and execute conversions, which can guide salvage efforts in these situations. Planning rescue strategies is an essential part of planning for any major operation. In robotically assisted surgery, it is essential that all team members in the room are part of the planning and execution of such a rescue strategy, in order to maximize team readiness to act and, more importantly, to maximize patient outcomes.

Emergent, Urgent, and Elective Conversion to Open Operation

Situations may arise during a robotically assisted procedure that requires urgent or emergent undocking of the robot without conversion to open surgery. For example, in cardiopulmonary arrest from a primary cardiac or pulmonary cause, rapidly obtaining close access for cardiopulmonary resuscitation including chest compression and cardioversion may be lifesaving. Paramount in urgent undocking are (1) the complete removal of all instruments from the patient before attempting to undock and (2) avoidance of entanglement or disconnection of power cords to each piece of robotic and OR equipment when personnel are rushing around the room. Failing to achieve either of these prior to attempted undocking can significantly delay the complete undocking or risk

A. J. B. Fong, MD, MBA
Department of Surgery, University of Washington Medical Center, Seattle, WA, USA

Y. Fong, MD (✉)
Department of Surgery, City of Hope National Medical Center, Duarte, CA, USA
e-mail: yfong@coh.org

Y. Fong et al. (eds.), *The SAGES Atlas of Robotic Surgery*, https://doi.org/10.1007/978-3-319-91045-1_9

further injury to the patient or staff. A more complete list of reasons for urgent and emergent undocking is presented in Table 9.1.

Other situations can arise that require not only urgent or emergent undocking but also conversion from robotically assisted to open surgery. Examples of such situations are presented in Table 9.2. A major cause of conversion is hemorrhage requiring open operation for repair. For urgent but not emergent causes, such as when visualization of the target structures is suboptimal, resulting in questions about the anatomy or the margins of tumors, immediate intraoperative consultation with a more experienced surgeon may be able to reorient and get the operative procedure back on track. In many cases, conversion is the most prudent course of action before inadvertent injury occurs.

It is also highly recommended that all needles, temporary clips, and other foreign objects utilized in the operation are removed as soon as possible. Leaving them inside a patient after use may save time in the moment but increases the risk of lost foreign objects that might require much time later to locate and remove. In such circumstances, loss of foreign objects can result in additional radiographs (additional radiation and time) or conversion (increased morbidity).

Table 9.1 Causes of undocking

Urgency	Cause
Emergent	Cardiac arrest
	Gas pulmonary embolism
	Tension pneumothorax
Urgent	Slippage of patient
Elective	Move to different anatomic location

Table 9.2 Causes for undocking and conversion to open operation

Urgency	Cause
Emergent	Uncontrollable hemorrhage
Urgent	Margin of cancer resection unclear
	Unsure of repair of injured vessel
	Anatomy unclear
	Inadvertent injury to adjacent organ not repairable by robotic assist
	Hemodynamic instability due to insufflation
Elective	Lost instrument (broken piece, needle, sponges, etc.)
	Poor visibility (habitus, port placement, quenching)
	Lack of progress, need for new technical approach

Preoperative Planning and Communications

Good communication among all members of the operative team allow for the greatest likelihood of safe, effective, and cost-effective delivery of patient care in the best possible work environment (Table 9.3). Good communication can help the operative team be prepared for and respond to all situations that they face in the OR. Additionally, strong communication can help appropriately set expectations for the operation.

The operative planning and team preparation and communication should begin long before the day of the operation. It starts with preoperative orders that include desired operative positioning of the patient (Fig. 9.1), equipment needed, and possible blood product needs. Setup of the room is particularly important, as the size of the robotic tower limits access to the patient. The multiple towers and consoles with the associated power and connection cords also limit the possible positions of anesthesia setup, the instrument

Table 9.3 Important communication items for the robotic surgery team

Preoperative orders	Position
	• Robot right or left
	• Supine, left lateral, right lateral
	• Trendelenburg, neutral, reverse Trendelenburg
	Equipment
	Blood products
Team briefing	Estimated time of operation
	Risk of hemorrhage
	Likelihood of conversion
Operating room equipment	Table and positioning equipment (e.g., footboard)
	Robotic instruments
	Laparoscopic instruments
	Open instruments
	• Retractors
	• Vascular instruments
	• Sutures
	• Staplers
	• Sealers
Associated medical risk analysis	Cardiac
	Lung
	Renal

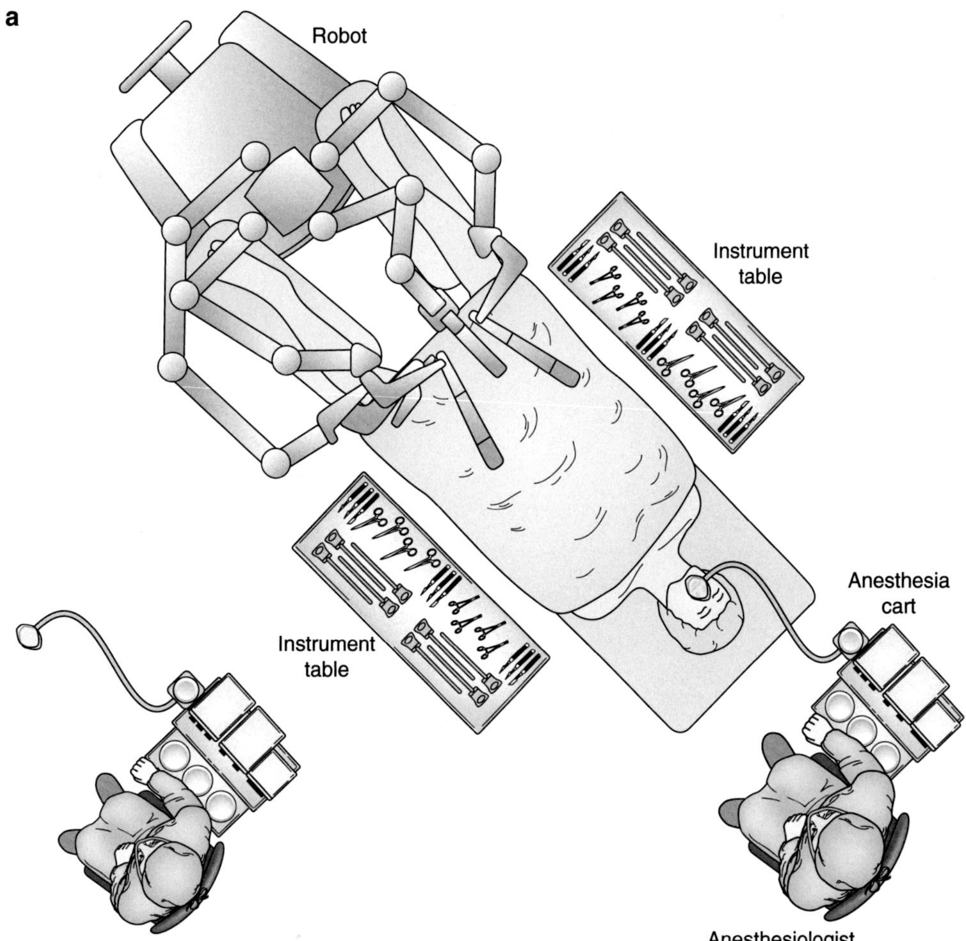

Fig. 9.1 Setup for Si robot. (**a**) *Setup for pelvic surgery*. In general, the patient is in lithotomy with steep Trendelenburg. In this position, slippage of the patient cephalad can produce traction injury to the lower extremities. Nursing needs include pads to prevent slippage of the patient, which may result in injury. The anesthesiologist is at the head of the table with good control of the airway and vascular access. The instrument tables can be to either side of the patient. (**b**) *Setup for upper abdominal surgery*. In general, the patient is in reverse Trendelenburg with the robot positioned over the head. Nursing needs include a footboard to prevent slippage of the patient, which may result in injury. The anesthesiologist is at the foot of the table with poor control of the airway and vascular access. Thus, a long anesthesia connector tube and long IV lines need to be set up. All needed vascular access lines must be placed before docking. It is nevertheless advisable to place a stopcock in the IV line at a position close to the patient for use if resuscitation medications are administered. This avoids having the medicine travel a long length of tubing before entering the patient to have effect. The instrument tables can be to either side of the patient. (**c**) *Setup for thoracic or flank surgery*. This is the position for thoracic, right liver, renal, and some adrenal operations. In general, the patient is positioned in a lateral position with the space between the costal margin and iliac crest positioned over the break in the table. A footboard is advisable to prevent slippage of the patient, which may result in injury. An arm tray is helpful in preventing upper extremity nerve injuries. The anesthesiologist is at the head of the table, but needs to plan the anesthesia machine placement to be facing the patient. There is generally a good control of airway and vascular access. The instrument table generally is at the foot of the bed facing the patient

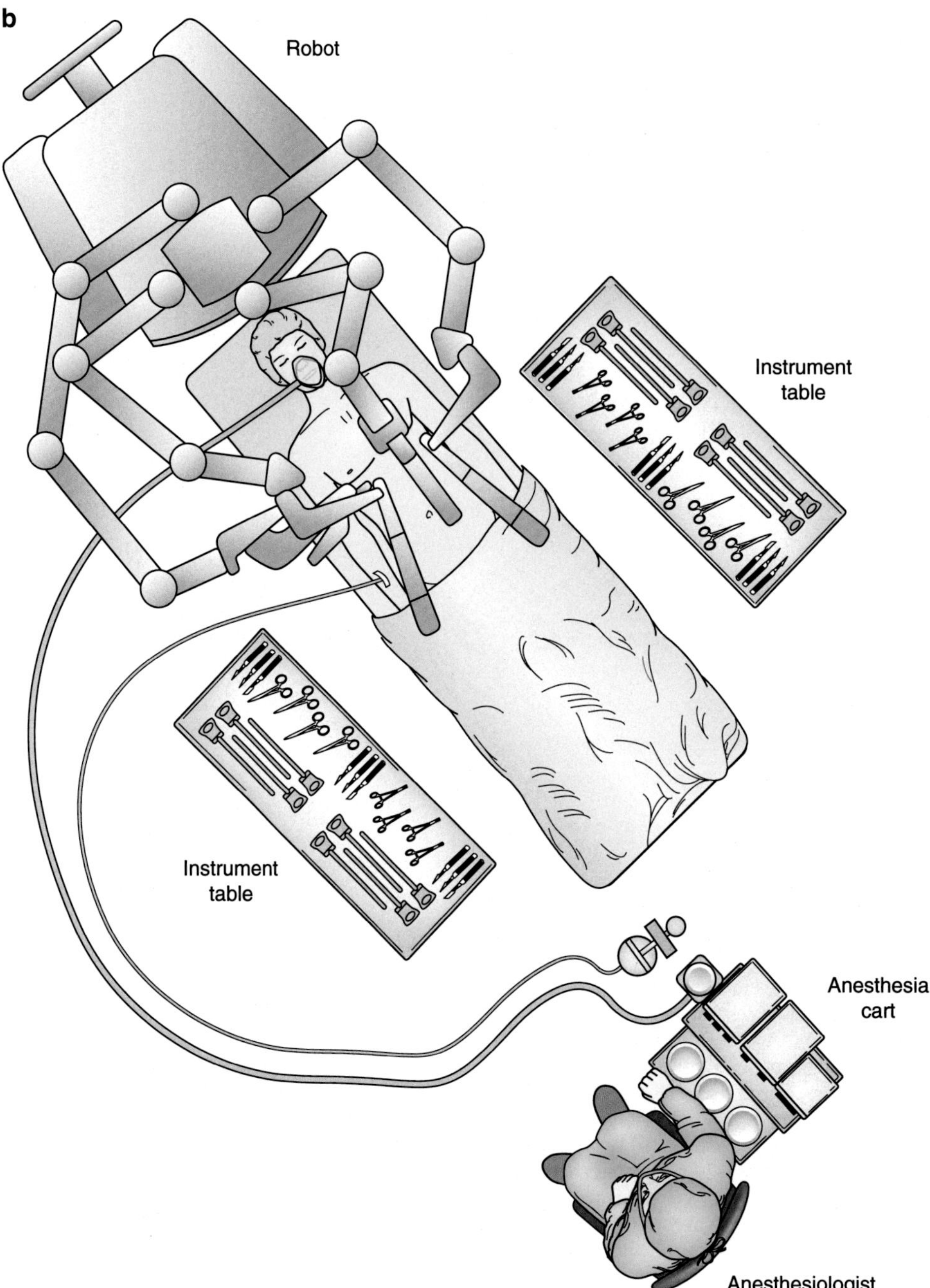

Fig. 9.1 (continued)

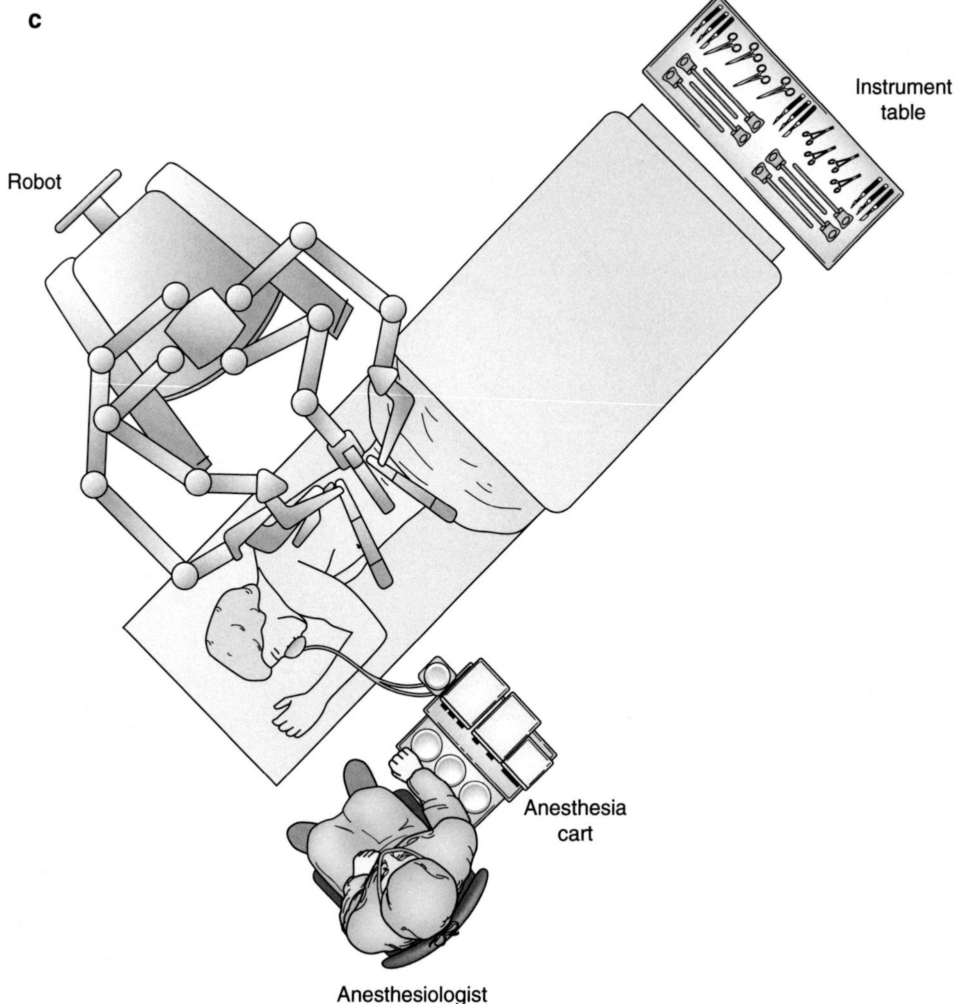

Fig. 9.1 (continued)

tables, and the positions of the bedside assistants. Additionally, OR workflow should be organized to allow IV access and other establishment of vitals monitoring before moving the robot into place and making access to the patient more difficult. Figure 9.1 shows three of the most common room setups for the da Vinci® Si system (Intuitive Surgical, Sunnyvale, CA) and illustrates the importance of communicating the correct position of the patient in the planning for all team members. Achieving the proper setup at the beginning of the case can save much time later in the operation by reducing equipment struggles and delays in navigating around the Si. As with any new setup in the OR, with continued use and experience, effective robotic positioning will become more efficient.

A team briefing should occur the day of surgery, to allow everyone participating in the procedure to be up to date on the operative plan and the emergency contingency planning and to open channels of communication among the operative team.

Figures 9.2 and 9.3 illustrate some common positioning of the da Vinci® Xi robot. The deployment of the Xi robot has greatly changed room setup and access to the patient, but the principles of conversion are the same. In particular, all instruments must be removed from the robot before undocking.

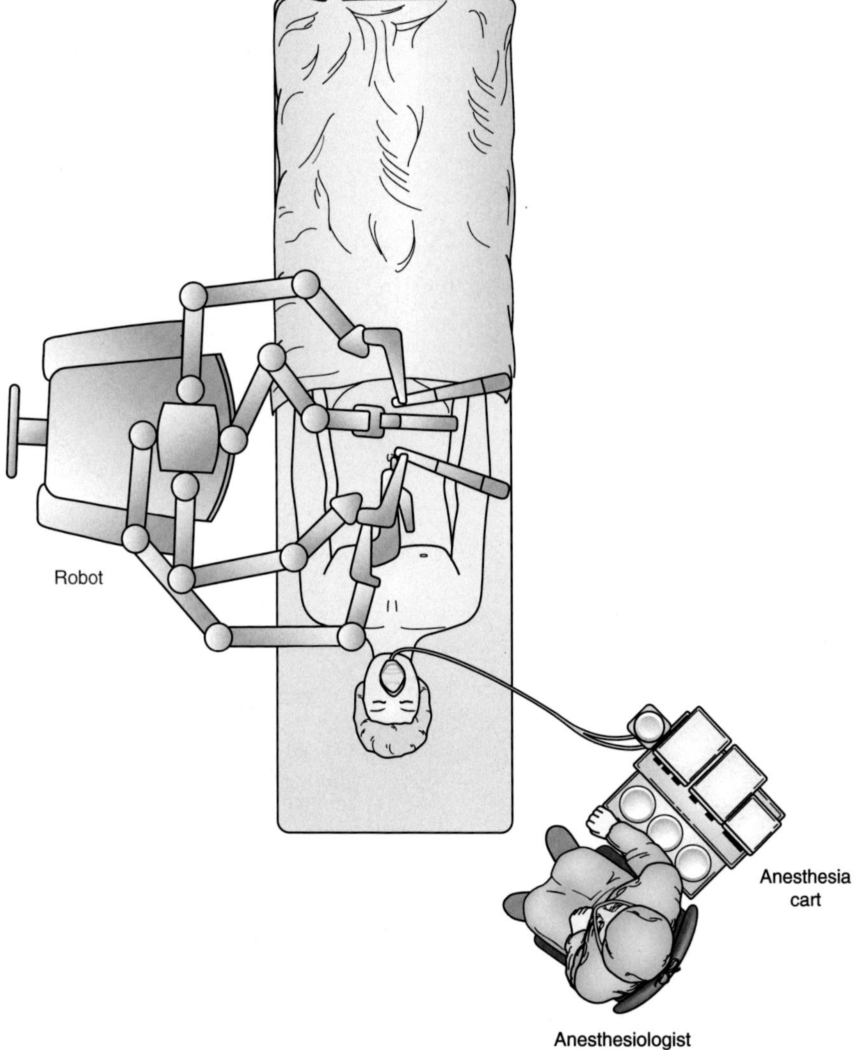

Fig. 9.2 Positioning of the Xi robot in an operating room. The arms of the Xi robot are mounted on a movable tower; this allows the tower to be positioned next to the patient and therefore permits very good access to the airway for the anesthesiologist

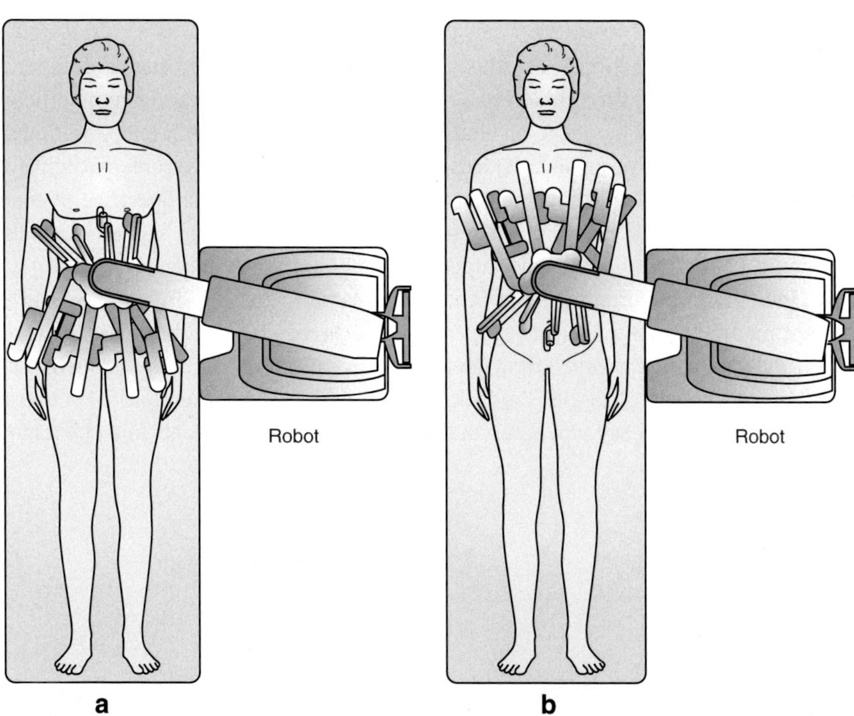

Fig. 9.3 (**a**, **b**) The arms of the Xi robot can be rotated en masse to optimize mechanical advantage when working at different parts of the body without moving the tower

Preparation and Personnel Roles During the Risk of Bleeding

Communicating the level of concern for hemorrhage, the cardiopulmonary risk level of the patient, and the likelihood of conversion is quite helpful in planning workflow. When prepared, team members can better react to unexpected circumstances. Table 9.4 lists likely actions by each member of the team as related to the level of concern for hemorrhage.

Table 9.4 Personnel roles with varying risks of bleeding

Team member	Preparation
High likelihood of bleeding	
Nurse	Open operation instruments open and ready for use, including vascular surgery instruments
	Robotic vascular sutures open and ready for use
	Have vascular staplers in room
Bedside assistant	Have accessory port for suction to allow best visibility if bleeding
	Have accessory ports ready for possible stapler use
Anesthesiologist	Large bore IV access ready
	Have stopcock close to patient for use with medications for resuscitation
	Blood products ready for transfusion
	Blood warmers ready
Console surgeon	Communicates constantly with team as to progress and risk
Blood bank	Blood products cross-matched and ready for transfusion
Moderate likelihood of bleeding	
Nurse	Open operation instruments, including vascular surgery instruments, in room but not necessarily open
	Open operation self-retaining retractors in room
	Robotic vascular sutures in room but not necessarily open
	Have vascular staplers in room
Bedside assistant	Have accessory port for suction to allow best visibility if bleeding
	Have accessory ports ready for possible stapler use
Anesthesiologist	Large bore IV access ready
	Have stopcock close to patient for use with medications for resuscitation
	Blood products ready for transfusion
	Blood warmers ready
Console surgeon	Communicates constantly with team as to progress and risk
Blood bank	Blood products cross-matched and ready for transfusion
Low likelihood of bleeding	
Nurse	Open operation instruments not open
	Open operation self-retaining retractors in room but not opened
	Robotic vascular sutures in room but not open
	Have vascular staplers in room
Bedside assistant	Ready to place accessory port for suction
	Have accessory ports for stapler use planned
Anesthesiologist	Large bore IV access ready
	Have stopcock close to patient for use with medications for resuscitation
	Blood typed but not cross-matched
Console surgeons	Communicates constantly with team as to progress and risk
Blood bank	Blood products typed but not cross-matched

Contingency Plans for Emergency Conversion

Planning and coordination of teamwork is important to maximize efficiency in the setting of necessary conversion. It generally will take longer to convert to open surgery from robotic than from laparoscopic surgery for several reasons:

- The robot is docked and is an obstacle to conversion.
- The primary surgeon is not at the surgical table or scrubbed in.
- Anesthesia personnel are generally more remote from the patient.
- The open surgical instrumentation may not be nearby and is not open for use.
- The OR environment must be reconfigured for open surgery.

Having a contingency plan for conversion to open surgery will increase the likelihood of a favorable outcome. Implementing and rehearsing such a plan is essential. Having a "robotic emergency time-out" as part of every robotic case ensures that emergency instruments and blood products are available and that all personnel involved understand the plan for emergency conversion, what their role will be in reconfiguring the operative setup if need be, and whom to call for help.

Instruments that may be needed urgently in case of unexpected conversion should be available:

- There should be an instrument set for emergency conversion, which should include standard open surgical instruments and vascular surgical instruments.
- There should be self-retaining retractors available to provide exposure, such as a Thompson or Goligher retractor.
- There should be a list of standard vascular sutures and staplers that are made immediately available when needed.

In cases where hemorrhage is likely, consideration should be given to placing a gel port at the beginning of the case to allow for rapid, manual tamponade of bleeding. Such a gel port insertion site can be used for specimen extraction. The gel port can also be used as an insertion site for additional trocars or can be used for manually assisted ultrasound assessment. (See chapter on hybrid procedures.)

An emergency conversion time-out should be performed at the beginning of each robotic surgical case and should include the following elements specific to circumstances of emergency conversion:

- Delineation of personnel responsibility, including who will maintain tamponade while conversion occurs
- Check to be sure emergency conversion instruments, retractors, vascular sutures, and staplers are readily available or in the room

- Check that necessary blood products for potential resuscitation are available
- Designation of who will perform resuscitation if needed
- Steps for undocking robot, including removing all instruments first
- Steps for making open incision, applying retractors, and controlling hemorrhage
- A list of other personnel who may be called to assist in an emergency, such as vascular surgeons

Lost Needle, Instrument, or Sponge

Conversion may also be required if instrument, needle, disposable, or sponge counts are incorrect. The usual course of action may involve a number of steps:

- Robotic sweep of the abdomen looking for the lost item
- Laparoscopic sweep of abdomen
- X-ray of cavity to assist in localization of item to decrease the size of incision needed even if conversion is the ultimate result
- Repeat robotic or laparoscopic sweep assisted by X-ray
- Conversion if required, or removal of the object robotically or laparoscopically when located

Simulation as Rehearsal for Emergency Conversion

Simulations have become part of the training for intensive care, trauma, and emergency room response to a severely hemodynamically unstable patient. To improve crisis management, simulator training scenarios have been developed [5, 6]. Some groups are now studying and advocating team simulation exercises as training for care of the patient undergoing robotic surgery who becomes hemodynamically unstable or has a cardiac arrest.

Huser et al. [5] performed a study on management of an acute emergency in an operating room setting, using a full-size simulator. The goal of their exercises was to shorten the time to resuscitation in a patient who suffers a cardiac arrest during robotically-assisted surgery. The exercise was set up to overcome the limited access to the patient during the start of a life-threatening emergency. In their study, six teams (each with three nurses, one anesthesiologist, and two urologists or gynecologists) were tested in a scenario of myocardial fibrillation. The investigators measured the time to first chest compression, removal of the robot, first defibrillation, and stabilization of circulation. The times to the start of chest compressions, removal of the robotic system, and first defibrillation were significantly improved at the second simulation ($P = 0.0054$). In particular, the sequence for emergency undocking was significantly faster when the rehearsal of the team's tasks was optimized. They concluded that with proper training, resuscitation can be started within seconds [6–10].

While undocking and beginning cardiac resuscitation is important for the patient with cardiac comorbidities who suffers a cardiac arrest, the most worrisome scenario during robotically assisted surgery remains the intraoperative hemorrhage that would require both undocking and conversion. For each anatomic location for which surgical hemorrhage can occur, a slightly different sequence for obtaining access and repair is in order. Working out these scenarios and setting up an emergency simulation with a multidisciplinary team in a real operating room setting can be strongly recommended.

Tricks of the Senior Surgeon

- Have in the room sutures that are commonly used for emergency repair of bleeding vessels.
- Have sutures and stapler ready to attempt repair in case of bleeding.
- Communicate immediately when worried about bleeding or possible need for conversion.
- Don't let "too few ports" be the cause of a conversion. When converting, don't let "too small incision" be the reason for a poor patient outcome.
- If you think conversion might be in the best interest of your patient, then conversion is the right thing to do.
- Do not view conversion as a failure; doing the right thing to maximize the patient's outcome is always more important than completing an operation robotically.
- Remember that robotic surgery conversion has some major differences from laparoscopic conversion, which need to be accounted for when planning for possible conversion:
  - The robot creates a physical obstacle to patient access.
  - The robot must be undocked and moved before conversion.
  - The surgeon is not scrubbed in at the table.
- In the operating room, all technology is a tool to help the patient. Use planning and communication to maximize the efficacy of the robot in helping the patient.

References

1. Sun V, Fong Y. Minimally invasive cancer surgery: indications and outcomes. Semin Oncol Nurs. 2017;33:23–36.
2. Thompson J. Myocardial infarction and subsequent death in a patient undergoing robotic prostatectomy. AANA J. 2009;77:365–71.
3. Mandal R, Duvvuri U, Ferris RL, Kaffenberger TM, Choby GW, Kim S. Analysis of post–transoral robotic-assisted surgery hemorrhage: frequency, outcomes, and prevention. Head Neck. 2016;38(Suppl 1):E776–82.
4. Yang CM, Chung HJ, Huang YH, Lin TP, Lin ATL, Chen KK. Standardized analysis of laparoscopic and robotic-assisted partial nephrectomy complications with Clavien classification. J Chin Med Assoc. 2014;77:637–41.
5. Huser AS, Muller D, Brunkhorst V, Kannisto P, Musch M, Kropfl D, Groeben H. Simulated life-threatening emergency during robot-assisted surgery. J Endourol. 2014;28:717–22.
6. Ziewacz JE, Arriaga AF, Bader AM, Berry WR, Edmondson L, Wong JM, et al. Crisis checklists for the operating room: development and pilot testing. J Am Coll Surg. 2011;213:212–7.
7. Holzman RS, Cooper JB, Gaba DM, Philip JH, Small SD, Feinstein D. Anesthesia crisis resource management: real life simulation training in operating room crisis. J Clin Anesth. 1995;7:675–87.
8. Yee B, Naik VN, Joo HS, Savoldelli GL, Chung DY, Houston PL, et al. Nontechnical skills in anesthesia crisis management with repeated exposure to simulation-based education. Anesthesiology. 2005;103:241–8.
9. Birkmeyer JD. Strategies for improving surgical quality—checklists and beyond. N Engl J Med. 2010;363:1963–5.
10. Arriaga AF, Bader AM, Wong JM, Lipsitz SR, Berry WR, Ziewacz JE, et al. Simulation-based trial of surgical-crisis checklists. N Engl J Med. 2013;368:246–53.

Hybrid Robot-Assisted Surgery

10

Aaron Lewis, Yanghee Woo, and Yuman Fong

Introduction

The robotically-assisted surgical approach offers the benefits of minimally invasive surgery to our patients, taking advantage of a sophisticated robotic system that provides a three-dimensional (3D) magnified operative view, wristed instruments, tremor filtering, control of four arms, and near-infrared imaging capabilities. While surgeons have reported performing various operative procedures from incision to closure using only the robotic surgical instruments, many of the more complex procedures are accomplished using some combination of open and laparoscopic methods along with robotic assistance. These hybrid approaches are usually conceived to address the two main concerns associated with robotic operations in certain circumstances: safety and speed.

Hybrid robotically-assisted surgery is a planned operative approach that combines the multiple access methods for various specific portions of a procedure to ensure safety and speed. It integrates a robot-assisted portion of an operation with other surgical methods (laparoscopy, hand-assisted laparoscopy, and mini-laparotomy) to offer the maximum advantages of the different approaches currently in surgical practice. The hybrid procedures can be broadly separated into the following approaches:

1. Hybrid robotic surgery with mini-laparotomy
   (a) Hybrid robotic surgery and open surgery
   (b) Hybrid laparoscopic surgery, robotic surgery, with open surgery
2. Hybrid laparoscopic surgery and robotic surgery
3. Hybrid hand-assisted, laparoscopic surgery in combination with robotic surgery

With early robotically-assisted surgical experiences, surgeons often use hybrid robotically-assisted surgery as a transition to a totally robotic procedure, using the hybrid method as a bridge. For very complex procedures, many surgeons have kept parts of the operations as open surgery or laparoscopic surgery when the tasks in those parts were best performed using conventional open or laparoscopic surgery. Using the tumor extraction sites to deliver bowel for extracorporeal anastomosis was a very natural choice for intestinal resections (Fig. 10.1) or radical cystectomies (Fig. 10.2)

A. Lewis, MD
Division of Surgical Oncology, Department of Surgery, City of Hope National Medical Center, Duarte, CA, USA
e-mail: alewis@coh.org

Y. Woo, MD
International Surgery, Department of Surgery, City of Hope National Medical Center, Duarte, CA, USA
e-mail: ywoo@coh.org

Y. Fong, MD (✉)
Department of Surgery, City of Hope National Medical Center, Duarte, CA, USA
e-mail: yfong@coh.org

Y. Fong et al. (eds.), *The SAGES Atlas of Robotic Surgery*, https://doi.org/10.1007/978-3-319-91045-1_10

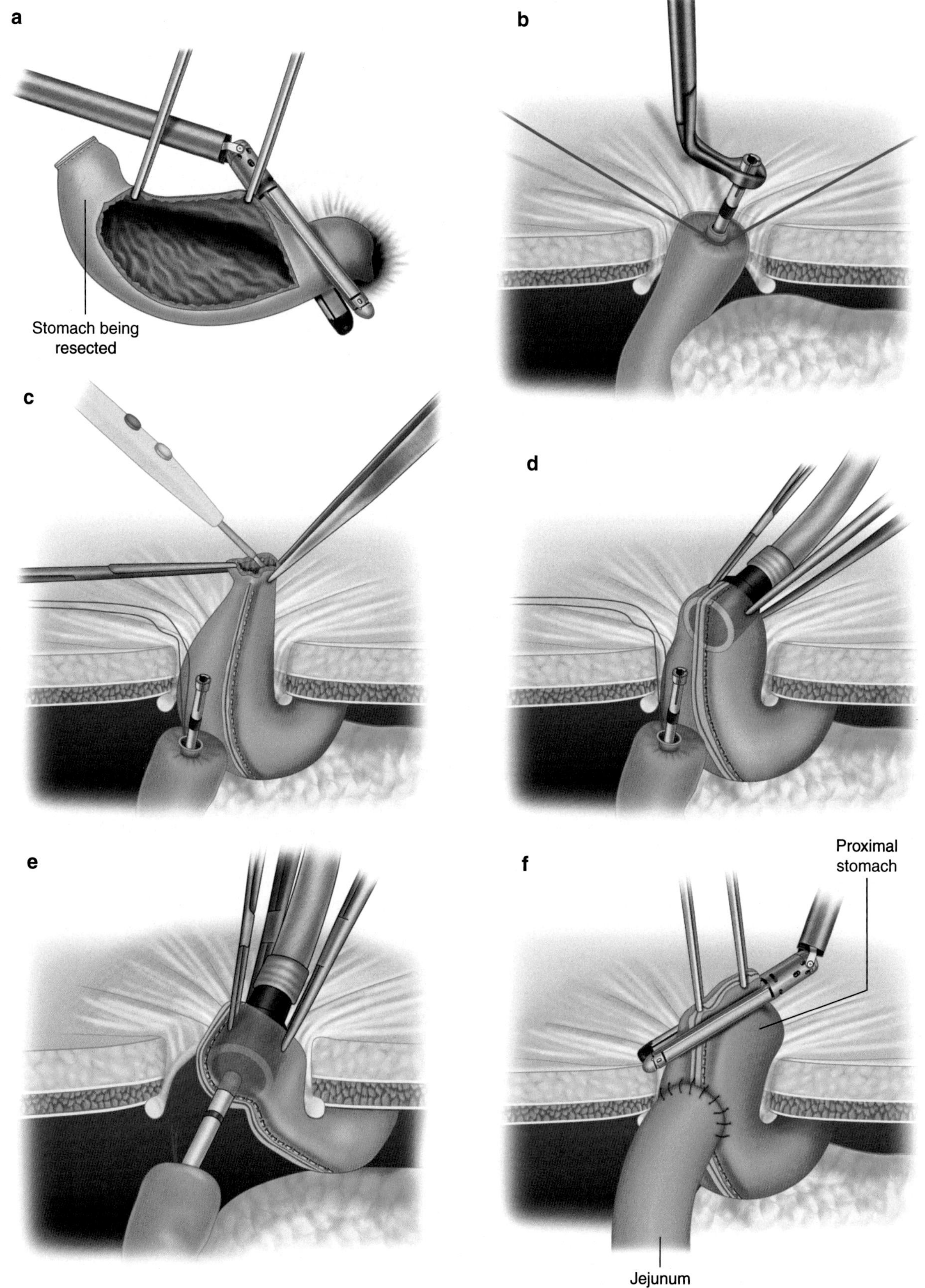

Fig. 10.1 Billroth-I reconstruction by the double stapling technique. (**a**) Confirmation of proximal resection line of the stomach. (**b**) Placement of the anvil at the duodenal stump. (**c**) Opening the nearest point of the greater curvature of the remnant stomach. (**d**) Insertion of a circular stapler. (**e**) Anastomosis on the staple line of the remnant stomach by the double-stapling technique. (**f**) Closure of the entry hole

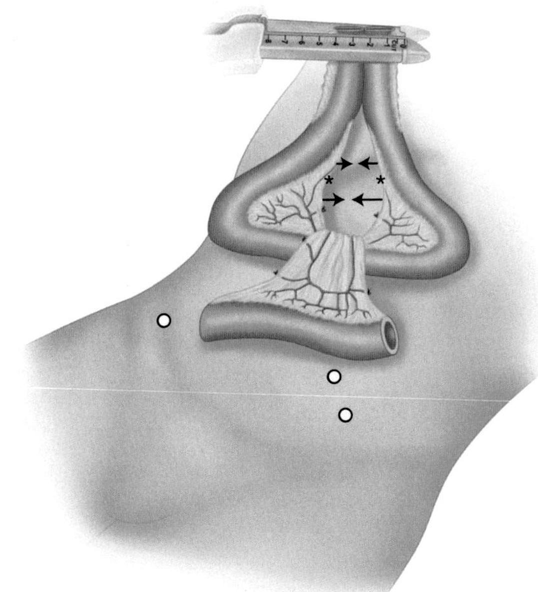

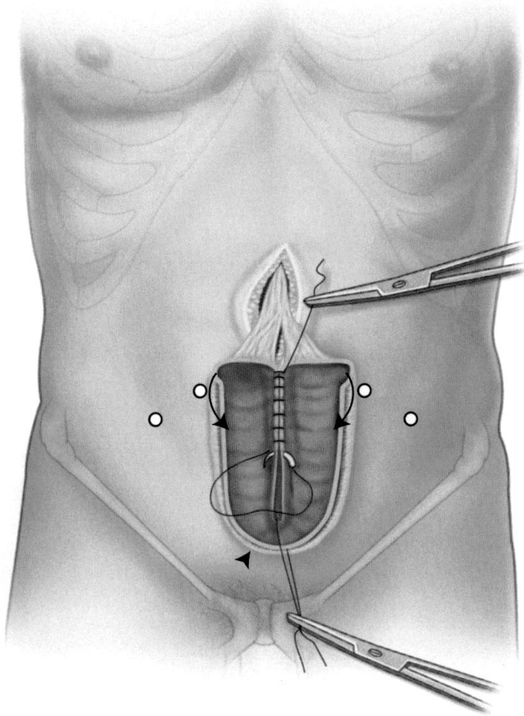

Fig. 10.2 External construction of a neobladder. An ileal segment is isolated with accurate preservation of its vascularization (**a**). Bowel ends are sutured antimesenterically in side-to-side anastomosis (arrows) using linear stapler, and mesenteric margins (asterisks) are reapproximated. A 20 cm detubularized ileal segment is modeled according to U configuration, (**b**) and posterior wall is completely sutured. Arrowhead indicates distal end of neobladder

before robotic staplers became available. In a patient with dense adhesions from previous surgery, using a mini-laparotomy or a traditional laparoscopic approach to take down adhesions prior to docking the robot for surgery often saves much time. A hand port placed in the planned specimen extraction site or in an ostomy takedown site can allow better staging for cancer by palpation or by use of a handheld ultrasound (Fig. 10.3).

Many factors play a role in the selection of a hybrid robot-assisted approach. Factors to consider include the surgeon's experience with each approach, surgical technique and complexity, necessary or available instruments, number of operative fields, expected length of the procedure, and goals of the operation. Hybrid robotically-assisted surgery has the potential advantage of optimizing the combined benefits of each of the platforms into one operation (Table 10.1).

With the introduction of new technology, such as the da Vinci Xi system or articulated laparoscopic instrument, hybrid surgery will continue to evolve. Ultimately, the most important driver for a new hybrid technique should be optimization of patient outcome. Hybrid approaches have already allowed for wider adoption of the MIS approach for complex operations. Many hybrid operations are currently considered the standard approach for various robotic procedures, and the details are described in other chapters within this book. The purpose of this chapter is also to discuss ways in which hybrid surgery has allowed minimally invasive, complex surgery not otherwise considered feasible or surgeries in which the approaches are enhanced by the combination of platforms. Both the novice and the expert robotic surgeon can benefit from concepts and operations developed in hybrid surgery.

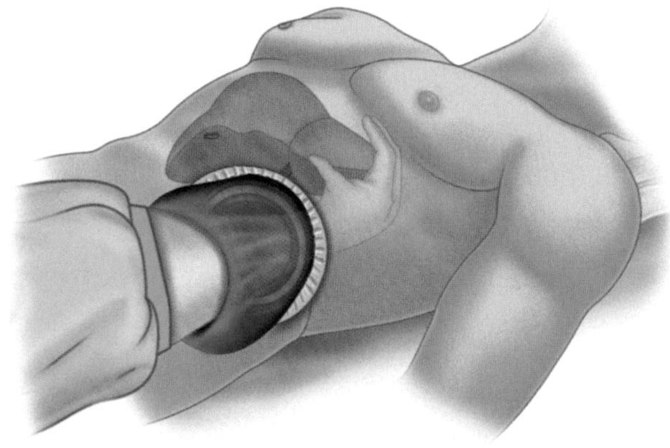

Fig. 10.3 A Gelport can be used for manual palpation of internal organs for cancer staging or for retraction

Table 10.1 Comparison of various minimally invasive approaches

	Laparoscopy	Robotics	Hand-assisted	Open	Hybrid approach
Pros	• Wide sweeping movements • Retraction • Minimal set up time	• Superior visualization • Instrument stabilization • Improved ergonomics • Degrees of freedom • Independent surgery • Complex movements • Less blood loss	• Tactile sensation • Superior retraction	• Immediate access • Tactile sensation • Most training	• Combined benefits of each platform • Speed of operation • Minimizes revenue losses • Useful after previous open operations
Cons	• Limited degrees of freedom • Requires expertise to perform complete operations	• Narrow focus of view • Instrument limitations • Lack of tactile sensation • Time restraints	• Cumbersome • Colliding of instruments with hand	• Large incision • Slower recovery • Large fluid shifts • Bowel edema	• Changes between techniques • Less independence than totally robotic
Techniques	• Division of lax tissues (i.e., omentum) • Running the bowel	• Fine motor dissections (i.e., lymphadectomy or vascular dissection) • Suturing • Anastomoses	• Tactile sensation • Extensive mobilization	• Extensive adhesions • Tactile sensation required	• Multiple field operations • Complex operations using various techniques

Hybrid Robotic Surgery with Mini-Laparotomy

Robotically-assisted surgery with mini-laparotomy is one of the most commonly used hybrid robot-assisted approaches. The mini-laparotomy is usually made at the end of the robotic portion of the operation to perform open, extracorporeal anastomoses or reconstruction after extirpative surgery. Complex gastrointestinal reconstructions (Fig. 10.1) or neobladder construction (Fig. 10.2) are often performed more quickly through a mini-laparotomy. Before the advent of the robotic stapler, intra-corporeal reconstruction was also often unwieldy. Hybrid robotic surgery with a mini-laparotomy significantly decreases operative time for surgeons not comfortable with intracorporeal anastomoses and decreases the concern for anastomotic complications in the beginning of the robotic learning curve for intracorporeal portions of the operation. In addition, surgical fluid losses and bowel edema associated with open surgery is minimized to a short portion of the operation [1].

There are times when a mini incision may be useful at the beginning of a case. Indications for early mini-laparotomy include lysis of adhesions or the need for tactile manipulation. Tactile sensation may improve tumor localization in patients with multiple liver tumors, potential carcinomatosis, or unmarked colon tumors (Fig. 10.3). If an ostomy is to be reversed as part of the robotic operation, first taking down the stoma allows wider access and provides an abdominal wall defect perfect for Gelport use (Fig. 10.4). Additionally, a hand port can be placed for assistance during technically difficult

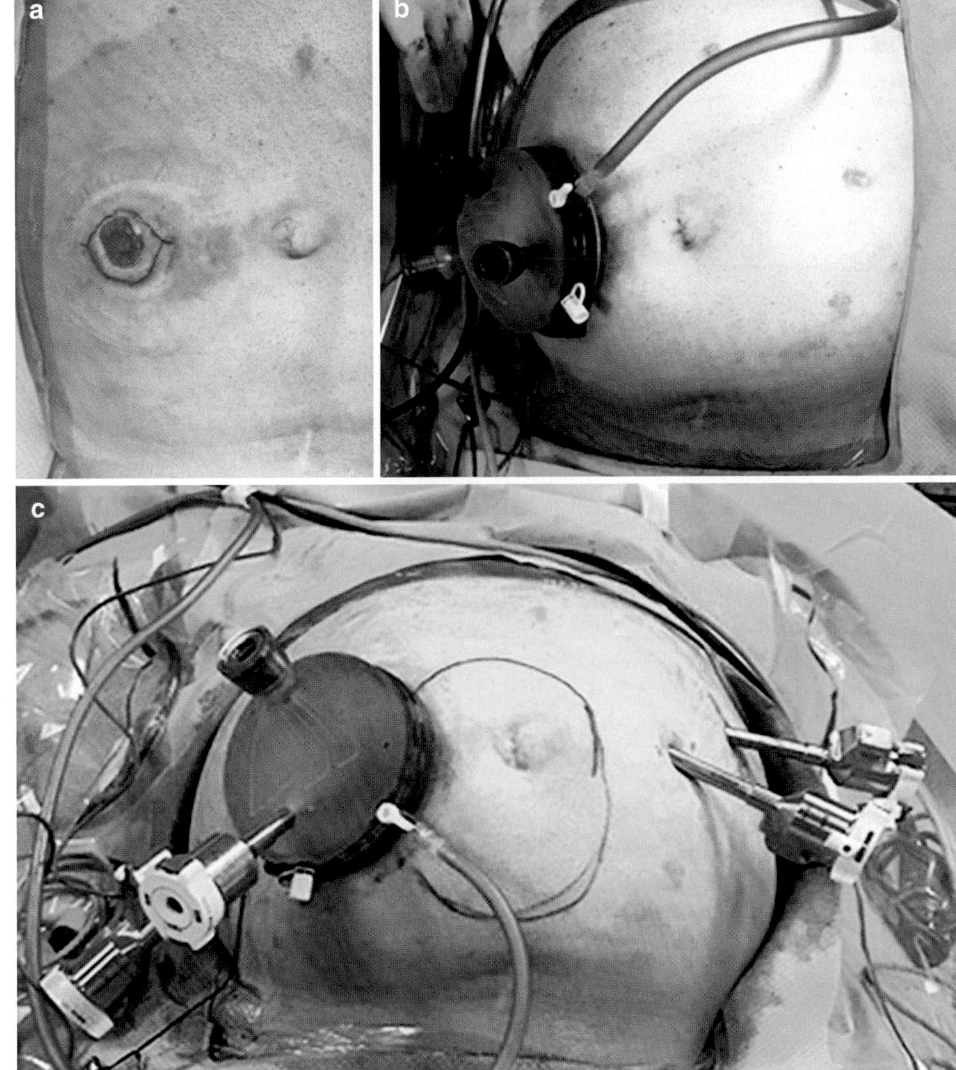

Fig. 10.4 In this patient with an ileostomy (**a**) that is to be reversed simultaneous with a bilateral liver resection, taking down and reversing the ileostomy first allows a site for Gelport placement (**b**). Through the Gelport, a robotic port as well as a 10-mm accessory port can be placed (**b**). Placing additional robotic ports then allows docking and robotic liver resection (**c**). The Gelport can be rotated to allow varied orientations of the robotic and accessory ports

maneuvers such as running the bowel or difficult retraction. Creation of a mini-laparotomy at any point during the case can sometimes prevent conversion to an open operation. A Gelport is used in the mini-laparotomy site to maintain insufflation during the robotic portion of the operation and for possible trocar placement (Fig. 10.5).

Examples of various combinations of mini-laparotomy and robotic operations include the following:

1. Gastrectomy with lymphadenectomy [2]
   (a) Laparoscopic gastrectomy with robotic lymphadenectomy and mini-laparotomy to perform the Roux-en-Y esophagojejunostomy and the jejunojejunostomy
   (b) Robotic total gastrectomy and lymphadenectomy with mini-laparotomy to perform the Roux-en-Y esophagojejunostomy and the jejunojejunostomy
2. Colectomy/Proctectomy
   (a) Robotic dissection and resection with mini-laparotomy and ileocolonic/colo-colonic/ileoanal anastomoses [3]
   (b) Laparoscopic takedown of splenic flexure, robotic dissection and resection, and open anastomosis through mini-laparotomy [4]
3. Pancreatectomy
   (a) Robotic dissection and resection of the head of the pancreas and duodenum with mini-laparotomy open reconstruction [5]
   (b) Robotic dissection and mobilization of the tail of the pancreas/spleen with mini-laparotomy for resection
4. Vascular reconstruction
   (a) Robotically-assisted laparoscopic dissection for aortobifemoral reconstruction with mini-laparotomy graft implantation [6]
5. Hepatectomy
   (a) Handport mini-laparotomy to pringle and retract, robotic resection, hand-assisted hepatic ultrasound localization of hepatic tumor with percutaneous ablations (Fig. 10.5) [7]
6. Cystectomy
   (a) Robotic bladder resection and open urinary diversion via a mini-laparotomy [8]
7. Hysterectomy
   (a) Robotic total abdominal hysterectomy and lymph node dissection and open staging operation via a mini-laparotomy (Fig. 10.6) [9]

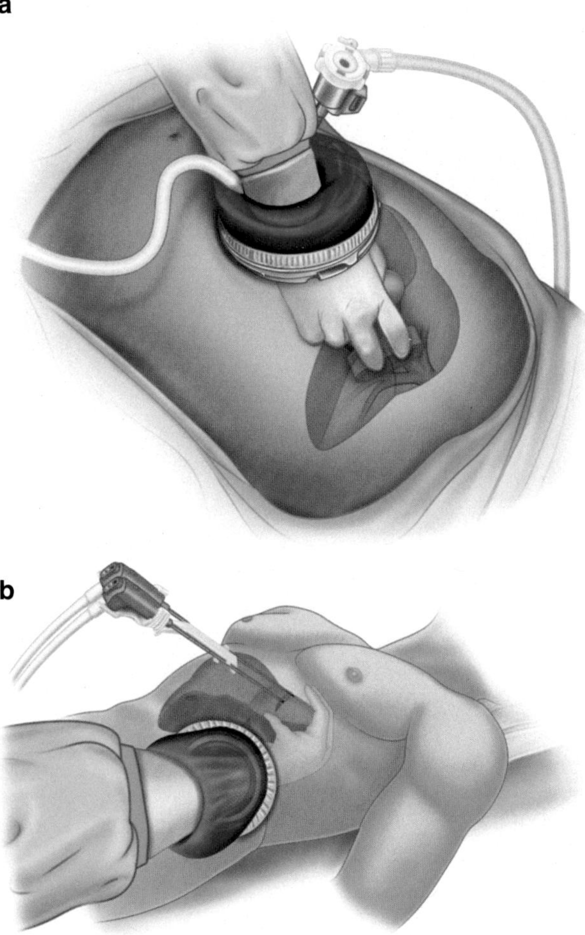

Fig. 10.5 An ultrasound T-probe can also be placed through the Gelport for ultrasound stage of liver (**a**) or for ultrasound-guided ablation of the liver (**b**)

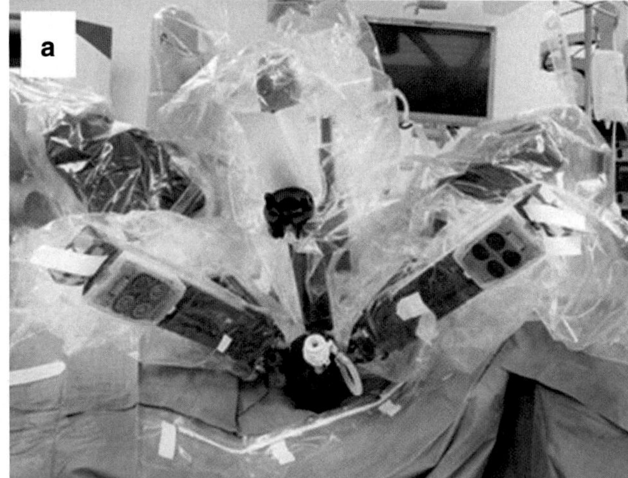

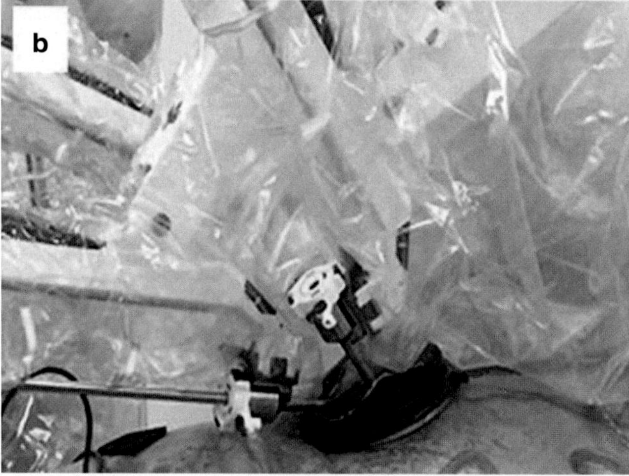

Fig. 10.6 Robotic ports can be placed through a Gelport for operative use while minimizing number of skin and facial incisions

While variations of the hybrid robotic combined with mini-laparotomy can be used across various fields, we will highlight its use in our own unpublished experience. The hand port has increased the possible candidates for robotic liver surgery. Liver surgery has changed over the last decade such that many of our operations are liver parenchymal, preserving non-anatomic operations in combination with ablation. Patients now undergoing liver surgery often have multiple tumors, which are amenable to a combined approach. In the past, these patients would all undergo an open operation. The hand port allows for easily placed pringle devices, palpation of liver for superficial tumor identification (Fig. 10.3), and hand-assisted intraoperative ultrasound for deep tumor localization with percutaneous tumor ablation (Fig. 10.5). This is done in combination with robotic resection of superficial lesions. Robotic ports can be placed through the Gelport to minimize the number of incisions needed (Fig. 10.6).

Robotically-assisted, Laparoscopic-Assisted, and Hand-Assisted Surgery

Hand-assisted surgery is a variation of hybrid robotic surgery with a mini-laparotomy, and it offers the perioperative advantages of minimally invasive surgery without the technical difficulty associated with a purely laparoscopic or robotic procedure. A larger incision notwithstanding hand assistance through a Gelport preserves the benefits associated with minimally invasive surgery, including lower blood loss, better control of fluid losses, and maintenance of normothermia. In addition, hand-assisted surgery has the added benefits of tactile feedback, gentle blunt dissection, and hand-assisted retraction during advanced minimally invasive procedures, including transcutaneous radiofrequency or microwave ablation (Fig. 10.6b). Conversion rates are lower than comparable minimally invasive operations [10].

Hand-assisted laparoscopic approaches have been described across most surgical specialties [11, 12]. However, hand-assist should not be used when the robot is docked and active. Hand-to-robotic arm collisions are potentially dangerous. The most common uses of the Gelport in robotic surgery may be to prevent conversion to open in a difficult robotic operation by providing a hand-assisted laparoscopic portion of the operation to bridge the operative impasse.

Traditional Laparoscopy Plus Robotic Surgery

Robotically-assisted surgery combined with conventional laparoscopy is a hybrid robotic method that has allowed for early adoption of the robot in many complex procedures. The benefits of laparoscopy include superior retraction with the use of four skilled surgeon hands, the ability to perform wide sweeping movements across multiple fields of view, and decreased time requirements in comparison to the robot alone. The use of laparoscopic instruments can facilitate taking down dense abdominal wall adhesions where insertions of robotic ports are prohibited by limited exposure. The robot may be best reserved in these hybrid operations for preoperatively determined focused portions of an operation, such as dissection around major vascular structures, difficult-to-access locations such as the pelvis or mediastinum, or tasks requiring fine motor skills such as suturing.

Hybrid laparoscopic-plus-robotic surgery may be beneficial across all surgical specialties. The following examples illustrate how hybrid laparoscopic-plus-robotic surgery has addressed some limitations of the robot.

1. Multi-field operations
   (a) Esophagogastrectomy
      (i) Hybrid robotically-assisted thoracoscopic esophagectomy and abdominal laparoscopic gastric mobilization and resection
   (b) Colectomy/proctectomy
      (i) Laparoscopic-assisted takedown of the splenic flexure and robotic pelvic dissection
      (ii) Laparoscopic-assisted total abdominal colectomy and robotic pelvic dissection
      (iii) Combined robotic rectosigmoid resection and laparoscopic segmental bowel resection (for severe endometriosis) [13]
2. Complex operations limited by time
   (a) Pancreaticoduodenectomy
      (i) Several variations of steps incorporating the laparoscope and robot
   (b) Esophagogastrectomy
      (i) Hybrid robotically-assisted thoracoscopic surgery and laparoscopy
3. Redo operations
   (a) Laparoscopy-assisted adhesiolysis prior to robotic operation

Evolution of Hybrid Operations

In many operations relatively new to robotics, the optimal approach has yet to be determined. This is a result of both evolving technology and the acquisition of experience.

The evolution of robotics in colon surgery demonstrates the transition from laparoscopic approach to totally robotic procedure through adoption of hybrid techniques. The difficult dissection in the narrow pelvis is ideally suited for the robot [14–16]. For colectomies, the need for multiquadrant surgery has prohibited widespread adoption of the robot despite its ubiquitous use in urologic [17] and gynecologic [18] pelvic operations. Naturally, early reports of robotic colon surgery described a hybrid approach in which the splenic flexure of the colon is taken down in a laparoscopic fashion and the more tedious total mesorectal excision (TME) is performed with the robot [4, 19, 20]. The extraction site can be adapted such that the incision used to remove the specimen is also used to assist with the colorectal anastomosis in an open fashion. Series reporting totally robotic low anterior resection with robotic takedown of the splenic flexure using the da Vinci S or Si systems are small, and the authors comment on the difficulty of the multiquadrant surgery [21, 22].

Total abdominal proctocolectomy offers an even greater challenge of a totally robotic approach. Evolution of technology has made multi-field surgery, such as total abdominal proctocolectomy, possible. The da Vinci Xi was developed to allow for repositioning and pivoting of the robotic arms without moving the base to accommodate multiple quadrant operations. Despite the advances, many surgeons may still find a hybrid approach more convenient. Many still prefer a hand-assisted approach for the abdominal colectomy portion of this operation.

Hepatobiliary surgery is another example of how hybrid approaches are leading to the implementation of minimally invasive surgery in a field historically resistant to MIS techniques. Reports of laparoscopic complex hepatobiliary procedures were described as far back as the 1990s [23, 24]. Limitations of the laparoscope and laparoscopic instruments have made hepatobiliary operations difficult to perform in a minimally invasive fashion, limiting its implementation to very few high-volume centers [25]. More recently, use of the robot has led to a greater acceptance of minimally invasive hepatobiliary procedures.

Robotic pancreaticoduodenectomy can be difficult to perform because it involves detailed dissection as well as three abdominal quadrant surgeries consisting of multiple steps. In addition, these operations can be prohibitively long. Operative times for robotic pancreaticoduodenectomy can often exceed 10 h [26]. Alternatively, a hybrid robotic laparoscopic technique can be done. The definition of hybrid surgery can be variable, which highlights the advantages of combining the various techniques to fit the needs of the surgeon. Examples of various hybrid approaches are listed in Table 10.2. The heterogeneity of approaches described in pancreatic robotic surgery represents the true potential of how the robot may be adopted as a tool to fit the surgeon's needs [27].

Table 10.2 Heterogeneous hybrid approaches to robotically-assisted pancreaticoduodenectomy

Laparoscopic resection and robotic reconstruction
Laparoscopic mobilization, robotic resection and reconstruction
Hand-assisted laparoscopic resection and robotic reconstruction
Laparoscopic-robotic resection and robotic reconstruction
Laparoscopic-robotic resection and reconstruction through mini-laparotomy

Hand-Assisted Robotic Surgery for Gynecologic Malignancies

Gynecologic malignancies are at high potential for peritoneal spread. Laparotomy has been the standard of care partly because of the complexity of staging, and of multi-field lymphadenectomy (pelvic, periaortic), and multi-field cytoreduction of peritoneal nodules. Laparotomy allows for palpation of small nodules not seen laparoscopically. In patients without evidence of carcinomatosis, a hand-assisted robotic surgery (HARS) for staging can be performed [9]. Total abdominal hysterectomy and lymphadenectomy are performed with the robotic in the usual fashion. A Gelport can be placed either before or after the robotic portion of the operation, depending on whether a diagnosis of cancer is known, through a 7–9 cm incision. The omentectomy or peritoneal biopsies can be performed using the hand-assisted technique. The small bowel is exteriorized and run through the Gelport to look for any implants (Fig. 10.7). Patients have a shorter hospital stay than laparotomy with this operation [9].

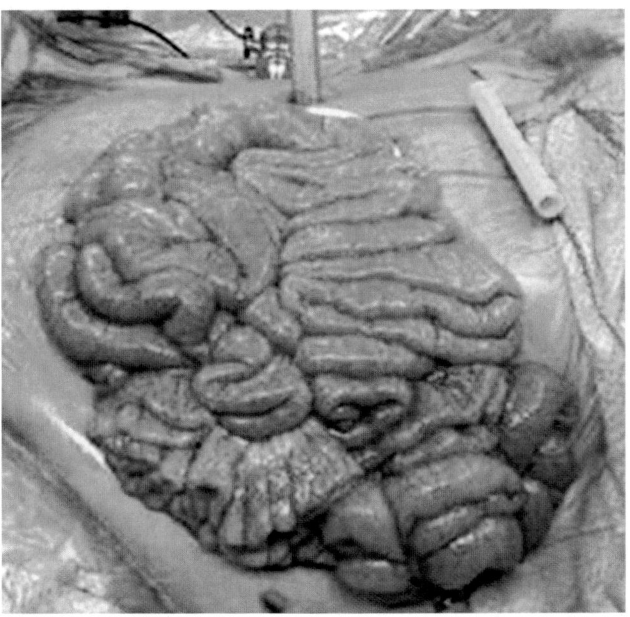

Fig. 10.7 Exteriorization of small bowel through a hand port for staging in gynecologic surgery

Robotically-assisted, Natural Orifice Transluminal Endoscopic Surgery

With the robot becoming more widely available, hybrid robotically-assisted natural orifice transluminal endoscopic surgery (NOTES) is being explored. Several hybrid robotically-assisted NOTES procedures have recently been reported. These include transrectal NOTES adrenalectomy [28]. A robotic trocar is passed through the rectum after creating a submucosal tunnel from below into the peritoneum, 1 cm above the pectinate line. The remaining trocars are placed transabdominally. Two additional laparoscopic ports are placed transabdominally for assistance in retraction of the liver. Either the adrenal gland or the kidney can be approached in this fashion. In women, the same approach can be done via the vagina rather than the rectum [29]. These procedures must be considered experimental, and a much larger experience needs to be reported before they are recommended for common use.

Combined Technologies

Hybrid operations are sometimes necessary to allow for the adoption of additional technologies that may exist only for open surgical or laparoscopic formats. Ablation is a technique that is being used more frequently to replace surgical dissection for smaller tumors and to be combined with treatment consisting of resection of larger tumors and ablation of smaller tumors [30]. Ablative techniques include radiofrequency ablation (RFA), microwave ablation (MWA), and irreversible electroporation (IRE). A combined approach allows the robot to be used for dissection or resection and ablation to be performed either laparoscopically or through a mini-laparotomy.

This approach has been described in urologic [31–33] and hepatic [7] operations. During robotic partial nephrectomy, RFA is used to ablate the tumor edge allowing for a bloodless plane of dissection. In liver surgery, patients with multiple liver lesions are treated with a combination of ablation and resection depending on size, location, and proximity to major vessels. Lesions amenable to resection can be removed robotically while deeper lesions are identified with the laparoscopic ultrasound probe or a T ultrasound probe placed by Gelport access, and percutaneous ablation is performed under ultrasound guidance (Fig. 10.6).

Summary

As with all procedures, there is a learning curve in adopting new techniques and technologies. Hybrid robotic surgery incorporates a broad range of non-robotic techniques that allow for optimization of robotic procedures and increased use of this technology. Thus, hybrid procedures combining robotics with traditional laparoscopic surgery, Gelport hand-assisted techniques, or open access through a mini-laparotomy incision were at first used to allow for earlier adoption of the surgical robot. These techniques were considered to be a bridge toward totally robotic surgeries. As the robot is used for increasingly complex procedures, hybrid approaches have taken on a different role. They now allow surgeons to use the robot as just another surgical tool, to be combined with other surgical approaches to provide the safest and fastest operation, rather than as a rigid single-modality technique.

References

1. Jacob M, Chappell D, Rehm M. The 'third space'—fact or fiction? Best Pract Res Clin Anaesthesiol. 2009;23(2):145–57.
2. Gholami S, Cassidy MR, Strong VE. Minimally invasive surgical approaches to gastric resection. Surg Clin North Am. 2017;97(2):249–64.
3. Bosio RM, Pigazzi A. Emerging and evolving technology in colon and rectal surgery. Clin Colon Rectal Surg. 2015;28(3):152–7.
4. Pigazzi A, Ellenhorn JD, Ballantyne GH, Paz IB. Robotic-assisted laparoscopic low anterior resection with total mesorectal excision for rectal cancer. Surg Endosc. 2006;20(10):1521–5.
5. Choi SH, Kang CM, Kim DH, Lee WJ, Chi HS. Robotic pylorus preserving pancreaticoduodenectomy with mini-laparotomy reconstruction in patient with ampullary adenoma. J Korean Surg Soc. 2011;81(5):355–9.
6. Lin JC, Reddy DJ, Eun D, Fumo M, Menon M. Robotic-assisted laparoscopic dissection of the infrarenal aorta and iliac artery: a technical description and early results. Ann Vasc Surg. 2009;23(3):298–302.
7. Nassour I, Polanco PM. Minimally invasive liver surgery for hepatic colorectal metastases. Curr Colorectal Cancer Rep. 2016;12(2):103–12.
8. Gudjonsson S, Hilmarsson R, Patschan O, Liedberg F. Does incision length matter? Robotic assisted extracorporeal urinary diversion via mini-laparotomy using the Alexis O-ring retractor. Eur Urol. 2015;67(1):179–80.
9. Fornalik H, Brooks H, Moore ES, Flanders NL, Callahan MJ, Sutton GP. Hand-assisted robotic surgery for staging of ovarian cancer and uterine cancers with high risk of peritoneal spread: a retrospective cohort study. Int J Gynecol Cancer. 2015;25(8):1488–93.
10. Moloo H, Haggar F, Coyle D, Hutton B, Duhaime S, Mamazza J, et al. Hand assisted laparoscopic surgery versus conventional laparoscopy for colorectal surgery. Cochrane Database Syst Rev. 2010;(10):CD006585.
11. Marcello PW, Fleshman JW, Milsom JW, Read TE, Arnell TD, Birnbaum EH, et al. Hand-assisted laparoscopic vs. laparoscopic colorectal surgery: a multicenter, prospective, randomized trial. Dis Colon Rectum. 2008;51(6):818–26. discussion 826–8
12. Zhang GT, Zhang XD, Xue HZ. Open versus hand-assisted laparoscopic total gastric resection with D2 lymph node dissection for adenocarcinoma: a case-control study. Surg Laparosc Endosc Percutan Tech. 2017;27(1):42–50.
13. Vitobello D, Fattizzi N, Santoro G, Rosati R, Baldazzi G, Bulletti C, et al. Robotic surgery and standard laparoscopy: a surgical hybrid technique for use in colorectal endometriosis. J Obstet Gynaecol Res. 2013;39(1):217–22.
14. Guillou PJ, Quirke P, Thorpe H, Walker J, Jayne DG, Smith AM, et al. Short-term endpoints of conventional versus laparoscopic-assisted surgery in patients with colorectal cancer (MRC CLASICC trial): multicentre, randomised controlled trial. Lancet. 2005;365(9472):1718–26.
15. van der Pas MH, Haglind E, Cuesta MA, Fürst A, Lacy AM, Hop WC, et al. Laparoscopic versus open surgery for rectal cancer (COLOR II): short-term outcomes of a randomised, phase 3 trial. Lancet Oncol. 2013;14(3):210–8.
16. Scarpinata R, Aly EH. Does robotic rectal cancer surgery offer improved early postoperative outcomes? Dis Colon Rectum. 2013;56(2):253–62.
17. Sohn W, Lee HJ, Ahlering TE. Robotic surgery: review of prostate and bladder cancer. Cancer J. 2013;19(2):133–9.
18. Orady M, Hrynewych A, Nawfal AK, Wegienka G. Comparison of robotic-assisted hysterectomy to other minimally invasive approaches. JSLS. 2012;16(4):542–8.
19. Bokhari MB, Patel CB, Ramos-Valadez DI, Ragupathi M, Haas EM. Learning curve for robotic-assisted laparoscopic colorectal surgery. Surg Endosc. 2011;25(3):855–60.
20. Park JS, Choi GS, Lim KH, Jang YS, Jun SH. Robotic-assisted versus laparoscopic surgery for low rectal cancer: case-matched analysis of short-term outcomes. Ann Surg Oncol. 2010;17(12):3195–202.
21. Park YA, Kim JM, Kim SA, Min BS, Kim NK, Sohn SK, et al. Totally robotic surgery for rectal cancer: from splenic flexure to pelvic floor in one setup. Surg Endosc. 2010;24(3):715–20.
22. Hellan M, Stein H, Pigazzi A. Totally robotic low anterior resection with total mesorectal excision and splenic flexure mobilization. Surg Endosc. 2009;23(2):447–51.
23. Farello GA, Cerofolini A, Rebonato M, Bergamaschi G, Ferrari C, Chiappetta A. Congenital choledochal cyst: video-guided laparoscopic treatment. Surg Laparosc Endosc. 1995;5(5):354–8.
24. Gagner M, Pomp A. Laparoscopic pancreatic resection: is it worthwhile? J Gastrointest Surg. 1997;1(1):20–5. discussion 25–6
25. Kendrick ML. Laparoscopic and robotic resection for pancreatic cancer. Cancer J. 2012;18(6):571–6.
26. Liao CH, Wu YT, Liu YY, Wang SY, Kang SC, Yeh CN, et al. Systemic review of the feasibility and advantage of minimally invasive pancreaticoduodenectomy. World J Surg. 2016;40(5):1218–25.

27. Cirocchi R, Partelli S, Trastulli S, Coratti A, Parisi A, Falconi M. A systematic review on robotic pancreaticoduodenectomy. Surg Oncol. 2013;22(4):238–46.
28. Eyraud R, Laydner H, Autorino R, Hillyer S, Long J-A, Panumatrassamee K, et al. Robot-assisted transrectal hybrid natural orifice translumenal endoscopic surgery nephrectomy and adrenalectomy: initial investigation in a cadaver model. Urology. 2013;81(5):1090–4.
29. Zou X, Zhang G, Xiao R, Yuan Y, Wu G, Wang X, et al. Transvaginal natural orifice transluminal endoscopic surgery (NOTES)-assisted laparoscopic adrenalectomy: first clinical experience. Surg Endosc. 2011;25(12):3767–72.
30. Leung U, Kuk D, D'Angelica MI, Kingham TP, Allen PJ, DeMatteo RP, et al. Long-term outcomes following microwave ablation for liver malignancies. Br J Surg. 2015;102(1):85–91.
31. Nadler RB, Perry KT, Smith ND. Hybrid laparoscopic and robotic ultrasound-guided radiofrequency ablation-assisted clampless partial nephrectomy. Urology. 2009;74(1):202–5.
32. Rimar K, Khambati A, McGuire BB, Rebuck DA, Perry KT, Nadler RB. Radiofrequency ablation-assisted zero-ischemia robotic laparoscopic partial nephrectomy: oncologic and functional outcomes in 49 patients. Adv Urol. 2016;2016:8045210.
33. Wu SD, Viprakasit DP, Cashy J, Smith ND, Perry KT, Nadler RB. Radiofrequency ablation-assisted robotic laparoscopic partial nephrectomy without renal hilar vessel clamping versus laparoscopic partial nephrectomy: a comparison of perioperative outcomes. J Endourol. 2010;24(3):385–91.

Part II

Urologic Procedures

11 Robot-Assisted Partial Nephrectomy

Jaspreet Singh Parihar and Clayton Lau

Background

In the United States, the annual incidence of renal cancers is approximately 61,560, and 14,080 die of the disease. The lifetime probability of developing invasive renal cancer is 2% in males and 1.2% in females [1]. Although recent advances in systemic and targeted immunotherapies have improved long-term survival in patients, surgical extirpation still offers the best chance for cure in localized disease. Other treatment approaches such as active surveillance, radiofrequency ablation, and cryotherapy may be appropriate for patients who are unfit for surgery or who have competing comorbidities. Surgical options for renal tumors include partial and radical nephrectomy. Nephron-sparing surgery (NSS), as allowed by the tumor characteristics and patient comorbidities, is the preferred approach for small renal masses. NSS may delay the onset of chronic kidney disease, associated cardiovascular events, and mortality, while providing equivalent oncologic results [2, 3]. Partial nephrectomy has become the standard of care for T1 tumors (≤7 cm in size).

Compared with traditional open surgery, minimally invasive techniques allow for reduced ischemia time, decreased intraoperative blood loss, and shorter length of hospitalization, while maintaining similar functional and oncologic outcomes [3–7]. Whereas pure laparoscopic approaches present technical challenges for tumor excision and subsequent renal reconstruction, robot-assisted techniques allow surgeons to overcome these limitations. In 2001, Guillonneau et al. [8] were the initial group of surgeons using a robot to perform nephrectomy. The feasibility of robot-assisted partial nephrectomy was reported by Gettman et al. [9] in 2004. Since then, wide adoption of robotic surgical systems has in turn facilitated an increase in the utilization of nephron-sparing techniques [10, 11].

J. S. Parihar, MD
Division of Urology and Urologic Oncology, City of Hope National Medical Center, Duarte, CA, USA
e-mail: jparihar@coh.org

C. Lau, MD (✉)
Department of Surgery, City of Hope National Medical Center, Duarte, CA, USA
e-mail: cllau@coh.org

Patient Selection

In general, patients must be able to tolerate pneumoperitoneum for several hours, typically in a modified lateral decubitus position. In cases of severe cardiopulmonary disease or prior surgeries suggesting a difficult surgical abdomen, any minimally invasive approach may be challenging, if not prohibitory. Any coagulopathies should be corrected prior to surgery. The tumor characteristics can be analyzed through objective parameters using renal scoring systems. One example is the RENAL nephrometry score, which measures the (R)adius (the maximal diameter in centimeters), (E)xophytic/Endophytic properties, (N)earness of the tumor to collecting system (in millimeters), (A)nterior/Posterior, and (L)ocation relative to polar lines. These strategies, patient preferences, and the surgeon's experience all help in selecting the optimal patient for the optimal operation.

Room Setup and Patient Positioning

For a safe and efficient setup, surgical equipment should be ideally positioned to facilitate the operating workflow. In general, the bedside assistant should have a clear view and access to the patient and to the scrub nurse, to facilitate passage of needles, instruments, etc. Additionally, an open surgical/vascular instrument tray should be readily available in case of an emergent conversion.

We describe our specific techniques of patient positioning. Following intubation on the operative table, a Foley catheter is placed. An oral gastric tube is selectively utilized; it may aid in surgical exposure, especially for left-sided upper pole lesions. The operative site is prepared, and any previous surgical scars or hernias are noted. The patient is then placed in a modified lateral decubitus position (approximately 70°)

Y. Fong et al. (eds.), *The SAGES Atlas of Robotic Surgery*, https://doi.org/10.1007/978-3-319-91045-1_11

with the operative side up. The patient is then well padded, with an axillary roll and two gel log rolls supporting the patient's back. The lower leg is flexed, with three pillows between the legs and additional padding placed at the lower knee and ankle joints. The ipsilateral arm remains on the patient's side and is supported with a log roll prepared with one or two rolled blankets. The patient is then flexed at the anterior superior iliac spine (ASIS) joint and gently secured to the operating table using tape/straps. A lower-body warmer such as a 3 M™ Bair Hugger™ is utilized.

Port Placement and Instruments

Pneumoperitoneum is routinely established using a Veress needle introduced at the umbilicus. We consistently use a SurgiQuest AirSeal insufflation system to maintain an intraperitoneal pressure of 15 mm Hg. Depending on surgeon preference, various port positioning setups can be used. We commonly use either a "Dice-5" configuration using the da Vinci standard four-arm approach (da Vinci Si) or a linear port placement in the pararectus space (da Vinci Xi) with all instruments more than 6 cm apart. After pneumoperitoneum is established, a 5-mm Visiport trocar (US Surgical) is introduced with a 0-degree lens and laparoscopic camera. This port is eventually exchanged for a 12-mm robotic camera port (8 mm if using da Vinci Xi). Subsequently, three robotic 8-mm trocars are inserted under direct vision: monopolar curved scissors in the right arm, fenestrated bipolar forceps in the left arm, and ProGrasp forceps or Tip-Up Fenestrated Grasper or Double Fenestrated Grasper (da Vinci Xi) in the fourth arm. Two assistant ports are typically used (two 10-mm ports or a 10-mm and a 5-mm port), with an additional 5-mm port used for a subxiphoid liver retractor for right-sided cases. The da Vinci Xi robot allows for more consistent and efficient docking and less arm clashing. This is especially true in those patients with short torsos.

Key Operative Steps

Reflection of the Colon

We describe our transperitoneal operative techniques. Posteriorly located renal tumors may also be approached via retroperitoneal access with the aid of dissector systems such as SpaceMaker™ (Covidien). Following placement of ports and instruments, the colon is identified and reflected medially over the kidney along the white line of Toldt. An avascular plane is further developed between the anterior Gerota's fascia and the mesenteric fat of the reflected colon. As a distinguishing feature, Gerota's fascia appears pale yellow, compared with the brighter yellow color of the mesentery. We prefer a wide reflection of the colon down to the iliac vessels in the pelvis, allowing for clear identification of gonadal vessels and the ureter. Furthermore, for right-sided cases, the duodenum is kocherized medially to identify the anterior surface of the inferior vena cava (Fig. 11.1).

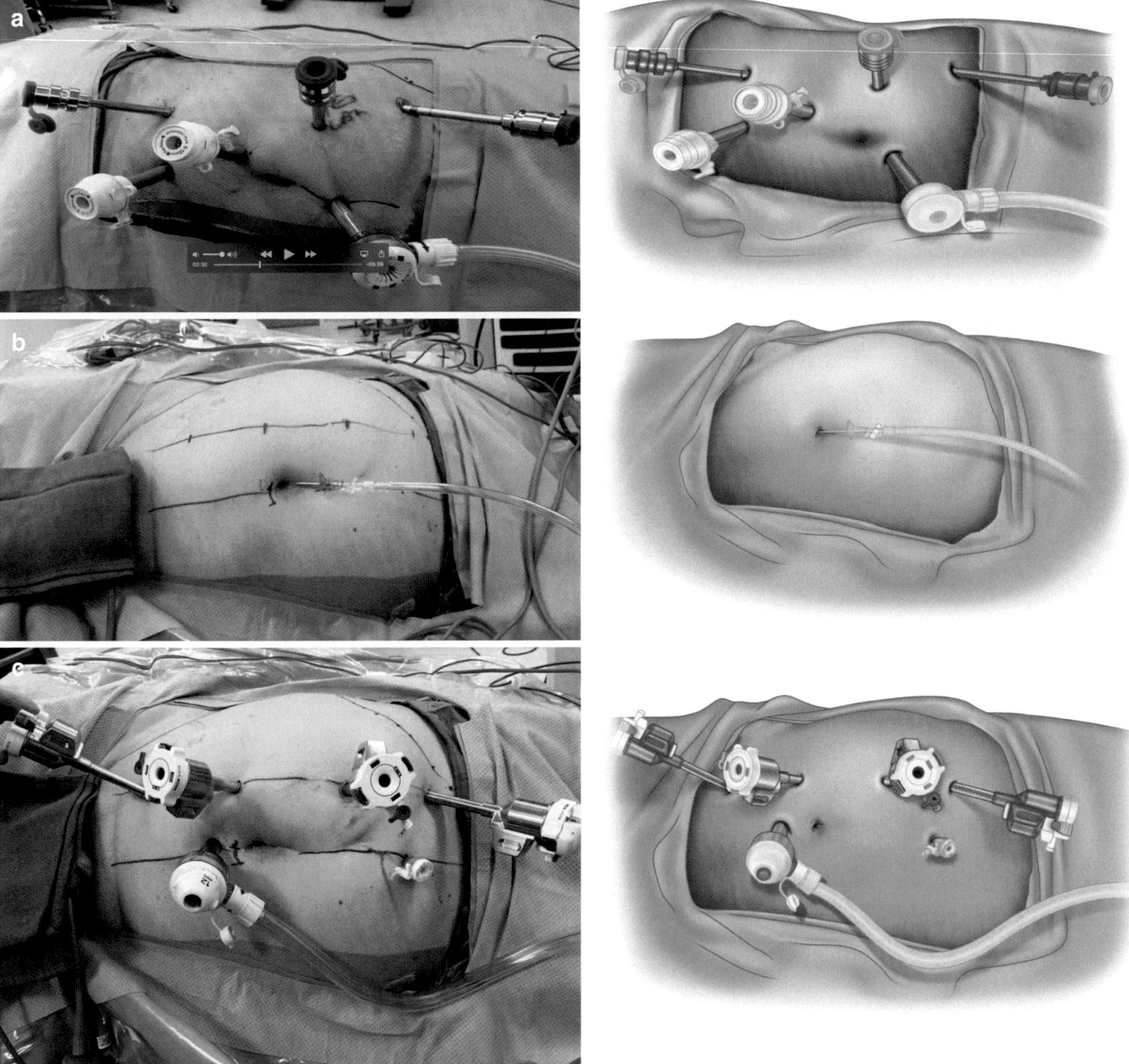

Fig. 11.1 (**a**) Dice-5 port placement for robot-assisted renal surgeries, with the patient's head toward the left. (**b**, **c**) Straight-line port placement for robot-assisted renal surgeries using the da Vinci Xi platform. The patient's head is toward the right

Hilar Exposure

One of the critical steps in obtaining safe and adequate exposure to the renal hilum is lateral and anterior retraction of the kidney, which can be achieved by starting dissection caudal to the inferior pole of the kidney to identify the ureter, gonadal vessels, and underlying psoas muscle. For left-sided cases, the ureter and gonadal vessels, both invested in Gerota's fascia, are retracted using the fourth arm instrument. In right-sided cases, the ureter is isolated, leaving behind the gonadal vein next to the inferior vena cava. This maneuver prevents inadvertent avulsion of gonadal vein from inferior vena cava (IVC). With appropriate hilar retraction, the gonadal vein (left-side cases) or the IVC (right-side cases) can be traced toward the renal vein. The renal vein is usually anterior to the artery and renal pelvis, although vascular variations may exist. An anatomical study of 100 embalmed kidneys revealed hilar variations in up to three fourths of cases, and variant patterns were more common on the left side [12]. The most common variation is multiple renal arteries, occurring in up to 25–30% of patients [13, 14]. With anterolaterally retraction of the kidney with the 4th arm, the renal hilum will be stretched and facilitate easier exposure of the renal artery posteriorly. On the left side the lumbar vein could hide the exposure of the left renal artery, therefore may need to be addressed with bipolar grasper and monopolar scissors or a vessel sealer.

Renal Dissection

Upper pole dissection of hepatorenal ligaments can be useful if further renal mobilization is required to access the tumor or to plan for reconstruction following excision. Division of splenorenal attachments also increases the working space at the upper pole and helps to identify the renal hilum. In general, unless adrenal tissue is grossly involved, it may be spared. The kidney is mobilized outside of Gerota's fascia, followed by defatting of perinephric fat around the tumor site. We routinely employ a drop-in ultrasound probe (Hitachi Aloka or BK ultrasound) to identify and isolate tumor lesion(s). Intraoperative ultrasound imaging provides excellent visualization and measurements of both exophytic and endophytic tumor configurations. Additionally, it may identify any satellite tumor lesions and help in planning the surgical resection.

Tumor Excision and Renorrhaphy

Prior to hilar clamping, the planned margin of excision is marked on the surface of the renal capsule using cautery. Intraoperative ultrasound may be used to define the margins of the tumor and its extent into the renal parenchyma. Intravenous mannitol may be administered to aid in osmotic diuresis. The renorrhaphy sutures can now be introduced and temporarily situated near the operative field. Alternatively, the sutures can be placed after the excision takes place if the surgeon feels that the suture may get in the way while extirpating the lesion. During excision, the assistant can help expose and maintain countertraction using a suction device and a laparoscopic peanut instrument (Fig. 11.2).

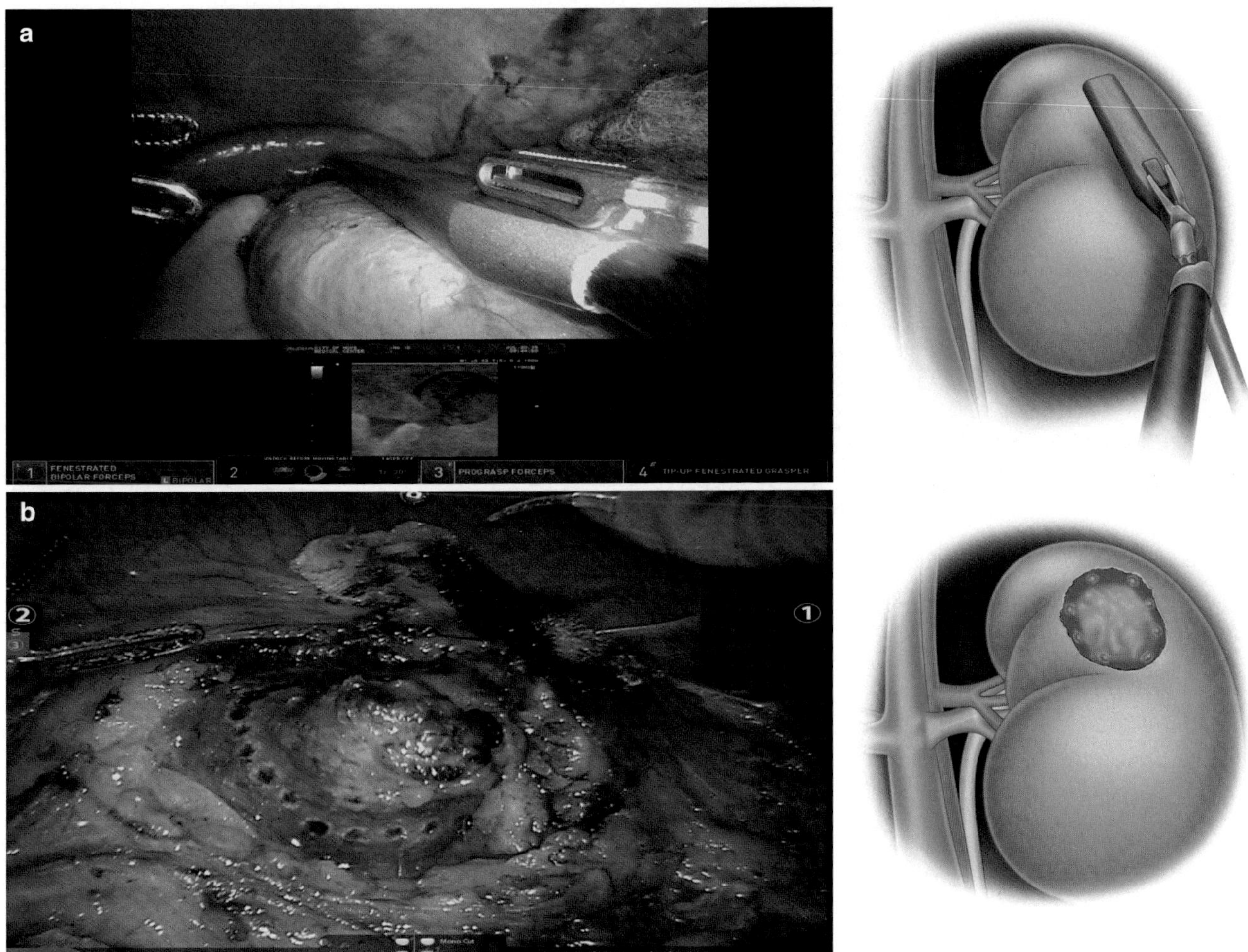

Fig. 11.2 Planning site of excision. (**a**) Using a drop-in ultrasound probe, the tumor lesion is identified. (**b**) Excision is planned, with marking of the margin around the tumor

Excision begins following the clamping of the renal hilum. Typically, the renal artery and vein are isolated individually, to allow individual clamping during temporary ischemia required for excision. Our practice is to commonly use a curved clamp followed by a straight bulldog vascular clamp on the artery alone, placed by the bedside assistant (Fig. 11.3).

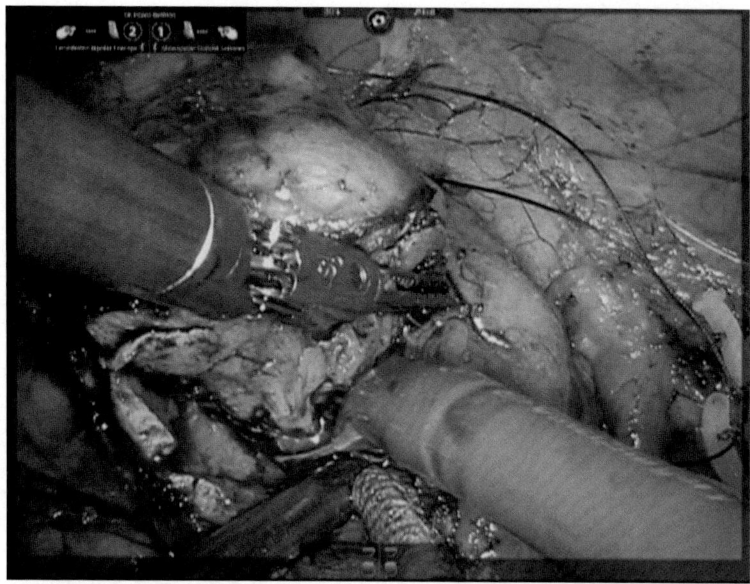

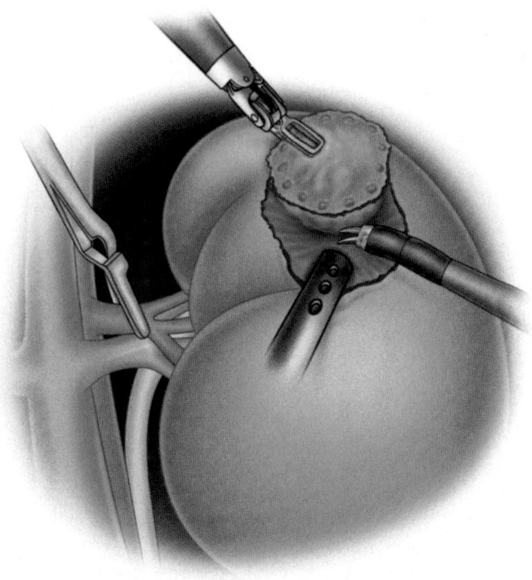

Fig. 11.3 Tumor excision. Tumor is excised using monopolar scissors, ensuring a margin of normal tissue

Tumor excision can be started using monopolar cautery through the renal cortex, followed by sharp excision around the tumor including a margin of normal tissue. Following tumor excision, the inner surface of the renal defect can be oversewn using a running suture such as 3-0 V-Loc V20 needle (Covidien) secured at the cortical edges using Weck® Hem-o-lok® clips on each end. The cortical layer is then reapproximated using an 0-Vicryl CT-1 needle or V-Loc GS-21 needle in simple or horizontal mattress fashion, with ends secured with Hem-o-lok® clips, using sliding renorrhaphy technique [7, 15]. After ensuring hemostasis, the vascular clamps are then removed. Additional cortical reapproximation sutures can be placed if necessary.

In some cases, selective vascular clamping or even off-clamp excisions may provide sufficient visualization to allow complete tumor resection. Near infrared fluorescence imaging following intravenous administration of indocyanine green (ICG) highlights the vasculature and may aid in surgical dissection of the vascular pedicle. Also it could be used to confirm ischemia, and in cases of selective clamping (Fig. 11.4) [16, 17].

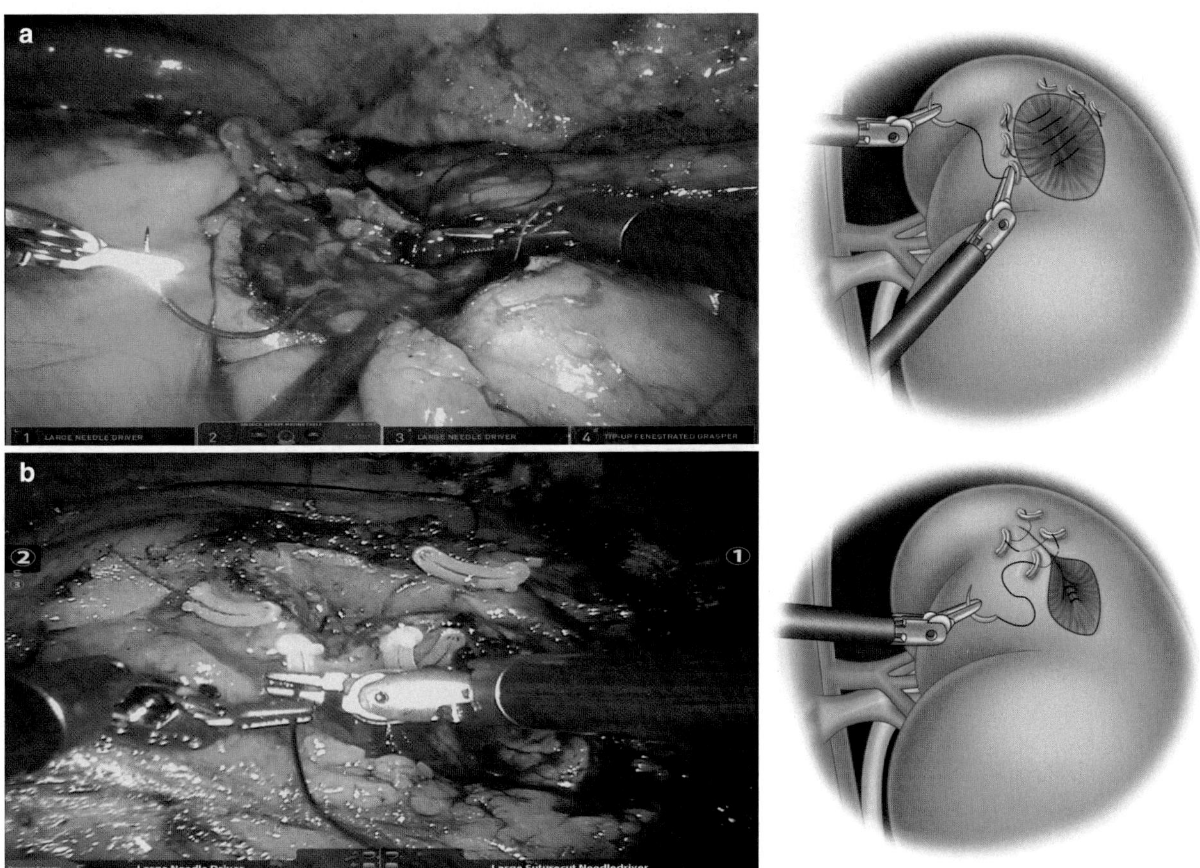

Fig. 11.4 Renorrhaphy. Following excision, renorrhaphy is completed using two-layer closure (**a**) and sliding renorrhaphy technique (**b**)

Specimen Extraction

The tumor specimen can be placed in an endoscopic retrieval bag and extracted through the 12-mm assistant port or the fourth arm port site. Following fascial closure, the abdomen may be reinsufflated to ensure hemostasis and to allow for perioperative drain placement, if appropriate. Hemostatic agents such as Surgiflo® (Ethicon), BioGlue® (CryoLife), or Evicel® (Ethicon) may be applied as per surgeon preference (Fig. 11.5).

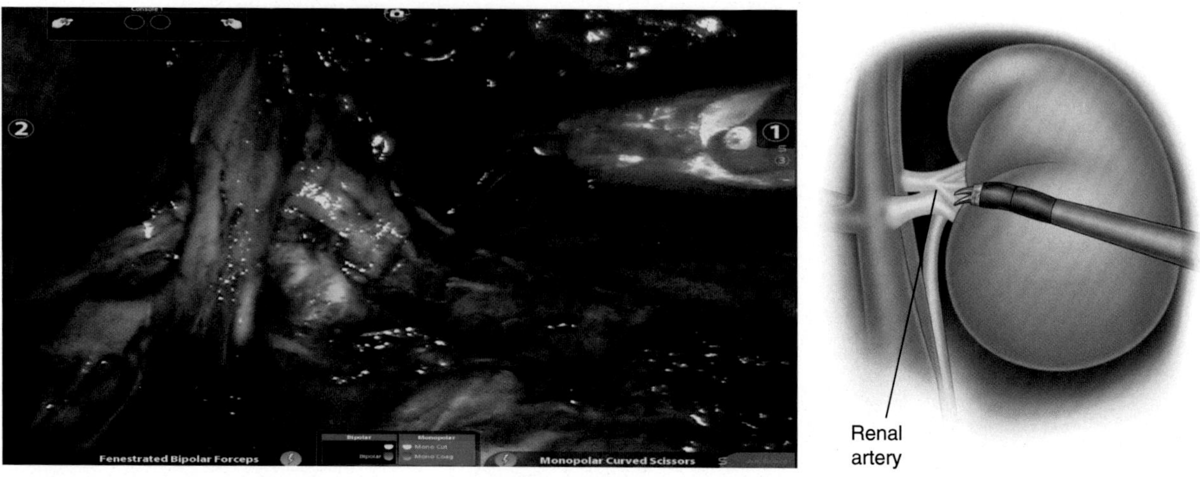

Fig. 11.5 Near infrared fluorescence imaging using indocyanine green (ICG). Following ICG administration, the renal hilar vasculature can be easily distinguished using the FireFly fluorescence imaging system

Outcomes

A 5-year periodic review after integrating robot-assisted partial nephrectomies into our institutional robotics program demonstrated acceptable operational, oncologic, and renal function outcomes. During the study period, we treated 92 patients with tumors ranging in size up to more than 8 cm. Despite increased complexity of tumors and treatment of multiple lesions, our operative and warm ischemia times were reduced [18]. With increasing surgical experience, our perioperative outcomes continue to improve. To this date we have done over 500 robotic partial nephrectomies.

Conclusion

This chapter has described the utility of robotically-assisted techniques in treating renal cancers. We described our specific techniques of robot-assisted partial nephrectomy and our perioperative measures to improve patient outcomes. We have found these techniques to be reliable and reproducible among surgeons across our institution. Regardless of the specific techniques used, sound surgical and oncologic principles should be followed to ensure patient safety and treatment success.

References

1. Siegel RL, Miller KD, Jemal A. Cancer statistics, 2015. CA Cancer J Clin. 2015;65:5–29.
2. Go AS, Chertow GM, Fan D, McCulloch CE, Hsu CY. Chronic kidney disease and the risks of death, cardiovascular events, and hospitalization. N Engl J Med. 2004;351:1296–305.
3. Mashni JW, Assel M, Maschino A, Russo M, Masi B, Bernstein M, et al. New chronic kidney disease and overall survival after nephrectomy for small renal cortical tumors. Urology. 2015;86:1137–45.
4. Gill IS, Kavoussi LR, Lane BR, Blute ML, Babineau D, Colombo JR Jr, et al. Comparison of 1,800 laparoscopic and open partial nephrectomies for single renal tumors. J Urol. 2007;178:41–6.
5. Lane BR, Gill IS. 7-year oncological outcomes after laparoscopic and open partial nephrectomy. J Urol. 2010;183:473–9.
6. Boylu U, Basatac C, Yildirim U, Onol FF, Gumus E. Comparison of surgical, functional, and oncological outcomes of open and robot-assisted partial nephrectomy. J Minim Access Surg. 2015;11:72–7.
7. Benway BM, Wang AJ, Cabello JM, Bhayani SB. Robotic partial nephrectomy with sliding-clip renorrhaphy: technique and outcomes. Eur Urol. 2009;55:592–9.
8. Guillonneau B, Jayet C, Tewari A, Vallancien G. Robot assisted laparoscopic nephrectomy. J Urol. 2001;166:200–1.
9. Gettman MT, Blute ML, Chow GK, Neururer R, Bartsch G, Peschel R. Robotic-assisted laparoscopic partial nephrectomy: technique and initial clinical experience with DaVinci robotic system. Urology. 2004;64:914–8.
10. Ghani KR, Sukumar S, Sammon JD, Rogers CG, Trinh QD, Menon M. Practice patterns and outcomes of open and minimally invasive partial nephrectomy since the introduction of robotic partial nephrectomy: results from the nationwide inpatient sample. J Urol. 2014;191:907–12.
11. Schiavina R, Mari A, Antonelli A, Bertolo R, Bianchi G, Borghesi M, et al. A snapshot of nephron-sparing surgery in Italy: a prospective, multicenter report on clinical and perioperative outcomes (the RECORd 1 project). Eur J Surg Oncol. 2015;41:346–52.
12. Trivedi SA, Kotgiriwar S. Normal and variant anatomy of renal hilar structures and its clinical significance. Int J Morphol. 2011;29: 1379–83.
13. Merklin RJ, Michels NA. The variant renal and suprarenal blood supply with data on the inferior phrenic, ureteral and gonadal arteries: a statistical analysis based on 185 dissections and review of the literature. J Int Coll Surg. 1958;29:41–76.
14. Boijsen E. Angiographic studies of the anatomy of single and multiple renal arteries. Acta Radiol Suppl. 1959;183:1–135.
15. Benway BM, Cabello JM, Figenshau RS, Bhayani SB. Sliding-clip renorrhaphy provides superior closing tension during robot-assisted partial nephrectomy. J Endourol. 2010;24:605–8.
16. Krane LS, Manny TB, Hemal AK. Is near infrared fluorescence imaging using indocyanine green dye useful in robotic partial nephrectomy: a prospective comparative study of 94 patients. Urology. 2012;80:110–6.
17. Tobis S, Knopf JK, Silvers C, Messing E, Yao J, Rashid H, et al. Robot-assisted and laparoscopic partial nephrectomy with near infrared fluorescence imaging. J Endourol. 2012;26:797–802.
18. Yuh B, Muldrew S, Menchaca A, Yip W, Lau C, Wilson T, Josephson D. Integrating robotic partial nephrectomy to an existing robotic surgery program. Can J Urol. 2012;19:6193–200.

12 Robot-Assisted Radical Prostatectomy

Bertram Yuh and Greg Gin

Radical prostatectomy (RP) is the surgical removal of the prostate and seminal vesicles for the treatment of prostate cancer. The National Comprehensive Cancer Network (NCCN) recommends RP as an option for men in all risk groups of localized disease. With an initial series dating back to 2001, robot-assisted radical prostatectomy (RARP) was one of the earliest robotic procedures to reach clinical practice and remains one of the most commonly performed [1]. From a technical and procedural standpoint, the transperitoneal approach to RARP represents a paradigm shift away from traditional open retropubic RP. Over time, refinements to the surgical technique have evolved, although basic principles of RARP have endured. The widespread dissemination of RARP worldwide has continued despite a scarcity of high-level evidence for its superiority compared to other surgical approaches. Outcomes exceeding 10 years post RARP have now been published reporting biochemical recurrence-free survival of 73% and cancer-specific survival of 99% [2]. A systematic review of the literature showed reduced blood loss and transfusion rates with RARP with possible improvements in continence and potency recovery [3–5].

Patient Selection

Patients who are candidates for other surgical approaches such as open or laparoscopic RP would generally also be considered candidates for RARP. However, since Trendelenburg positioning is typically used for the procedure, patients with certain neurologic or cardiopulmonary comorbidities may not be ideal candidates. Cases that can present more of a technical challenge include patients with morbid obesity, patients with previous prostate surgery such as transurethral resection of the prostate (TURP), those with a large median lobe or bulky high-stage tumors, and those who have had previous pelvic surgery or radiation.

Room Setup and Positioning

Antibiotic prophylaxis is recommended with first- or second-generation cephalosporins, if possible. Patients are placed on the operating room table supine with legs in stirrups or in the split-leg position. Sequential compression devices are used, and the buttocks are positioned at the very end of the table. Foam padding secured to the table can help prevent the patient from sliding cephalad. The arms are tucked to the side and padded. The table is then shifted into the Trendelenburg position to allow the bowel to fall away from the pelvis and increase instrument working space. Patients are prepped from the chest to the mid-thigh and then draped. A Foley catheter is inserted sterilely. Because patients in the extreme Trendelenburg position for prolonged periods of time develop increased intraocular pressure, an alternative that may reduce this risk is a modified Z-Trendelenburg position [6].

Port Placement

Port placement depends on whether a transperitoneal or extraperitoneal approach is used. Figure 12.1 depicts some examples of port placements, depending on approach and assistant side preference. While either approach is suitable in experienced hands, the transperitoneal technique is more commonly performed. The extraperitoneal approach may reduce operative time but is associated with higher CO_2 reabsorption and risk of acidosis [7, 8]. Trocars are typically placed at least a handbreadth apart in order to prevent internal and external clashing of instruments. Since the bedside assistant is a critical member of the operative team, optimization of assistant ports is also important. Assistant ports may be placed either on the right or left side of the patient.

B. Yuh, MD, MSHCPM, MISM (✉)
Division of Urology and Urologic Oncology, City of Hope Comprehensive Cancer Center, Duarte, CA, USA
e-mail: byuh@coh.org

G. Gin, MD
VA Long Beach Healthcare System, Long Beach, CA, USA

Y. Fong et al. (eds.), *The SAGES Atlas of Robotic Surgery*, https://doi.org/10.1007/978-3-319-91045-1_12

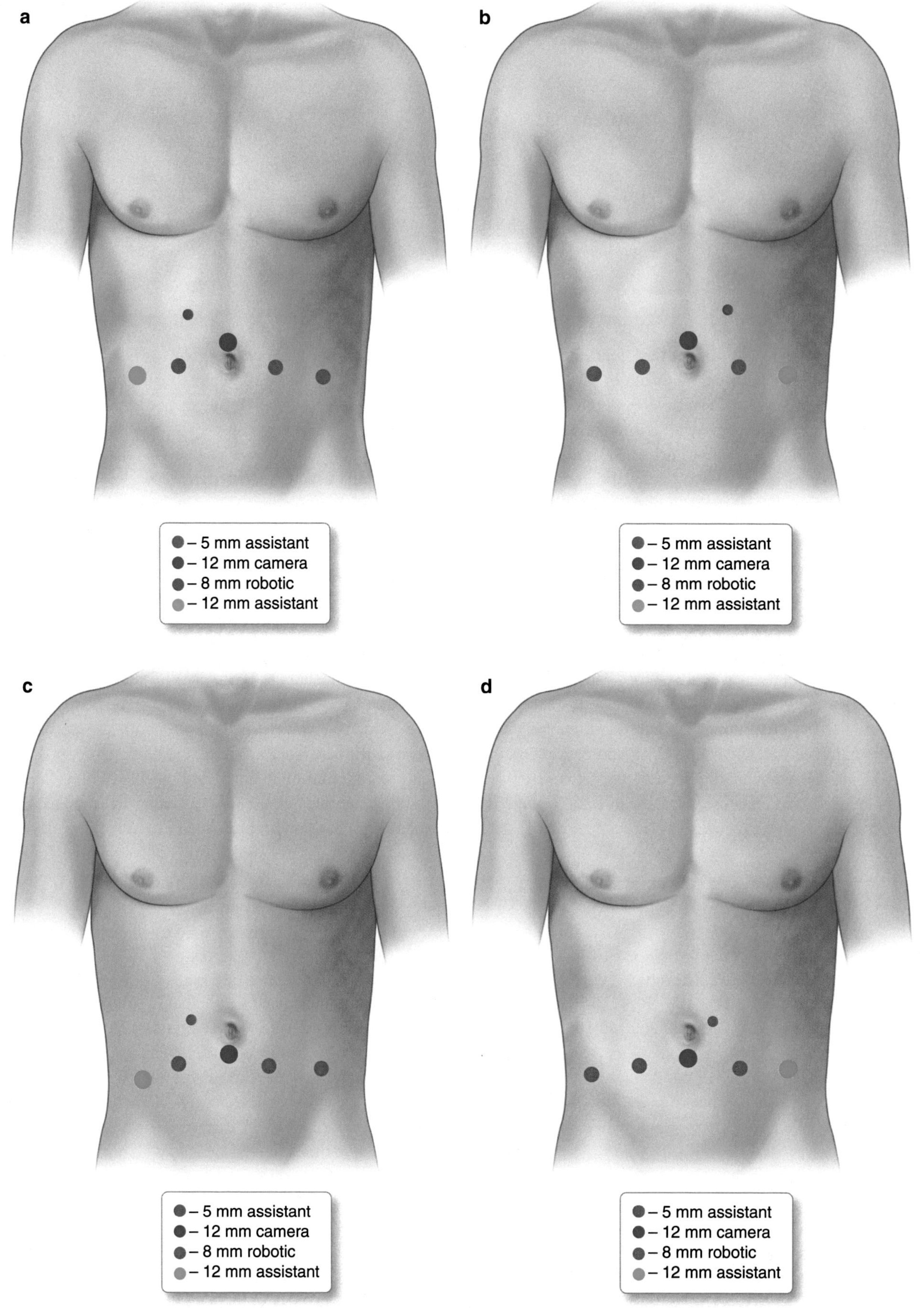

Fig. 12.1 Port placements for robot-assisted radical prostatectomy. (**a**) Transperitoneal with right assistant ports. (**b**) Transperitoneal with left assistant ports. (**c**) Extraperitoneal with right assistant ports. (**d**) Extraperitoneal with left assistant ports (Camera ports may also be 8 mm if Da Vinci Xi robot is used)

Transperitoneal

Pneumoperitoneum can be attained using a Veress needle or with the open access Hassan technique. Generally the camera port is placed above the umbilicus except in patients with excessive distance between the pelvis and umbilicus (>25 cm). Once the camera is inserted, the other ports are placed under direct vision. Three robotic ports and two assistant ports are placed as indicated (Fig. 12.1a, b). For the suction to reach the pelvis from the upper assistant port, an extra-long suction tube is needed. The view of the pelvis from a transperitoneal approach can be seen in (Fig. 12.2).

Extraperitoneal

Extraperitoneal access is first obtained through a skin incision routinely made below the umbilicus. Through this incision, the posterior rectus sheath is developed and the preperitoneal space is further expanded using blunt dissection and a balloon dissector. Once the space is sufficient, robotic ports are placed similarly under direct vision (Fig. 12.1c, d).

For both transperitoneal and extraperitoneal surgeries, the pneumoperitoneum is usually maintained at 15 mm Hg but can be increased during active or anticipated bleeding or decreased in order to monitor for hemostasis or prevent cardiopulmonary effects of pneumoperitoneum. The robot is then docked between the legs or alternatively alongside the patient [9]. When using the Xi robot, side docking is used. Also an 8-mm robotic cannula is substituted for the camera port.

Steps of Operation

Dissection of the Vas Deferens, Seminal Vesicles, and Posterior Prostate

This stage of the procedure involves dissection and removal of the vas deferens and seminal vesicles as well as mobilizing the prostate off the rectum. It can be performed initially or after bladder neck transection. Of importance is complete or partial removal of the seminal vesicles, depending on disease stratification.

Posterior Approach

If performed initially, an incision is made in the peritoneum at the rectovesical pouch a few centimeters above the visualized rectum (Fig. 12.3). This starting point often can be confirmed by following the course of the vas deferens as it courses behind the peritoneum. The incision is deepened through areolar tissue following a plane below the vas deferens and seminal vesicles. The posterior plane can be developed superficial to

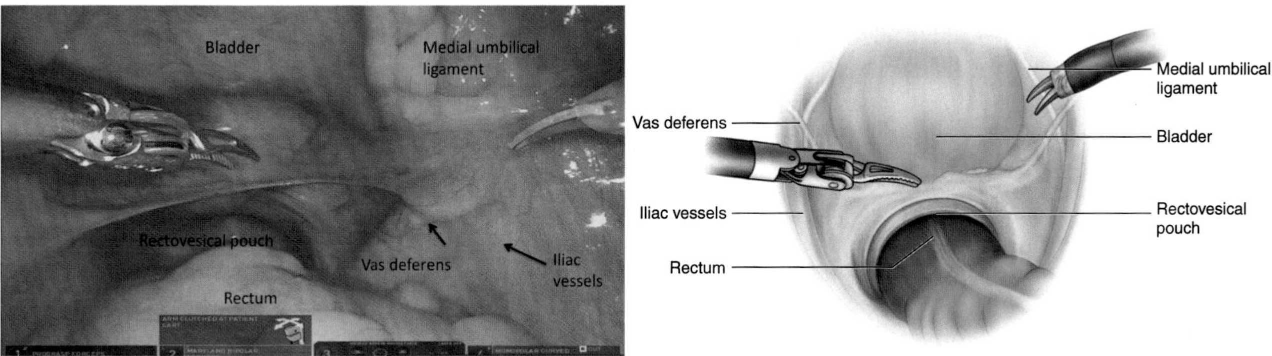

Fig. 12.2 Initial anatomic view of the pelvis with transperitoneal robot-assisted radical prostatectomy

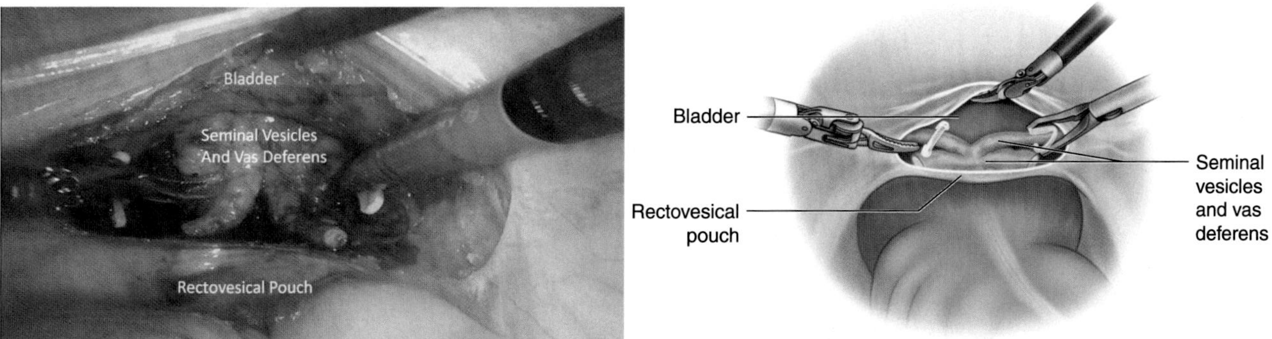

Fig. 12.3 Dissection of the vas deferens and seminal vesicles through a posterior approach

the posterior layer of Denonvilliers fascia in lower-risk disease or completely below the fascia in higher-risk disease. Once the posterior plane is sufficiently created, the anterior surface of the ampulla of the vas deferens and seminal vesicles is dissected in order to clearly visualize the anatomic boundaries of the seminal vesicles. The vas deferens is divided laterally, and the dissection continues around the tip and lateral border of the seminal vesicles up toward the base of the prostate. This dissection can be performed without cautery with the aid of clips to prevent thermal injury to adjacent structures.

Anterior Approach

If not performed initially but instead approached after bladder neck transection, the anterior layer of Denonvilliers fascia covering the vas deferens and seminal vesicles is incised. This exposes the structures for dissection. Upward traction of the prostate using the fourth robotic arm or assistant allows for dissection around the edges of the seminal vesicles. Once the vasa are dissected and mobilized, they can also be used as a handle for the seminal vesicle dissection. After division of the vasa, dissection proceeds around the lateral edge of the seminal vesicles, continuing toward the base of the prostate.

Dissection behind the Prostate

The dissection posterior to the prostate is a critical step of RARP, in particular when treating high-volume, bulky tumors or patients who have had previous radiation therapy. Since the intent is to avoid inadvertent injury to the rectum, limited use of cautery to optimize visualization of the perirectal fat plane is prudent. The plane posteriorly is developed sharply and bluntly all the way to the apex of the prostate. Changing back to the zero degree lens for this portion of the operation improves the ability to dissect toward the apex. This dissection also aids in setting up the prostate pedicles and preservation of neurovascular bundles.

Development of the Retzius Space

In transperitoneal RARP, extended pelvic lymph node dissection (see Section "Pelvic Lymph Node Dissection") can be performed next; otherwise the operation proceeds with the development of the space of Retzius in patients at low risk for nodal metastases. The space is initially entered by incising the peritoneum above the dome of the bladder and lateral to the medial umbilical ligaments. This is carried down following the shape of the pelvis to the level of the pubic symphysis. Once the bladder is mobilized enough to drop below the pubic bone, the endopelvic fascia as well as the anterior prostatic fat should be easily visible. The superficial dorsal vein can be controlled with bipolar cautery and the anterior prostate fat cleared off the surface of the prostate because it occasionally harbors lymph nodes. Excising this fatty tissue also improves visualization for the subsequent dissection of the bladder neck. The endopelvic fascia can be opened at this point, although this this is optional. When opened, the incision is followed toward the puboprostatic ligaments. In up to 30% of patients, an accessory pudendal artery can be encountered during this dissection; its preservation may assist with erectile function recovery [10]. The dorsal venous complex (see Section "Dorsal Venous Complex Control") can be controlled at this time or alternatively prior to urethral transection.

Bladder Neck Dissection

Preoperative imaging with computed tomography, magnetic resonance imaging (MRI), or ultrasound can provide information about the volume and shape of the prostate as well as the presence of asymmetric lobes or an enlarged median lobe. A 30-degree down lens can assist with bladder neck dissection and in identifying the junction between the prostate and bladder. During this step, the primary goal is separation of the prostate from the bladder. The optimal dissection leaves no prostate behind so as to avoid a positive margin, cancer recurrence, or postoperative detectable prostate-specific antigen (PSA). Although magnified visualization is superb with RARP, bladder neck dissection can present challenges in that tactile feedback commonly used to identify the prostatovesical junction during open RP is lacking robotically. Also in high-risk disease or in patients with large median lobes or asymmetric prostates, determining the exact plane between prostate and bladder can be challenging.

Initially, the shape and size of the prostate is visually gauged, and the Foley balloon can be deflated to show where the collapsed bladder ends and the prostate begins. Alternatively, lifting up the bladder anteriorly with careful observation of where the catheter balloon seats when pulled back and forth can also show the junction. Early high anterior release of the neurovascular bundles is another way to prospectively identify the prostate border. Visual cues and tissue feedback are important during dissection to provide assurance of the correct dissection plane. Continued and active cranial retraction of the bladder with frequent repositioning using the fourth robotic arm also helps delineate prostate glandular tissue from the muscular bladder fibers. If the correct plane is not entered, entry into the bladder, injury to the ureters, or cutting into the prostate can occur.

Anterior Bladder Neck Dissection

Dissection is begun anteriorly through the bladder neck using cautery with a transverse incision that is deepened along the junction between bladder and prostate until the catheter is reached (Fig. 12.4). The catheter can then be deflated and retracted anteriorly using the fourth robotic arm or the assistant. The posterior bladder neck is thus identified, which allows incision through the remainder of the bladder. Identification of the trigone and ureteral orifices is important to confirm absence of injury to the ureters. Carrying this dissection through the posterior bladder neck reveals the anterior Denonvilliers fascial layer that covers the vas deferens and seminal vesicles (see Section "Dissection of the Vas Deferens, Seminal Vesicles, and Posterior Prostate") or the posterior space if dissection of the vas deferens and seminal vesicle has already been performed. In situations in which there is a large median lobe, a stitch can be used to retract the lobe out of the bladder [11].

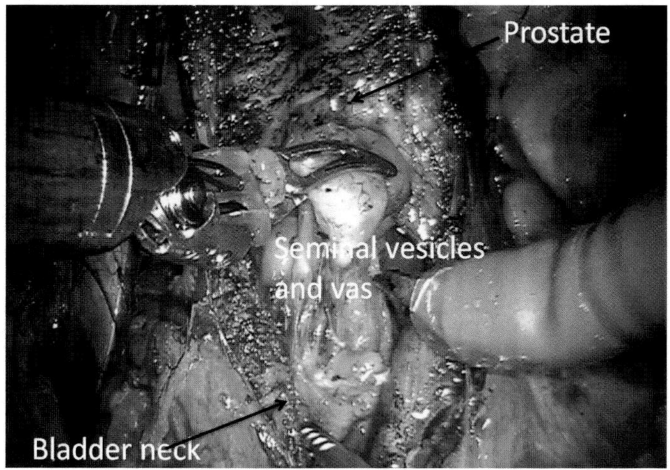

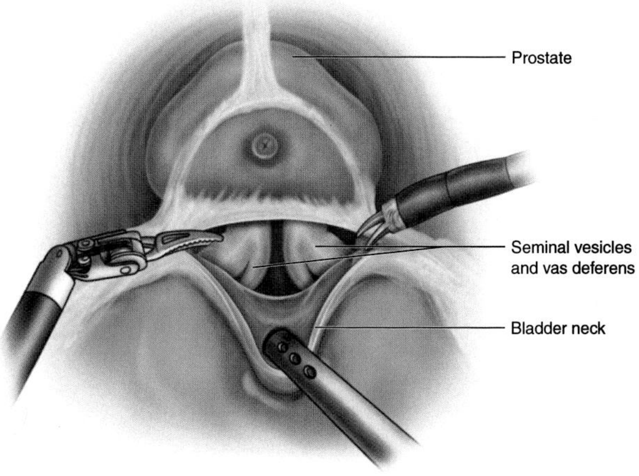

Fig. 12.4 Dissection of the vas deferens and seminal vesicles after bladder neck dissection

Perivesical Fat Space Dissection Technique

An alternative technique used for bladder neck dissection approaches the prostatovesical junction from the anterolateral direction. This blunt dissection through the perivesical fat allows for preservation of the bladder neck as it funnels into the prostate and for preemptive detection of large median lobes. The bladder is retracted with the fourth arm to the contralateral side and cephalad to expose the angle of dissection. The perivesical tissue lateral to the bladder neck is developed bluntly under direct vision until the posterior space created during seminal vesicle dissection is encountered. Laparoscopic traction to separate the prostate and bladder tissue is provided by the assistant. Next, the plane funneling to the bladder neck between the base of the prostate and the bladder neck is developed with a combination of cautery and blunt dissection. The junction of the prostate and bladder neck can be identified by the tissue differences between the bladder neck fibers and the firmer more defined prostatic tissue. The same technique is applied to the contralateral side as shown in (Fig. 12.5). Once the dissection is completed laterally and posteriorly on both sides, the anterior bladder neck is opened. The Foley catheter is retracted back into the prostatic urethra, and the posterior bladder neck is transected. This technique preserves the anatomic bladder neck. In the case of a large median lobe, the posterolateral plane can be developed around the median lobe and the bladder neck can still be preserved.

Neurovascular Bundle Preservation

Anatomic nerve sparing has been shown to improve continence and potency after surgery [12, 13]. Nerve sparing can be variably performed depending on preoperative cancer risk and stratification, patient age, and preoperative functional status. Clinical staging and tumor appearance on MRI may guide the surgeon to perform wider dissection in order to achieve an oncologic resection. While the importance of nerve sparing to functional outcomes has been well reported, preservation of the bundle should not supersede performing an oncologically sound operation.

Numerous descriptions of nerve sparing during RARP have been reported in the literature. Savera and colleagues described the neurovascular bundles as not just posterolateral nerve bundles but as a "Veil of Aphrodite" that incorporates the lateral prostatic fascia [14]. This supports using a high anterior release of the prostatic fascia to preserve the nerves in this location. Tewari described a graded nerve-sparing technique that corresponded to postoperative return of sexual function. Risk stratification by nomograms, MRI, and clinical staging can be used to determine the extent of nerve sparing for the individual patient [15].

The cavernous nerves may be injured by transection, use of the cautery, and excessive traction. Therefore the delicate nature of this portion of the operation supports minimizing handling of the bundle tissue, avoiding excessive traction on the bundle and cautery in order to prevent thermal injury to

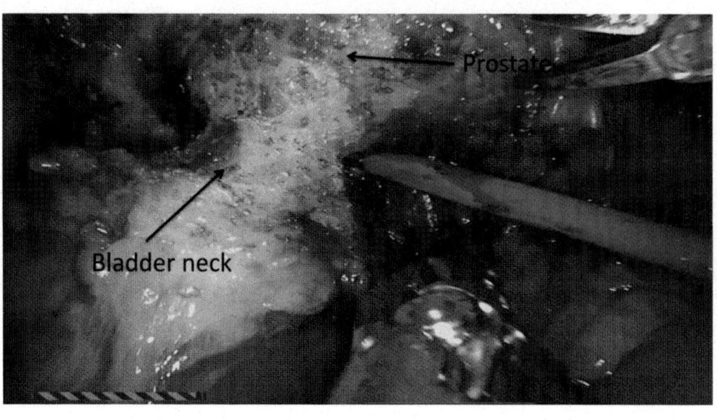

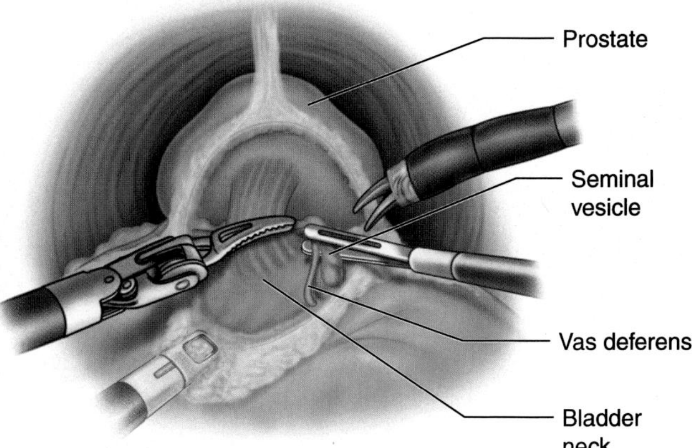

Fig. 12.5 Bladder neck dissection using a perivesical fat space dissection technique

the bundle. Nerve sparing can be performed in antegrade fashion from the bladder to the prostatic apex or in retrograde fashion from the prostatic apex to the bladder [16]. During either form of nerve sparing, intraoperative frozen sectioning, as described in the NeuroSAFE technique (Martini-Klinik, Hamburg, Germany), has been used to maximize nerve sparing while minimizing positive margins [17].

Antegrade Nerve Sparing

Using a zero-degree lens, the vasa and seminal vesicles are retracted anteriorly by the fourth arm or the assistant. The pedicles should be seen posterior and lateral with the prostate retracted anteriorly as in (Fig. 12.6). These prostate pedicles can be controlled with plastic or metallic clips. At this point, if a nerve-sparing procedure is performed, the prostatic fasciae are released high on the lateral prostate with sharp dissection. Depending on the patient's risk factors, graded nerve sparing may be performed leaving little to no tissue on the prostatic capsule. The neurovascular bundle is dropped with a combination of blunt and sharp dissection as shown in (Fig. 12.7). The dissection is continued following the contour of the prostate while continuously assessing for tissue irregularities that could suggest extracapsular disease. Toward the apex, the neurovascular bundle can be gently teased off the prostate. The lateral edge of the urethra is then visualized.

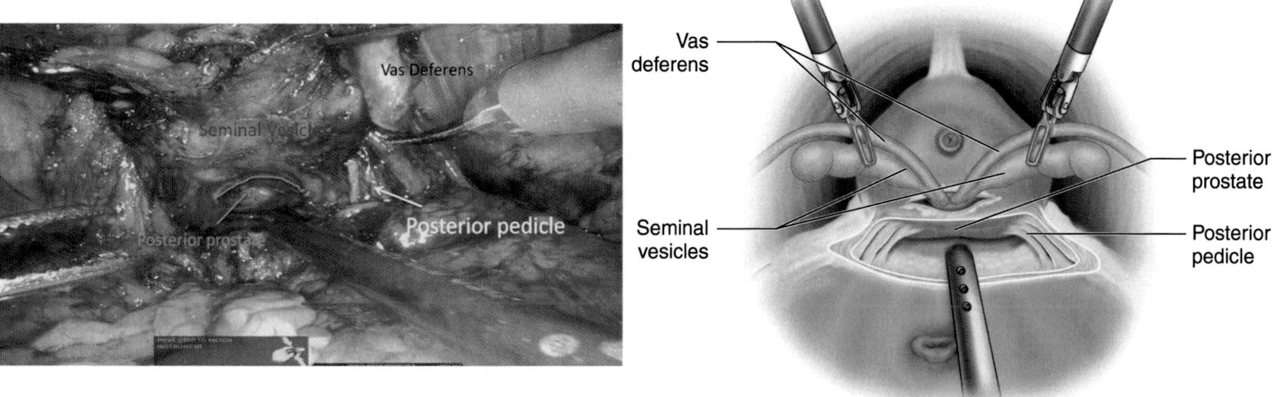

Fig. 12.6 Anterior retraction of the seminal vesicles and vas deferens in order to expose the posterior prostate and posterolateral pedicles

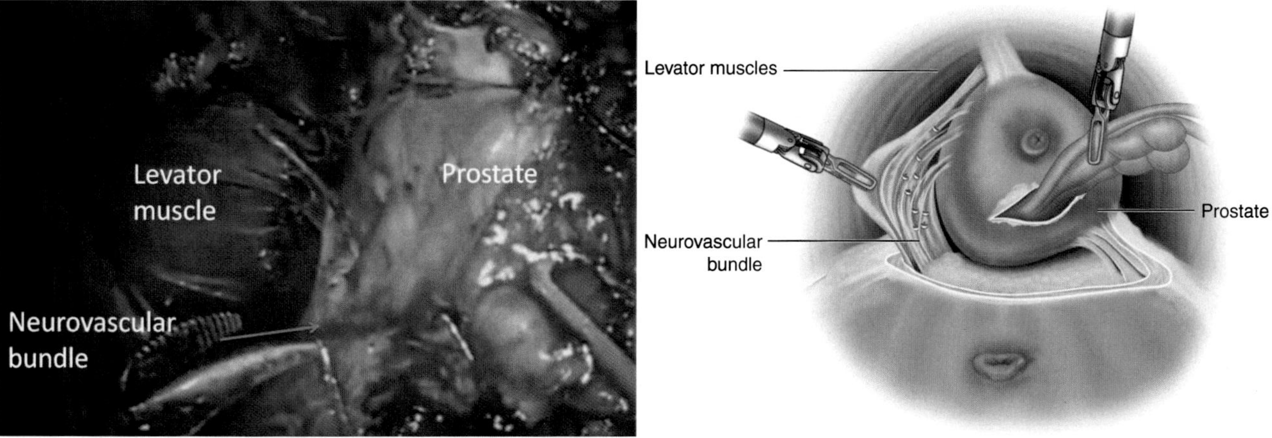

Fig. 12.7 Nerve-sparing procedure performed on the left side showing the location of the bundle relative to the levator muscles and prostate

Retrograde Nerve Sparing

With the retrograde approach, the neurovascular bundle is released anteriorly and near the apex, and the urethra is incised. Through the open urethra, the transected catheter is delivered into the pelvis and used for traction. The distal end of the catheter is cut to shorten its length. The prostate is then freed off the rectum using sharp dissection from the apex toward the base. Once the prostate pedicles are reached, these can be divided using plastic or metallic clips.

Lymph Node Dissection (LND)

Removal of lymph nodes during RP is the most accurate means of lymph node staging and assessment. Such data are important for prognosis and guiding additional therapy. In addition, LND often removes metastatic cancer, particularly with more aggressive disease. Whether this contributes to survival is as yet unknown.

The NCCN recommends that a pelvic LND be performed concomitantly if predicted probability of lymph node metastasis from nomograms is greater than or equal to 2%. The European Association of Urology guidelines recommend a LND if predicted probability is greater than 5%. Both guidelines suggest that an extended LND be performed if dissection is indicated, although the optimal extent of LND for prostate cancer also remains unknown. Balancing the real and theoretical benefits of LND against the time and comorbidity to perform the procedure is important.

Commonly used boundaries for extended LND include the common iliac artery and ureteral crossing proximally, the lateral border of the external iliac artery laterally, the bladder medially, the node of Cloquet distally, and the pelvic floor inferiorly. The use of cautery and clips may decrease the risk of lymphatic leak. A stepwise dissection from proximal to distal involves first prospectively identifying the course of the ureter as it crosses over the iliac vessels [18]. This is noted as the proximal extent of dissection. In thinner patients this may be visible through the peritoneum, but in others it may require incising the peritoneum to identify this landmark. The peritoneal incision is then carried alongside the lateral border of the external iliac artery, keeping the vas deferens tented up anteriorly. The crossing of the circumflex iliac vein over the artery is used as a distal limit. Larger lymphatics can be clipped and divided. The lymphatic tissue is then mobilized in order to skeletonize the external iliac vessels. The internal iliac artery is identified with the obliterated umbilical artery retracted medially to mark the medial extent of dissection. Lymphatic tissue along the internal iliac (hypogastric) artery is similarly removed. Retraction using the fourth arm of the obliterated umbilical artery allows blunt dissection between this and the obturator packet. This blunt sweeping is carried down to the endopelvic fascia. The node of Cloquet is then clipped and used as a handle to dissect beneath the external iliac vein and in the obturator fossae. The obturator vessels and nerve are preserved with hemostatic control of the surrounding lymphatic tissue. Similar dissection is carried out on the contralateral side. Completed bilateral anatomic extended LND is shown in (Fig. 12.8a, b).

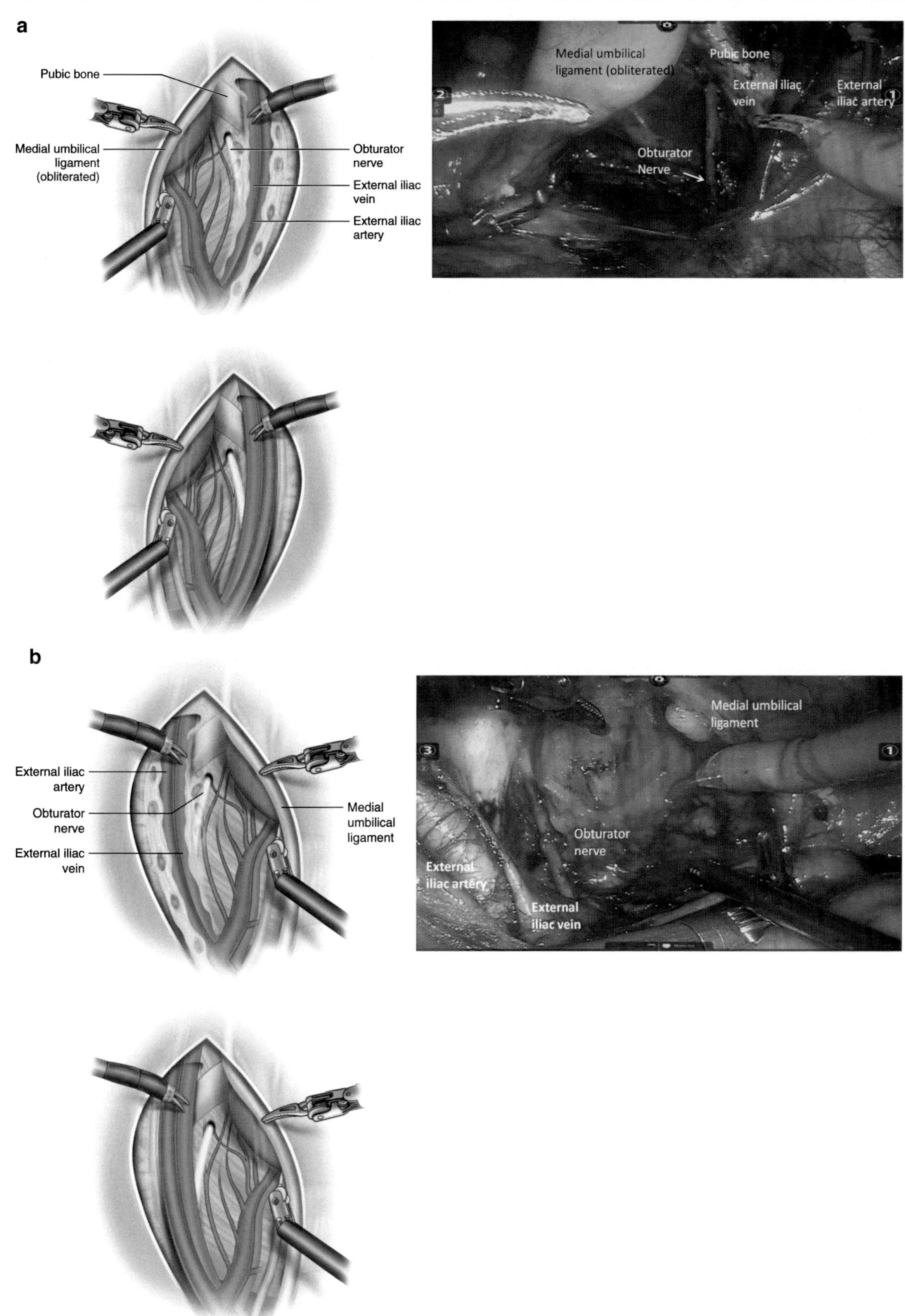

Fig. 12.8 Completed extended pelvic lymph node dissection. (**a**) Right side. (**b**) Left side

Dorsal Venous Complex Control

The deep dorsal veins drain deoxygenated blood away from the penis and can present a troublesome source of bleeding during RP. Venous complex control can be performed at various time points during RARP such as after the endopelvic fascia incision or just prior to apical dissection. During RARP the pneumoperitoneum, especially if temporarily increased, may reduce active bleeding during this step of the operation. Control of the dorsal venous complex (DVC) during RARP may be achieved in various ways. Reports have described suture ligation, cutting the complex followed by suturing, or cautery or stapling of the complex. A zero-degree lens is used for this portion of the procedure. Dissection on either side of the DVC in order to isolate it by endopelvic fascia opening or nerve sparing prepares the anatomy for DVC ligation. Sharp and blunt dissection drop the levator muscles away from the DVC so that what remains attached anteriorly is this venous complex.

Staple Control

When stapling, an Endo GIA stapler (Medtronic-Covidien, Minneapolis, MN) is brought through the lateral assistant port and articulated to straddle the grooves along either side of the DVC. The orientation of the stapler is adjacent to the course of the pubic bone in order to leave some anterior tissue on the prostate. Once the stapler traverses the DVC for a few centimeters, it can be closed, as seen in (Fig. 12.9). Care is taken to ensure that the Foley catheter and urethra are not caught in the staple line by moving the catheter in and out of the urethra freely after the stapler is clamped. Once just the DVC is within the jaws of the stapler, the complex is stapled and divided.

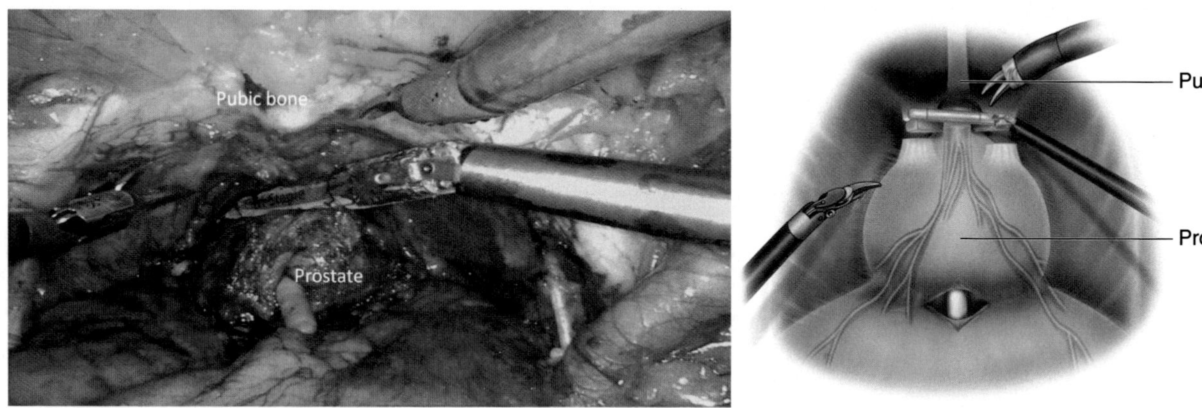

Fig. 12.9 Dorsal venous complex control using an Endo GIA stapler

Suture Control

When suturing, a large absorbable stitch such as 1 or 2-0 Vicryl (Ethicon, Cincinnati, OH) on a CT needle can be used. The needle is carefully passed anterior to the urethra so as not to injure the urethra or sphincter mechanism. The trajectory for passing the needle from side to side is completely horizontal. An additional pass of the suture more anteriorly is used to secure the complex before tying down. Once adequately suture ligated, the complex can be divided sharply or with cautery. Alternatively, the DVC can also be transected sharply and then similarly oversewn with an absorbable suture with the pneumoperitoneum turned up briefly to 20 mmHg.

After division of the DVC and completion of nerve sparing, the urethra is prepared and divided beyond the apex of the prostate. Functional urethral length can be important for recovery of continence. However, division of the urethra too close to the prostate may lead to positive apical margins. The anterior portion of the urethra is first divided, maximizing the urethral stump. A holding stitch of 3-0 Vicryl can be placed in the posterior urethra at 6 o'clock before posterior division in order to allow easier identification of the posterior urethral stump and prevent urethral retraction. This time point provides an excellent opportunity for the entire operative field to be examined for hemostasis.

Vesicourethral Anastomosis

After the prostate is removed and the specimen bagged, the bladder must be sutured down to the urethra in order to allow for normal micturition. Similar to open RP, the key principle of creating a watertight anastomosis that is not under tension is important to prevent anastomotic leak. A difference of RARP is that the visualization is superb in the deep pelvis, which assists with accurate suture placement and visual assurance of tissue apposition.

Prior to urethral suturing, posterior reconstruction can be considered for hemostasis and to assist with performing the vesicourethral anastomosis. Initially described by Rocco [19], the posterior musculofascial reconstruction helps to reduce tension of the anastomosis and may aid in early recovery of continence. A 3-0 barbed or Vicryl suture is used to bring the posterior musculofascial plate behind the urethra to the cut edge of the Denonvilliers fascia as shown in (Fig. 12.10). An additional suture from the plate to the midline posterior bladder can reduce tension between the urethra and bladder.

Once again, inspection of the bladder trigone and ureteral orifices is important to identify possible ureteral injuries. The vesicourethral anastomosis is then performed. If a previous 6 o'clock posterior urethral stitch was used, it is placed in the corresponding 6 o'clock position of the bladder neck. Next,

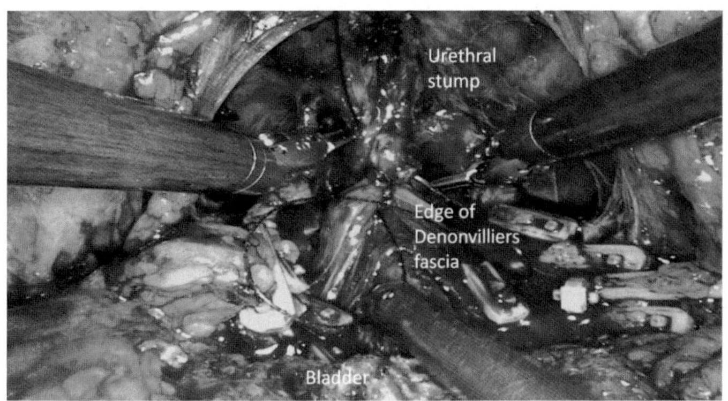

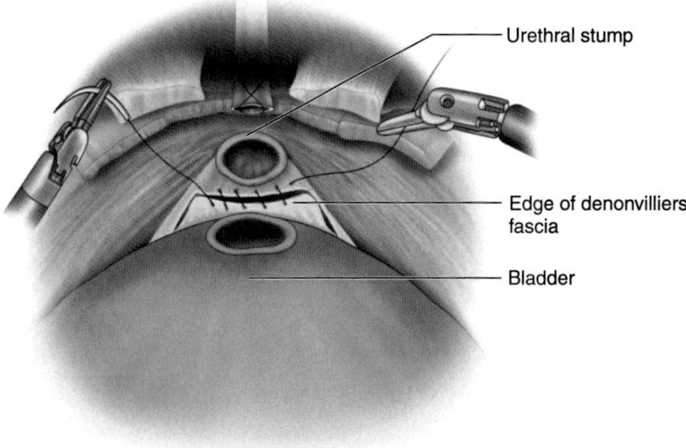

Fig. 12.10 Posterior reconstruction with suture connecting the posterior musculofascial plate of the urethra to the cut edge of Denonvilliers fascia

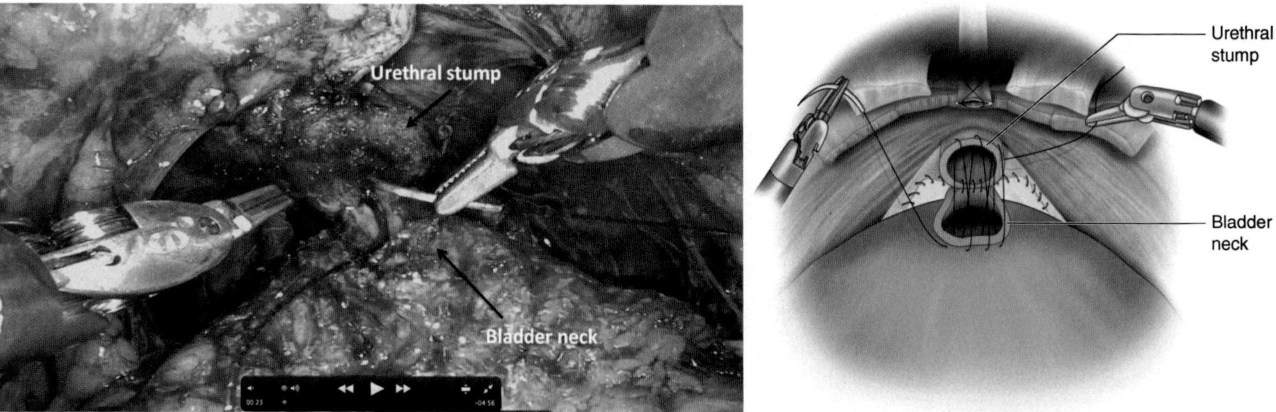

Fig. 12.11 Vesicourethral anastomosis using barbed suture (posterior urethral stitch already complete)

the anastomosis can be completed with absorbable suture in running or interrupted fashion as shown in (Fig. 12.11). The Van Velthoven is a common anastomotic technique wherein double 3-0 Vicryl or barbed sutures are tied together to run the anastomosis from 6 to 12 o'clock in both counterclockwise and clockwise fashion with the sutures tied at the 12 o'clock position [20]. A Foley catheter or sound is used to identify the lumen of the urethra in order to assist with accurate urethral stitch placement. Tensioning of the suture in between needle passes brings the mucosal edges of the urethra and bladder together. Recently, several meta-analyses examining the use of barbed suture for completion of the vesicourethral anastomosis found similar complication and continence rates with reduced operative time [21, 22].

In patients with a wide bladder, it may be necessary to reduce its caliber to sew down to the urethra. Posterior or anterior tennis racket closure with sutures in the midline posterior and anterior bladder away from the trigone can reduce the size of the bladder neck. Alternatively, approximation of the bladder edges lateral to the ureteral orifices with absorbable suture achieves reduction in the aperture of the bladder neck. Once the anastomosis is finished, the bladder is filled with saline to test for an anastomotic leak. A new urethral catheter or suprapubic catheter is then inserted into the bladder and inflated [23]. A temporary pelvic drain can then be inserted into the pelvis through one of the lateral port sites if desired.

Extraction and Closure

The 12-mm assistant port is closed under direct vision or with a laparoscopic closure device. The remainder of the ports can be removed under vision in order to inspect for internal bleeding from the port tract. The specimen is then extracted through the midline camera port by extending the skin and fascial incisions. After the specimen is removed, the fasciae and skin are closed.

Conclusions

RARP is a reproducible, effective treatment option for prostate cancer. The operation can be divided into logical steps in order to produce consistent outcomes. Complete dissection of the seminal vesicles is particularly important in aggressive disease. Bladder neck dissection separates the prostate from the bladder and relies heavily on visual cues to preserve a functional bladder neck. Nerve sparing is a meticulous dissection wherein the surgeon continually differentiates prostate tissue from nonprostate tissue. Keen knowledge of prostate anatomy is important to assess for variations that could be related to extraprostatic tumors. Lymph node dissection is essential for staging purposes and removes micrometastatic disease. Finally the vesicourethral anastomosis reconstitutes the urinary tract to allow for physiologic micturition.

References

1. Pasticier G, Rietbergen JB, Guillonneau B, Fromont G, Menon M, Vallancien G. Robotically assisted laparoscopic radical prostatectomy: feasibility study in men. Eur Urol. 2001;40:70–4.
2. Diaz M, Peabody JO, Kapoor V, Sammon J, Rogers CG, Stricker H, et al. Oncologic outcomes at 10 years following robotic radical prostatectomy. Eur Urol. 2015;67:1168–76.
3. Novara G, Ficarra V, Rosen RC, Artibani W, Costello A, Eastham JA, et al. Systematic review and meta-analysis of perioperative outcomes and complications after robot-assisted radical prostatectomy. Eur Urol. 2012;62:431–52.
4. Ficarra V, Novara G, Rosen RC, Artibani W, Carroll PR, Costello A, et al. Systematic review and meta-analysis of studies reporting urinary continence recovery after robot-assisted radical prostatectomy. Eur Urol. 2012;62:405–17.

5. Ficarra V, Novara G, Ahlering TE, Costello A, Eastham JA, Graefen M, et al. Systematic review and meta-analysis of studies reporting potency rates after robot-assisted radical prostatectomy. Eur Urol. 2012;62:418–30.
6. Raz O, Boesel TW, Arianayagam M, Lau H, Vass J, Huynh CC, et al. The effect of the modified Z Trendelenburg position on intraocular pressure during robotic assisted laparoscopic radical prostatectomy: a randomized, controlled study. J Urol. 2015;193:1213–9.
7. Soncin R, Mangano A, Zattoni F. Anesthesiologic effects of transperitoneal versus extraperitoneal approach during robot-assisted radical prostatectomy: results of a prospective randomized study. Int Braz J Urol. 2015;41:466–72.
8. Lee JY, Diaz RR, Cho KS, Choi YD. Meta-analysis of transperitoneal versus extraperitoneal robot-assisted radical prostatectomy for prostate cancer. J Laparoendosc Adv Surg Tech A. 2013;23:919–25.
9. Uffort EE, Jensen JC. Side docking the robot for robotic laparoscopic radical prostatectomy. JSLS. 2011;15:200–2.
10. Secin FP, Touijer K, Mulhall J, Guillonneau B. Anatomy and preservation of accessory pudendal arteries in laparoscopic radical prostatectomy. Eur Urol. 2007;51:1229–35.
11. Abreu AL, Chopra S, Berger AK, Leslie S, Desai MM, Gill IS, Aron M. Management of large median and lateral intravesical lobes during robot-assisted radical prostatectomy. J Endourol. 2013;27:1389–92.
12. Walsh PC, Lepor H, Eggleston JC. Radical prostatectomy with preservation of sexual function: anatomical and pathological considerations. Prostate. 1983;4:473–85.
13. Srivastava A, Chopra S, Pham A, Sooriakumaran P, Durand M, Chughtai B, et al. Effect of a risk-stratified grade of nerve-sparing technique on early return of continence after robot-assisted laparoscopic radical prostatectomy. Eur Urol. 2013;63:438–44.
14. Savera AT, Kaul S, Badani K, Stark AT, Shah NL, Menon M. Robotic radical prostatectomy with the “veil of Aphrodite” technique: histologic evidence of enhanced nerve sparing. Eur Urol. 2006;49:1065–73. discussion 1073–4.
15. Tewari AK, Srivastava A, Huang MW, Robinson BD, Shevchuk MM, Durand M, et al. Anatomical grades of nerve sparing: a risk-stratified approach to neural-hammock sparing during robot-assisted radical prostatectomy (RARP). BJU Int. 2011;108(6 Pt 2):984–92.
16. Ko YH, Coelho RF, Sivaraman A, Schatloff O, Chauhan S, Abdul-Muhsin HM, et al. Retrograde versus antegrade nerve sparing during robot-assisted radical prostatectomy: which is better for achieving early functional recovery? Eur Urol. 2013;63:169–77.
17. Beyer B, Schlomm T, Tennstedt P, Boehm K, Adam M, Schiffmann J, et al. A feasible and time-efficient adaptation of NeuroSAFE for da Vinci robot-assisted radical prostatectomy. Eur Urol. 2014;66:138–44.
18. Yuh BE, Ruel NH, Mejia R, Wilson CM, Wilson TG. Robotic extended pelvic lymphadenectomy for intermediate- and high-risk prostate cancer. Eur Urol. 2012;61:1004–10.
19. Rocco B, Cozzi G, Spinelli MG, Coelho RF, Patel VR, Tewari A, et al. Posterior musculofascial reconstruction after radical prostatectomy: a systematic review of the literature. Eur Urol. 2012;62:779–90.
20. Van Velthoven RF, Ahlering TE, Peltier A, Skarecky DW, Clayman RV. Technique for laparoscopic running urethrovesical anastomosis: the single knot method. Urology. 2003;61:699–702.
21. Li H, Liu C, Zhang H, Xu W, Liu J, Chen Y, et al. The use of unidirectional barbed suture for urethrovesical anastomosis during robot-assisted radical prostatectomy: a systematic review and meta-analysis of efficacy and safety. PLoS One. 2015;10:e0131167.
22. Bai Y, Pu C, Yuan H, Tang Y, Wang X, Li J, et al. Assessing the impact of barbed suture on vesicourethral anastomosis during minimally invasive radical prostatectomy: a systematic review and meta-analysis. Urology. 2015;85:1368–75.
23. Ghani KR, Trinh QD, Sammon JD, Jeong W, Simone A, Dabaja A, et al. Percutaneous suprapubic tube bladder drainage after robot-assisted radical prostatectomy: a step-by-step guide. BJU Int. 2013;112(5):703.

Robot-Assisted Adrenalectomy

13

Jaspreet Singh Parihar and Clayton Lau

Background

Diseases of the adrenal gland have been treated surgically since the nineteenth century. Since the first planned adrenalectomy by Sargent in 1914 for a large adenoma, various approaches to this operation have been developed. Open techniques have paved the way for less invasive approaches. In 1992, Gagner et al. [1] reported their initial experience with transperitoneal laparoscopic adrenalectomy. Since then, minimally invasive techniques have gained wide adoption, partly due to decreased postoperative pain, lessened morbidity, and quicker patient recovery. The advent of robot-assisted techniques has overcome many of the limitations of traditional laparoscopy. In 2001, Horgan et al. [2] first reported their experience using a da Vinci® robotic system to perform adrenalectomy. Contemporary literature continues to support the use of robotically-assisted techniques to treat adrenal pathology [3–6]. When planning for surgeries of the adrenal gland, complete imaging and endocrine workup is warranted to achieve an accurate preoperative clinical diagnosis.

Patient Selection and Preparation

Similar to any laparoscopic case, the patient's cardiac and pulmonary health must be assessed prior to the operation. Patients must be able to tolerate prolonged pneumoperitoneum in a modified lateral decubitus position. Any coagulopathy should be addressed and corrected. Relative contraindications to minimally invasive approaches include obesity, previous surgeries, tumor size, vena cava involvement, and adrenal cortical carcinoma.

Prior to surgery, an adrenal mass should be subjected to comprehensive endocrine testing to assess for hormonal functionality. In hormonally active adrenal lesions, both preoperative and intraoperative coordination among the endocrinologist, surgeon, and anesthesiologist is crucial to ensure treatment success. In cases of pheochromocytoma, it is critical to achieve adequate alpha-adrenergic blockade, ensure intravascular volume hydration, and perform further beta-adrenergic blockade if necessary. Intraoperative hypertension may be controlled by short-acting beta-blockers or nitroprussides. In Cushing's syndrome, correction of hyperglycemia and electrolyte disturbances is necessary. Cases of aldosteronomas (Conn's syndrome) may require pretreatment with spironolactone. Postoperatively, adrenal insufficiency may ensue, particularly in Cushing's syndrome, owing to contralateral cortisol suppression.

Room Setup and Patient Positioning

Patient and operative equipment setup can be similar to the setup for robot-assisted kidney cases. We describe our specific techniques of patient positioning. Following intubation on the operative table, a Foley catheter is placed, and an oral gastric tube can be inserted for left adrenal cases. The operative site is prepared and assessed for any previous surgical scars or hernias. The patient is then positioned in a modified lateral decubitus position (approximately 70°) with the operative side up. The patient is then well padded, with an axillary roll and two gel log rolls supporting the patient's back. The lower leg is flexed, with three pillows between the legs and additional padding placed at the knee and ankle joints. The ipsilateral arm remains on the patient's side and is supported with a log roll prepared with one or two rolled blankets. The patient is then flexed at the anterior superior iliac spine (ASIS) joint and gently secured to the operating table using tape/straps. A lower-body warmer such as a 3 M™ Bair Hugger™ is utilized.

J. S. Parihar, MD
Division of Urology and Urologic Oncology, City of Hope National Medical Center, Duarte, CA, USA
e-mail: jparihar@coh.org

C. Lau, MD (✉)
Department of Surgery, City of Hope National Medical Center, Duarte, CA, USA
e-mail: cllau@coh.org

Y. Fong et al. (eds.), *The SAGES Atlas of Robotic Surgery*, https://doi.org/10.1007/978-3-319-91045-1_13

Port Placement and Instruments

We describe our transperitoneal operative techniques. Adrenal tumors may also be approached via retroperitoneal access, with the aid of dissector systems such as Spacemaker™ (Covidien). Pneumoperitoneum is established using a Veress needle introduced at the umbilicus. We use a SurgiQuest AirSeal insufflation system to maintain an intraperitoneal pressure of 15 mmHg. We use a "Dice-5" configuration using the daVinci standard four-arm approach. After pneumoperitoneum is established, a 5-mm Visiport trocar (US Surgical) is introduced with a 0-degree lens and laparoscopic camera. This port is eventually exchanged for a 12-mm robotic camera port (8 mm if using da Vinci XI) with a 30-degree down lens. Subsequently, three robotic 8-mm trocars are inserted under vision: monopolar curved scissors in the right arm, fenestrated bipolar forceps in the left arm, and ProGrasp forceps in the fourth arm. Two assistant ports are typically used (two 10-mm ports or a 10-mm and a 5-mm port), with an additional 5-mm port used for a subxiphoid liver retractor for right-sided cases (Fig. 13.1).

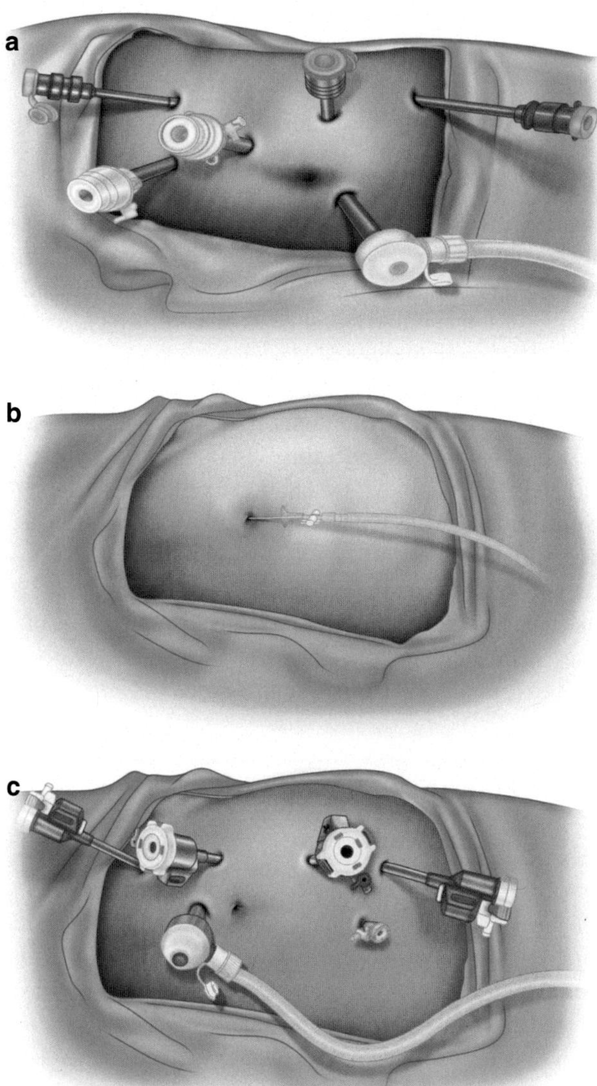

Fig. 13.1 (**a**) Dice-5 port placement for robot-assisted adrenal surgeries. The patient's head is toward the left. (**b**, **c**) Straight-line port placement for robot-assisted adrenal surgeries using the da Vinci Xi platform. The patient's head is toward the right

Key Operative Steps

Landmarks

When approaching the adrenal gland, it is important to recognize and expose the key surgical landmarks, including the superior pole of the kidney, the renal vein, the adrenal vein, the inferior vena cava (IVC) or aorta, and the underlying psoas muscle. The right adrenal gland is typically more cephalad than the left and thus will require liver retraction with a subxiphoid grasper instrument. The adrenal gland often has a variable network of arterial blood supply arising from the renal artery, aorta, and inferior phrenic artery, whereas venous drainage is more consistent. The left adrenal vein usually drains into the left renal vein, and the right renal vein enters the posterolateral IVC. The key is the dissect around the adrenal gland to maximize it's visual exposure before dissecting the adrenal gland free. On the right side, that includes opening up the Coronary Ligament and taking down the Triangular ligament to mobilize the liver more anterolaterally to give access to the most cranial portion on the adrenal gland. On the left the splenorenal ligament has to be taken down, exposing the lateral limit o the pancreas and splenic vessels. Then dissection should be carried to the crus of the diaphragm to exposure the medially extent of the left adrenal gland.

Reflection of the Colon

The colonic flexure is identified and reflected medially over the kidney along the white line of Toldt. An avascular plane is further developed between the anterior Gerota's fascia and the mesenteric fat of the reflected colon. Often, the right colon may be well away from the area of dissection and may not require further mobilization. For right-sided cases, the duodenum needs to be kocherized to identify the underlying IVC. On the left side, it is important to dissect away splenorenal ligaments toward the greater curvature of the stomach to expose the diaphragm and the medial aspect of the adrenal gland. The fourth robotic arm instrument can be used for caudal retraction of the kidney.

Adrenal Dissection

When establishing surgical exposure, care must be taken not to inadvertently avulse the delicate adrenal vasculature, especially the right adrenal vein. A posterior IVC tear may become difficult to identify and control. As manipulation of the adrenal tissue is undertaken, early control of venous drainage, especially in cases of pheochromocytoma, is critical to minimize catecholamine release into the systemic circulation (Fig. 13.2). Traditionally, Weck® Hem-o-lok® clips or Endo GIA stapler has been utilized to ligate the adrenal vasculature. We prefer da Vinci® EndoWrist One

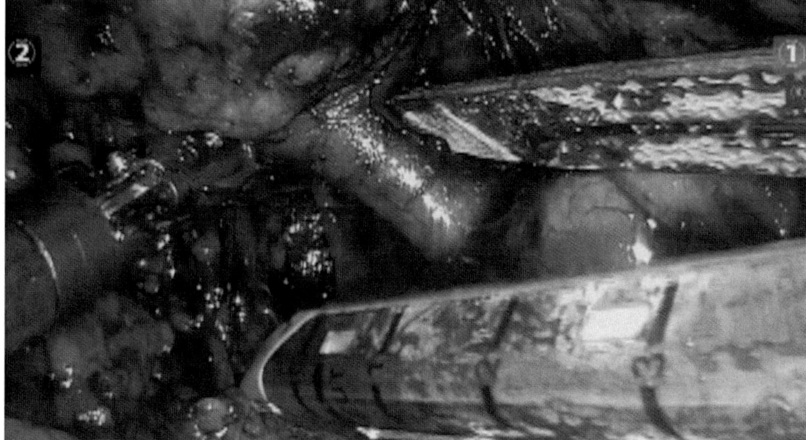

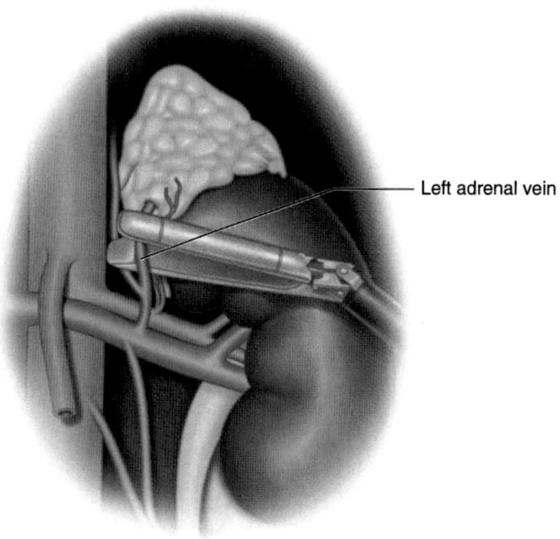

Fig. 13.2 Ligation of left adrenal vein. (**a**, **b**) The left adrenal vein is identified and ligated using an Endo GIA® (Covidien) stapler

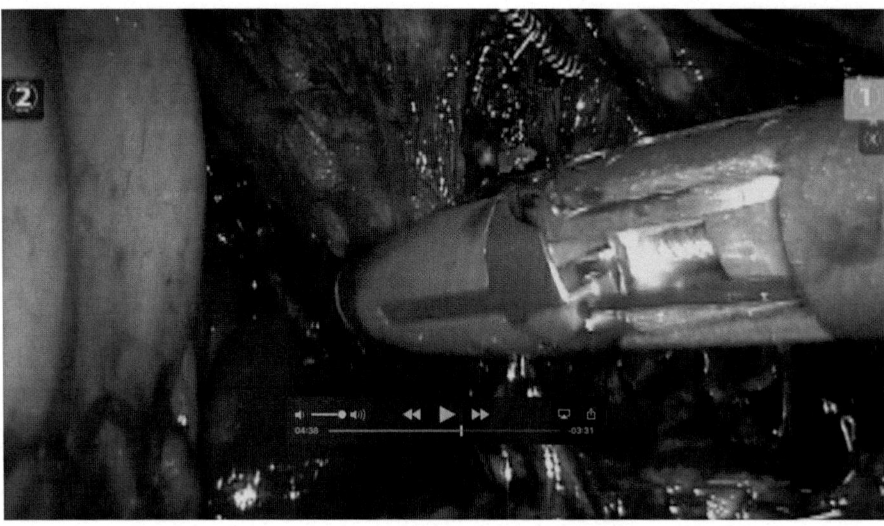

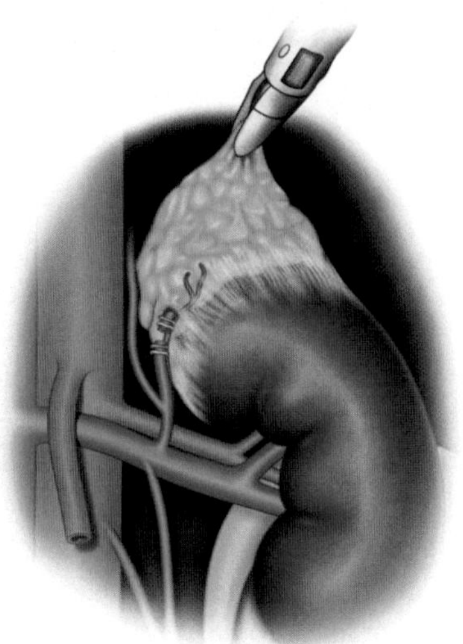

Fig. 13.3 Adrenal dissection. (**a**, **b**) Adrenal gland dissection using the da Vinci® EndoWrist One Vessel Sealer

Vessel Sealer instrument to circumferentially ligate and divide around the adrenal lesion of interest (partial adrenalectomy) or, more frequently, the entire gland (Fig. 13.3). In our experience, the Vessel Sealer instrument allows for more precise and angulated dissections in control of the console surgeon. Lymph node dissection, if indicated, can also be accomplished using this instrument.

Specimen Extraction

The tumor specimen can be placed in an endoscopic retrieval bag and extracted through the 12-mm assistant port or the fourth arm port site. Following fascial closure, the abdomen may be reinsufflated to ensure hemostasis and to allow for perioperative drain placement, if appropriate. Hemostatic agents such as Surgiflo® (Ethicon), BioGlue® (CryoLife), or Evicel® (Ethicon) can be applied as per surgeon preference.

Conclusion

Minimally invasive approaches have reduced the morbidity associated with adrenal surgical pathology. This chapter has described our robotic surgical techniques in approaching surgical diseases of the adrenal gland. Preoperative and intraoperative patient planning is crucial for hormonally active lesions. Sound oncologic and surgical principles should be followed to ensure patient safety and treatment success.

References

1. Gagner M, Lacroix A, Bolte E. Laparoscopic adrenalectomy in Cushing's syndrome and pheochromocytoma. N Engl J Med. 1992;327:1033.
2. Horgan S, Vanuno D. Robots in laparoscopic surgery. J Laparoendosc Adv Surg Tech A. 2001;11:415–9.
3. Brandao LF, Autorino R, Laydner H, Haber GP, Ouzaid I, De Sio M, et al. Robotic versus laparoscopic adrenalectomy: a systematic review and meta-analysis. Eur Urol. 2014;65:1154–61.
4. Yiannakopoulou E. Robotic assisted adrenalectomy: surgical techniques, feasibility, indications, oncological outcome and safety. Int J Surg. 2016;28:169–72.
5. Taskin HE, Berber E. Robotic adrenalectomy. Cancer J. 2013;19:162–6.
6. Desai MM, Gill IS, Kaouk JH, Matin SF, Sung GT, Bravo EL. Robotic-assisted laparoscopic adrenalectomy. Urology. 2002;60:1104–7.

14 Robotically-Assisted Laparoscopic Radical Cystoprostatectomy and Anterior Exenteration

Ali Zhumkhawala, Jonathan N. Warner, and Kevin Chan

Introduction

Despite advances in nonsurgical treatments and noninvasive surgical techniques, radical cystectomy and pelvic lymph node dissection remains the gold standard treatment for urothelial and non-urothelial carcinoma of the bladder with invasion into the muscularis propria [1]. Radical cystectomy is also frequently employed in the setting of high-risk, non-muscle-invasive disease refractory to less-invasive therapies.

Menon et al. initially described robot-assisted laparoscopic radical cystectomy in 2003, and this method has expanded its footprint internationally since that time [2]. A thorough pelvic lymph node dissection is critical and is directly related to survival outcomes [3, 4].

This chapter explores robot-assisted laparoscopic radical cystectomy with bilateral extended pelvic lymph node dissection in both male and female patients, describing the sparing of the cavernosal nerve in the male patient and the reproductive organs in the female patient. Common extracorporeal and intracorporeal urinary diversion techniques are also described.

Patient Selection and Preoperative Preparation

Oncologic indications for radical cystectomy include urothelial and non-urothelial carcinoma of the bladder with invasion into the muscularis propria, as well as high-risk, non-muscle-invasive disease refractory to less-invasive techniques and intravesical medical therapies.

All patients should undergo appropriate cardiac and medical clearance. Patients must be physiologically able to tolerate pneumoperitoneum and prolonged Trendelenburg positioning. Prior abdominopelvic surgery is rarely a contraindication, and the decision to convert to an open procedure based on adhesions can be made intraoperatively. The decision to perform a cavernosal nerve-sparing procedure in the male patient or a reproductive organ-sparing procedure in the female patient should rely heavily on the patient's disease characteristics, as a positive surgical margin should be avoided. The choice of urinary diversion type is a complex decision based on multiple factors including the patient's desires, manual dexterity, cognitive function, age, medical comorbidities, renal function, prior malignancies, and intestinal disease.

Patient Positioning and Port Placement

The patient should be placed in the dorsal lithotomy or split-leg position when the da Vinci® standard, S, or Si robotic platform is employed. Male patients can remain in the supine position when the da Vinci® Xi robotic platform is employed. An exaggerated Trendelenburg position is utilized to allow for adequate exposure of the pelvis and lower retroperitoneum. Care should be taken to adequately pad all pressure points, especially the posterior lower extremity, to avoid a peroneal nerve palsy.

Port placement is similar to that for robot-assisted laparoscopic radical prostatectomy, with the ports placed further cephalad to allow for a more extended lymph node dissection. The robotic camera port (12 mm or 8 mm depending on platform) is placed in the supraumbilical position, approximately 25 cm away from the pubic symphysis. Two 8 mm robotic ports are then placed in the pararectus location

A. Zhumkhawala, MD · J. N. Warner · K. Chan (✉)
Division of Urology and Urologic Oncology, Department of Surgery, City of Hope Comprehensive Cancer Center, Duarte, CA, USA
e-mail: azhumkhawala@coh.org; KChan@coh.org

Y. Fong et al. (eds.), *The SAGES Atlas of Robotic Surgery*, https://doi.org/10.1007/978-3-319-91045-1_14

approximately 20–21 cm from the pubic symphysis. An additional 8 mm robotic port is placed cephalad to the left anterior superior iliac spine, approximately 23 cm away from the pubic symphysis. Two 12 mm laparoscopic assistant ports are then placed, one in the right subcostal location and another cephalad to the right anterior superior iliac spine, approximately 23 cm away from the pubic symphysis. Port placement can be varied according to surgeon preference. The assistant surgeon may also be positioned on the patient's left to allow for a more natural path for a laparoscopic stapler for use in intracorporeal urinary diversions (Fig. 14.1).

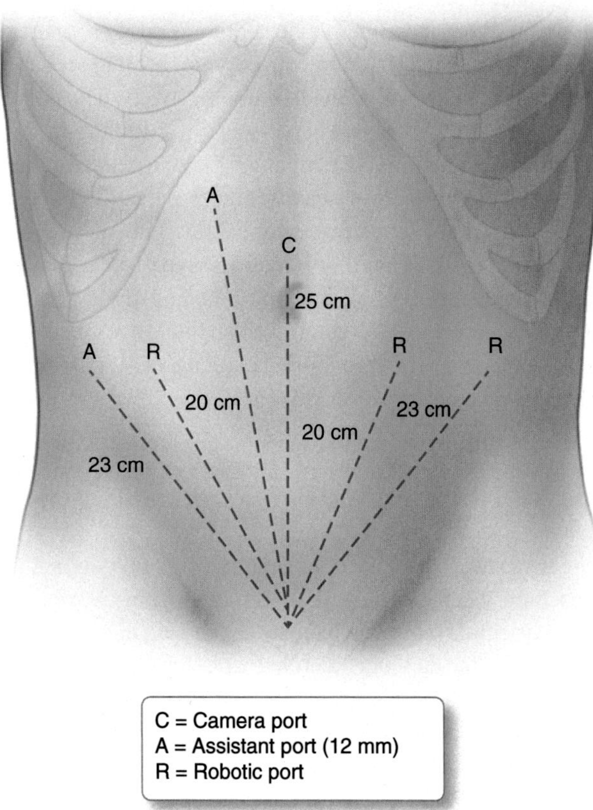

Fig. 14.1 Port placement. *A* assistant port, *C* camera port, *R* robotic port

Technique and Steps of Radical Cystoprostatectomy in the Male Patient

Bowel Mobilization

The sigmoid colon should be mobilized to allow for adequate access to the left retroperitoneum. The peritoneum lateral to the sigmoid colon is incised at the line of Toldt. The sigmoid colon and its mesentery are then dissected medially. This dissection can be accomplished with sharp dissection to avoid thermal enteric injury. The sigmoid colon should be mobilized nearly to the splenic flexure to allow for adequate lymph node dissection and to create a large window under the inferior mesenteric artery to avoid kinking the left ureter as it crosses under the sigmoid mesentery.

Seminal Vesicle/Posterior Dissection

The peritoneum overlying the seminal vesicle complex is incised deep in the pouch of Douglas. The vasa deferentia and posterior seminal vesicles are then dissected free. The posterolateral aspects of the seminal vesicles, including their tips, should be dissected free and identified. In the nerve-sparing patient, care should be taken to avoid the use of cautery lateral to the tips of the seminal vesicles; clips can be used to ligate small blood vessels at this location.

In the non-nerve-sparing or high-risk patient, the posterior dissection should be performed in the perirectal fat plane. This plane can be entered by incising through both layers of Denonvilliers' fascia lateral to the rectum. The perirectal fat is identified, and the incision in Denonvilliers' fascia is carried across the midline just anterior to the rectum. The dissection is continued with blunt and sharp dissection in this plane distally to the apex of the prostate and laterally out to the neurovascular bundles.

In the nerve-sparing patient, the posterior dissection can be performed in the plane between the two leaflets of Denonvilliers' fascia. The anterior leaflet of Denonvilliers' fascia is incised in the midline, and the plane between the two leaflets is developed bluntly and sharply toward the apex of the prostate and laterally to the neurovascular bundles.

Ureteral Dissection

Each ureter is identified where it crosses over the common iliac artery. The peritoneum is incised on either side of the ureter sharply. The ureter is then dissected away from the common iliac artery. A shortened Penrose drain can be used to encircle the ureter and allow for ease of manipulation of the ureter. (The ureter is never handled with instruments.) The ureter is then mobilized proximally for a short distance. Care should be taken to avoid stripping the ureter of its vascular supply, and much of the fatty tissue adjacent to the ureter should be left in place. The ureter should then be mobilized distally down to its insertion in the posterior aspect of the bladder. A large clip is then applied on the ureter just proximal to its insertion. This is performed in a right-to-left manner in order to give orientation to the ureter later during the urinary diversion. The clip has a long suture attached to it for ease of identification and atraumatic manipulation of the ureter during urinary diversion. A second clip is applied along the bladder side of the ureter, and the ureter is divided between the clips. A frozen-section pathologic analysis of the distal ureter can be performed to evaluate for carcinoma at the ureteral margin. The identical procedure is then replicated for the contralateral side (Fig. 14.2). The long dyed and undyed sutures on the ureteral clip identify the left and right ureters, respectively.

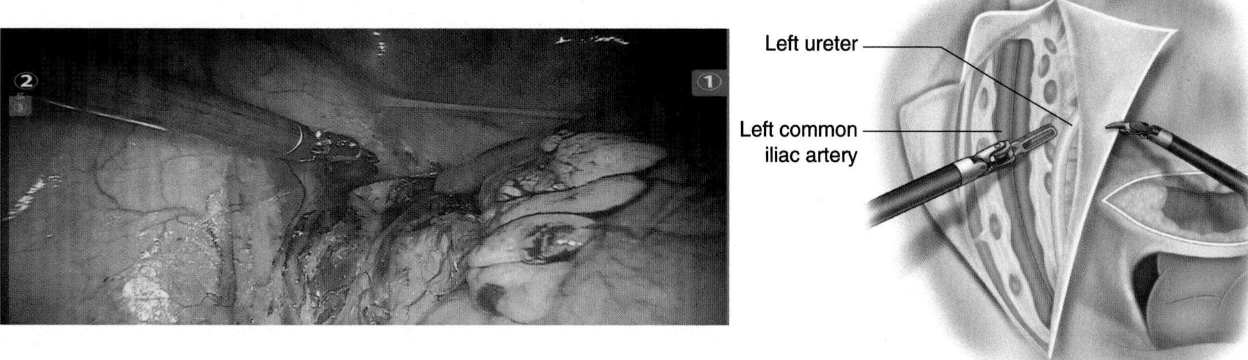

Fig. 14.2 Left ureteral dissection

Extended Pelvic Lymph Node Dissection

A systematic approach and exposure of key anatomic landmarks are the hallmarks of a safe and adequate lymph node dissection. The distal limit of lymph node dissection is the circumflex iliac vein and Cloquet's node. The lateral limit of dissection is the genitofemoral nerve. The medial limit of dissection is contiguous with the bladder. The posterior limit of dissection is the posterior obturator fossa and presciatic fat pad. The proximal limit of an extended pelvic lymph node dissection is debated; this atlas focuses on the takeoff of the inferior mesenteric artery on the aorta as the proximal limit.

The lymph node dissection is initiated by incising the peritoneum lateral to the common and external iliac artery. The genitofemoral nerve is identified and preserved. The peritoneal incision is continued distally until the circumflex iliac vein is identified. The lymphatic tissue lateral to the iliac vessels is then mobilized medially off of the genitofemoral nerve and pelvic sidewall. This tissue can be bluntly dissected away from the pelvic sidewall musculature. Perforating vessels can be easily identified and ligated using bipolar cautery. This dissection is continued posteriorly into the fossa of Marseille. In this location, the obturator nerve can be identified. A split-and-roll technique is then used to split the fatty and lymphatic tissue off of the anterior common and external iliac vessels. The lymphatic tissue is then mobilized off of the lateral aspect of the iliac artery and vein. This dissection is continued posteriorly into the fossa of Marseille. The internal iliac vein can be identified in this location, and care should be taken to avoid an injury here. The lymphatic tissue can then be carefully dissected off of the proximal obturator nerve in the fossa of Marseille and swept distally into the pelvis. This tissue will be easily removed from the medial aspect of the vessels later. Monopolar cautery should be avoided in the fossa of Marseille, as it may stimulate the obturator nerve and cause adduction of the ipsilateral leg.

Next, the medial border of dissection is identified using the lateral edge of the medial umbilical ligament as a landmark. The bladder is then mobilized medially away from the iliac vessels until the endopelvic fascia is identified. The bladder can be retracted medially using the robotic fourth arm. At this point, the lymphatic tissue is mobilized off the medial aspect of the external and common iliac vessels. Distally, clips or cautery should be used to ligate lymphatic vessels stemming from the leg, for lymphostasis. The distal limit of dissection is the crossing of the circumflex iliac vein over the external iliac artery.

The internal iliac artery is identified at its takeoff from the common iliac artery. Lymphatic tissue is then mobilized off of the anterior surface of the internal iliac artery. This dissection is continued distally, and the obturator artery and vein are identified at their takeoffs from the internal iliac vessels. This lymph node packet is dissected free distally to the endopelvic fascia. Much of this dissection can be done by bluntly sweeping the lymphatic tissue anteriorly and distally, with care taken to cauterize perforating vessels and avoid traction injury to the obturator vessels.

The lymph node of Cloquet is then identified posterior to the external iliac vein. The lymphatics distal to Cloquet's node should be ligated using clips or cautery. Cloquet's node is then dissected off the pubis and the posterior aspect of the external iliac vein. The node is then retracted posteromedially to expose the obturator lymph node chain. The obturator nodes are dissected off of the posterior surface of the vein. The obturator nerve and vessels are identified as they course into the obturator foramen. The lymph node packet is dissected away from the obturator nerve and vessels, with care taken to avoid the use of monopolar cautery in this location. Once the obturator packet is freed distally, the packet can be removed, as the proximal attachments were already divided during the dissection of the fossa of Marseille. An identical node dissection is completed on the contralateral side in similar fashion (Fig. 14.3).

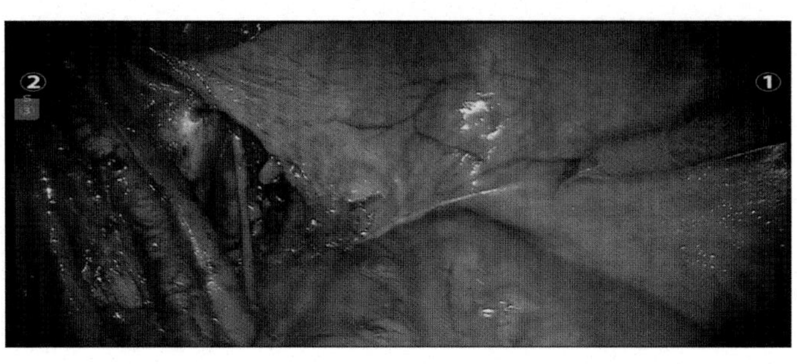

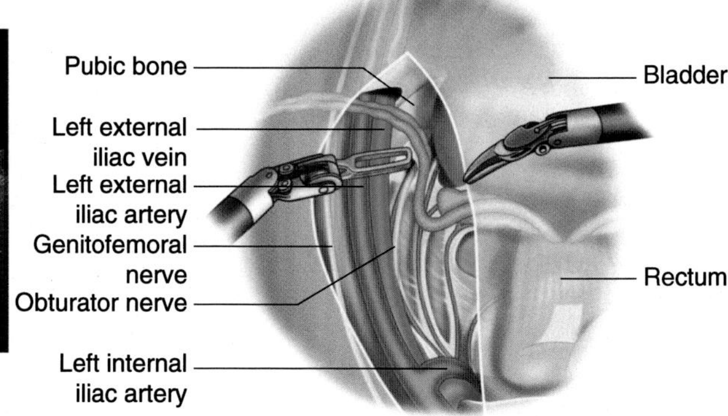

Fig. 14.3 Completed left pelvic lymph node dissection

The sigmoid colon is then retracted to the left using the robotic fourth arm. The more proximal lymph node dissection is then completed. The peritoneum overlying the right common iliac artery is then incised until the aortic bifurcation is exposed. The sigmoid colon is retracted anteriorly so that the plane between the sigmoid mesentery and the para-aortic lymph node tissue can be identified and incised. A large sigmoid window should be created to allow adequate room for the left ureter to be transposed to the right abdomen without kinking later. A split-and-roll technique is used to expose the anterior surface of the aorta. This dissection is continued proximally until the takeoff of the inferior mesenteric artery is identified. The lymphatic tissue along the aorta is then gently dissected off the surface of the aorta. Just distal to the aortic bifurcation, care must be taken to avoid damage to the left common iliac vein as it crosses below the left common iliac artery. All lymphatic channels proximally should be sealed with either clips or cautery. The lymphatic tissue is dissected distally until it is contiguous with the previous pelvic dissections. The presacral nodal tissue is then retracted anteriorly and dissected off the inferior border of the left common iliac vein and off the anterior surface of the sacral periosteum. The sacral veins must be adequately cauterized at this location (Fig. 14.4). A split-and-roll technique is used to expose the vena cava, and the paracaval and precaval lymph nodes are excised. Care should be taken to adequately cauterize the small anterior branch of the vena cava at this location. The proximal border of the precaval and paracaval lymph node dissection is the level of the takeoff from the aorta of the inferior mesenteric artery.

Ligation of the Vascular Pedicles

The robotic fourth arm is then used to retract the bladder and prostate anteriorly to expose the posterior space. The lateral and posterior pedicles are then bluntly separated. A laparoscopic stapler with a vascular load is brought in through the subcostal assistant port and used to ligate and divide the lateral and posterior pedicles on each side. If a nerve-sparing procedure is planned, the pedicles should be stapled up to the tips of the seminal vesicles. If nerve sparing is not planned, the pedicle to the prostate and neurovascular bundle can also be stapled, extending to the apex of the prostate (Fig. 14.5).

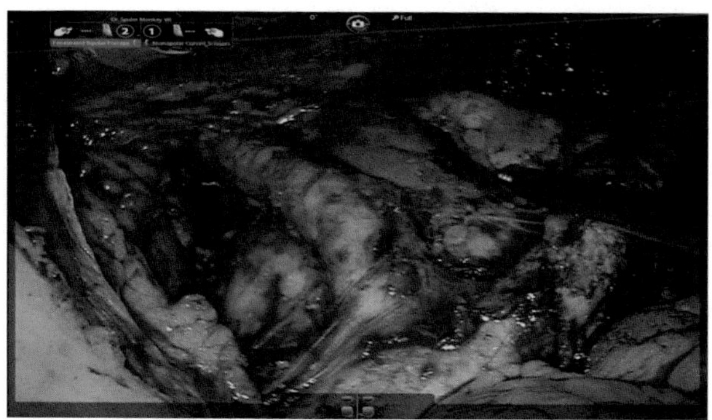

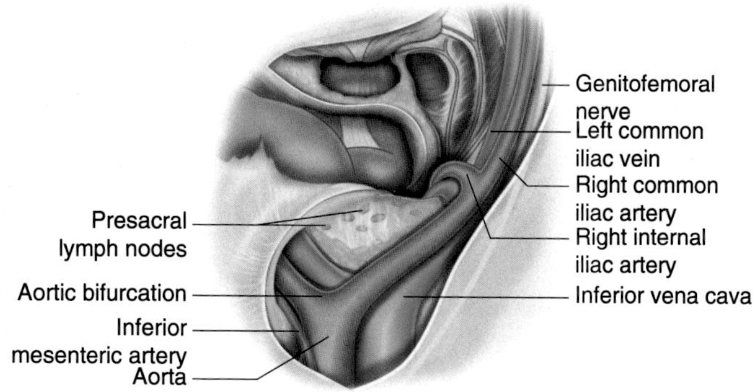

Fig. 14.4 Completed para-aortic and paracaval lymph node dissection

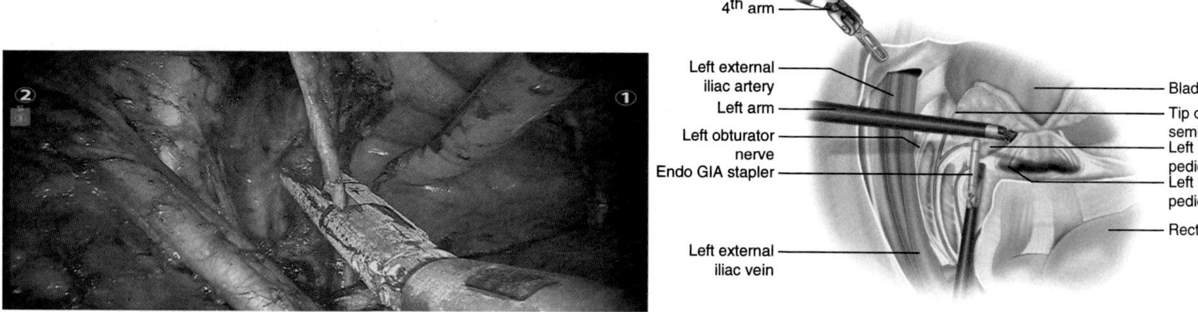

Fig. 14.5 Ligation of the left lateral and posterior pedicles

Bladder Mobilization

The peritoneum lateral to the medical umbilical ligaments is incised, and the space of Retzius is developed using blunt dissection and cautery. The vasa deferentia are clipped and divided adjacent to their insertion in the deep inguinal ring. The medial umbilical ligaments and urachus are divided using cautery proximally along the anterior abdominal wall. The bladder is mobilized down to the endopelvic fascia. The anterior prostatic fat pad is then mobilized off of the anterior surface of the prostate to aid in exposure. Care should be taken to ligate the superficial dorsal venous complex with bipolar cautery prior to its division.

If an orthotopic continent diversion is planned, the endopelvic fascia should be spared to improve continence outcomes. Otherwise, the endopelvic fascia is incised sharply bilaterally. The levator muscles are bluntly dissected away from the prostate. This dissection is continued up to the apex of the prostate.

Nerve-Sparing Neurovascular Bundle Dissection

The bladder and prostate are retracted to the left and posteriorly. The lateral prostatic fascia is incised over the right anterior prostate, at the level of the puboprostatic ligaments (Fig. 14.6). The lateral prostatic fascia and neurovascular bundle are then dissected away from the prostate in an interfascial plane. This dissection is continued distally to the apex and, in retrograde fashion, back toward the base. The bladder and prostate are then retracted to the left and anteriorly. The right vascular pedicle to the prostate is clipped and divided using permanent Weck® clips or absorbable Lapra clips. The neurovascular bundle is then gently dissected away from the posterolateral surface of the prostate. This dissection is continued anteriorly up to the dorsal venous complex. The entire dissection should be completed athermally and with minimal traction on the neurovascular bundle, to avoid long-standing postoperative neurapraxia.

An identical procedure is replicated on the left side.

The puboprostatic ligaments are divided sharply. The dorsal venous complex is stapled and divided using a laparoscopic stapler (Fig. 14.7). The catheter should be mobile prior to sta-

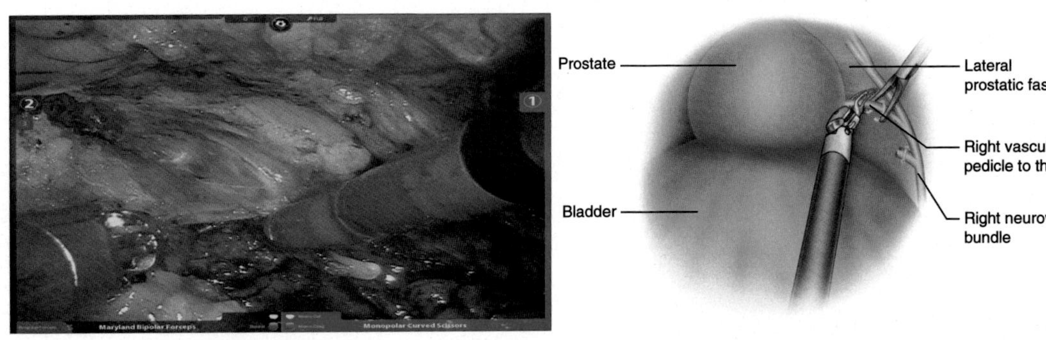

Fig. 14.6 Right cavernosal nerve sparing

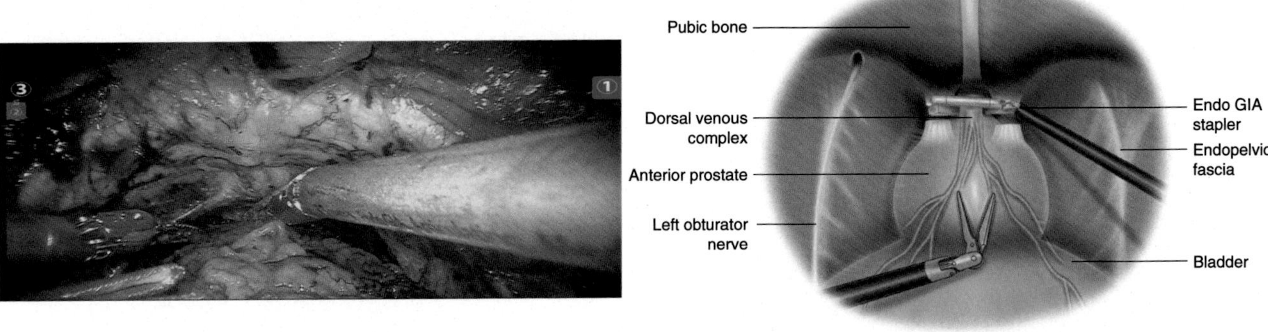

Fig. 14.7 Stapled division of the dorsal venous complex

pling, ensuring that the urethra is not ensnared in the stapler. The urethra is dissected free. The Foley catheter is then withdrawn, and a large clip is then placed on the urethra at its entrance into the prostatic apex, to avoid spillage of urine. The urethra is divided along its anterior aspect sharply, distal to the clip. If an orthotopic neobladder diversion is planned, a 3-0 polyglactin suture should be placed in the 6 o'clock position in the posterior urethral stump prior to division of the posterior urethra. A segment of the urethra is then taken from the prostatic portion and sent for frozen-section pathologic analysis. The bladder and prostate are then placed in a specimen retrieval bag to be removed at the time of urinary diversion (Fig. 14.8).

If a nerve-sparing procedure is not planned, the neurovascular bundle is divided using the laparoscopic stapler, and the endopelvic fascia is opened as described above. The division of the dorsal venous complex and urethra are the same as in the nerve-sparing technique.

Techniques and Steps of Anterior Exenteration/Radical Cystectomy in the Female Patient

Bowel Mobilization

The sigmoid colon should be mobilized to allow for adequate access to the left retroperitoneum. The peritoneum lateral to the sigmoid colon is incised at the line of Toldt. The sigmoid colon and its mesentery are then dissected medially. This dissection can be accomplished with minimal use of cautery to avoid enteric injury. The sigmoid colon should be mobilized nearly to the splenic flexure to allow for adequate lymph node dissection and to avoid kinking the left ureter as it crosses under the sigmoid mesentery.

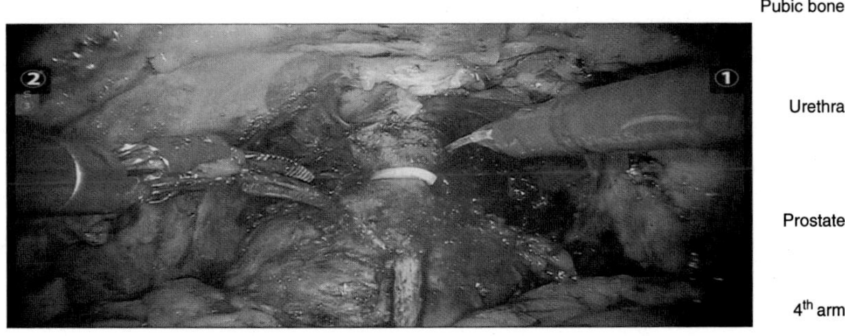

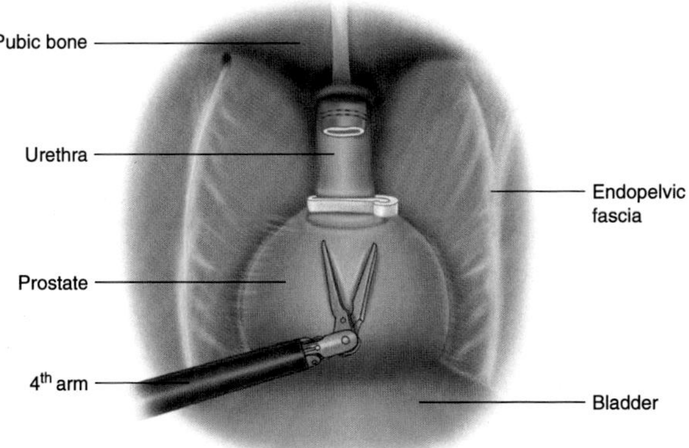

Fig. 14.8 Apical prostatic and urethral dissection

Ureteral Dissection

The ureter is identified where it crosses over the common iliac artery. The peritoneum is incised on either side of the ureter sharply. The ureter is then dissected away from the common iliac artery. A shortened Penrose drain can be used to encircle the ureter and allow for ease of manipulation of the ureter. The gonadal vessels (infundibulopelvic ligament) are separated away from the ureter. They are ligated and divided at this time, using either clips, LigaSure bipolar cautery or the robotic vessel sealer device. The ovary and fallopian tube are then mobilized medially toward the uterus. It can be secured to the uterus using clips, to improve exposure of the remainder of the pelvis. The ureter is then mobilized proximally for a short distance. Care should be taken to avoid stripping the ureter of its vascular supply, and much of the fatty tissue adjacent to the ureter should be left in place. The ureter should then be mobilized distally down to its insertion in the posterior aspect of the bladder. A large clip is then applied on the ureter just proximal to its insertion. The clip has a long suture attached to it for ease of identification and atraumatic manipulation of the ureter during urinary diversion. A second clip is applied along the bladder side of the ureter, and the ureter is divided between the clips. A frozen-section pathologic analysis of the distal ureter can be performed to evaluate for carcinoma at the ureteral margin. The identical procedure is then replicated for the contralateral side.

Extended Pelvic Lymph Node Dissection

The lymph node dissection for the female patient is performed in similar fashion as for the male patient, as detailed in the prior section.

Division of the Vascular Pedicles

The uterus is retracted anteriorly, using the robotic fourth arm. A robotic tenaculum can be useful to assist with adequate exposure. The peritoneum overlying the posterior uterus is incised at the pouch of Douglas. This space is then bluntly developed to mobilize the posterior vaginal wall off of the rectum. Care should be taken to avoid a rectal injury at this location, and the use of cautery should be judicious. The superior vesical arteries on both sides are then clipped at their takeoffs from the internal iliac artery and divided distally using the robotic vessel sealer device. The vessel sealer is also used to divide the remainders of the broad and cardinal ligaments to the level of the cervix (Fig. 14.9).

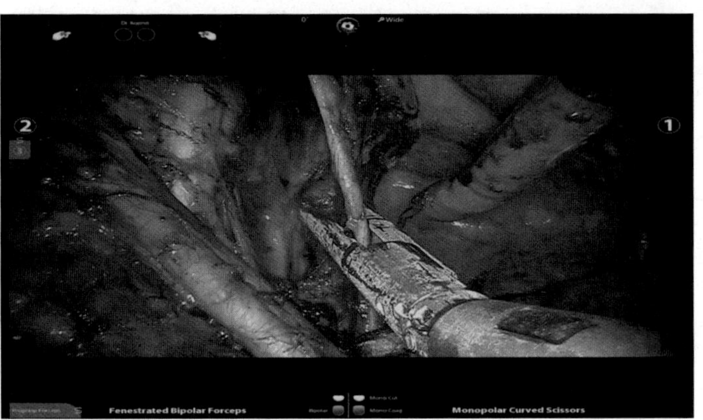

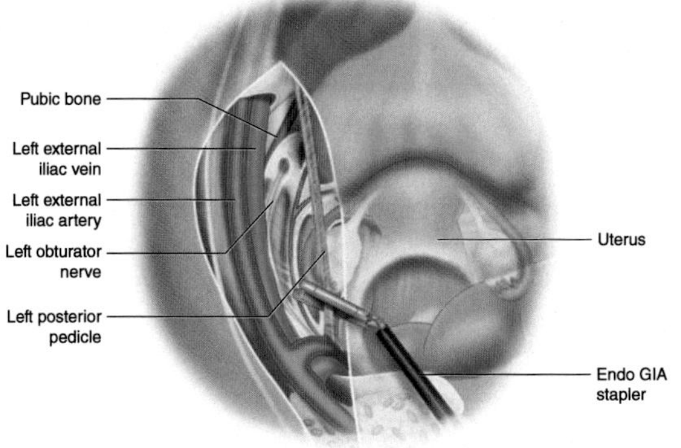

Fig. 14.9 Ligation of the left lateral and posterior pedicles

A betadine-impregnated sponge stick or vaginal manipulator is then placed in the vagina by the bedside assistant and used to manipulate the vagina anteriorly. The posterior vaginal wall is incised just distal to the cervix, using cautery. A laparotomy pad can be placed at the introitus to avoid loss of pneumoperitoneum. This vaginal incision is then carried distally anterolaterally along each side of the vaginal wall using the robotic vessel sealer device. Care should be taken to avoid excising more of the vaginal wall than is necessary, while being mindful of the posterior wall of the bladder on either side of the vagina. This incision is carried as distally as feasible (Fig. 14.10).

Bladder Mobilization

The peritoneum lateral to the medial umbilical ligaments is incised, and the space of Retzius is developed using blunt dissection and cautery. Cautery is used to divide the round ligaments adjacent to their insertion in the deep inguinal ring and to divide the medial umbilical ligaments and urachus proximally along the anterior abdominal wall. The bladder is mobilized down to the endopelvic fascia. The endopelvic fascia is incised sharply bilaterally. The levator muscles are bluntly dissected away from the bladder. This dissection is continued distally up to the urethra. The dorsal venous complex is then ligated using the vessel sealer device.

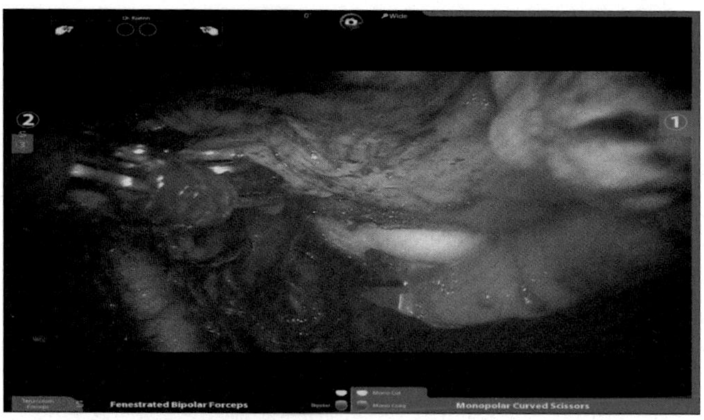

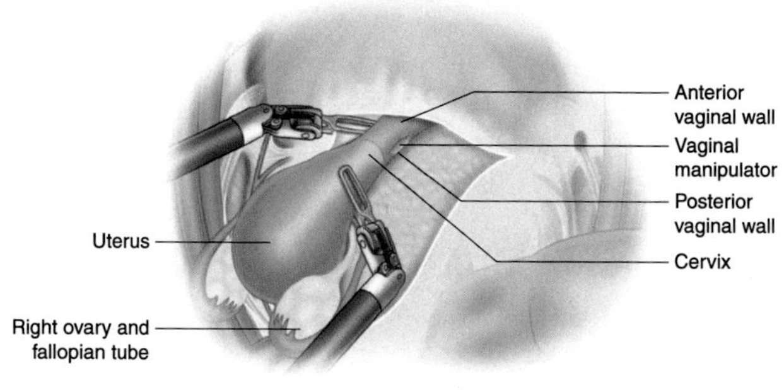

Fig. 14.10 Incision of the vaginal wall

Completion of the Anterior Exenteration

The Foley catheter is then capped and delivered through the vaginal opening into the abdominal cavity. The Foley catheter is then retracted superiorly, exposing the urethral meatus, which should now be visible through the vaginal opening. The entire urethra and urethral meatus with a cuff of vaginal mucosa is then excised using cautery. The uterus, ovaries, fallopian tubes, cervix, anterior vaginal wall, bladder, and urethra are then placed en bloc in a specimen retrieval bag.

Vaginal Closure

The posterior vaginal wall is then rotated anteriorly, and the vaginal opening is closed in clamshell fashion using either two continuous #0 barbed, absorbable sutures or polyglactin or monofilament absorbable sutures.

Uterine-Sparing Cystectomy

After completion of the extended pelvic lymph node dissection, the uterus is retracted anteriorly using the robotic fourth arm. A robotic tenaculum can be useful to assist with adequate exposure. The superior vesical arteries on both sides are then clipped at their takeoff from the internal iliac artery and divided distally using the robotic vessel sealer device.

The uterus is then retracted posteriorly. The bladder is then filled with saline to allow for identification of the plane between the bladder and the anterior vaginal wall. The peritoneum along the anterior cervix is incised with cautery. The bladder is then carefully dissected away from the anterior cervix and anterior vaginal wall using cautery (Fig. 14.11). Care must be exercised to avoid a positive margin at this location, and some vaginal musculature can be left on the bladder to avoid entry into the bladder. The bladder is then lifted superiorly off of the anterior vagina. In doing this, the vascular supply to the bladder will be exposed and can be ligated using bipolar cautery. This dissection is continued distally to the urethra.

The peritoneum lateral to the medial umbilical ligaments is incised and the space of Retzius is developed using blunt dissection and cautery. The medial umbilical ligaments and urachus are divided using cautery proximally along the anterior abdominal wall. The bladder is mobilized down to the endopelvic fascia. The endopelvic fascia is incised sharply bilaterally. The levator muscles are bluntly dissected away from the bladder. This dissection is continued distally up to the urethra. The dorsal venous complex is then ligated using the vessel sealer device.

The urethral meatus should be completely excised unless an orthotopic neobladder is planned. Once the bladder is completely mobile, it is placed in a specimen retrieval bag. The vaginal opening at the urethral meatus can be closed with a 2-0 polyglactin suture in figure-of-eight fashion.

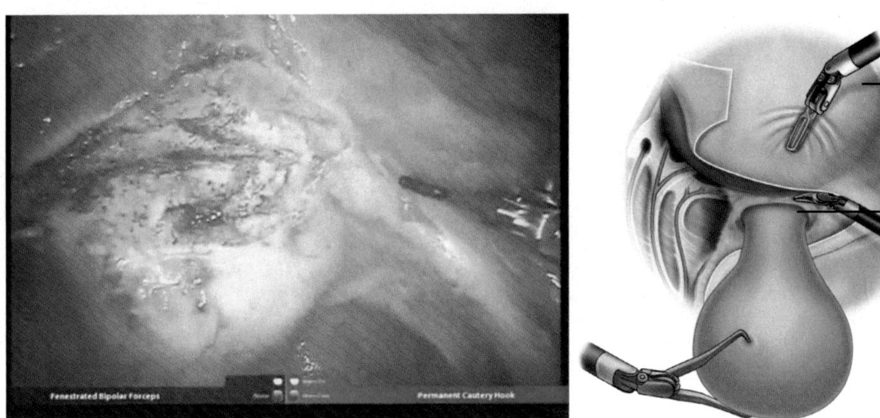

Fig. 14.11 Separation of the bladder from the anterior vaginal wall

Technique of Extracorporeal Urinary Diversion

Extracorporeal urinary diversion mirrors open surgical technique regardless of the type of urinary diversion being performed. However, in the setting of robotic cystectomy, there are maneuvers that can aid in allowing the incision to remain the size of the extraction site, as well as optimize efficiency of the surgery by utilizing the advantage of the robotic and laparoscopic exposure for key portions of the operation. This allows for a minimal learning curve and expeditious operative times.

In this chapter, we describe the extracorporeal technique of the ileal conduit, the Studer orthotopic neobladder, and the Indiana pouch continent cutaneous urinary diversions. There are various other types of orthotopic and continent cutaneous urinary diversions that can easily be applied and translated to the extracorporeal techniques we describe.

Ileal Conduit Extracorporeal Urinary Diversion

Robotic Preparation

The left ureter is transposed to the right abdomen through the sigmoid mesenteric window. A 2-0 silk suture is placed through the Veil of Treves at the terminal ileum. The robotic instruments are then removed, and the robot is undocked.

Ileal Harvest

A 6-cm midline incision is then made just below the umbilicus, and the rectus fascia and peritoneum are opened. An Alexis wound retractor is then placed for aid in exposure (Fig. 14.12). The sutures for the right ureter, left ureter, and terminal ileum are delivered through the incision. The terminal ileum is then stapled and divided using a GIA stapler approximately 15 cm proximal to the ileocecal valve. The mesentery at this location is divided toward the root of the mesentery for a distance of approximately 8–10 cm at the

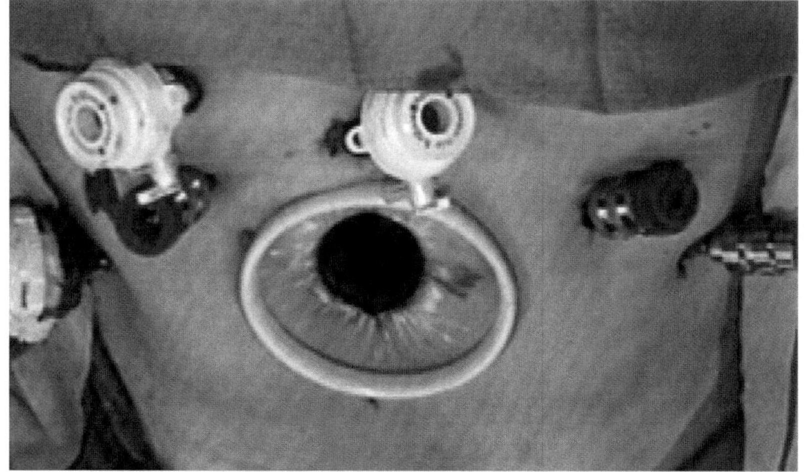

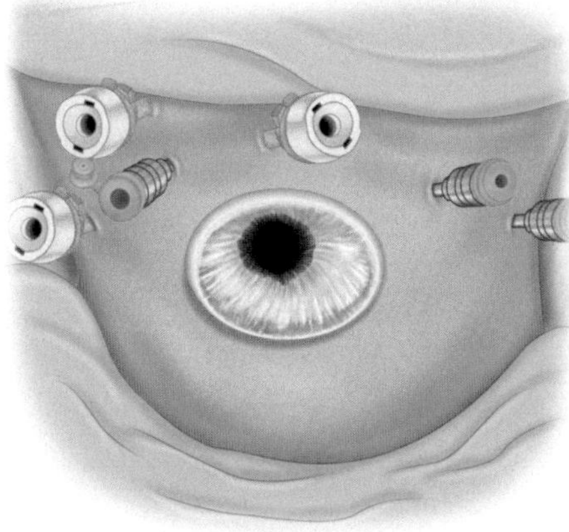

Fig. 14.12 Placement of Alexis wound retractor

bloodless plane of Treves. This can be performed with the LigaSure device or suture ligations of crossing mesenteric vessels with 3-0 silk sutures. A segment of ileum is then measured to create the conduit. An appropriate length can be obtained by placing the distal end of the harvested segment on the skin at the planned stomal site and measuring the length of ileum needed to perform tension-free uretero-enteric anastomoses (Fig. 14.13). An additional 5-cm segment of ileum is then marked, which will be excised to reduce mesenteric tension and to keep the bowel anastomoses farther away from the ureteroileal anastomoses. A GIA stapler is used to staple and divide the ileum at this location. The ileum is then divided, using cautery at the proximal end of the conduit. The proximal 5-cm segment is then excised and discarded. The proximal end of the conduit is closed using absorbable 3-0 polyglactin sutures in continuous fashion. The closure is reinforced with 3-0 silk Lembert sutures, which are left long for future identification in the event of reoperation.

The ileum is then brought back into continuity. With the conduit placed inferiorly, a stapled side-to-side bowel anastomosis is then performed using the GIA stapler. The crossing staple lines and the base of the anastomosis are reinforced with interrupted 3-0 silk sutures. The mesenteric defect is then closed using 3-0 polyglactin suture in continuous fashion.

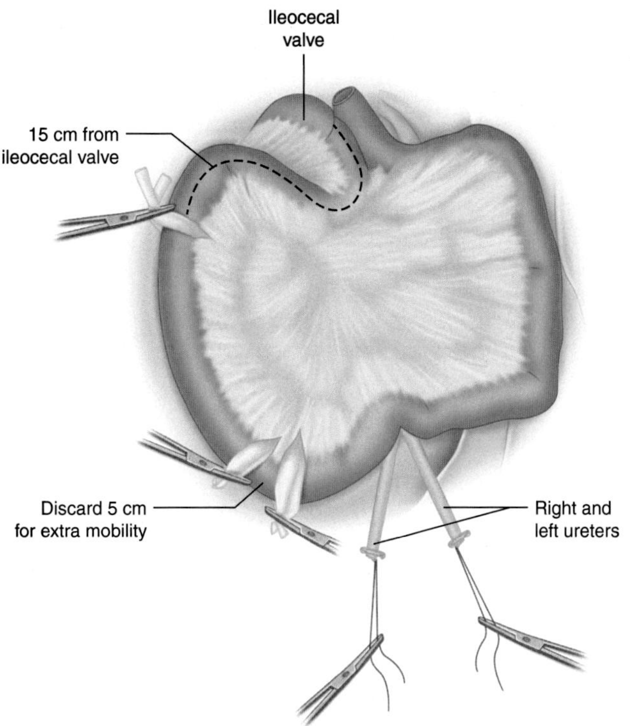

Fig. 14.13 Ileal harvest for ileal conduit

Uretero-Enteric Anastomoses

For the left ureter, a small enterotomy is made sharply, adjacent to the proximal end of the conduit. The mucosal edges are then everted using 4-0 chromic sutures in the four quadrants of the enterotomy. The left ureter is then brought adjacent to the planned anastomosis site. The excess ureter is excised and sent as a specimen. The uretero-enteric anastomosis is then performed in end-to-side, spatulated fashion using interrupted or continuous 4-0 polyglactin or monofilament absorbable suture. Halfway through the anastomosis, a single-J urinary diversion stent is placed across the anastomosis and brought out the distal end of the conduit. The anastomosis is then completed. Care should be taken to create a watertight anastomosis, with a "no touch" technique on the ureteral mucosa. The procedure is then replicated for the right uretero-enteric anastomosis.

Ileal Conduit Stoma Creation

A disk of skin is excised at the previously marked planned stoma site. The subcutaneous tissue is divided using cautery, and a cruciate incision is made in the anterior rectus fascia. The peritoneum is then incised. To avoid strangulation of the conduit, the fascial incision should be wide enough to accommodate two fingerbreadths. If the small bowel mesentery is pliable, a rosebud stoma can be created, but if the small bowel mesentery is not pliable, a modified Turnbull stoma should be created.

For a rosebud stoma, the distal end of the conduit is brought through the incision with the mesentery along the superior aspect (Fig. 14.14). The conduit is secured to the

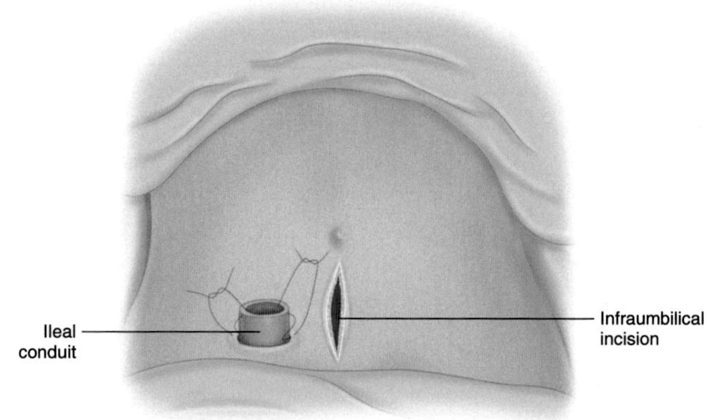

Fig. 14.14 Rosebud stoma creation

fascia at four locations using a 0 polyglactin suture through a seromuscular layer of the conduit. The distal staple line is then excised. The stoma is then matured using 2-0 polyglactin sutures through the distal edge of the stoma, seromuscular along the conduit at the level of the skin, and then subcuticular at the skin. The stomal mucosa is everted as these sutures are tightened. The intervening gaps can then be filled in with additional 2-0 polyglactin sutures.

For a modified Turnbull stoma, a segment of conduit several centimeters proximal to the distal end is brought through the incision. The conduit is secured to the fascia at four locations using 0 polyglactin suture through a seromuscular layer. A semilunar incision is then created through the conduit. The stoma is then matured at the functional limb using 2-0 polyglactin sutures through the distal stoma edges, including a seromuscular bite along the conduit at the level of the skin and then subcuticular at the skin. The stomal mucosa is everted as these sutures are tightened. The defunctionalized limb can simply be sutured to the skin, and the intervening gaps can then be filled in with additional 2-0 polyglactin sutures.

A red Robinson catheter is placed into the conduit and secured at the stomal level, along with the two ureteral stents. A 19-Fr round Blake drain is then placed through the left pararectus port site into the pelvis and ending next to the ureteroileal anastomoses adjacent to the proximal end of the conduit. The incisions are irrigated thoroughly. The fascia and skin are then closed at the midline incision, and all port sites are closed. A urostomy appliance is placed over the stoma.

The stents and red Robinson catheter are removed 1 day before discharge. The drain is removed when the output is less than 400 mL/24 h.

Studer Orthotopic Ileal Neobladder Formation

Robotic Preparation

Several key steps performed with the robot still docked facilitate an expeditious creation of the orthotopic urinary diversion. A 3-0 polyglactin suture has been placed at the 6 o'clock position of the urethra at the time of urethral division. The left ureter is transposed to the right abdomen through the sigmoid mesenteric window. A 2-0 silk suture is placed on the terminal ileum. A red Robinson catheter is placed into the urethra with a 0 silk suture secured to the end. A grasper secures the ureteral, ileal, and red Robinson catheters prior to undocking the robot. The robotic instruments are then removed and the robot is undocked.

Ileal Harvest and Neobladder Formation

A 7-cm midline incision is then made below the umbilicus, and the rectus fascia and peritoneum are opened. The specimen is removed, and an Alexis wound retractor is then placed for aid in exposure. The sutures for the right ureter, left ureter, terminal ileum, and the red Robinson catheter that had previously been secured on the grasper are now delivered through the incision. The ureters and ileum are oriented in their correct anatomic position. Care is taken to ensure that the ureters are traveling along their anatomic course. A GIA stapler is then used to staple and divide the terminal ileum approximately 15 cm proximal to the ileocecal valve. The mesentery at this location is divided toward the root of the mesentery for a distance of approximately 8–10 cm at the bloodless plane of Treves. This can be performed with the LigaSure device or suture ligations of crossing mesenteric vessels with 2-0 or 3-0 silk sutures. A 60-cm segment of ileum is then measured proximally to create the neobladder

(Fig. 14.15). An additional 5-cm segment of ileum is then marked, which will be excised to reduce mesenteric tension and to separate the end of the afferent limb of the neobladder from the bowel anastomosis. The GIA stapler is then used to staple and divide the ileum at this location. The ileum is then divided using cautery at the proximal end of the afferent limb of the neobladder. The 5-cm segment is then excised and discarded. The afferent limb of the neobladder is closed using absorbable 3-0 polyglactin sutures in continuous fashion. The closure is reinforced with 3-0 silk Lembert sutures, which are left long for future identification in the event of reoperation.

The ileum is then brought back into continuity. With the ileal segment used for neobladder placed inferiorly, a stapled side-to-side bowel anastomosis is then performed using the GIA stapler. The crossing staple lines and the base of the anastomosis are reinforced with interrupted 3-0 silk sutures. The mesenteric defect is then closed using 3-0 polyglactin suture in continuous fashion.

A 15-cm afferent limb segment is marked in the ileal segment of the neobladder. The remaining ileum for the neobladder is then detubularized using cautery along the antimesenteric edge. The detubularized segment is then placed in a U-shaped configuration and the medial edges are sewn together using continuous 3-0 polyglactin sutures. These sutures should incorporate a larger seromuscular bite and a smaller mucosal bite to allow for adequate inversion of the mucosa. The sutures should be placed in close enough proximity to ensure a watertight closure. The pouch is then folded on itself in Heineke-Mikulicz fashion, and the remaining edges are sewn to close the pouch using 3-0 polyglactin suture, with the same technique as described above (Fig. 14.16).

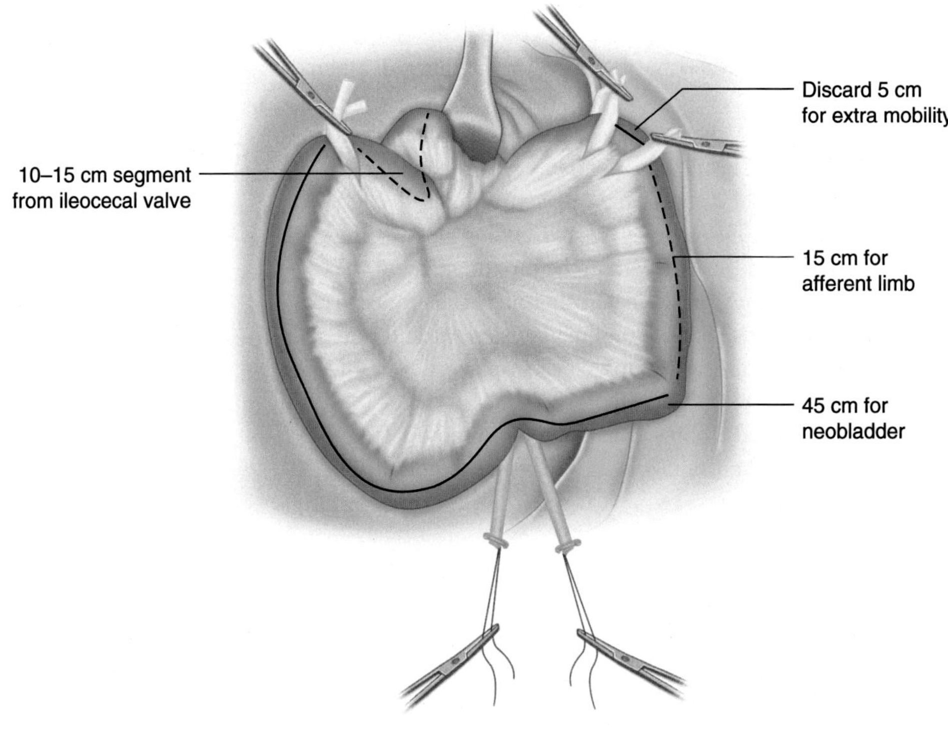

Fig. 14.15 Ileal harvest for orthotopic neobladder

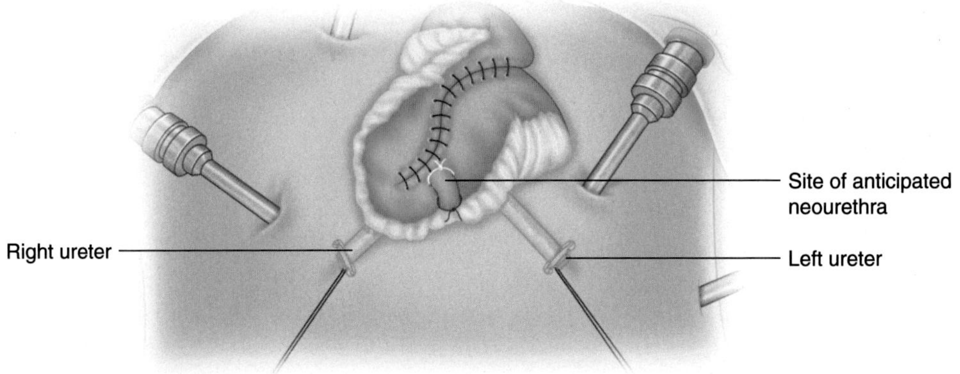

Fig. 14.16 Completed neobladder, prior to the uretero-enteric anastomoses

A 0 polyglactin suture is then placed at the 6 and 12 o'clock positions of the anticipated urethra-neovesical anastomosis site. It should be noted that no opening in the neobladder for the urethral anastomosis is made until after the robot is redocked so that we can choose an optimal location on the pouch for the anastomosis based on the exposure. An additional 6 o'clock polyglactin suture at the neobladder is tied to the tip of the urethral red Robinson catheter, which can act as a handle for the bedside assistant.

Uretero-Enteric Anastomoses

The uretero-enteric anastomoses are then performed in the same way as for ileal conduit urinary diversion, detailed above. The two ureters are stented with single-J urinary diversion stents that are brought out through a 1-mm incision in the distal afferent limb of the neobladder and placed beside the right robotic port site. A 3-0 plain gut purse-string suture is used to secure the stents at the afferent limb.

Posterior Plate Reconstruction and Urethra-Neovesical Anastomosis

Once the uretero-enteric anastomoses are completed, the midline incision is closed and the abdomen insufflated. The robot is redocked to the ports, and the robotic instruments are replaced. The posterior urethral plate reconstruction is then performed in similar fashion to a Rocco reconstruction (Fig. 14.17). First, the musculofascial plate of the rectourethralis is approximated to the cut edge of Denonvilliers' fascia in figure-of-eight fashion using 3-0 polyglactin suture. The neobladder is brought down to the pelvis by applying gentle pressure on the red Robinson catheter and the 6 o'clock suture in the neobladder. Once in the pelvis, the neobladder is held in place using the robotic fourth arm on the 0 polyglactin 6 o'clock suture. Care should be taken to ensure that the fourth arm of the robot is not compressing the external iliac vessels while it is holding the neobladder down in the pelvis for the urethral anastomosis. Next, the musculofascial plate of the rectourethralis is approximated to the posterior neobladder, approximately 2 cm posterior to the planned urethral aperture, using 3-0 polyglactin suture. The suture on the red Robinson catheter is cut, and this catheter is removed. The urethral aperture is then created sharply or with cautery using the cutting current. The previously placed 3-0 polyglactin 6 o'clock posterior urethral suture is then placed in its corresponding location in the urethral aperture and is tied down. If there is significant tension on this initial 6 o'clock suture, additional interrupted sutures can be used to reapproximate the posterior urethral plate. Two 3-0 absorbable barbed sutures that are looped together are then brought in and are placed in the neobladder neck on each side of the 3-0 polyglactin suture and then in their corresponding location in the posterior urethra. Each suture is used to complete the urethra-neovesical anastomosis along each side, up to the 12 o'clock position. An 18-Fr two-way hematuria Foley catheter is then inserted per urethra and into the bladder. The anastomosis is then tested by irrigating the Foley catheter. The balloon is then inflated with 15 mL of sterile water.

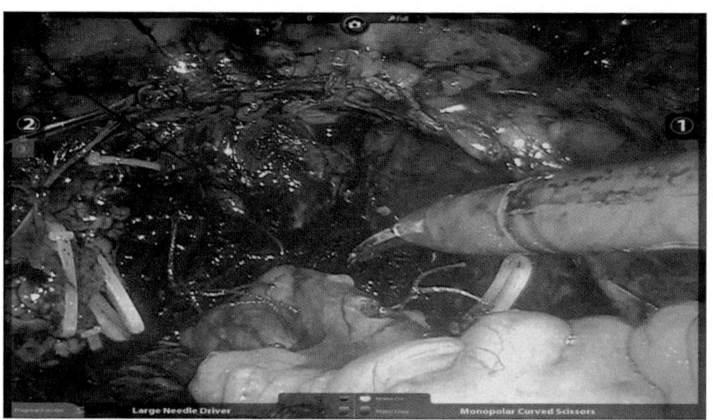

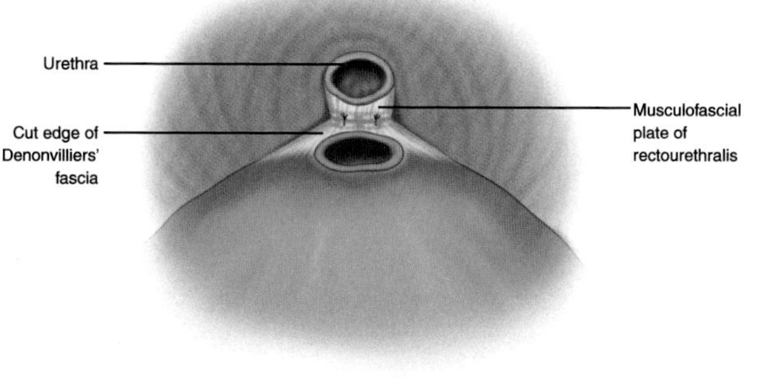

Fig. 14.17 Rocco reconstruction

A 19-Fr round Blake drain is brought through the left pararectus port site and placed along the urethral anastomosis and adjacent to the ureteroileal anastomoses. The drain and stents are secured to the skin. The remaining robotic instruments are removed, and the robot is undocked. All ports are irrigated thoroughly. The fascia at the 12-mm robotic port sites are closed, and the skin is closed at all incisions. The stents are cut short and an ostomy appliance is placed over them.

Postoperative Care

Hospital stay typically ranges from 5 to 7 days. The stents are removed when the patient has full return of bowel function. The drain is removed when the output is less than 400 mL/24 h. The Foley catheter is hand-irrigated every 4 h and kept in place for 3 weeks. A cystogram is performed to ensure no leakage before catheter removal.

Indiana Pouch Formation

Robotic/Laparoscopic Preparation

Before undocking the robot, the left ureter is transposed to the right abdomen underneath the sigmoid mesentery. The sutures on the two ureters are secured with a grasper that is in the right iliac port. At this point, the robot is undocked and the patient is positioned flat, with the right side up. Using the existing port configuration, a hand-assist gel port and the Alexis wound retractor are placed in the 7-cm incision used for specimen retrieval, and the abdomen is re-insufflated. A hand-assisted, laparoscopic mobilization of the right colon is then performed.

Using monopolar shears, the ascending colon is then mobilized by continuing the peritoneal incision lateral to the colon along the white line of Toldt. The colon and colonic mesentery are then dissected medially. The hepatic flexure is taken down using cautery. This mobilization is continued to the mid transverse colon.

Ileocolonic Harvest

The abdomen is desufflated and the gel port is removed. The Alexis wound retractor is kept in place for exposure. The sutures for the left ureter and right ureter are delivered through the incision. A GIA stapler is then used to staple and divide the terminal ileum approximately 15 cm proximal to the ileocecal valve. The mesentery at this location is divided toward the root of the mesentery for a distance of approximately 8–10 cm at the bloodless plane of Treves. This can be performed with the LigaSure device or suture ligations of crossing mesenteric vessels with 2-0 or 3-0 silk sutures. A 31-cm segment of ascending colon is then measured starting at the appendix; this segment will be used to create the colonic reservoir. The colon is then stapled and divided at this location using a GIA stapler (Fig. 14.18).

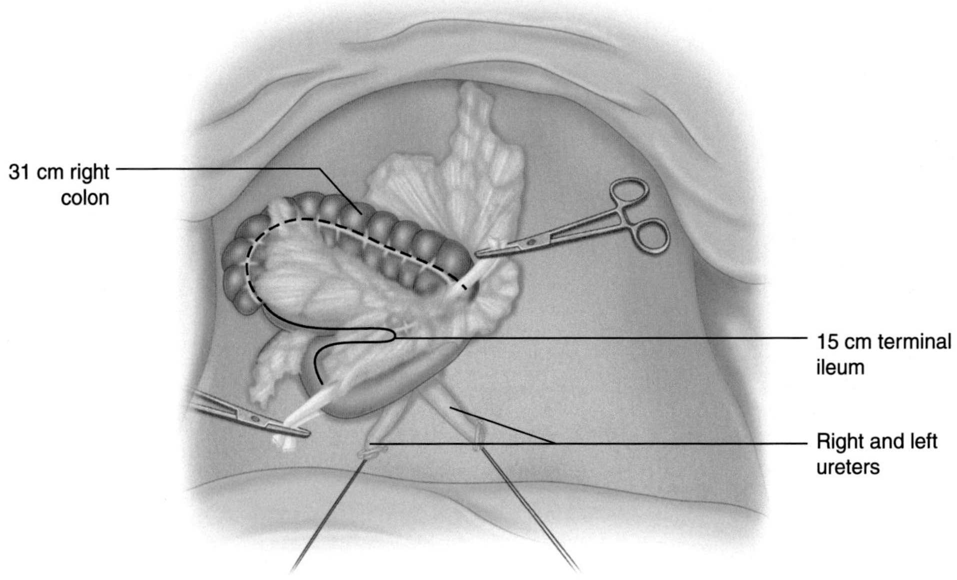

Fig. 14.18 Ileocolonic harvest for Indiana pouch

The ileocolonic anastomosis is then performed with the ileal-colonic segment inferior to the bowel anastomosis. A stapled side-to-side bowel anastomosis is performed using the GIA stapler and a TA-60 stapler. The crossing staple lines and base of the anastomosis are reinforced with interrupted 3-0 silk sutures. The mesenteric trap is then closed using a 3-0 polyglactin suture in continuous fashion.

The colonic portion of the Indiana pouch is then detubularized using cautery along its antimesenteric edge. This incision is continued around the appendix. The mesoappendix is then divided using the LigaSure device or serial 3-0 silk suture ligations. The appendix is removed. The detubularized colonic segment is then folded on itself in Heineke-Mikulicz fashion, and the edges are sewn together using 3-0 polyglactin suture, with the same technique as described above. These sutures should incorporate a larger seromuscular bite and a smaller mucosal bite to allow for adequate inversion of the mucosa. The sutures should be placed in close enough proximity to create a watertight closure.

Catheterizable Limb Formation

The staple line on the ileal segment of the Indiana pouch is excised. A 14-Fr red Robinson catheter is then advanced through the ileal segment and into the pouch itself, to facilitate tapering the ileal segment. Allis clamps are used to tension the ileal segment against the catheter along its antimesenteric edge. A GIA stapler is then used to excise this excess ileum along the catheter, continuing up to the ileocecal valve; multiple staple loads may be required (Fig. 14.19). The base of the ileocecal valve is imbricated, using Lembert style 3-0 silk sutures in a seromuscular layer in three locations equally spaced around the ileocecal valve, superiorly, anteriorly, and inferiorly. The catheter is then removed and replaced, ensuring ease of catheterization.

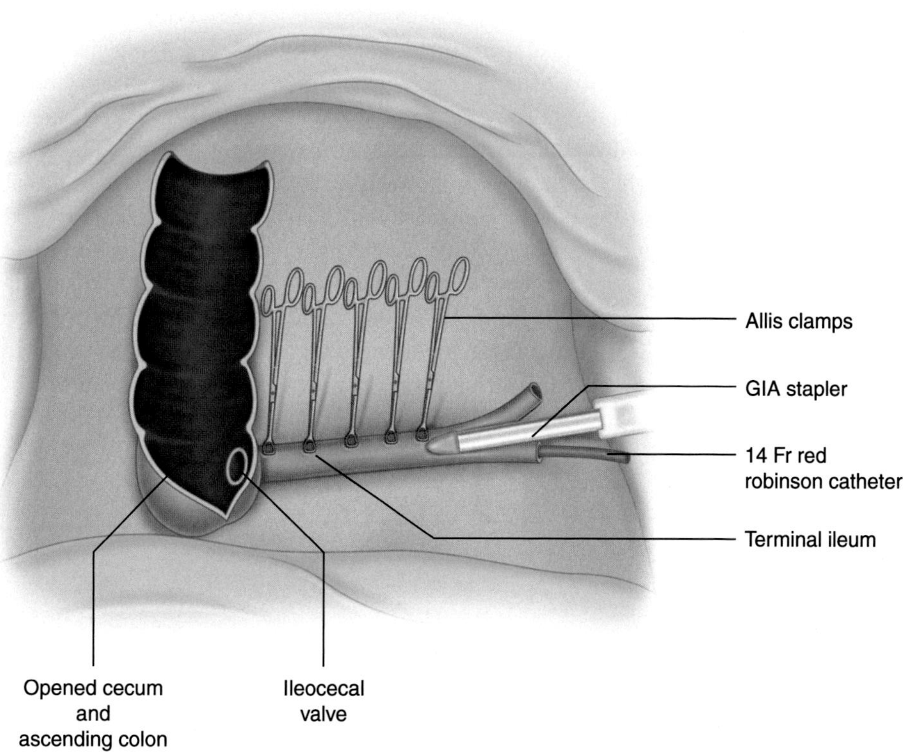

Fig. 14.19 Stapling and tapering of catheterizable limb

Pouch Formation

The detubularized colonic segment is then folded on itself in Heineke-Mikulicz fashion, and the edges are sewn together using 3-0 polyglactin suture, with the same technique as described above. These sutures should incorporate a larger seromuscular bite and a smaller mucosal bite to allow for adequate inversion of the mucosa. The sutures should be placed in close enough proximity to create a watertight closure. The pouch is then filled with 300 mL of normal saline to confirm no extravasation as well as continence at the ileal segment and subsequently emptied.

Uretero-Enteric Anastomoses

Once the pouch is created and the continence mechanism is completed, we proceed with the ureteral anastomoses. The right side of the Indiana pouch is then rotated counterclockwise 90°. A small enterotomy is made sharply along the left aspect of the Indiana pouch, at least 1 cm away from any suture line. The mucosal edges are then everted using 4-0 chromic sutures in four quadrants of the enterotomy. The left ureter is then brought adjacent to the planned anastomosis site. The excess ureter is excised and sent as a specimen. The uretero-colonic anastomosis is then performed in either interrupted or continuous fashion using 4-0 polyglactin or monofilament absorbable suture. Halfway through the anastomosis, a single-J urinary diversion stent is placed across the anastomosis and brought out through a stab incision in the right anterior aspect of the pouch. The anastomosis is then completed. Care should be taken to create a watertight anastomosis, using a "no touch" technique on the ureteral mucosa. The procedure is then replicated for the right uretero-enteric anastomosis. The stents are then secured to the pouch using a 4-0 plain gut purse-string suture and are externalized at the right iliac port site.

Suprapubic Catheter Placement

A 24-Fr Foley catheter is brought into the abdomen through the right upper quadrant port site, or a separate 1-cm incision if the port site is too cranial. The term *suprapubic* is a historical term for this catheter and not at the true suprapubic region. The key to placement of the suprapubic site and the future stoma site is that the distance and orientation between two sites on the pouch match the corresponding sites on the skin. The catheter is placed into the Indiana pouch in a Stamm fashion using two rows of purse string 2-0 polyglactin sutures. Ten milliliters of sterile water is placed into the balloon. The suprapubic catheter is pulled taut and the pouch anchored to the anterior abdominal wall using the two Stamm polyglactin sutures. The catheter is secured at the skin using a 0 silk suture.

Creation of Stoma

A small disk of skin is then excised at the right pararectus port site. The fascia at this location is bluntly dilated to one fingerbreadth. The limb is then brought through this incision and is pulled anteriorly until the excess limb is outside the skin. The excess is then excised and discarded using cautery. Our goal is to excise as much redundant ileal segment as possible to create an easily catheterizable channel. Catheterization is then performed again to ensure ease. The stoma is secured to the skin using interrupted 3-0 polyglactin sutures, full thickness through the stoma and subcuticular at the skin. A 19-Fr Blake drain is placed in the pelvis and adjacent to the uretero-colonic anastomoses and externalized at the left pararectus port site. The fascia and skin are then closed at the midline incision and all remaining port sites (Fig. 14.20). The suprapubic tube and stents are placed to gravity drainage. A Vaseline gauze is used to cover the stoma which is left uncatheterized.

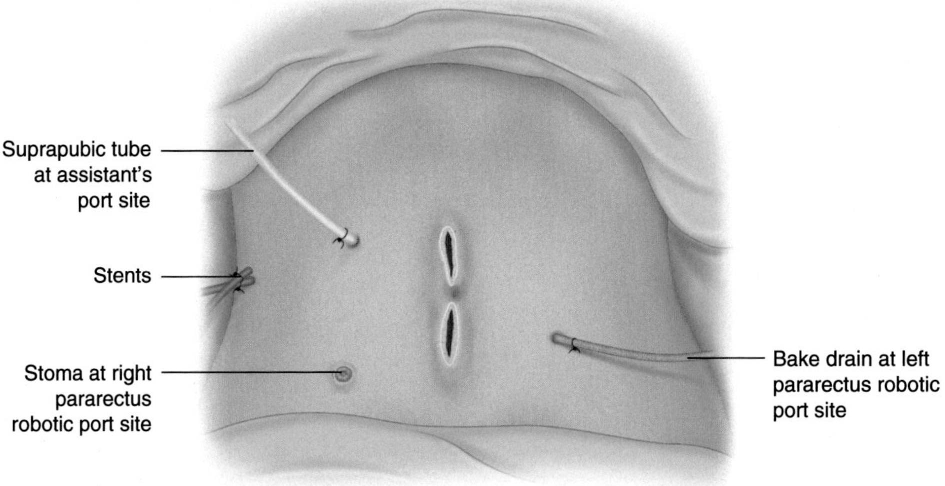

Fig. 14.20 Completed Indiana pouch incision and drain sites

Postoperative Care

Similar to the neobladder, hospital stay ranges between 5 and 7 days. The suprapubic catheter is hand-irrigated every 4 h. The stomal dressing is changed daily. Stents are removed when the patient has had full return of bowel function. The drain is removed when the output is less than 400 mL/24 h. The suprapubic catheter is removed at 3 weeks when a pouchogram confirms no extravasation.

Intracorporeal Urinary Diversion

More than any other portion of the cystoprostatectomy, the manipulation of the bowel requires careful planning, proper instrumentation, and an expert bedside assistant. Having the assistant perform the stapling, clipping, and cutting can save valuable time over the course of the case.

Port Placement

To adequately staple the bowel via the assistant ports, it is best to have the assistant ports on the left-hand side. For this reason, it is preferred to have two working robot arms on the patient's right and one working arm on the patient's left, with the lateral-most right-sided port 2–3 cm above the anterior superior iliac spine (ASIS) at the anterior axillary line. On the left-hand side, a 12-mm port is placed in a similar position 2–3 cm above the ASIS. Of note, instead of a 12-mm port at this assistant site, a hybrid 15-mm port can be used, which can enable node removal during the case directly through the port. Alternatively if the operative surgeon prefers to have the third robot working arm on the patient's left, he or she can telescope a robotic port through the 15-mm port for the cystectomy portion of the case. A second left-sided assistant port (also 12 mm) can be placed either at the level of the umbilicus in the anterior axillary line or triangulated between the camera and the robotic arm serving the surgeon's left hand.

Patient Positioning

If a neobladder is planned, it is beneficial to remove the robotic instruments when the cystectomy is completed and level the patient from steep Trendelenburg to approximately 10°. A good rule of thumb is to place the camera in the abdomen as the patient is leveled, and continue the leveling of the patient until the bowel starts to fall into the pelvis.

Instrumentation

To minimize changing instruments repeatedly throughout the case, it is useful to have two Cadiere graspers in the left-hand port and the most lateral right-hand port, with a large needle driver in the medial right-hand port. Arm 1 will be the only instrument that is changed over the course of the case, except to perform the urethral or ureteral anastomoses.

Isolating the Bowel

A piece of precut umbilical tape 20 cm long is placed into the abdomen. The ileocecal valve is identified, and the umbilical tape is used to identify the point 20 cm proximal to the valve (Fig. 14.21). This can be accomplished while holding the umbilical tape and the bowel simultaneously, performing a hand-to-hand motion as if running the bowel.

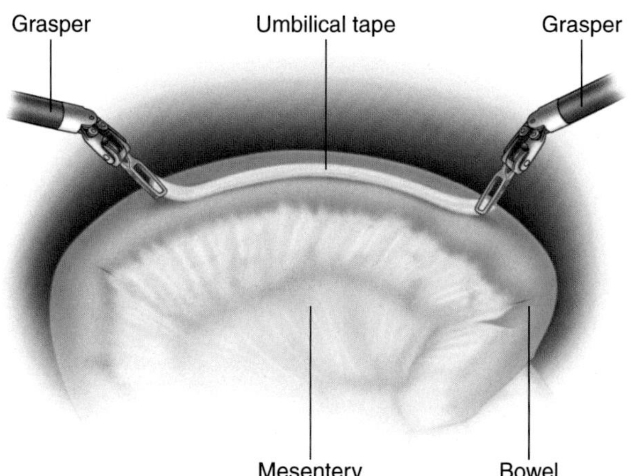

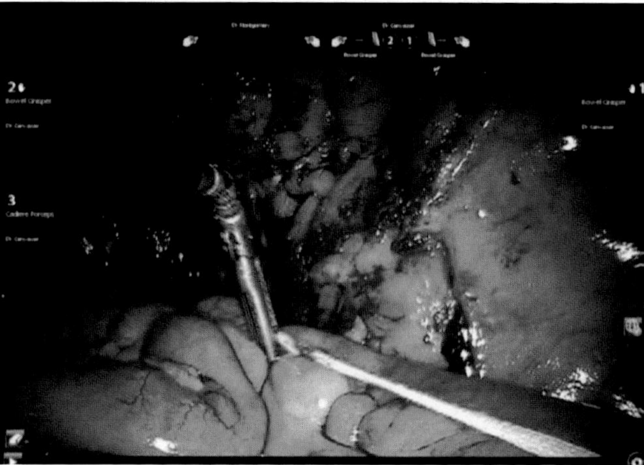

Fig. 14.21 Umbilical tape cut to 20 cm is used to measure the segments of the bowel, 20 cm proximal to the terminal ileum and 20 cm for conduit length. Ensure the bowel and tape are held simultaneously to ensure an accurate measurement

Once the point 20 cm proximal is identified, the left hand continues to hold the bowel, while the right-hand needle driver is used to throw two stay sutures at the 20-cm mark, each just over 1 cm apart, with 3-0 silk. These stay sutures should be air knots and cut by the assistant to be 3 cm in length. To save time, use the Cadiere forceps in the left hand to help throw the suture, rather than putting a second needle driver in the left hand. Using the umbilical tape, an additional 20 cm proximally on the ileum is measured out, and here two 3-0 Vicryl stay sutures are thrown, 1 cm apart (Fig. 14.22).

If more bowel is needed, as is necessary for a neobladder, the umbilical tape can be reset to allow more bowel to be isolated. Using the Cadiere graspers to hold the two most distal stay sutures, a 60-cm articulating Endo-GIA stapler is brought in through the lower assistant port. For the initial division, a tan load for the Tri-Staple™ (Covidien; Dublin, Ireland) is recommended, or a 2.5-mm vascular load. This will ensure that the mesenteric vasculature is sufficiently secured. The luminal intestine is not separated from the mesentery for an isolated staple fire. Rather, the stapler is fired across the bowel, including a portion of the mesentery. When stapling the distal bowel (between the paired silk sutures), two staple loads should be used to facilitate an additional "bite" of mesentery to help the stoma to pass through the abdominal wall. The stapler is directed toward the root of the mesentery, not at an angle, with careful attention paid to mesenteric vascular arcades, to avoid devascularization (Fig. 14.23). When stapling the proximal bowel (between the paired Vicryl sutures), only one staple load is needed. The ileal loop is placed into the pelvis.

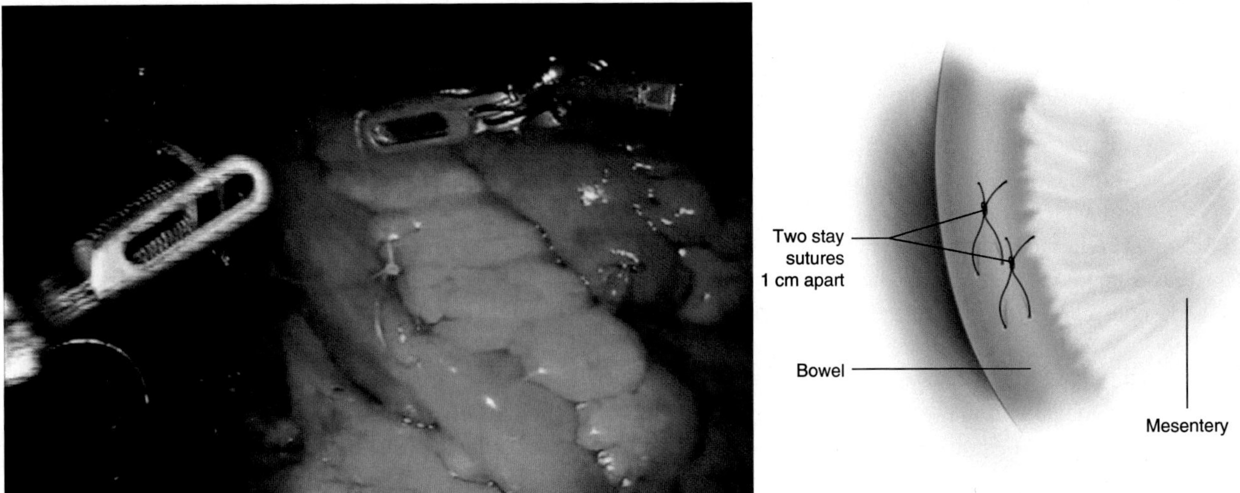

Fig. 14.22 The stay sutures are placed 1 cm apart to allow the stapler to pass between them

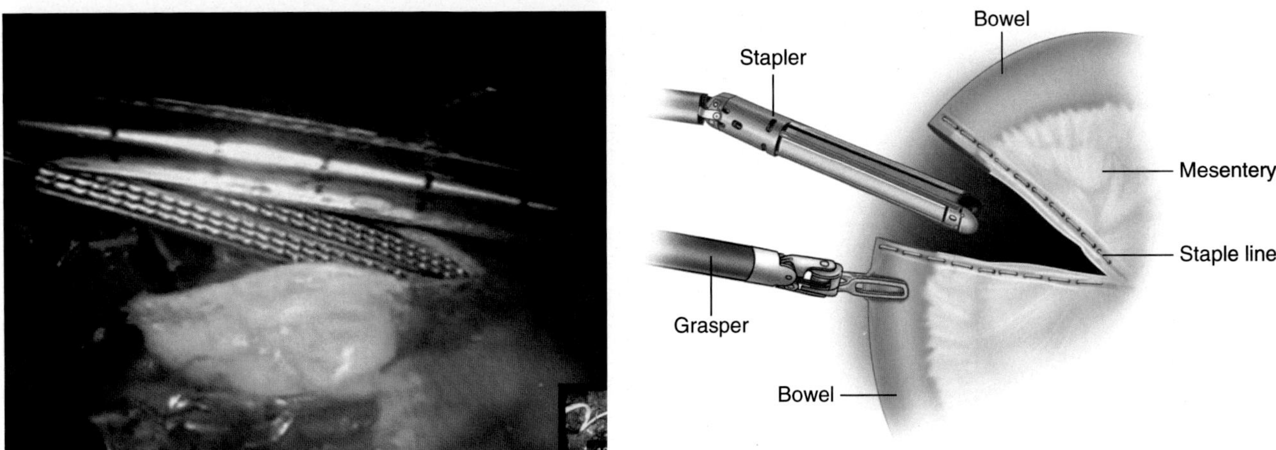

Fig. 14.23 The staple load is directed toward the root of the mesentery to avoid devascularization during division of the ileal loop. Proximally, only one load is needed; distally, two loads should be used to allow passage through the abdominal wall

Using the left-hand Cadiere grasper, the stapled ends of the bowel to be reanastomosed are held. In the medial right hand, the needle driver is exchanged with a scissor. The corner of each staple line is incised and removed, leaving an approximate 1-cm enterotomy. The scissor is replaced with a needle driver. The assistant now brings in a 60-cm purple load for the Endo-GIA Tri-Staple™, or a 3.5-mm blue load, and both the arm 2 and arm 3 graspers are used on the bowel to fit the stapler blades into the defects that were created. This is best accomplished through the lower assistant port. Close the blades of the stapler, and use the graspers to gently pull the mesentery away from the stapler to ensure an antimesenteric staple fire (Fig. 14.24).

A second stapler load is passed into the bowel lumen to create a larger communication between the two bowel segments. After the second load is fired, the needle driver is used to throw a secure "crotch" stitch at the end of the staple line. The assistant cuts the suture.

Next, a final 60-cm staple load is used to staple close the common enterotomy (Fig. 14.25). This is also a purple Tri-Staple™ load or a blue small-bowel Endo-GIA load. Passing this stapler load through the upper-most assistant port typically gives the best angle.

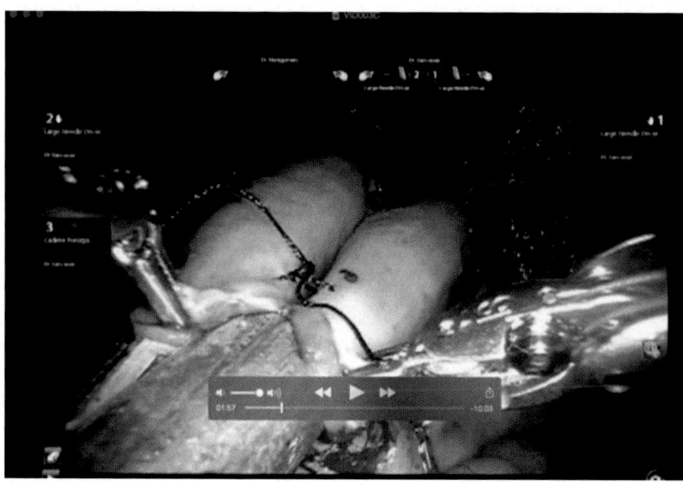

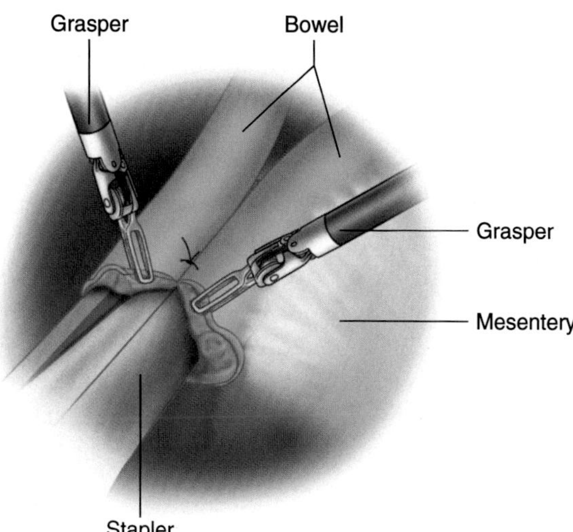

Fig. 14.24 The Endo-GIA stapler is inserted in the two bowel ends, oriented antimesenteric, to initiate the side-to-side bowel anastomosis

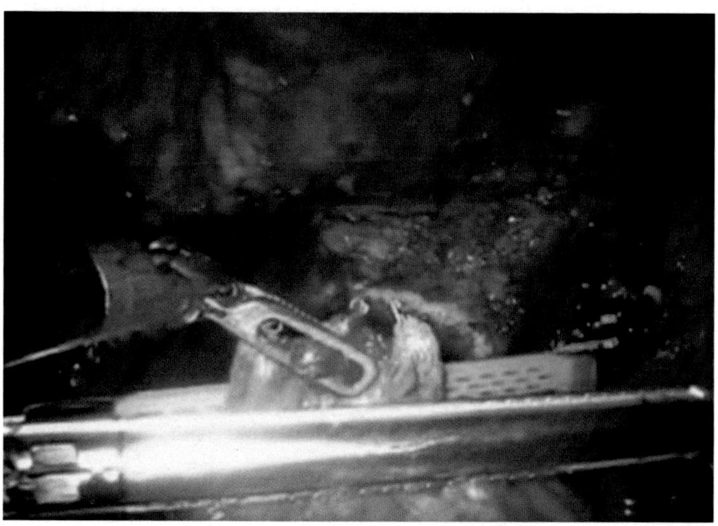

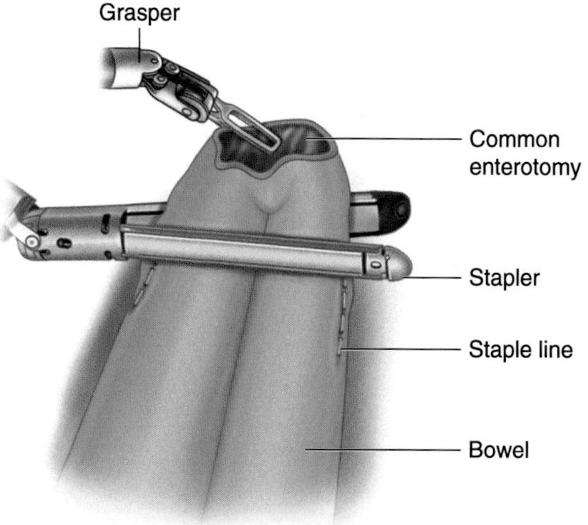

Fig. 14.25 Once the two side-to-side staple loads have been fired, a final staple load completes the bowel anastomosis, passed through the left upper assistant's port

Intracorporeal Ileal Conduit

A Keith needle with a 30-cm-long, 2-0 silk suture attached is passed through the abdominal wall 2 cm inferior to the medial right-hand port. Once inside the abdomen, the Keith needle is passed through the staple line at the distal end of the ileal loop. The suture is passed close to the mesenteric side of the bowel. The Keith needle is passed back out of the abdomen near the entry site. The assistant secures the suture outside the body with a hemostat. During the case, the tension can be adjusted as needed.

Generally, the left ureter is attached first. Sometimes it is necessary to secure the proximal end of the conduit to the retroperitoneum in order to stabilize the bowel for the anastomosis. This can be done with a single Vicryl suture passed through the proximal bowel, close to the staple line, and then to the psoas muscle just above the common iliac artery. This maneuver will also aid in stent passage later in the case.

The left ureter is placed over the bowel near the proximal end in an appropriate location. Select the length of the ureter that will be divided and spatulated. The ureter is manipulated only using the previously placed clip and suture, or the excess ureter. When the appropriate point is selected, the ureter is held up toward the abdominal wall on tension. To initiate the spatulation process, a scissor is placed into the medial right-hand port. The ureter is cut at an angle with a robotic Potts scissor or standard scissors, pointing the tips of the scissors toward the distal ureter. Do not fully divide the ureter; leave a small amount of ureter attached for a handle. If needed, the ureter can be incised more proximally to increase the amount of spatulation. We suggest at least 1.5 cm total spatulation. An equal defect is created in the bowel in the appropriate location.

A needle driver is placed in the right medial port and the left port. Two separate 4-0 Monocryl sutures (some prefer Vicryl) on an RB-1 needle are brought into the abdomen. The first suture is passed out-to-in on the bowel side, then in-to-out on the ureteral apex. The second needle is passed in a similar fashion at the same location. Once the sutures are passed, each is tied down. One will be used for the posterior wall (furthest from the camera), and one will be used for the anterior wall (closest to the camera). First, the entire posterior wall is approximated. Once the distal ureter is approached, the excess ureter is excised by the assistant. Once the wall is complete, the suture is tied to itself.

A needle driver is placed in the medial right arm, and a Cadiere grasper in the remaining arms. A 75-cm single-J stent with 20 cm of the noncoiled end removed is placed over a wire, and 2–3 cm of the wire is exposed (enough to take the curl out of the 'J'). The assistant grabs the end of the wire with a laparoscopic needle driver and passes it in through one of the assistant ports. It is grabbed with the robotic needle driver, and the tip is placed into the left ureter, using the Cadiere grasper to aid the passage. The resistance and the measurements are noted. The stent is passed 15–20 cm on the left and 10–15 cm on the right. Once in location, the needle driver is used to pinch the stent next to the wire, not including the wire in the grasp, which will allow the assistant to pull the wire while leaving the stent in place. With the lateral right grasper, the stent is held close to the anastomosis site.

A scissor is used to cut off 1 cm of the distal staple line close to the abdominal wall. The ileal conduit is tensioned using the transabdominal stitch to pull the bowel straight. This allows the needle driver to pass uninhibited through the lumen of the bowel (Fig. 14.26). Once the tips are seen at the level of the anastomosis, the left-hand grasper is used to place the end of the stent into the jaws of the needle driver, which pulls it through the bowel. The lateral right hand is held until the stent is pulled through the bowel.

The anterior portion of the ureteral anastomosis is completed with the previously placed suture. The process is repeated on the right side. The right ureter can be passed lateral or medial to the conduit. If lateral, the tension that is holding the bowel to the abdominal wall often must be released to allow access to the anastomosis.

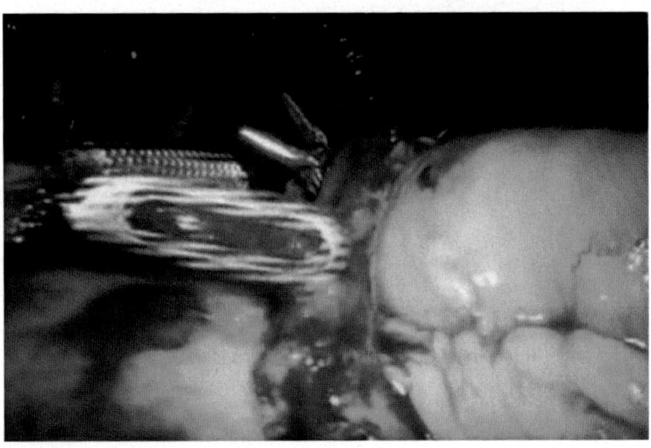

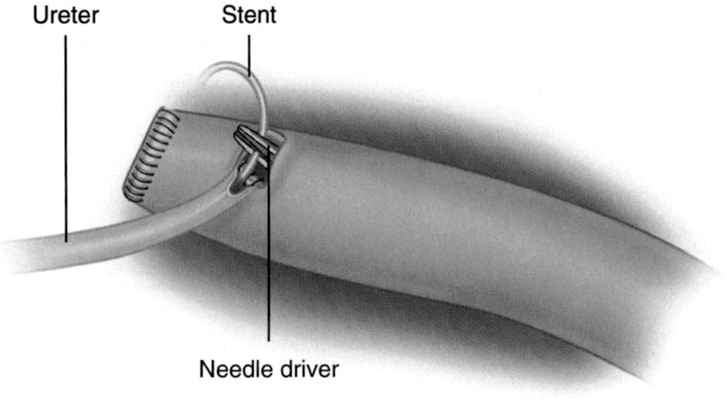

Fig. 14.26 The needle driver is passed through the lumen of the bowel to grab the end of the ureteral stent after it has been placed into the ureteral lumen

Preparing for Stoma Maturation and Specimen Removal

The assistant passes a small bowel grasper through the upper port. The grasper is used to hold the bowel and stents near the distal end. The transabdominal stitch is removed from the bowel and pulled through the abdominal wall. In the lower port, the assistant passes a laparoscopic needle driver and secures the suture of the specimen bags.

The skin incision is made in the midline, far enough away from the selected stoma site that the ostomy appliance will not interfere but close enough that a hand can be used to create the defect in the abdominal wall. Once the abdomen is entered, the needle driver holding the specimen bag is passed to the incision. The incision is made as small as necessary to remove the specimen. All ports not in use are removed, except those holding the ileal conduit and stents. The conduit and stents are delivered to the incision and secured with a Babcock clamp. All ports can be removed.

Next, the defect in the abdominal wall at the stoma site is created in a standard fashion. A Babcock clamp is passed through the defect to grab the bowel and stents from the laparoscopic bowel grasper and is pulled through the stoma site. At this point all ports can be removed. The stoma is matured in a standard fashion, and all 12-mm ports and the specimen extraction port are closed.

Intracorporeal Studer Orthotopic Neobladder

The most dependent portion of the ileum that will easily reach to the level of the urethra is identified and marked with a stay suture. The stay suture is held in arm 3 to keep the ileum pulled into the pelvis, and 20 cm is measured both proximally and distally. The distal marking is made with 2-0 silk stay sutures as detailed in the above description of ileal conduit creation. Proximally, however, an additional 15–20 cm is measured and marked with two 3-0 Vicryl stay sutures. The bowel is divided, and the anastomosis is performed as described previously.

Urethral Anastomosis

The initially preplaced stay suture at the most dependent portion of the ileum is used as a handle in arm 3. The suture is held close to the urethra. A scissor in the medial right port is used to create a 1–2-cm enterotomy on the antimesenteric border of the ileum. A suture is placed from the rectourethralis to just posterior to the enterotomy. This suture is tied down. The ileum should stay in place if arm 3 is removed. If not, secure the ileum on either side of the previous suture until arm 3 can be removed.

The urethral-ileal anastomosis is then performed in a van Velthoven fashion, with either a barbed suture or two 4-0 Monocryl sutures that have been tied together (Fig. 14.27). A 20-French catheter is passed as the anastomosis is almost complete. After completing the anastomosis, additional stay sutures are placed lateral and anterior to the anastomosis site to hold the bowel to the pelvis.

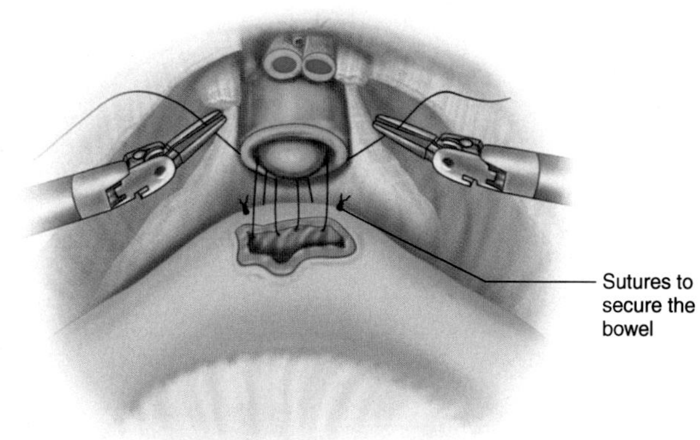

Fig. 14.27 The urethral-ileal anastomosis is then performed in a van Velthoven fashion, with either a double-armed 3-0 absorbable, barbed suture or two running 4-0 Monocryl sutures

Creating the Pouch

After the urethral anastomosis is complete, the distal staple line is removed. An antimesenteric incision is then made, beginning at the distal end of the loop and moving toward the site of the urethral anastomosis. A sucker can be passed into the lumen for traction to ease the incision.

Once near the urethra, the incision deviates to the mesentery, to keep the urethral anastomosis away from the incision. Next, an enterotomy is created 20 cm proximal to the urethral anastomosis. The assistant passes a laparoscopic sucker through the enterotomy, and the antimesenteric border is incised to communicate with the previous enterotomy.

Place a stay suture at the medial edge of the exposed afferent limb to the medial edge of the distal loop. This will allow traction for the posterior closure. The posterior wall of the neobladder can be performed in a running, single-layer fashion with a self-retaining barbed suture, 2-0 or 3-0, which is run from the urethra to the afferent limb (Fig. 14.28).

The assistant can use a laparoscopic hook to help pull the suture through after each pass, expediting the tying process. Once the posterior wall is complete, the lateral edges of the bowel closest to the urethral margin are closed in a running fashion for approximately 10 cm (Fig. 14.29). Next, the lateral edge of the distal margin of detubularized lumen is folded down to the apex of the anterior edge of the enterotomy. This

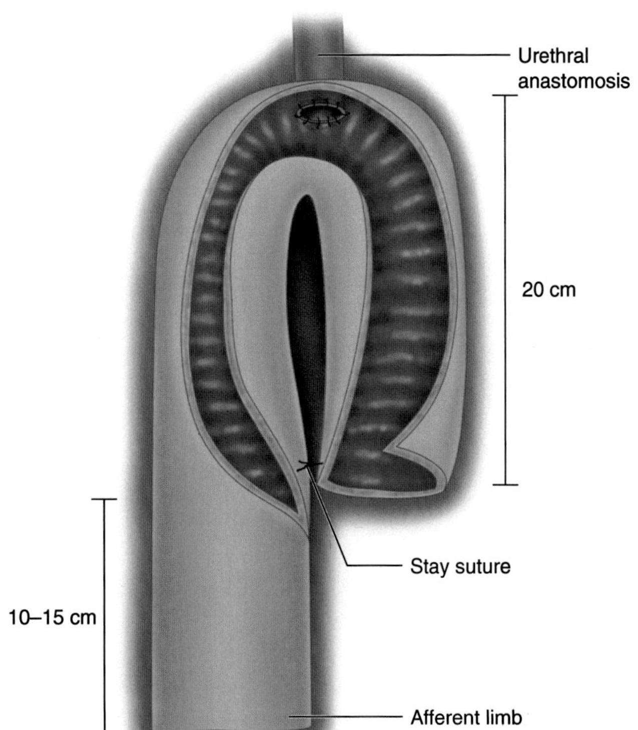

Fig. 14.28 After the urethral anastomosis is complete, the distal staple line is removed and the ileal segment is opened on the antimesenteric border. The posterior wall of the neobladder is constructed using a running, single-layer absorbable, barbed suture

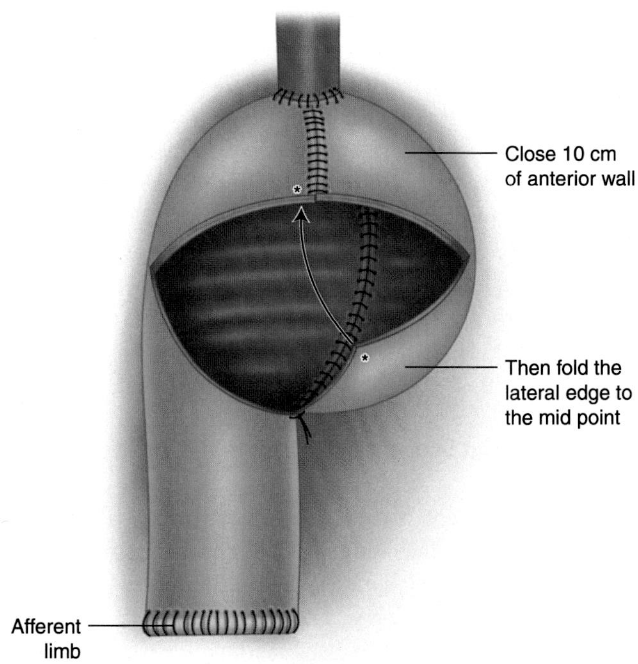

Fig. 14.29 Once the posterior wall is complete, the lateral edges of the bowel closest to the urethral margin are closed in a running fashion for approximately 10 cm

creates dog-ears of equal length, which can then be closed in a running fashion, first the right and then the left. Do not finish the left-sided closure until stents have been passed (Fig. 14.30).

As the left dog-ear is closed, leave 5 cm open to allow passage of the stents. This is performed in a similar fashion as previously described. The ureteral anastomosis is started once the wall furthest away from the camera is complete. The needle driver is passed through the ureteral anastomosis into the defect in the suture line; the stent is grasped, pulled through the afferent limb, and then passed into the ureter. The wire is removed. A wide enterotomy and spatulation on the ureter are necessary to pass the needle driver through the enterotomy in order to grab the stent. Ensure that the afferent limb is held on tension by holding the end with arm 2 or arm 3.

Once the stents are in place, there are several options. The stents can be inserted through the inner lumen of a large catheter through the urethra and then passed into the ureters. Alternatively, double-J stents can be passed and removed later, at the time of catheter removal via cystoscopy, or the stents can be tied to the Foley catheter so they are removed at the 3-week post-op visit. Finally, the stents can be externalized through the abdominal wall.

Wiklund Neobladder

The Wiklund neobladder described by Jonsson et al. [5] uses a similar approach to the previous neobladder with a slight modification in the detubularization process. In addition, a Wallace-style ureteral anastomosis is performed on the afferent limb.

In this approach, 50–60 cm of bowel is isolated. The urethral anastomosis is performed, and 20 cm total bowel is incised along the antimesenteric border. The posterior wall of the neobladder is performed in a similar fashion. Then the lateral edge of the distal ileal edge is secured to the lateral edge of the opposite lateral edge, 7–10 cm proximal to the urethral anastomosis (Fig. 14.31). The two dog-ears are then closed (again, the right and then the left). The left is not completed until stents are passed (Fig. 14.32).

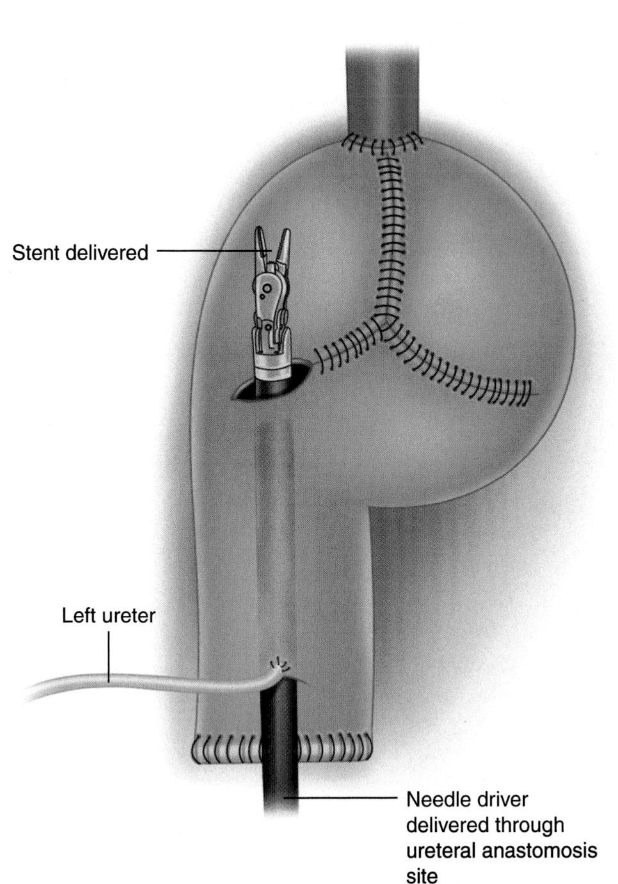

Fig. 14.30 The left-sided suture line is completed after the stents are brought through the enterotomy for the ureteral anastomoses. The needle driver is carefully passed through the ureteral anastomosis site through the afferent limb and into the opening in the pouch to pull the stent to the ureteral anastomosis. The left side is shown here

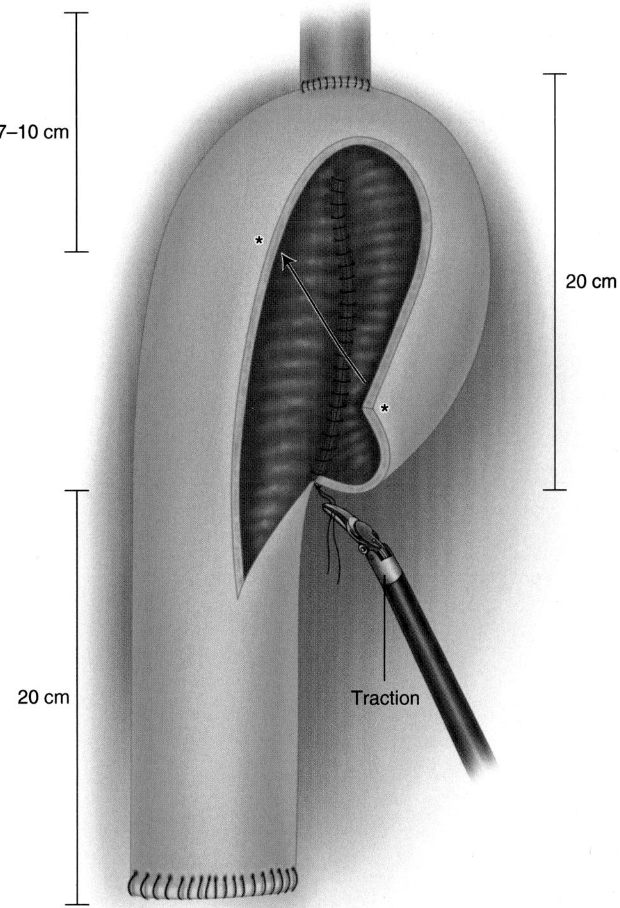

Fig. 14.31 Closure of the neobladder is initiated by reapproximating the distal ileal corner to an edge 7–10 cm proximal to the urethral anastomosis

Y-Pouch Neobladder

More recently, the Y-pouch neobladder, as described by Sim et al. [6], was applied in the robotic arena. In total, 40 cm of bowel is isolated, and the urethral anastomosis is performed as described. Ten centimeters of the bowel in either direction from the urethral anastomosis is incised along the antimesenteric border. The posterior wall is reapproximated in a similar fashion as previously described, but rather than folding the anterior wall, it is simply reapproximated (Fig. 14.33). The ureteral anastomosis is performed before completing the anterior wall. The left ureter is not passed under the sigmoid colon, but is anastomosed to the left limb, and the right ureter is anastomosed to the right limb (Fig. 14.34). The limb may be secured to the retroperitoneum to simplify the anastomosis and stent placement.

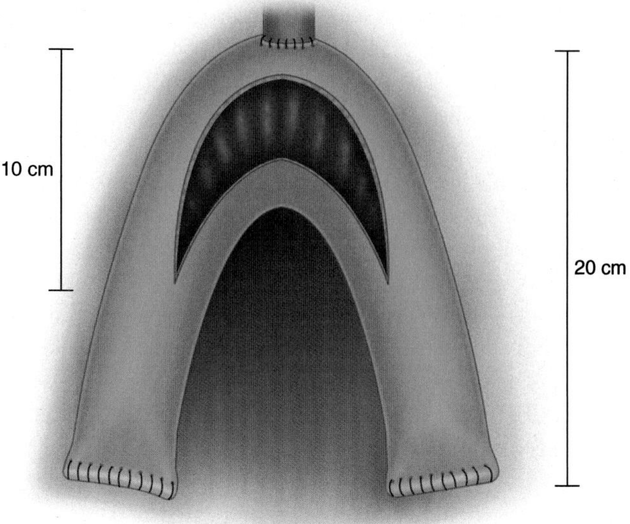

Fig. 14.33 The Y neobladder is created after the urethral anastomosis by opening the bowel 10 cm proximal and distal to the urethral anastomosis

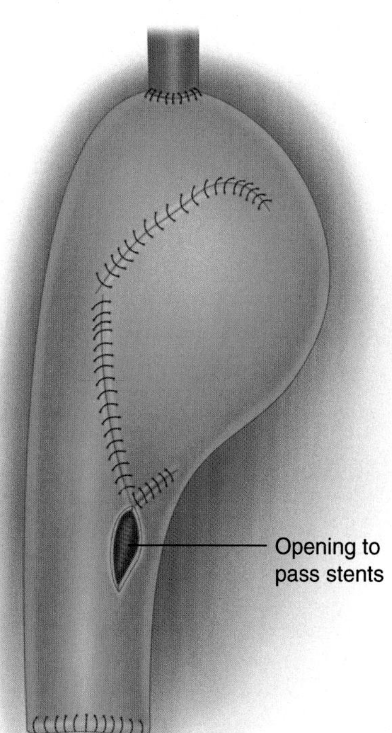

Fig. 14.32 An opening remains in the anterior closure to facilitate stent passage for the ureteral anastomoses

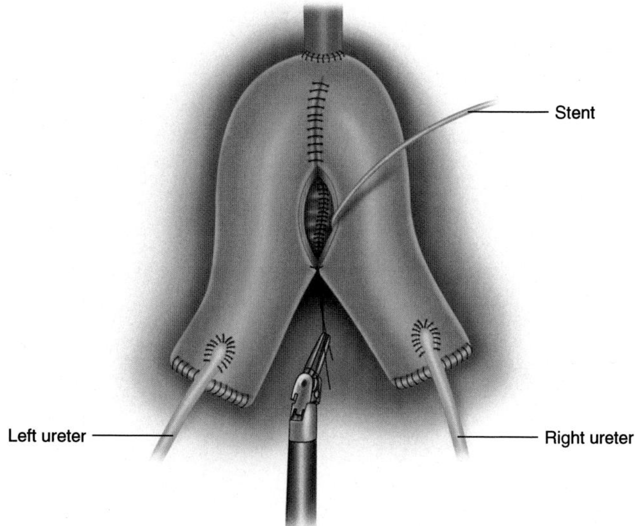

Fig. 14.34 For the Y neobladder, the left ureter is not passed under the sigmoid colon but is anastomosed to the left limb, which passes anterior to the sigmoid

References

1. Shariat SF, Karakiewicz PI, Palapattu GS, Lotan Y, Rogers CG, Amiel GE, et al. Outcomes of radical cystectomy for transitional cell carcinoma of the bladder: a contemporary series from the bladder cancer research consortium. J Urol. 2006;176:2414–22; discussion 2422.
2. Menon M, Hemal AK, Tewari A, Shrivastava A, Shoma AM, El-Tabey NA, et al. Nerve-sparing robot-assisted radical cystoprostatectomy and urinary diversion. BJU Int. 2003;92:232–6.
3. Stein JP, Lieskovsky G, Cote R, Groshen S, Feng AC, Boyd S, et al. Radical cystectomy in the treatment of invasive bladder cancer: long-term results in 1,054 patients. J Clin Oncol. 2001;19:666–75.
4. Siemens DR, Mackillop WJ, Peng Y, Wei X, Berman D, Booth CM. Lymph node counts are valid indicators of the quality of surgical care in bladder cancer: a population-based study. Urol Oncol. 2015;33:425.e15–23.
5. Jonsson MN, Adding LC, Hosseini A, Schumacher MC, Volz D, Nilsson A, et al. Robot-assisted radical cystectomy with intracorporeal urinary diversion in patients with transitional cell carcinoma of the bladder. Eur Urol. 2011;60(5):1066–73.
6. Sim A, Todenhöfer T, Mischinger J, Halalsheh O, Fahmy O, Boettge J, et al. Y pouch neobladder-a simplified method of intracorporeal neobladder after robotic cystectomy. J Endourol. 2015;29(4):387–9.

Robotic Pelvic and Retroperitoneal Lymph Node Dissection

15

Steven V. Kardos and Jonathan Yamzon

Introduction

Pelvic lymph node dissection (PLND) and retroperitoneal lymph node dissection (RPLND) remain critical components of many urologic disease processes and procedures. Dissection may provide accurate lymph node staging and confer potential therapeutic benefit. For prostate cancer management, lymph node dissection at prostatectomy provides an opportunity for staging and, when compared with other treatment options, has been shown to have a possible therapeutic benefit by lower cancer-specific death rates [1–3]. In the management of testicular cancer, RPLND is considered an established treatment option, depending on the histologic subtype and clinical stage of the disease. The robotic platform allows for a full therapeutic dissection with equivalent oncologic outcomes and shorter convalescence when compared with open RPLND [4, 5]. Finally, in the management of patients with locally advanced renal masses (T3–T4) or unfavorable clinical and/or pathologic features, a template lymph node dissection may offer improved survival [6–8].

Pelvic Lymph Node Dissection for Prostate Cancer

Patient Selection

Depending on risk stratification based on either D'Amico criteria or validated nomograms, a limited or extended PLND can provide accurate staging and perhaps therapeutic benefit. An extended lymph node dissection (ELND) can be performed safely with minimal additional morbidity, but the extent of dissection must be individualized for each patient [9, 10].

Room Setup, Positioning, and Port Placement

Please refer to Chapter 12.

S. V. Kardos, MD (✉)
Urology and Urologic Oncology, Northeast Medical Group, Yale New Haven Health, Fairfield, CT, USA

J. Yamzon, MD
Department of Surgery, City of Hope National Medical Center, Duarte, CA, USA

Y. Fong et al. (eds.), *The SAGES Atlas of Robotic Surgery*, https://doi.org/10.1007/978-3-319-91045-1_15

Technique and Steps of Pelvic Lymph Node Dissection

The boundaries of limited lymph node dissection (LLND) encompass the tissue in the obturator fossa as well as the area overlying the external iliac vein. On the other hand, an ELND includes the boundaries of the common iliac bifurcation proximally, the lateral border of the external iliac artery laterally, and the node of Cloquet distally, as well as the obturator fossa. Figure 15.1 highlights the anatomic regions in both an LLND and ELND [9].

A systematic approach must be applied in either lymph node dissection by using anatomic landmarks throughout the dissection to avoid iatrogenic injury of structures including the genitofemoral nerve laterally, the ureter medially, and the obturator nerve. Throughout the dissection, cautery is utilized for meticulous hemostasis, and clips are used judiciously at both the proximal and distal limits to prevent lymphatic leakage.

For an ELND, prospective identification of landmarks remains the most critical component of a thorough, anatomic dissection. First, the proximal limit of the dissection is identified as the ureter crosses over the iliac vessels, which can often be seen through the peritoneum or by incising the peritoneum lateral to the obliterated umbilical artery. The peritoneal incision can then be carried along the lateral border of the external iliac artery, serving as the lateral aspect of the dissection and preventing inadvertent injury to the genitofemoral nerve. The distal extent of the lateral border of dissection is the crossing of the circumflex iliac vein over the external iliac artery. The distal lymphatic tissue is meticulously controlled with a series of clips for lymphostasis.

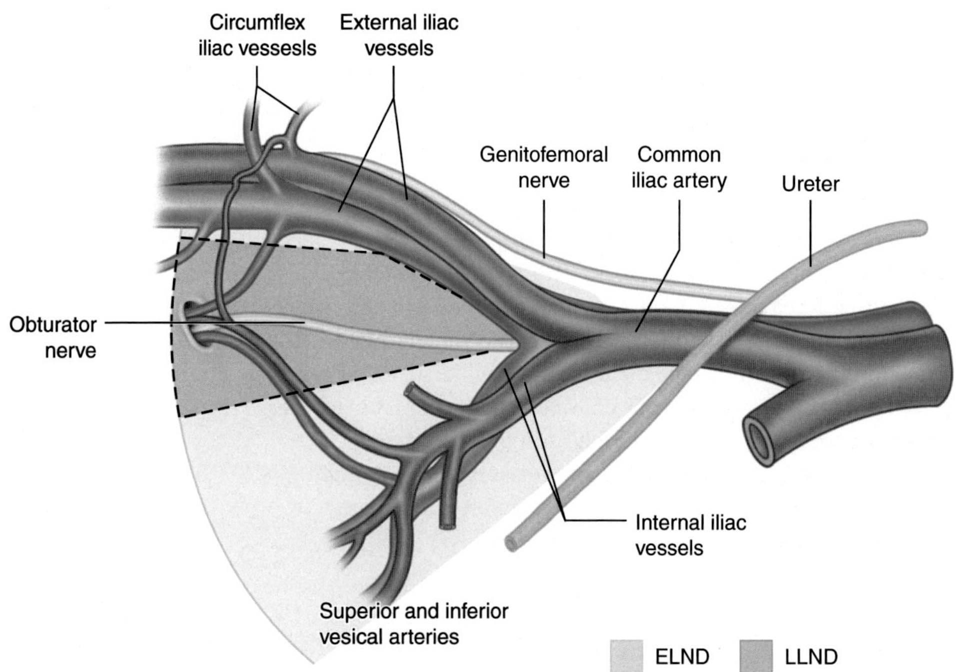

Fig. 15.1 Anatomic landmarks for a limited lymph node dissection (LLND) and extended lymph node dissection (ELND) for prostate cancer [9]

Next, the medial border of the dissection is identified as the lateral edge of the obliterated umbilical artery, over which the peritoneum is initially incised to identify the proximal margin of the dissection. Using the fourth arm to retract the obliterated umbilical artery medially, the medial edge of the lymph node packet is developed by bluntly sweeping the tissue laterally and coursing down to the endopelvic fascia. The lymphatic tissue is then mobilized in a split-and-roll technique off of the external iliac vessels, using a combination of cautery and clips. The external iliac vessels are gently retracted laterally to dissect the lymphatic tissue posterior to the vessels. Importantly, meticulous hemostasis is achieved with bipolar cautery of the perforating vessels off of the psoas muscle and pelvic sidewall. With gentle medial retraction of the obliterated umbilical artery, following its course and insertion into the hypogastric artery can identify the hypogastric lymph node packet. Lymphatic tissue is similarly removed off of the hypogastric artery. Finally, the node of Cloquet is clipped distally and used as a handle for exposure beneath the external iliac vessels and into the obturator fossa. The lymphatic tissue is dissected off of the obturator vessels and nerve, paying close attention to minimize the use of monopolar cautery around the obturator nerve. A contralateral dissection is done in a similar fashion. Complete bilateral extended pelvic lymph node dissection (EPLND) can be seen in Figs. 15.2 and 15.3.

Similar surgical technique and principles are applied to an LLND. The peritoneum overlying the external iliac vein is incised and used as the lateral extent of the dissection. The lymphatic tissue is dissected off, utilizing a split-and-roll technique. The obturator vessels and nerve are prospectively identified, and the lymphatic tissue is dissected off with meticulous hemostatic and lymphatic control, using bipolar electrocautery and Hem-o-lok® clips.

For an LLND, lymph nodes can be sent in four separate packets: right and left external iliac and right and left obturator. In an ELND technique, 11 packets are sent: right and left common iliac, right and left external iliac, right and left internal iliac, right and left obturator, right and left node of Cloquet, and anterior bladder fat. The greater number of packets allows for a more thorough pathologic evaluation [11].

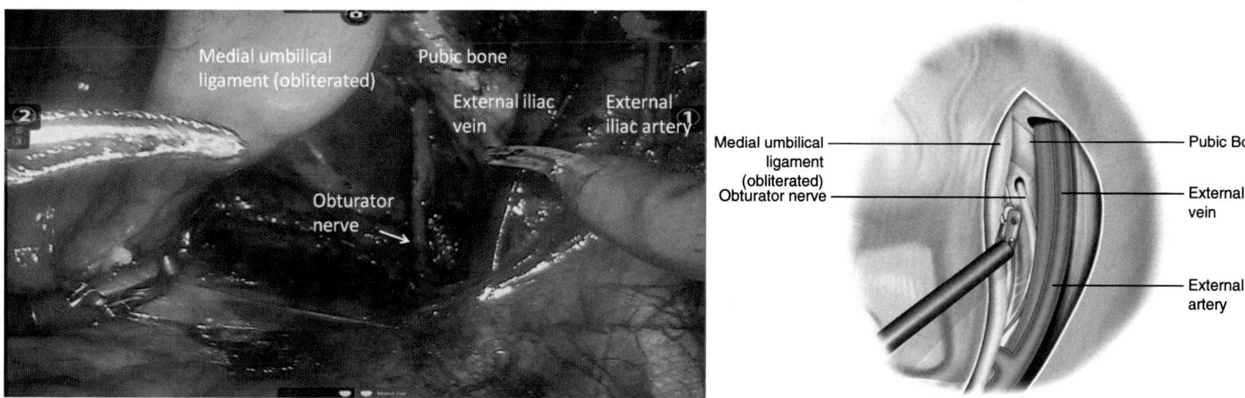

Fig. 15.2 Extended right pelvic lymph node dissection

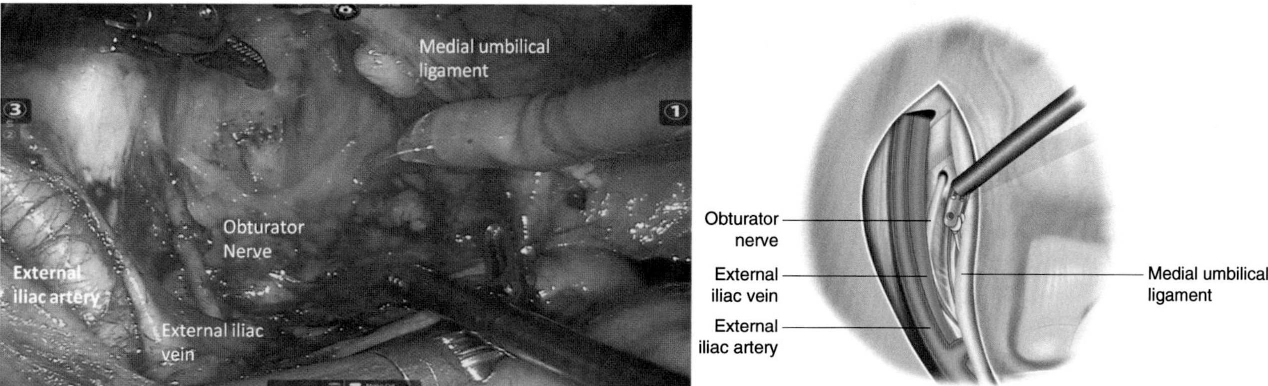

Fig. 15.3 Extended left pelvic lymph node dissection

Retroperitoneal Lymph Node Dissection for Testicular Cancer

Patient Selection

Testicular cancer is the most common solid organ malignancy in young men with a therapeutic principle of curative intent. Given that most germ cell tumor metastases (except choriocarcinoma) occur via lymphatic spread, its course is relatively predictable, and advanced disease can be treated with multimodal therapy, including both chemotherapy and surgery [4, 5]. As such, RPLND is considered to be an appropriate treatment option for clinical stages I–IIB as well as for post-chemotherapy residual masses in those with clinical stages IIC–III [12, 13]. Even though the patient population is young and healthy, those who received bleomycin should have appropriate preoperative pulmonary function testing as well as judicious intraoperative fluid management, owing to the risk of postoperative pulmonary edema [14]. It is the practice of our institution to place all Stage I patients on active surveillance. Post-chemotherapy robotic RPLND is seldom performed except in patients with good-risk small residual masses after chemotherapy, in whom it is felt that the desmoplastic fibrotic tissue response would be minimal.

Robotic RPLND should be performed only by high-volume surgeons prepared to convert to an open approach. Severe desmoplastic response after chemotherapy, or intraoperative vascular injuries, may require conversion. Thoroughness of dissection should never be compromised for a minimally invasive approach, and appropriate patient selection is paramount in achieving oncologic outcomes equivalent to those of the open approach without increased morbidity.

Room Setup, Positioning, and Port Placement

A single dose of a first-generation or second-generation cephalosporin is recommended as antibiotic prophylaxis. Sequential compression devices are used for deep vein thrombosis prophylaxis. A Foley catheter is then inserted under sterile technique. An orogastric tube is placed to maximize bowel decompression.

Two options exist for the approach. The first is a lateral approach similar to positioning for a radical nephrectomy, except with more medial port placement (see Chapter 11 "Robot-Assisted Partial Nephrectomy" for details on positioning). The ports are placed in a similar configuration, only slightly more medial to allow access across the midline. Another approach is with the patient in supine position [15]. Briefly, the patient is positioned supine with both arms tucked. The patient is placed in Trendelenburg position, and the robot is docked over the head (Si robot) or from the side (Xi robot). The ports are placed in the lower abdomen in an arc, with slight favoring to the side of disease. This approach allows for ease of bilateral retroperitoneal access, though both approaches have their advantages.

Port placement begins by achieving insufflation using a 15-cm Veress needle through the umbilicus. Port sites are then placed according to the approach seen in (Fig. 15.4).

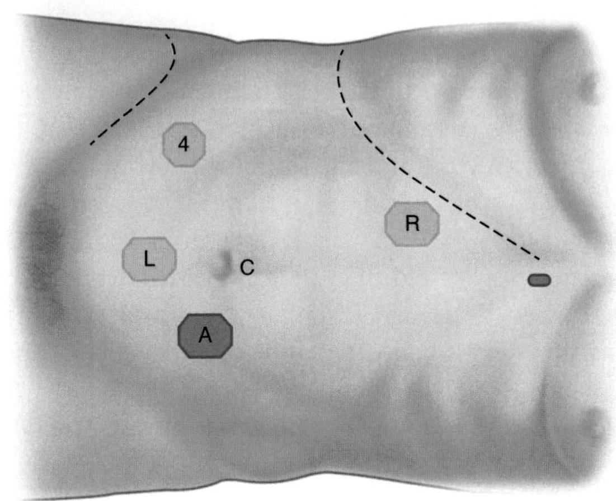

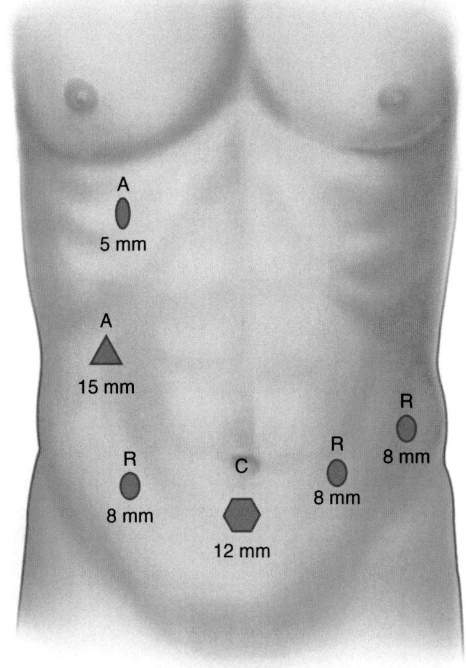

Fig. 15.4 (**a**) Standard port placement for a robotic retroperitoneal lymph node dissection in lateral position [16]. (**b**) Standard port placement for a robotic retroperitoneal lymph node dissection in supine position [15]

Technique and Steps of Retroperitoneal Lymph Node Dissection

For the paracaval lymph node dissection, the procedure begins with reflection of the right colon medially along the avascular white line of Toldt, achieving elevation of the root of the mesentery and kocherization of the duodenum to expose the great vessels up to the renal hila. The dissection is done in a caudal-to-cephalad direction, using the split-and-roll technique. Identification of the right ureter as it courses along the bifurcation of the right common iliac artery serves as the lateral and caudal margin of dissection, as can be seen in (Fig. 15.5). For a right-sided tumor, the right gonadal vein is identified, ligated, and divided between Hem-o-lok® clips. It is then mobilized caudad toward the internal inguinal ring and completely excised distally. The lymph node dissection is carried cephalad from the bifurcation of the right common iliac artery to the level of the renal hilum. It is then followed medially to the great vessels.

The inferior vena cava (IVC) is identified as the fibrofatty tissue over the IVC is divided in a split-and-roll fashion. The paracaval lymph node packet is dissected off the IVC laterally where the lumbar vessels and sympathetic branches coursing medially are identified prospectively. Lumbar vessels are identified and can be ligated with Hem-o-lok® clips at this time, as seen in (Fig. 15.6). Caution should be taken to ensure adequate clip placement, as the lumbar veins can retract if divided unsecured. The fibrofatty tissue is cleared medially along the IVC into the interaortocaval location. The IVC can be rolled/retracted by the assistant to expose the retrocaval lymph node packet. The fibrofatty tissue is cleared off posterior to the IVC, exposing the anterior spinous ligament. The sympathetic branches previously identified are preserved as dissection is performed in the interaortocaval location.

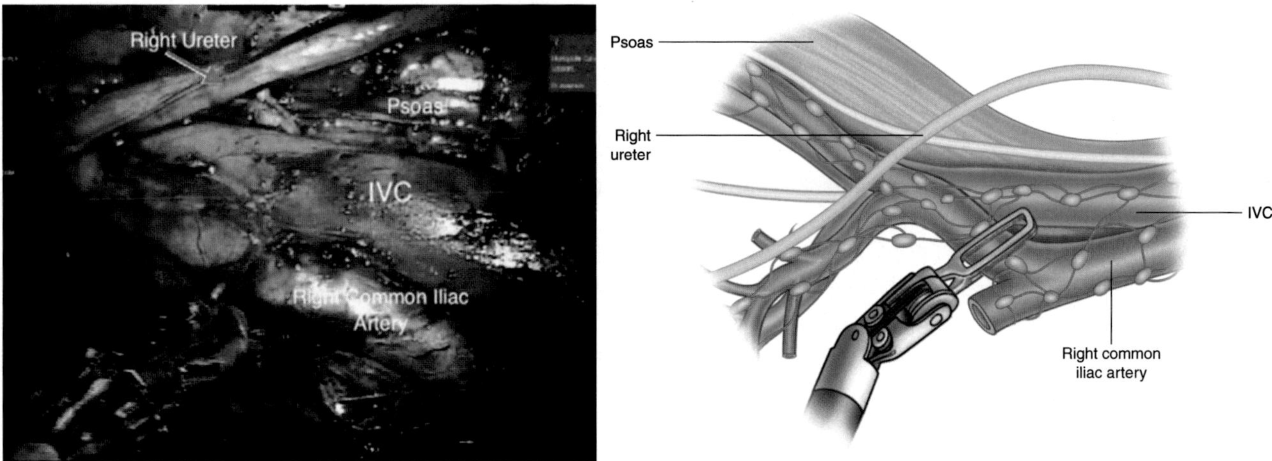

Fig. 15.5 Identification of the right ureter as it courses along the bifurcation of the right common iliac artery serves as the right and caudal margin of dissection [16]

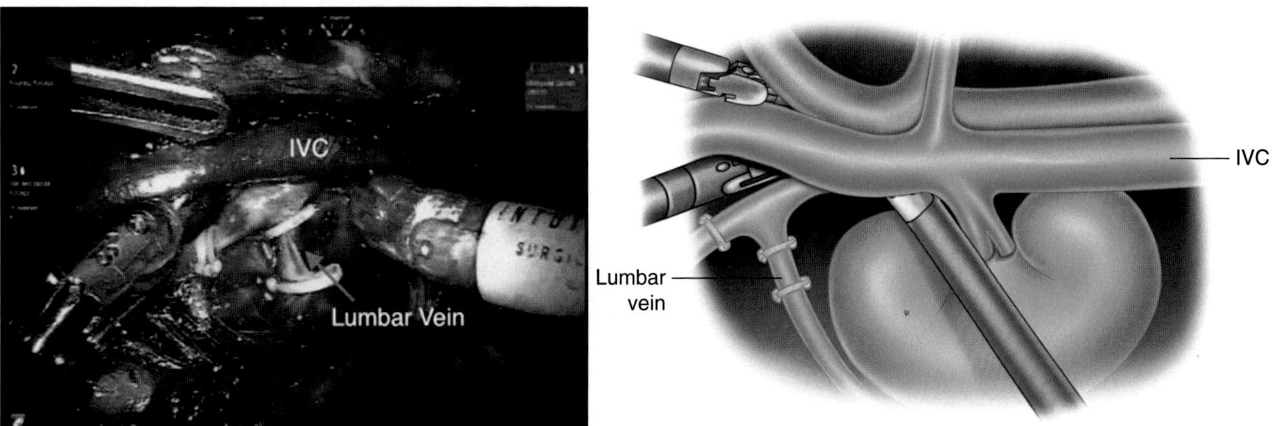

Fig. 15.6 Lumbar vessels off the inferior vena cava (IVC) are prospectively identified and controlled [16]

Next, mobilizing the lymph nodes off of the right common iliac artery delineates the medial edge of the aorta. This is carried proximally to expose the aortic bifurcation and the inferior mesenteric artery (IMA); it stops at the cephalad aspect of the left renal vein. The dissection is carried over the aorta in a cephalad manner, encountering lumbar arteries that are controlled with clips. The right renal artery should be prospectively identified prior to ligation of the lumbar arteries to ensure that it is not inadvertently ligated. The retro-aortic and para-aortic lymph node packets are then dissected lateral to the IMA toward the left ureter, crossing over the left common iliac artery. The combination of gravity and retraction by the fourth robotic arm allows exposure of the aorta and left common iliac vessels. This tissue is then dissected cephalad up to the left renal hilum. Care is also taken to preemptively identify the left renal artery prior to ligation of lateral lumbar arteries.

Throughout the dissection, meticulous hemostasis and lymphostasis are preserved using clips and the split-and-roll technique. Clips are applied to the cisterna chyli, which is located just posterior to the right renal artery. We routinely apply hemostatic agents (Evicel® and Surgicel®) into the interaortocaval and para-aortic regions. An intraperitoneal drain is placed via a robotic port and secured with a 2-0 silk suture. A Carter-Thomason device is used to close the 12-mm ports with 0 Vicryl under direct visualization. The overlying incisions are closed with 4-0 Monocryl suture and skin glue, and 0.25% Marcaine is infiltrated into the incisions. The patient is returned to supine position and extubated. Postoperatively, tachycardia can be expected secondary to autonomic dysreflexia and sympathetic discharge from the RPLND and should not be confused with hypovolemia [15–17].

Lymph Node Dissection for Renal Cell Carcinoma and Upper Tract Urothelial Carcinoma

Patient Selection

The role of lymphadenectomy in the management of renal cell carcinoma remains controversial, but it is used in the management of patients with locally advanced renal masses (T3–T4), unfavorable clinical and/or pathologic features, or bulky adenopathy on cross-sectional imaging or intraoperative evaluation [6, 7]. Crispen et al. identified five intraoperative pathological features considered high risk for nodal metastasis, including nuclear grade 3 or 4, sarcomatoid components, tumor size >10 cm, tumor stage pT3 or pT4, and coagulative necrosis with two features yielding lymphadenectomy [18]. In patients with upper tract urothelial carcinoma, regional lymph nodes are frequently involved and represent the most common metastatic locations. Lymphadenectomy not only improves disease staging and identification of patients for adjuvant therapy but also can have a potential therapeutic role by improving both local control and cancer-specific survival [19, 20].

Room Setup, Positioning, and Port Placement

Please refer to the "Robotic Radical Nephrectomy and Nephroureterectomy" chapter.

Technique and Steps for Pelvic and/or Retroperitoneal Lymph Node Dissection for Renal Cell Carcinoma and Upper Tract Urothelial Carcinoma

Surgical technique and steps for both pelvic and retroperitoneal lymph node dissections can be found above. The standard template for lymphadenectomy in a radical nephrectomy is contingent upon the laterality of the procedure. For left-sided tumors, a standard dissection includes the para-aortic and preaortic lymph nodes, as well as interaortocaval nodes for an ELND. For right-sided tumors, a standard dissection includes paracaval and precaval lymph nodes with the addition of interaortocaval nodes for an ELND [21].

Similarly, the role of lymphadenectomy in the management of upper tract urothelial carcinoma is predicated by the location of the tumor. In patients with tumors in the renal pelvis or proximal ureter, a modified retroperitoneal lymphadenectomy (as found above) can be performed contingent on laterality. For those with tumors in the mid to distal ureter, a pelvic lymphadenectomy (as above) can be performed.

References

1. Kibel AS, Ciezki JP, Klein EA, Reddy CA, Lubahn JD, Haslag-Minoff J, et al. Survival among men with clinically localized prostate cancer treated with radical prostatectomy or radiation therapy in the prostate specific antigen era. J Urol. 2012;187:1259–65.
2. Joslyn SA, Konety BR. Impact of extent of lymphadenectomy on survival after radical prostatectomy for prostate cancer. Urology. 2006;68:121–5.
3. Hyndman ME, Mullins JK, Pavlovich CP. Pelvic node dissection in prostate cancer: extended, limited, or not at all? Curr Opin Urol. 2010;20:211–7.
4. Siegel R, Ma J, Zou Z, Jemal A. Cancer statistics, 2014. CA Cancer J Clin. 2014;64:9–29.

5. National Comprehensive Cancer Network. Testicular cancer. (Version 2. 2016).
6. Capitanio U, Becker F, Blute ML, Mulders P, Patard JJ, Russo P, et al. Lymph node dissection in renal cell carcinoma. Eur Urol. 2011;60:1212–20.
7. Pantuck AJ, Zisman A, Dorey F, Chao DH, Han KR, Gitlitz BJ, et al. Renal cell carcinoma with retroperitoneal lymph nodes: role of lymph node dissection. J Urol. 2003;169:2076–83.
8. Liebovich BC, Blute ML. Lymph node dissection in the management of renal cell carcinoma. Urol Clin North Am. 2008; 35:673–8.
9. Yuh BE, Ruel NH, Mejia R, Novara G, Wilson TG. Standardized comparison of robot-assisted limited and extended pelvic lymphadenectomy for prostate cancer. BJU Int. 2013;112:81–8.
10. Yuh B, Artibani W, Heidenreich A, Kimm S, Menon M, Novara G, et al. The role of robot-assisted radical prostatectomy and pelvic lymph node dissection in the management of high-risk prostate cancer: a systematic review. Eur Urol. 2014;65:918–27.
11. Stein JP, Penson DF, Cai J, Miranda G, Skinner EC, Dunn MA, et al. Radical cystectomy with extended lymphadenectomy: evaluating separate package versus en bloc submission for node positive bladder cancer. J Urol. 2007;177:876–81.
12. Nicolai N, MIceli R, Artusi R, Piva L, Pizzocaro G, Salvioni R. A simple model for predicting nodal metastasis in patients with clinical stage 1 nonseminomatous germ cell testicular tumors undergoing retroperitoneal lymph node dissection only. J Urol. 2004;171:172–6.
13. Weissbach L, Bussar-Maatz R, Flechtner H, Pichlmeier U, Hartmann M, Keller L. RPLND or primary chemotherapy in clinical stage IIA/B nonseminomatous germ cell tumors? Results of a prospective multicenter trial including quality of life assessment. Eur Urol. 2000;37:582–94.
14. Donat SM, Levy DA. Bleomycin associated pulmonary toxicity: is perioperative oxygen restriction necessary? J Urol. 1998;160:1347–52.
15. Abdul-Muhsin HM, L'Esperance JO, Fischer K, Woods ME, Porter JR, Castle EP. Robot-assisted retroperitoneal lymph node dissection in testicular cancer. J Surg Oncol. 2015;112:736–40.
16. Williams SB, Lau CS, Josephson DY. Initial series of robot-assisted laparoscopic retroperitoneal lymph node dissection for clinical stage 1 nonseminomatous germ cell testicular cancer. Eur Urol. 2011;60:1299–302.
17. Cheney SM, Andrews PE, Leibovich BC, Castle EP. Robot assisted retroperitoneal lymph node dissection: technique and initial case series of 18 patients. BJU Int. 2015;115:114–20.
18. Crispen PL, Breau RH, Allmer C, Lohse CM, Cheville JC, Leibovich BC, Blute ML. Lymph node dissection at the time of radical nephrectomy for high-risk clear cell renal cell carcinoma: indications and recommendations for surgical templates. Eur Urol. 2011;59:18–23.
19. Roscigno M, Brausi M, Heidenreich A, Lotan Y, Margulis V, Shariat SF, et al. Lymphadenectomy at the time of nephroureterectomy for upper tract urothelial cancer. Eur Urol. 2011;60:776–83.
20. Seisen T, Shariat SF, Cussenot O, Peyronnet B, Renard-Penna R, Colin P, Rouprêt M. Contemporary role of lymph node dissection at the time of radical nephroureterectomy for upper tract urothelial carcinoma. World J Urol. 2017;35(4):535–48.
21. Jamal JE, Jarrett TW. The current role of lymph node dissection in the management of renal cell carcinoma. Int J Surg Oncol. 2011;2011:816926.

Part III

Gynecologic Procedures

Hysterectomy with Bilateral Salpingo-Oophorectomy

16

Ernest S. Han and Stephen J. Lee

Introduction

Hysterectomy is one of the most commonly performed gynecologic procedures. Historically, an abdominal, vaginal, or laparoscopic approach was utilized. With the advent of robotic technology, a new approach to hysterectomy is available to the surgeon. Although recent studies suggest that there are minimal differences in complications and outcomes between a laparoscopic approach compared to a robotically-assisted laparoscopic approach, potential advantages of robotic surgery include its wristed instrumentation, three-dimensional immersive visualization, and increased surgical precision. This chapter discusses a robotic laparoscopic approach to hysterectomy with or without bilateral salpingo-oophorectomy. We will describe the technique and discuss issues that can arise during robotic surgery.

Indications

Indications for performing hysterectomy with or without bilateral salpingo-oophorectomy vary from the most benign conditions, such as leiomyomas, to malignancy. The surgeon must decide on the most appropriate route (laparotomy, laparoscopy, vaginal) to accomplish the surgery, and this may be determined in part by multiple factors such as indication for surgery, prior surgical history, and patient comorbidities. Compared to an abdominal approach, laparoscopic hysterectomy has the potential benefits of faster return to normal activities, reduced wound or abdominal wall infections, fewer febrile episodes, shorter hospital stay, and less intraoperative blood loss [1]. However, laparoscopic hysterectomy is associated with longer operating time and a higher rate of lower urinary tract injuries compared to abdominal approach. The American Congress of Obstetrics and Gynecology has stated that a vaginal hysterectomy approach should always be considered if feasible and indicated, as this is still the least invasive procedure available [1, 2].

Recently, robot-based procedures for gynecologic surgeries have been steadily increasing. The robotic platform may allow the surgeon to potentially tackle increasingly difficult cases that ordinarily would have required a laparotomy incision. Such cases can include severe endometriosis, uterine leiomyomas, and pelvic malignancies such as cervical, uterine, and even ovarian cancers. Robotic technology has the added benefit of wristed instruments, which increases the range of motion for accessing difficult areas in the pelvis. The wristed component for robotic instruments allows for additional angles and rotations, not easily achieved by standard laparoscopic techniques [3]. Other potential benefits include a three-dimensional immersive view, better ergonomics for the operating surgeon, and a steady camera controlled by the operating surgeon.

Despite the potential advantages of robotic surgery, several studies have recently compared robotically-assisted and laparoscopic hysterectomy for treatment of benign disease and found no significant benefits in outcome and higher costs for robotic surgery [4–6]. The perceived benefits of robotic surgery over laparoscopic surgery are still controversial, and there is currently a lack of data comparing the laparoscopic versus robotic approach to complex pelvic surgery. One study suggested that the robotic surgical approach to endometrial cancer treatment was faster than traditional laparoscopic surgery, but no difference in cancer outcomes was seen [7].

Recognizing the potential benefits and current controversies over the role of robotic technology in gynecologic surgery, our goal in this chapter is to provide insight into performing a hysterectomy and/or bilateral salpingo-oophorectomy utilizing a robotically-assisted laparoscopic approach. We will focus on the setup and the detailed procedures and discuss approaches for dealing with certain complex circumstances encountered during robotic surgery.

E. S. Han, MD, PhD (✉) · S. J. Lee, MD
Division of Gynecologic Oncology,
City of Hope National Medical Center, Duarte, CA, USA
e-mail: ehan@coh.org

Y. Fong et al. (eds.), *The SAGES Atlas of Robotic Surgery*, https://doi.org/10.1007/978-3-319-91045-1_16

Setup

Patient Setup

Patient setup is critical to performing a smooth, successful operation and to avoid potential complications. Just like a pilot who checks the airplane prior to takeoff, the surgeon and/or his designee should be present to ensure that the patient is properly prepared for robotic surgery. As the patient is typically in steep Trendelenburg position (45° position) to minimize obstruction of view to the pelvis from the small bowel, the surgeon must ensure that the patient's body remains in position and does not shift during surgery. This is particularly of concern in morbidly obese patients in steep Trendelenburg position, where the patient's body may tend to shift cephalad, toward the head of the bed. This can lead to straightening of the legs and nerve damage, difficulties with uterine manipulation, and alterations in the relationship of the ports/instrumentation within the abdominal cavity. The authors recommend utilizing the least amount of Trendelenburg possible without compromising the surgeon's view of the pelvis. Steep Trendelenburg has also been shown to increase intraocular pressure, but may not lead to significant visual changes [8, 9]. Lithotomy position is utilized in order to gain access to the vaginal opening. The legs should be positioned in such a way to avoid hyperflexion of the knees and maintain a comfortable neutral position. We like to maintain a 90-degree angle at the knee area with slight flexion at the hip. Each leg is typically aligned with the opposite shoulder. However, depending on how the robot is docked to the patient, the legs may need to be adjusted to prevent potential collision of the robot arms/base to the patient's leg. Some surgeons consider removing the legs from lithotomy position temporarily to avoid prolonged flexion and to reduce the risk of well leg compartment syndrome [10]. The surgeon should also ensure that there is adequate space underneath the robot arms, which is necessary to avoid collision with the patient's legs and torso, and potential injury to the patient, during surgery. The bedside assistant should always be mindful of the relationship between the robot arms.

Another important consideration is to secure the patient's position during surgery. Although the rate of position-related injury was found to be low (0.8%) in one institution's experience [11], one should not ignore this important consideration for injury prevention. Being in steep Trendelenburg position, the patient can sometimes slide toward the head side. This has the potential to straighten the legs and alter the robot arm positioning during the operation. There are several options that are available to prevent slippage on the operating room (OR) table. The patient can lie on nonslip surfaces (e.g., foam padding, The Pink Pad-Pigazzi Patient Positioning System™) or on a beanbag to maintain positioning. We have typically avoided shoulder padding devices as these may lead to brachial plexus injuries. It is important to ensure that the patient's gluteus is just off the edge of the OR table padding to help minimize slippage. However, one must make sure that the patient is not too far off the table, which can cause pressure sores and/or complications to the lower back. When patient slippage is a particular concern (e.g., morbidly obese patient), one can place the patient in steep Trendelenburg position prior to prepping and draping her, to ensure that the patient is secure on the table. Adjustments can then be made accordingly. The surgeon and/or surgical team should also occasionally check the positioning of the patient during surgery to confirm that no significant changes have occurred.

The arms are typically tucked to the patient's side using sheets underneath the patient. Foam padding is typically used to avoid pressure underneath the arms. The surgeon should also ensure that any components of IV lines and other monitoring devices that may impinge into the patient are well padded to avoid injury to the skin. One should avoid using excessive force when tucking the arms to the side (don't make them too tight) and also avoid excess tension to the shoulder area. Immediately after tucking the arms, the surgeon should make sure that IV lines and all anesthesia monitoring equipment are functioning properly. For obese patients, extensions to the bed such as arm sleds may need to be utilized as there may not be enough space on the bed to have the patient's arms to the side. The hands and fingers should also be well protected, as often they lie near the joint area of the stirrups.

Uterine Manipulators and Vaginal Occluders

The use of a uterine manipulator device can help to facilitate a hysterectomy procedure. This allows the assistant to position the uterus in a way that gives access to various areas around the uterus during the dissection of surrounding tissues. There are numerous devices available to the surgeon. A detailed discussion regarding various uterine manipulators was recently reviewed [12]. Each device has certain pros and cons. We typically utilize the RUMI II uterine manipulator device as it allows the assistant to easily position the uterus into an anteverted and retroverted configuration. A vaginal occluder will be important to use to minimize CO_2 gas loss through the vagina after colpotomy incision. This sudden loss of gas can lead to an acute reduction in exposure to the surgical field. Another option to consider is utilizing a device that provides a stable pneumoperitoneum (e.g., AirSeal® system by Conmed).

Port Placement and Instrumentation Considerations

Port placement is critical for the performance of a smooth surgery. Suboptimal placement can lead to collisions between the robot arms and between the robot instruments and assistant instrumentations. This can also lead to arm motion constraints during the surgery, which can limit access to certain areas.

Port placements will vary depending on the robot platform utilized. The camera port is typically placed along the midline of the patient. For benign cases, we typically place the camera port 20–22 cm from the symphysis pubis (Fig. 16.1a). For patients undergoing cancer surgeries requiring lymphadenectomy, the camera port will be placed higher, at 25–27 cm from the symphysis pubis, when using the Si or S platform. For the Xi robot platform, the camera port can be placed lower, at 20–22 cm from symphysis pubis, during cancer operations. This allows for 180-degree rotation of the Xi arms to provide access to the upper abdominal regions. In patients with large pannus, utilization of the pubic symphysis as a landmark may underestimate the distance required for proper port placement. We typically will account for this by identifying the pubic symphysis and measuring from a straight line above this point (Fig. 16.1b).

Non-camera robot ports may be placed about 10 cm lateral and 15° down angle to each side when using the S or Si robot platform (Fig. 16.2). For the Xi robot platform, we typically place ports about 6–8 cm lateral to the midline port.

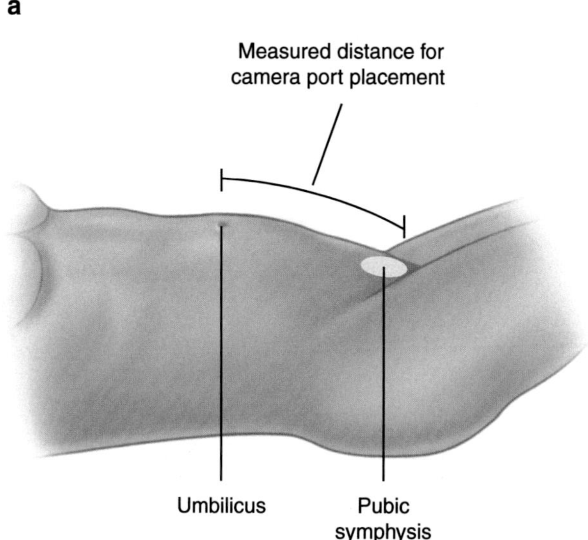

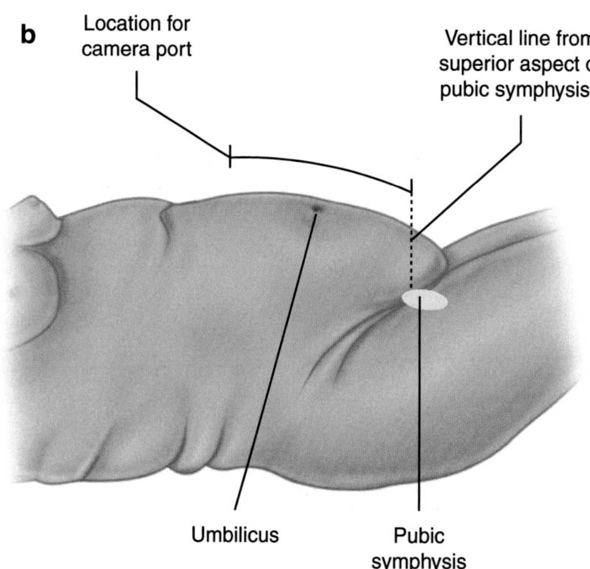

Fig. 16.1 Placement of camera port along midline. (**a**) Typical measurement from the superior aspect of the symphysis pubis to the camera port site (20–22 cm for benign cases, 25–27 cm for cancer cases) with a tape measure. (**b**) For obese patients with a pannus, we will measure from an imaginary line vertically from the superior edge of the symphysis pubis to the camera port site. Note that the port placement is usually well above the umbilicus

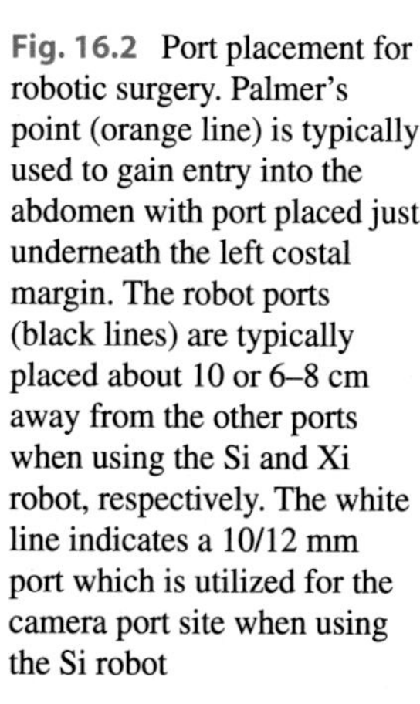

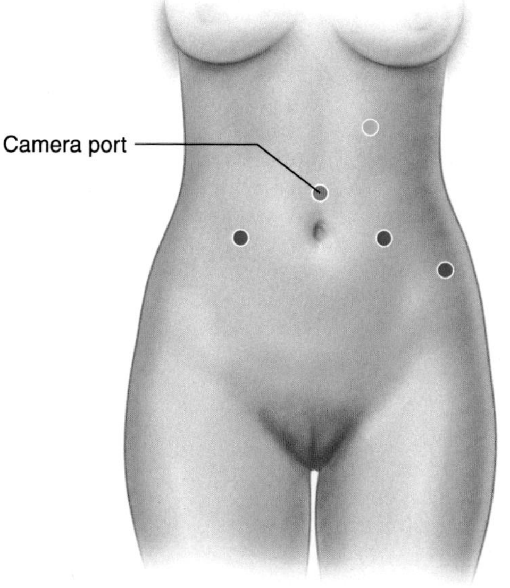

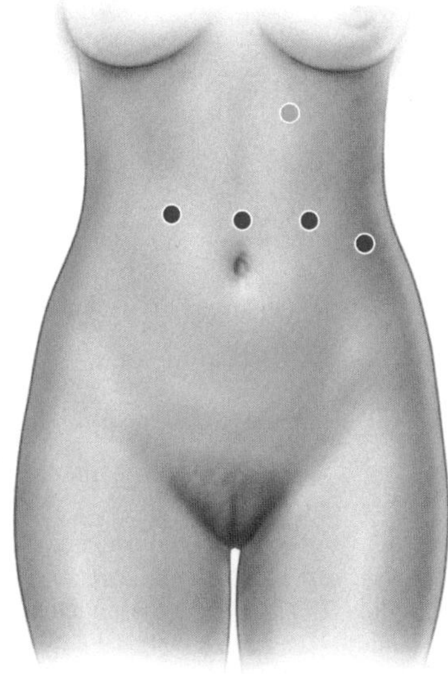

Fig. 16.2 Port placement for robotic surgery. Palmer's point (orange line) is typically used to gain entry into the abdomen with port placed just underneath the left costal margin. The robot ports (black lines) are typically placed about 10 or 6–8 cm away from the other ports when using the Si and Xi robot, respectively. The white line indicates a 10/12 mm port which is utilized for the camera port site when using the Si robot

Additional ports may be added further a 6–8 cm or 10 cm lateral for the Xi and Si robot, respectively, but should be about 2 cm superior from the anterior-superior iliac spine. For patients with low body mass index, placement of the lateral-most port can be challenging since the positioning can be close to the tucked arm. In these situations, we have shifted all the ports about 2 cm lateral and away from the side that has the port affected by the tucked arm (Fig. 16.3).

Port positioning should be determined prior to making an incision. We typically have achieved CO_2 insufflation and placed the patient in steep Trendelenburg position prior to determining port positioning. We will measure the approximate position and mark them with a marking pen. Proper positioning should also be confirmed intraabdominally, as well by visualization with a diagnostic laparoscope, to avoid potential port placement into areas with significant adhesions of the bowel to the anterior abdominal wall. Lysis of adhesions may need to be performed prior to port insertion to avoid injury to the underlying tissue.

The assistant port is typically placed in the lower abdomen opposite the fourth arm port site. Alternatively, we like to utilize Palmer's point to enter the abdomen, and we use this port as the assistant port as well. However, care must be taken to ensure proper spacing of this port to avoid collision of the assistant instrumentation with the robot arms/port. When placing this port, we like to anticipate the port placements by making a triangular-shaped pattern over the potential port site prior to insufflation (Fig. 16.4). The assistant port is usually more medial in its position. We typically have anesthesia place an oral gastric tube to decompress the stomach and tent the abdomen while placing a Veress needle for CO_2 insufflation. After insufflation, we like to insert the port under direct visualization using trocars that allow for insertion of a laparoscope to the tip (e.g. Visiport™ optical trocar by Covidien, Endo-path XCEL® trocars with OPTIVIEW® technology by Ethicon). If utilizing Palmer's point trocar as the assistant port, bariatric-length instruments will

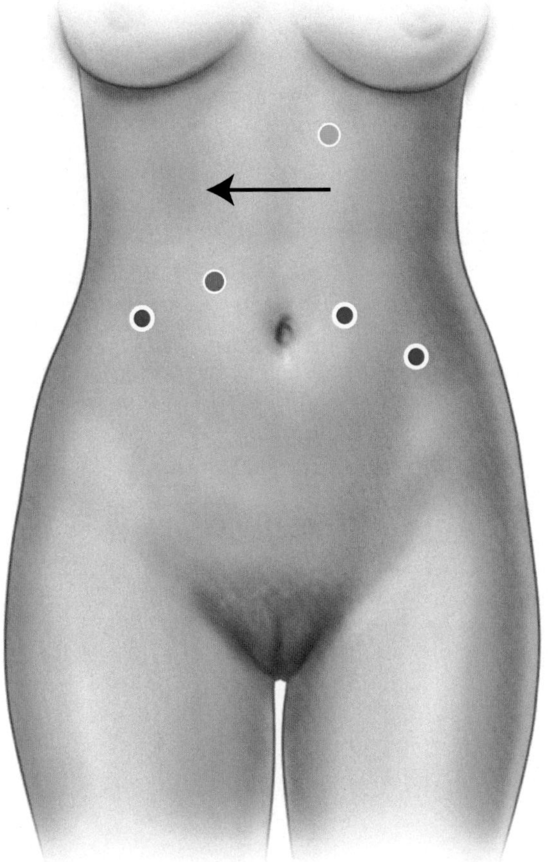

Fig. 16.3 Port placement in patients with low body mass index. The robot ports and 10/12 camera ports are shifted about 2 cm away from the midline. This allows for the left lateral robot port to be placed closer to the midline and avoid potential collisions with the patients left arm and avoid close proximity to the descending colon

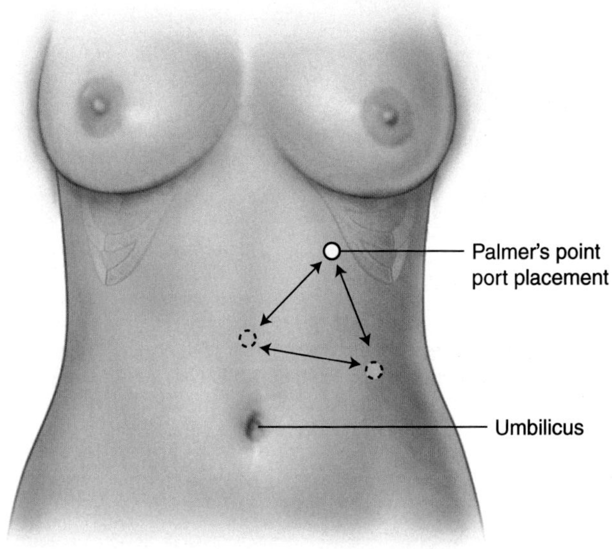

Palmer's point port placement

Umbilicus

Fig. 16.4 Proper placement of the assistant port at Palmer's point. Prior to creating incision, we will simulate a triangular-shaped position of the camera port, left robot port, and Palmer's point assistant port. This prevents potential collision of instruments from the Palmer's point assistant port with the other two ports during the case

need to be utilized in order to gain access to the pelvis during surgery.

Insertion of the robot trocars should occur under direct visualization. The use of blunt-tip robot trocars can help to minimize trauma to intraabdominal organs. However, in some patients with thick or tough fascia, the blunt-tip trocar may require significant force and compression of the abdomen for insertion. Care should be taken to ensure that the tip of the trocar does not injure intraabdominal contents. The disposable bladeless obturator for the robot trocars may give some advantage by avoiding the use of excessive pressure and force during trocar insertion, as compared to the blunt-tip obturator. Regardless, care must always be taken to avoid contact of the trocar tip with intraabdominal contents.

After the surgery is concluded, the fascia for port sites that are 10 mm or larger should be closed in order to avoid incisional hernias. We use the Carter-Thomason® (CooperSurgical) laparoscopic closure device to close the fascia from these port sites. If a port is placed at Palmer's point, we typically will not close this port site (even for 10/12 trocars) as hernias to this area are quite rare. As the Xi robot platform utilizes an 8-mm port for the camera, we commonly do not close these ports after surgery.

Standard CO_2 gas insufflation can be used during surgery. Some additional equipment can aide in smoke evacuation during surgery (e.g., PlumePort® by Buffalo Filter, SeeClear® by CooperSurgical). We like to utilize the AirSeal® system (Conmed) insufflation device. This facilitates maintaining CO_2 gas pressure after colpotomy and also assists with smoke evacuation during the case.

Docking Robot

There are several ways to position or dock the robot to the patient (Fig. 16.5). Initial considerations were for docking between the legs of the patient, but this limited access to the vaginal area for manipulation or removal of specimen. With the S and Si robot platforms, the robot can typically be docked in a position at an angle to or parallel to the patient. In the angled position, the patient's leg may need to be moved medially to avoid collision of the leg with the robot arm base. Parallel docking helps to avoid this problem. However, proper arm configuration will help to ensure that limitations with robot arm and instrument mobility can be avoided. For the Xi robot platform, the robot may be docked perpendicular to the patient, a position with fewer issues related to collision of the base of the robot to the patient. Once the robot is docked to the patient, the patient position cannot be changed. Thus, the patient should be in adequate Trendelenburg positioning prior to docking. One should utilize the minimum amount of Trendelenburg positioning tolerated to perform a safe surgery (*see* section "Patient Setup").

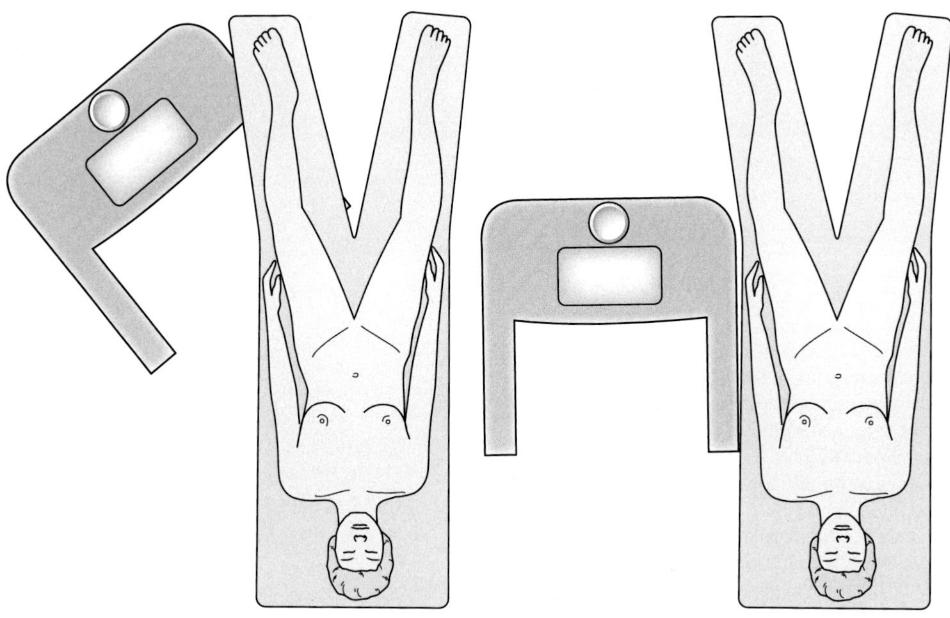

Fig. 16.5 Docking configurations for the Si da Vinci robot system. We typically favor a side-docking approach as shown on the right. This helps to facilitate access to the vaginal area for uterine manipulation and tissue extraction. In addition, there are less conflicts of the patient's legs with the base/arms of the robot

Robotic Hysterectomy and Bilateral Salpingo-Oophorectomy Procedure

Bilateral Salpingo-Oophorectomy

When performing a bilateral salpingo-oophorectomy by robotic approach, the technical aspects do not change. The robot platform is a "tool" used to help facilitate this procedure. As there is a lack of haptic feedback, the surgeon must utilize visual cues to determine when tissues are under too much tension. As in open surgery, the surgeon must utilize all of the robotic arms to help maintain traction and countertraction at all times. This facilitates the dissection of tissues during robotic surgery.

When removing the left ovary and tube, the procedure is initiated by placing the infundibulopelvic (IP) ligament and round ligament under tension (Fig. 16.6). This is accomplished by using a robotic arm to grasp the medial aspect of the round ligament and tenting the arm anteriorly and medially. This would be analogous to tenting the uterus up out of an open abdomen during laparotomy-based hysterectomy. Physiologic adhesions between the rectosigmoid colon and the left pelvic sidewall and adnexal tissues should be taken down. By placing the IP ligament under tension, the ureter will be dropped away from the IP ligament, thus avoiding potential injury to the ureter. The peritoneum overlying the psoas muscle is incised just 1–2 cm lateral to IP ligament, which is usually visible to the naked eye. The incision is taken up to the level of the round ligament and continued at the left paracolic gutter along the line of Toldt. Care must be taken to avoid critical structures underneath the peritoneum (e.g., external iliac artery and vein). With adequate exposure, the course of the ureter should be identified. This is facilitated by gently tenting the IP ligament medially and carefully dissecting the areolar tissue in the retroperitoneal space until the ureter is identified. Care must be taken to avoid injury to the infundibulopelvic ligament and/or the ureter. A window is

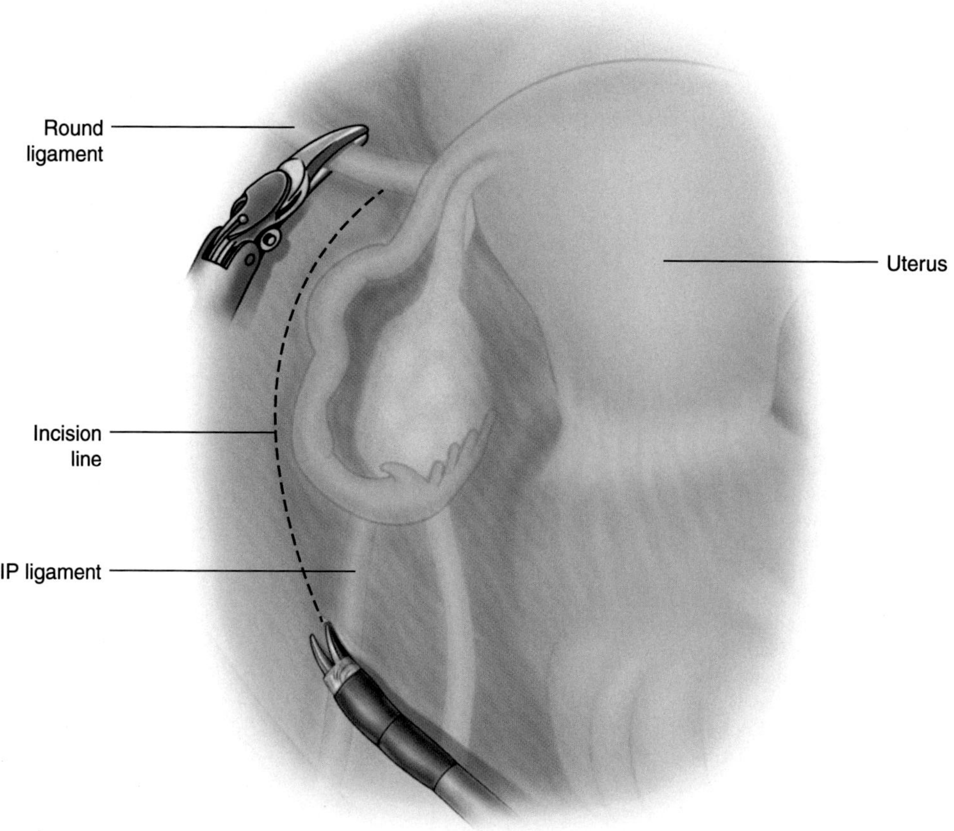

Fig. 16.6 Gaining access to the retroperitoneal space in the pelvis. Tension is placed on the round ligament near the cornu region of the uterus in an anterior and slightly caudal direction. This provides appropriate tension on the infundibulopelvic ligament (IP). An incision is created about 1–2 cm lateral to the IP ligament to gain access into the retroperitoneal space

created between the IP ligament and the ureter. The IP ligament should then be tented away from the ureter by using the monopolar scissor. Bipolar cautery can be used to coagulate the IP ligament (Fig. 16.7). As the IP ligament contains a major blood supply to the ovary that comes from the aorta, care should be taken to ensure adequate coagulation of the IP ligament. We typically cauterize sequentially with bipolar cautery and then partially transect the IP pedicle using a combination of the scissors and electrocautery with the monopolar scissors. This sequence is repeated several times until the entire pedicle is transected. Once the IP ligament is completely transected, the proximal IP ligament stump can easily retract. If any bleeding occurs from the proximal IP ligament stump, one risks potential injury to the ureter when trying to cauterize this stump as it courses just under the IP ligament.

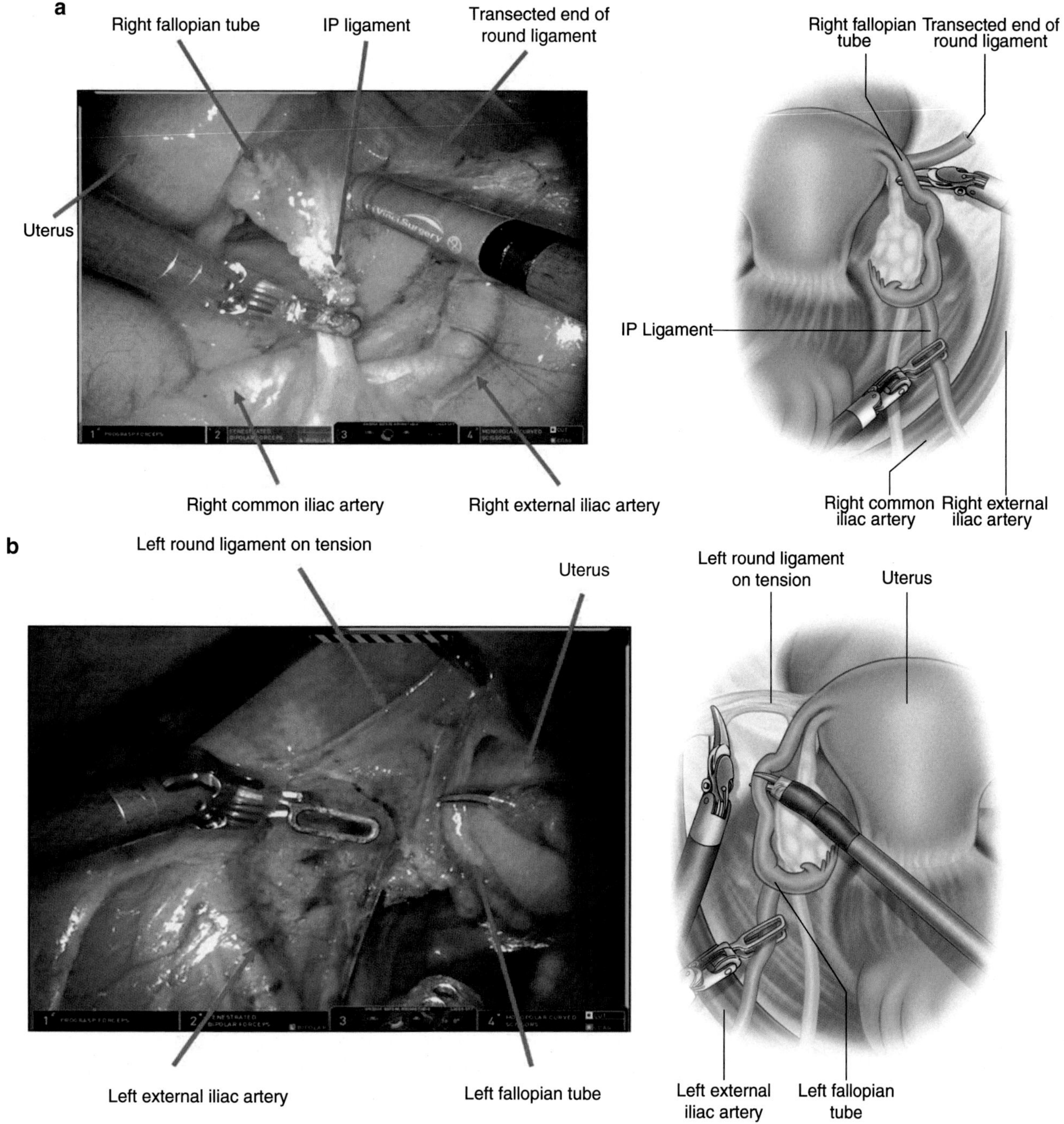

Fig. 16.7 Isolation of the ovary and fallopian tube. (**a**) Isolation of the right infundibulopelvic ligament. (**b**) After transection of the left infundibulopelvic ligament

The distal stump is carefully mobilized medially and anteriorly by taking down the pelvic peritoneum just underneath the adnexa. Care should be taken to avoid dissection of the peritoneum in the anterior/posterior plane as one can potentially injure the ureter that is attached to the peritoneum. The adnexa should be mobilized just up to the level of the uterus. The posterior peritoneum can then be excised. Careful dissection needs to be performed at the uterus as one can potentially injure the uterine vessels located just behind the peritoneum. Sharp dissection should be performed to first separate the peritoneum from the adjacent structures and to gain proper exposure to the posterior and lateral aspects of the uterus; during this time the assistant should always place gentle pressure of the uterine manipulator into the patient with a slightly anteverted position. The peritoneum overlying the posterior KOH cup ring can be dissected at this time. If the uterus is not to be removed, the utero-ovarian ligament is isolated, cauterized, and transected in order to completely remove the ovary and tube.

Hysterectomy

Steps for performing a robotically-assisted laparoscopic hysterectomy are essentially not different from an abdominal approach. Key steps that are required for both approaches include mobilizing the bladder away from the cervix and uterus, isolating the uterine vessels, taking down the cardinal ligaments, and amputating across the vagina. If the ovaries and fallopian tubes are being spared, one must also first isolate the utero-ovarian ligament. The main differences between a robotic and abdominal approach, however, involve how the tissues are dissected and blood vessels ligated. Similar care is needed to achieve the appropriate tension to the tissues to facilitate tissue dissection. Without proper tension to the tissue, excessive cauterization to the tissues can occur. With a robotic approach, proper tension will need to be applied to the uterus by utilizing a uterine manipulator and either an assistant port or one of the robot arms to grasp the tissue to apply the necessary tissue tension. For the uterus, a uterine manipulator can be positioned by the assistant to adjust the position of the uterus according to the specific part of the surgery. The surgeon can utilize one of the robot arms with a grasper (e.g., ProGrasp™ Forceps) that assist with manipulating the uterus in the proper position. At the beginning of the hysterectomy, it is critical to maintain an anteverted position, with slight angling away from the side that the surgeon is working (Fig. 16.6). This places tension on the round ligament and the infundibulopelvic ligament and allows the surgeon to gain safe access to the retroperitoneal space. In an abdominal approach, Pean clamps placed along the cornu region of the uterus are used to achieve this similar positioning. The surgeon can then safely divide the round ligaments and develop the retroperitoneal spaces. When the bladder must be separated away from the uterus and cervix, the uterus should be in a neutral-to-slightly retroverted position to facilitate this dissection. After the bladder peritoneum is incised just below the junction of the bladder and the cervix/uterus, the bladder peritoneum is gently tented anteriorly and caudally so that the plane between the bladder and cervix/uterus can be carefully developed (Fig. 16.8). It is critical to ensure that the assistant is also placing gentle pressure on the uterine manipulator in a cephalad direction. This

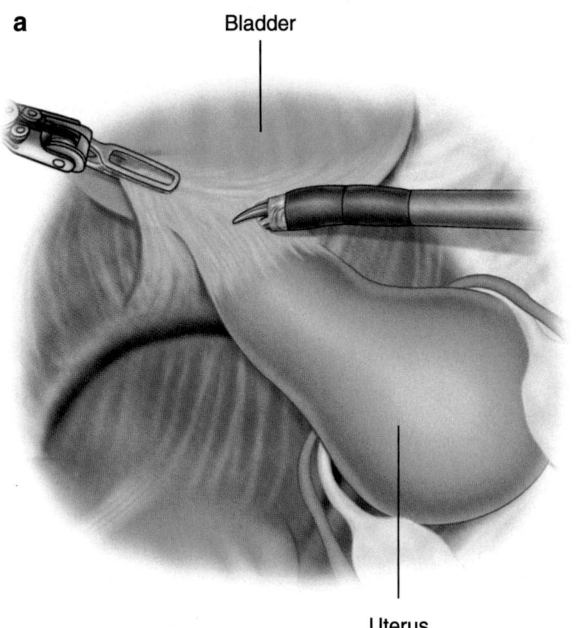

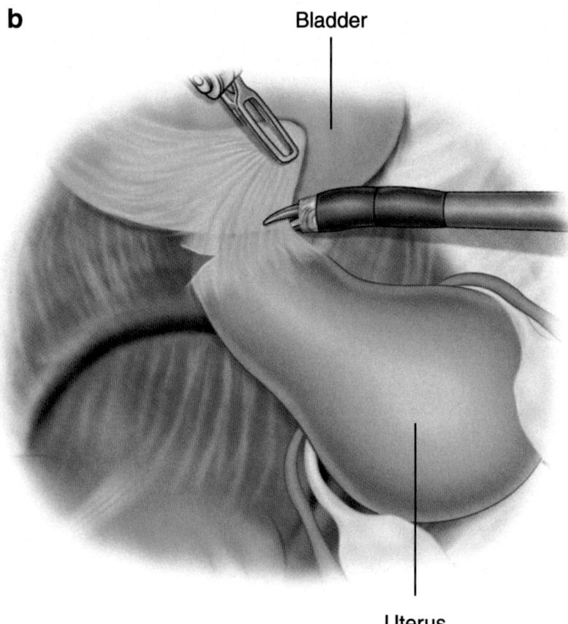

Fig. 16.8 Mobilization of bladder away from the uterus/cervix. (**a**) Bladder peritoneum is incised near the cervix/uterine junction. (**b**) The bladder is being carefully dissected away from the uterus/cervix

helps the surgeon with dissecting the tissues and avoiding injuries to the ureter, bladder, and other surrounding tissues. In patients who have prior cesarean sections, the plane between the bladder and the cervix/uterus may be difficult to identify. In difficult cases, the bladder can be retrograde filled with a dye-containing fluid (e.g., methylene blue in sterile saline solution) to distend the bladder. This can help the surgeon better identify the plane between the bladder and the cervix/uterus. This may help to facilitate identifying this plane. Sharp dissection can be accomplished with the robotic scissors to develop this plane and avoid thermal injury to the bladder. A KOH cup or device that delineates the cervical/vaginal junction will then assist the surgeon as to how far the bladder needs to be mobilized. The bladder should be well cleared from this junction by about 1–1.5 cm to avoid developing a vesicovaginal fistula.

The uterine vessels are then carefully skeletonized. Visualization of these vessels is greatly facilitated by the optics on the robotic machine. Once the uterine vessels are clearly identified, the vessels must be cauterized and transected (Fig. 16.9). We typically use the fenestrated bipolar cautery to accomplish ligation of the uterine vessels. From our experience, even after the vessels are well cauterized and transected, bleeding can still occur from the vessels. Several iterations of cauterization and transection may need to be employed to gain complete hemostasis. Taking some time to skeletonize the uterine vessels may help to reduce the tissue thickness and improve cauterization of the uterine vessel. It is important to have a suction-irrigator device readily available to ensure a clean surgical field and to potentially facilitate smoke evacuation. There are several smoke evacuation devices available that can be used to help maintain excellent visualization throughout this process (*see* section "Port Placement and Instrumentation Considerations"). Next, the cardinal ligaments are isolated and transected. The fenestrated bipolar cautery can be again used to first cauterize and then transect the tissues with the monopolar scissors. Although tactile feedback is blunted with robotic surgery, the KOH device or instrument that is used to delineate the cervicovaginal junction can still be readily identified by gently pressing against the tissue until the instrumentation (e.g., KOH cup) is palpated. The cardinal ligament is transected until this boundary is identified. Finally, a colpotomy incision can be created either with the monopolar scissor

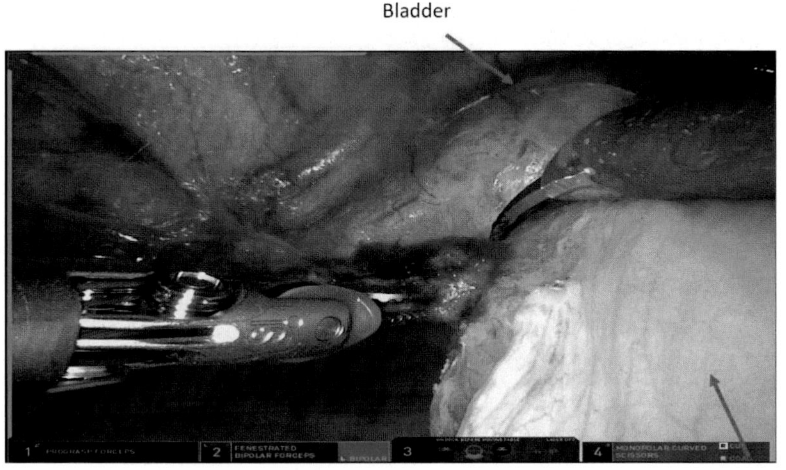

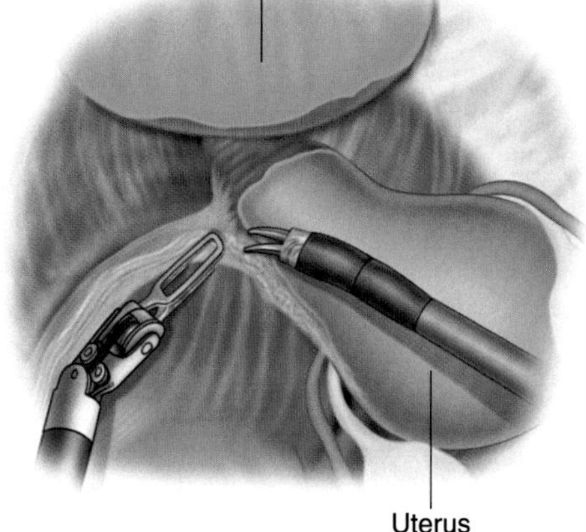

Fig. 16.9 Isolation of uterine vessels with the fenestrated bipolar forceps

cautery or an instrument suitable to the surgeon (Fig. 16.10). Once the uterus/cervix, with or without the ovaries/fallopian tubes, have been amputated, the entire specimen is brought through the vagina intact. In our experience, the specimen may require extraction through the abdomen due to its large size in less than 5% of cases (see section "Special Circumstances Encountered During Robotic Surgery").

Vaginal cuff closure can be performed by various techniques. This can involve a running closure with an absorbable 0 polyglactin suture. Closure with a figure of eight technique can also be used with a similar suture at a length of 6 in. There have been concerns in regard to vaginal cuff dehiscence rates with closure type. Overall, the rates are very low (<1–2% [13]). There has not been one technique that has clearly demonstrated benefit in reducing vaginal cuff dehiscence [14, 15]. However, there was some suggestion that a transvaginal closure approach may be better than a robotic approach [13]. The authors feel that the rates of dehiscence are small and the time spent converting to a transvaginal closure would unnecessarily increase operating room time. The robotic instrumentation facilitates suturing. Recently, a locking, barbed, suture was introduced and facilitates vaginal cuff closure without having to perform knot-tying. There may be some potential benefit to preventing vaginal cuff dehiscence [16], but additional studies are needed to support this.

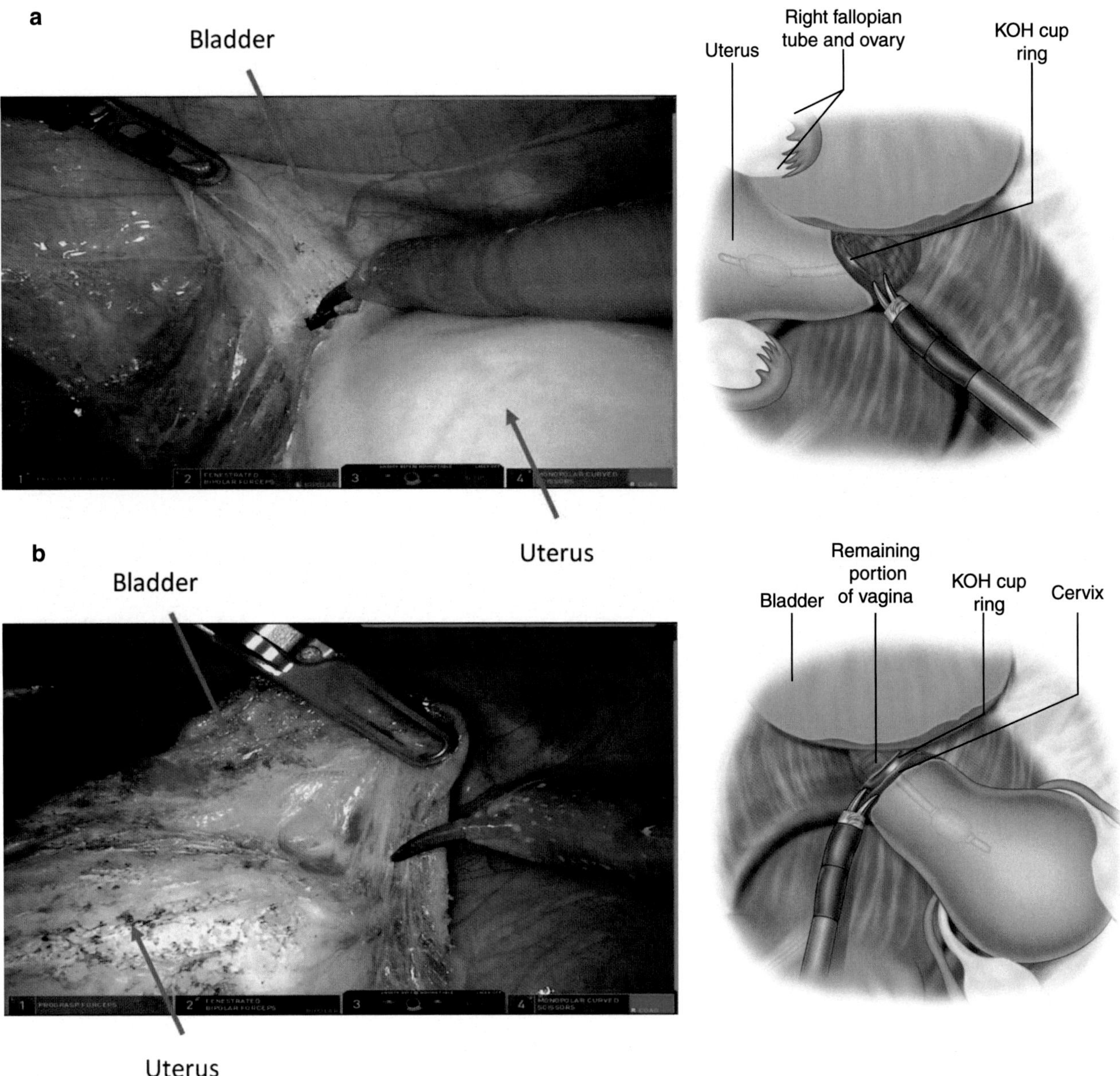

Fig. 16.10 Creation of colpotomy incision. Monopolar scissors are used like a Bovie cautery device over the KOH cup ring (blue) to transect the entire specimen from the vagina. (**a**) Posterior view. (**b**) Lateral view

Special Circumstances Encountered During Robotic Surgery

During surgery, certain circumstances can arise that make robotic surgery more challenging. This can also lead to conversion to open laparotomies. Careful thought and clinical judgment is always needed in making these decisions. We will be discussing issues of an enlarged uterus/mass that is unable to be extracted via the vagina, visualization concerns, and robotic surgery on morbidly obese patients.

In the situation where the specimen is too large to fit through the vaginal canal, the surgeon should ensure that the legs are well flexed at the hip. One can also corkscrew the specimen through the vaginal canal. If the specimen does not still pass through the vaginal canal, the surgeon must decide upon either an alternate route for or means of extraction. There have been recent concerns about uterine morcellation to facilitate removal of the tissues from the body. In patients where an occult or unsuspected cancer exists (in the uterus), uterine morcellation has the potential to spread cancerous cells into the abdominal cavity and decrease survival [17]. There have been descriptions of alternate techniques of morcellating the tissue in a bag [18, 19]. We will typically place the specimen in an appropriate fitting Endo Catch bag and bring the specimen through one of the abdominal port incisions, which was extended to accommodate the specimen. Obviously, the robot must be undocked from the patient, at least at the port site that will be used for extraction. Alternatively, a separate Pfannenstiel incision can be created.

In some patients, visualizing the pelvic organs can be made difficult by certain patient factors. This can include a large mass filling the pelvis (e.g., leiomyomata, ovarian mass), redundant rectosigmoid colon, obliteration of the posterior cul-de-sac, narrowed pelvis, and a short torso/abdomen in the cranial/caudal direction leading to small bowel filling the pelvis. The use of a 30-degree camera can help improve visualization around large uterus/mass in the pelvis. Attention to port placement will be critical to optimize access to pelvic structures. In cases of severe endometriosis, the posterior cul-de-sac can be obliterated. Placement of a rectal probe can help to delineate the rectosigmoid colon from other pelvic structures such as the vagina, uterus, and/or ovaries. In cases where the redundancy of the rectosigmoid colon obscures the surgeon's view of pelvic structures, the rectosigmoid colon may be mobilized and fixed in place with the aid of an assistant or by fixating the colon to the abdominal wall by means of a stitch.

Morbid obesity is becoming more prevalent in the USA, and these patients can present unique challenges during robotic surgery. The robotic technique offers significant advantage over an open approach to hysterectomy. Visualization of the uterus is often facilitated by robotic surgery. The instruments are of bariatric length, allowing the surgeon to gain access and exposure to the pelvis without having to pack the bowel with sponges or use extra-long instruments. There is less wound complication and bleeding, and return to presurgical function is greatly aided by robotic surgery [20]. For morbidly obese patients who have a significant pannus, we typically like to secure the pannus to the thigh with a strong tape (Fig. 16.11). We apply tape across the pannus as far caudally as possible and secure the tape to the table/Allen stirrups. Then we tape the pannus to the thigh and place reinforcing tape to prevent the tape from coming apart during the case. Morbidly obese patients often require the most

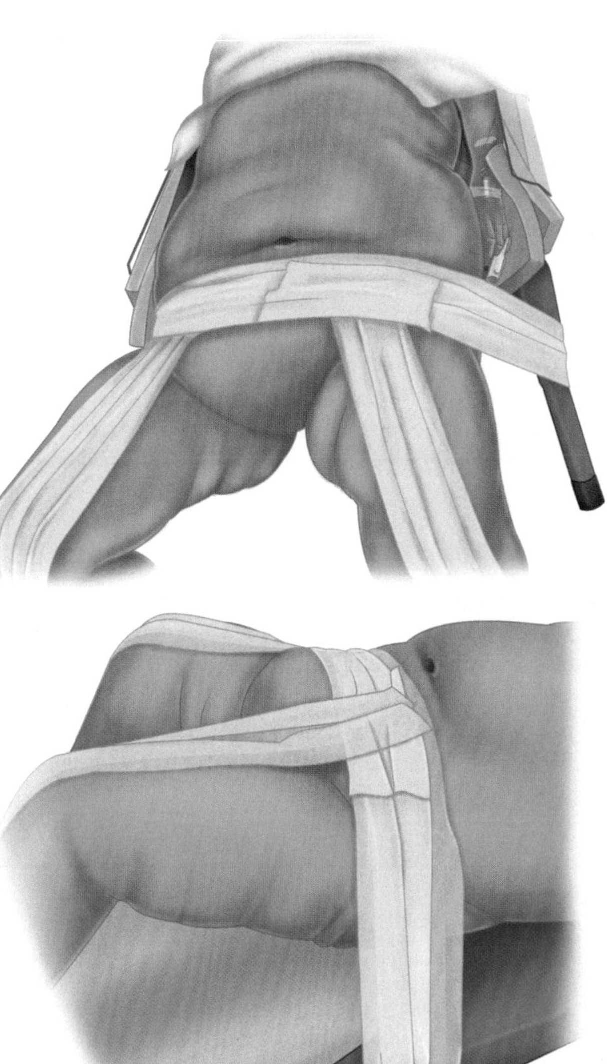

Fig. 16.11 Robotic surgery positioning in morbidly obese patients with large pannus. The pannus is secured with tape to the patient's thighs and stirrups. This helps to prevent the pannus from moving cranially during steep Trendelenburg positioning

significant amount of Trendelenburg position as possible to keep the bowels away from the pelvis, so the pannus/abdomen can often shift or move toward the chest. By fixing the pannus to the thigh, we can prevent this. It is our experience that this also allows improved ventilation by anesthesia and allows port placement in the upper abdomen, which usually contains the thinnest portion of the abdomen and facilitates port placement. There are extra-long robotic trocars that can be used, but generally, we can use the regular-sized robot trocars with this approach. There is always the possibility that one must convert to an open approach due to other factors (e.g., extensive adhesions, metastatic cancer). Staying above the tape, and thus the pannus, also facilitates open surgery. If necessary, however, the laparoscopic incisions can be closed, the tape removed, and the abdomen re-prepared for surgery (antiseptic wash and draping).

Summary

A robotic approach to performing a hysterectomy offers a safe and effective means to accomplish surgery. Although there are potentially cost-related issues, robotic surgery gives the surgeon another tool to perform complex operations. The surgical steps of the robotic and the open approach to accomplishing a hysterectomy are very similar. The same principles of surgery (e.g., appropriate tissue tension, traction, and countertraction) are applied to robotic surgery and are critical to a smooth and efficient operation. The surgeon must, however, understand some of the issues unique to robotic surgery, such as proper port placement and loss of haptic and tactile feedback. The surgeon must rely on visual cues and knowledge of the anatomic landscape. Further advances in robotic technology will continue to push the surgeon's boundaries of performing efficient and effective minimally invasive gynecologic surgeries.

References

1. ACOG Committee opinion no. 444: choosing the route of hysterectomy for benign disease. Obstet Gynecol. 2009;114(5):1156–8.
2. Aarts JW, Nieboer TE, Johnson N, Tavender E, Garry R, Mol BW, et al. Surgical approach to hysterectomy for benign gynaecological disease. Cochrane Database SystRev. 2015;8:CD003677. https://doi.org/10.1002/14651858.CD003677.pub5.
3. Maeso S, Reza M, Mayol JA, Blasco JA, Guerra M, Andradas E, et al. Efficacy of the Da Vinci surgical system in abdominal surgery compared with that of laparoscopy: a systematic review and meta-analysis. Ann Surg. 2010;252(2):254–62.
4. Albright BB, Witte T, Tofte AN, Chou J, Black JD, Desai VB, et al. Robotic versus laparoscopic hysterectomy for benign disease: a systematic review and meta-analysis of randomized trials. J Minim Invasive Gynecol. 2016;23(1):18–27.
5. Swenson CW, Kamdar NS, Harris JA, Uppal S, Campbell DA Jr, Morgan DM. Comparison of robotic and other minimally invasive routes of hysterectomy for benign indications. Am J Obstet Gynecol. 2016;215(5):650.
6. Wright JD, Ananth CV, Lewin SN, Burke WM, Lu YS, Neugut AI, et al. Robotically assisted vs laparoscopic hysterectomy among women with benign gynecologic disease. JAMA. 2013;309(7):689–98.
7. Mäenpää MM, Nieminen K, Tomás EI, Laurila M, Luukkaala TH, Mäenpää JU, Maenpaa MM, Nieminen K, Tomas EI, Laurila M, Luukkaala TH, Maenpaa JU. Robotic-assisted vs traditional laparoscopic surgery for endometrial cancer: a randomized controlled trial. Ame J Obstet Gynecol. 2016;215(5):588.
8. Blecha S, Harth M, Schlachetzki F, Zeman F, Blecha C, Flora P, et al. Changes in intraocular pressure and optic nerve sheath diameter in patients undergoing robotic-assisted laparoscopic prostatectomy in steep 45 degrees Trendelenburg position. BMC Anesthesiol. 2017;17(1):40.
9. Hoshikawa Y, Tsutsumi N, Ohkoshi K, Serizawa S, Hamada M, Inagaki K, et al. The effect of steep Trendelenburg positioning on intraocular pressure and visual function during robotic-assisted radical prostatectomy. Br J Ophthalmol. 2014;98(3):305–8.
10. Raman SR, Jamil Z. Well leg compartment syndrome after robotic prostatectomy: a word of caution. J Robot Surg. 2009;3(2):105–7.
11. Ulm MA, Fleming ND, Rallapali V, Munsell MF, Ramirez PT, Westin SN, et al. Position-related injury is uncommon in robotic gynecologic surgery. Gynecol Oncol. 2014;135(3):534–8.
12. van den Haak L, Alleblas C, Nieboer TE, Rhemrev JP, Jansen FW. Efficacy and safety of uterine manipulators in laparoscopic surgery: a review. Arch Gynecol Obstet. 2015;292(5):1003–11.
13. Uccella S, Ghezzi F, Mariani A, Cromi A, Bogani G, Serati M, et al. Vaginal cuff closure after minimally invasive hysterectomy: our experience and systematic review of the literature. Am J Obstet Gynecol. 2011;205(2):119.e1–12.
14. Tsafrir Z, Palmer M, Dahlman M, Nawfal AK, Aoun J, Taylor A, et al. Long-term outcomes for different vaginal cuff closure techniques in robotic-assisted laparoscopic hysterectomy: a randomized controlled trial. Eur J Obstet Gynecol Reprod Biol. 2017;210:7–12.
15. Landeen LB, Hultgren EM, Kapsch TM, Mallory PW. Vaginal cuff dehiscence: a randomized trial comparing robotic vaginal cuff closure methods. J Robot Surg. 2016;10(4):337–41.
16. Rettenmaier MA, Abaid LN, Brown JV 3rd, Mendivil AA, Lopez KL, Goldstein BH. Dramatically reduced incidence of vaginal cuff dehiscence in gynecologic patients undergoing endoscopic closure with barbed sutures: a retrospective cohort study. Int J Surg. 2015;19:27–30.
17. Raine-Bennett T, Tucker LY, Zaritsky E, Littell RD, Palen T, Neugebauer R, et al. Occult uterine sarcoma and Leiomyosarcoma: incidence of and survival associated with Morcellation. Obstet Gynecol. 2016;127(1):29–39.
18. Spagnolo E, Bassi E, Ferrari S, Rossitto C, Campagna G, Scambia G, et al. Extra-corporeal in-bag manual Morcellation for uterine specimen extraction: analysis of 350 consecutive cases. J Minim Invasive Gynecol. 2015;22(6S):S107–8.
19. Serur E, Zambrano N, Brown K, Clemetson E, Lakhi N. Extracorporeal manual Morcellation of very large uteri within an enclosed endoscopic bag: our 5-year experience. J Minim Invasive Gynecol. 2016;23(6):903–8.
20. Iavazzo C, Gkegkes ID. Robotic assisted hysterectomy in obese patients: a systematic review. Arch Gynecol Obstet. 2016;293(6):1169–83.

Radical Hysterectomy

17

Brooke A. Schlappe, Mario M. Leitao Jr., and Yukio Sonoda

Introduction

Radical hysterectomy has been a mainstay in the management of early-stage cervical cancer. With the advent of laparoscopy, and subsequently robotic surgery, more radical hysterectomies are now performed in a minimally invasive fashion. Minimally invasive radical hysterectomies entail greater complexity compared to simple hysterectomies. However, the robotic platform (the da Vinci Si® or Xi®; Intuitive Surgical, Sunnyvale, CA) offers improved visualization, dexterity, and better ergonomics for the surgeon. The robotic platform has some significant advantages compared with conventional laparoscopy. The instruments used in laparoscopy lack flexibility, and the surgeon must operate while standing and looking at a two-dimensional monitor. In the robotic system, the surgeon may remain seated; visualization is provided by a high-definition, three-dimensional camera; and wristed instruments are operated by movement of the surgeon's hands through use of the EndoWrist® instrument, which affords extraordinary dexterity. In addition, three robotic arms may be used simultaneously. For the practiced clinician, utilization of the robot is advantageous in both simple and complex cases. This chapter will address the data supporting the use of the robotic platform for radical hysterectomy. We will also describe the procedure in a step-by-step fashion.

Background

Robotic Radical Hysterectomy for Cervical Cancer

Robotic radical hysterectomy in the management of cervical cancer has been shown to be feasible and is increasingly popular among gynecologic surgeons [1–6]. Soliman et al. [7] compared operative and oncologic outcomes in 95 consecutive patients undergoing radical hysterectomy and pelvic lymph node (LN) dissection via a robotically-assisted, conventional laparoscopic or open approach. Short-term peri- and postoperative outcomes favored the minimally invasive procedures, with less blood loss ($p < 0.001$) and fewer infectious complications ($p < 0.01$) in both robotically-assisted and conventional laparoscopy groups, compared to the open laparotomy group. Length of stay was shorter for the robotic group (1 day, $p < 0.001$) compared to both the conventional laparoscopy (2 days) and laparotomy groups (4 days). Total number of LNs removed, parametrial size, and vaginal cuff length were used as surrogate oncologic outcomes, and no differences were found among the three groups [7]. In a smaller series, Estape et al. [8] compared 32 patients undergoing robotic radical hysterectomy, matched by stage and histology, to 17 patients undergoing conventional laparoscopic radical hysterectomy and 14 undergoing open radical hysterectomy. Each of the patients in this series also had a pelvic and para-aortic lymphadenectomy during the procedure. Estimated blood loss was similar in the robotic and laparoscopic cohorts (130 mL ± 119.4 vs. 209.4 mL ± 169.9, $p = 0.09$) but was much higher in the laparotomy group compared to the robotic group (621.4 mL ± 294.0 vs. 130 mL ± 119.4, $p < 0.0001$). The positive margin rate was similar across all groups (15.6% for robotic cases, 17.7% for laparoscopic cases, and 21.4% for open cases), but a greater number of LNs were retrieved robotically (32.4 ± 10.0) than laparoscopically (18.6 ± 5.3, $p < 0.001$) or via laparotomy (25.7 ± 11.5, $p < 0.05$) [8]. These data suggest that robotic radical hysterectomy in the management of cervical cancer is safe and feasible and may be advantageous in some ways.

Oncologic outcomes do not appear to be poorer when using the robotic platform. Chen et al. [9] evaluated disease-free survival (DFS) in a series of 100 patients. They found no difference in DFS between women undergoing radical hysterectomy by robotically-assisted laparoscopy, conventional laparoscopy, or laparotomy. Cantrell et al. [10] compared a cohort of patients undergoing robotic radical hysterectomy

B. A. Schlappe, MD · M. M. Leitao Jr., MD · Y. Sonoda, MD (✉)
Department of Surgery, Memorial Sloan Kettering Cancer Center, New York, NY, USA
e-mail: schlappb@mskcc.org

Y. Fong et al. (eds.), *The SAGES Atlas of Robotic Surgery*, https://doi.org/10.1007/978-3-319-91045-1_17

for cervical cancer to a historic cohort of patients who underwent open radical hysterectomy and found no difference in progression-free survival (PFS) ($p = 0.27$) or overall survival (OS) ($p = 0.47$). These series support the conclusion that, in early-stage cervical cancer, PFS and OS are no worse after robotic surgery.

Given its demonstrated feasibility and oncologic safety, the use of the robotic platform in radical hysterectomies has increased over the past several years. Conrad et al. reported the results of two surveys of members of the Society of Gynecologic Oncology (SGO) regarding their use of minimally invasive surgery, including the robotic platform. Conducted in 2007 and 2012, each survey contained questions specifically addressing robotic surgery. The number of respondents who thought that minimally invasive surgery was appropriate for radical hysterectomy and pelvic lymphadenectomy in the setting of cervical cancer increased from 36.7% in 2007 to 81.6% in 2012. When asked specifically about the robotic platform, the number of respondents who felt that its use was appropriate increased from 60.2% in 2007 to 89.1% in 2012. Respondents were then asked which procedures they performed with the robotic platform rather than with conventional laparoscopic equipment, and 75% indicated that they performed radical hysterectomy and pelvic lymphadenectomy with the robotic platform but not with conventional laparoscopic equipment [6]. The improved visualization and dexterity afforded by the robot make it an ideal tool in the surgical treatment of cervical cancer.

Several classification systems exist to describe the radicality of a radical hysterectomy, including the Piver-Rutledge-Smith [11] and the Querleu-Morrow [12] systems. A full description of these systems is beyond the scope of this chapter. However, the radicality of a procedure must be tailored to the spread of disease; a common procedure in early-stage cervical cancer is a Querleu-Morrow type B, or modified radical hysterectomy. The steps in performing this procedure robotically are described below. Any of these may be done robotically; therefore, even a laterally extended resection is not necessarily an indication for laparotomy.

Sentinel Lymph Node Detection

Sentinel lymph node (SLN) assessment has gained popularity in the setting of cervical cancer. SLN mapping has demonstrated feasibility, with acceptable sensitivity and negative predictive value shown in several trials [13–16]. SENTICOL was a large, prospective, multicenter trial of SLN mapping and utilized technetium 99 lymphoscintigraphy and patent blue dye in patients, ranging from stage IA1 with lymphovascular invasion to stage IB1 disease. Only two women were discovered to have metastases in non-SLNs, resulting in a sensitivity and negative predictive value of 92.0–98.2%, respectively [13]. One of the women with false-negative SLNs had a non-mapping hemi-pelvis; this highlights the necessity of a full lymphadenectomy in a non-mapping hemi-pelvis, as previously described by Cormier et al. [14].

The Cormier group also highlighted the importance of an SLN algorithm (Fig. 17.1), which includes pathologic ultrastaging of all SLNs, excision of any enlarged or suspicious non-SLNs, full lymphadenectomy on any non-mapping hemi-pelvis, and parametrectomy performed en bloc with primary tumor resection. Using this algorithm, they found a side-specific sensitivity and negative predictive value of 92.6–98.9%, respectively, in women with stage IA1 with lymphovascular invasion, to stage IIA disease [14]. In our institution, SLN assessment has become standard surgical practice in early-stage cervical cancer.

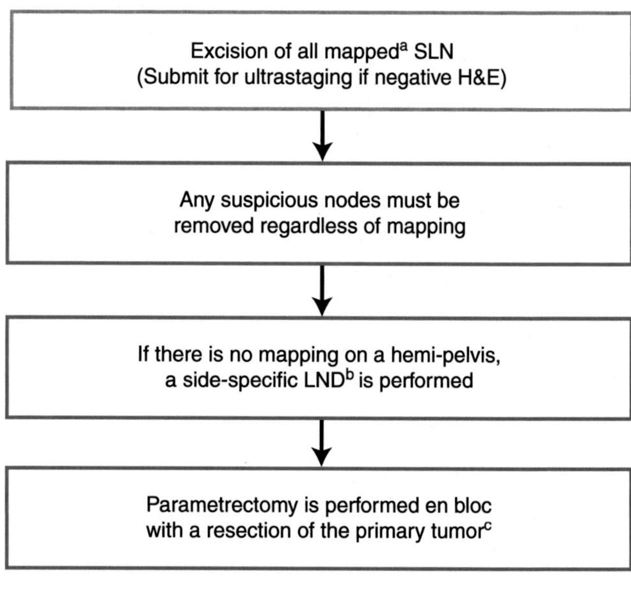

Fig. 17.1 Excision of all mapped sentinel lymph nodes. Submit for ultrastaging if hematoxylin and eosin (H&E) is negative. (**a**) Intracervical injection of dye. (**b**) Including interiliac/subaortic node. (**c**) Exceptions made in select cases

Cost-Effectiveness

As with many novel treatments in the field of oncology, the costs associated with incorporating a robotic platform in the operating room are of significant concern. Several studies have tried to address this issue. The cost-effectiveness of robotically-assisted radical hysterectomy has been compared to both the open and laparoscopic approaches. Using the perspective database, Wright et al. [17] evaluated patients undergoing radical hysterectomy with these three approaches. The median cost of the laparoscopic and robotic radical hysterectomy was significantly higher compared to abdominal radical hysterectomy (laparoscopic, $11,774; robotic, $10,176; abdominal, $9618). In a multivariate model, laparoscopic radical hysterectomy was associated with higher costs than abdominal radical hysterectomy, but the robotic procedure was not statistically different from the abdominal approach.

In a study comparing hospital costs for robotic radical hysterectomy with open radical hysterectomy, Reynisson et al. [18] evaluated 231 consecutive women (180 robotic and 51 open) who underwent radical hysterectomy with lymphadenectomy in a Western European public hospital. The estimated mean cost for an open radical hysterectomy was $12,986. For the first 30 robotic procedures, the cost was $18,382; however, this dropped to $12,759 for the subsequent 30 cases. The break-even cost for robotic radical hysterectomy came after 90 cases. The cost savings for the final 30 cases were due to shorter OR time and decreased length of stay. The authors concluded that, with an established institutional robotic program, and after a period of substantial, active implementation, robotic radical hysterectomy could be performed with comparable costs. Minimally invasive radical hysterectomy with pelvic lymphadenectomy can be safely performed as same-day surgery [19], which may further decrease costs.

Procedure

Patient Positioning

The patient should be positioned in dorsal lithotomy, with arms tucked at her sides, with careful attention paid to protecting the hands from inadvertent injury under the sterile drapes. For safe positioning of larger women, bed extenders or arm sleds may be required. A variety of pads are available in the OR to prevent sliding. These include pink foam, egg crate, beanbag, and gel. Patients should also be strapped to the table at the level of the shoulders, to prevent sliding when in deep Trendelenburg.

Sentinel Lymph Node Dye Injection

If SLN detection is planned, the cervical injection of dye should be done prior to placement of a uterine manipulator. A variety of dyes may be used, including both colorimetric (methylene blue and isosulfan blue) and immunofluorescent (indocyanine green). SLN detection rates vary according to the dye, with the best rates reported for indocyanine green (detection of 88–100% compared to 75–92% for methylene blue and 75–84% for isosulfan blue) [20, 21]. The da Vinci Si® and Xi® are equipped with Firefly™ Fluorescence Imaging, which allows the use of indocyanine green. When operating with the da Vinci S® system, a colorimetric dye must be used.

Cervical stromal dye injection is most commonly utilized and involves injecting a total of 4 mL of either immunofluorescent or colorimetric dye into the cervical stroma. A speculum is first inserted to obtain adequate visualization of the cervix. One milliliter of dye is then injected into four locations in the cervical stroma, using a spinal needle. This can be done either superficially and 1 cm deep into the stroma at the 3–9 o'clock positions (Fig. 17.2a), or superficially into the four quadrants of the cervix (Fig. 17.2b). Injection of dye at the 3–9 o'clock positions allows adequate detection of SLNs without staining of the bladder flap [22].

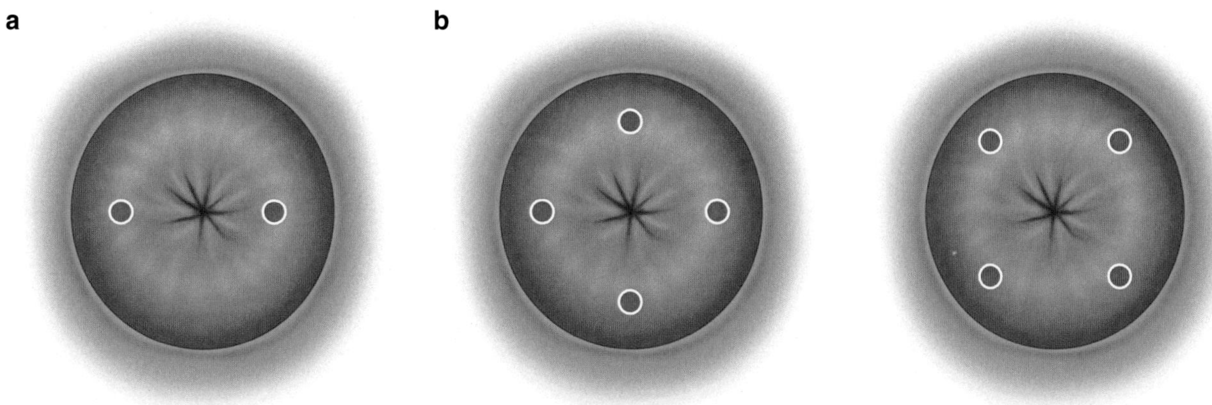

Fig. 17.2 Options for cervical stromal dye injections for sentinel lymph node mapping. (**a**) Deep and superficial injections, 3–9 o'clock. (**b**) Four quadrant injections

Placement of a Uterine Manipulator

A uterine manipulator is frequently used in radical hysterectomies and can facilitate visualization during the procedure, as well as demarcating the vaginal margin during colpotomy. A larger vaginal margin is required in radical hysterectomy; this can be obtained by using a uterine manipulator with a cervical cup and cutting on the cup's base, or making other modifications to existing uterine manipulators as previously described [23]. Alternatively, vaginal probes, EEA™ Sizers (Medtronic Minimally Invasive Therapies, Minneapolis, MN), or a sponge stick may be used to make the colpotomy if uterine manipulation is not felt to be necessary, or if a large cervical tumor prohibits placement of a manipulator.

Trocar Placement and Docking

Entry into the abdomen should be performed in a manner consistent with the surgeon's preference and comfort level. When using the da Vinci S® and Si®, the trocars should be arranged in an arc concave toward the operative field, with the camera port at or slightly cranial to the umbilicus. The camera port should be a minimum of 15 cm from the pubic symphysis. The trocars should be at least 10 cm apart and at an approximately 30° angle. When using the da Vinci Xi®, the trocars should be arranged in a more linear fashion and need to be only 8 cm apart (Fig. 17.3). An accessory port may be placed to facilitate LN removal and the passing of suture in and out of the abdomen. The accessory port may be placed in either the left upper quadrant or in the suprapubic region.

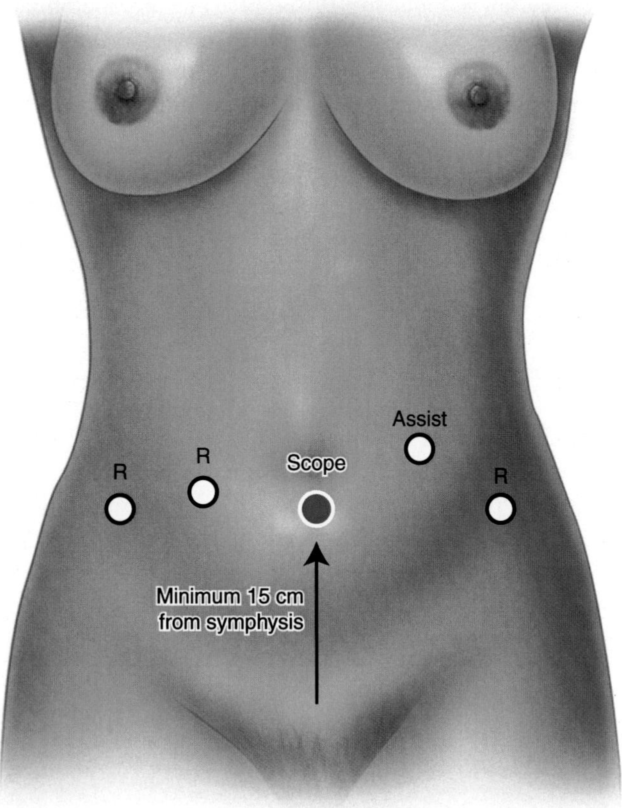

Fig. 17.3 Trocar placement for radical hysterectomy using da Vinci Xi®

To dock the robot, the patient should be placed in steep Trendelenburg with the operating table as low as possible. The da Vinci S® or Si® can be docked either in the center (between the patient's legs (Fig. 17.4a) or on the side (generally the patient's right side) in either a parallel (Fig. 17.4b) or angled position (Fig. 17.4c). The da Vinci Xi® should be docked on the patient's side in an angled (Fig 17.4c) or perpendicular position.

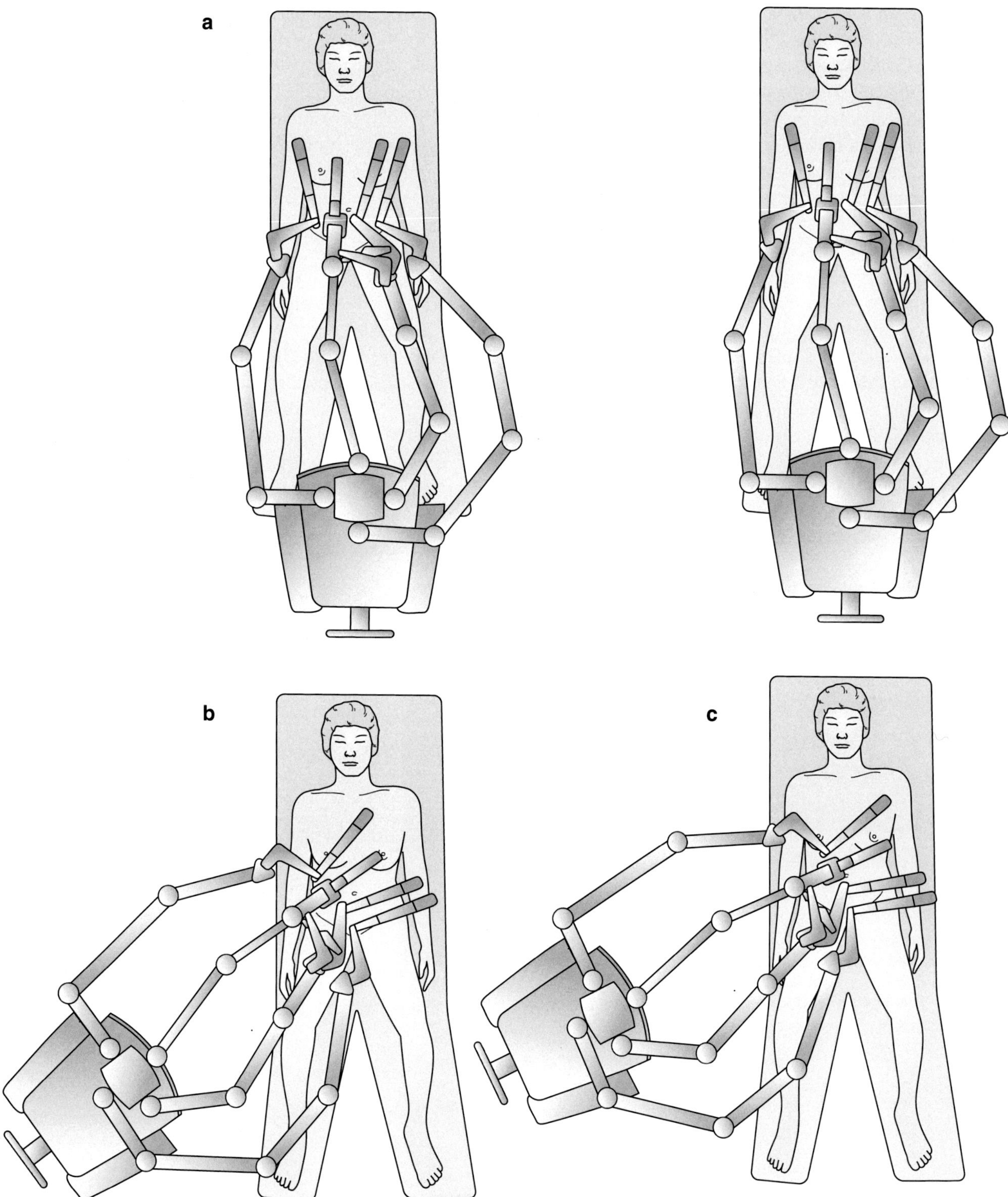

Fig. 17.4 Options for docking da Vinci robot for radical hysterectomy. (**a**) Center docking option for da Vinci S® or Si®. (**b**) Parallel side docking option for da Vinci S® or Si®. (**c**) Angled side docking option for da Vinci S®, Si®, or Xi®. The da Vinci Xi® may also be docked perpendicular to patient

Instrument Selection

Instrument selection is based on surgeon preference. A monopolar and a bipolar instrument are commonly selected and are generally placed in arms 3 and 1, respectively, for a right-handed surgeon. The available monopolar instruments include the EndoWrist® Hot Shears™ Monopolar Curved Scissors, the Permanent Cautery Hook, and the Permanent Cautery Spatula (Intuitive Surgical). The Monopolar Curved Scissors allow the most versatility because they can be used to cut tissue without cautery and, when closed, are useful in blunt dissection as well. A variety of bipolar instruments are also available, the most commonly used being the Maryland Bipolar Forceps or the Fenestrated Bipolar Forceps. The Fenestrated Bipolar Forceps have more grasping strength and a broader area of cautery, whereas the Maryland Bipolar Forceps possess a finer tip that facilitates better dissection. In the fourth arm, non-cautery forceps are generally recommended to aid in retraction; these include the ProGrasp™ Forceps and the Cadiere Forceps. The ProGrasp™ Forceps (Intuitive Surgical) have more grasping force and are better for use in tough tissue, whereas the Cadiere Forceps are better for more delicate tissue. The procedure can be performed with any combination of these instruments, depending upon surgeon preference and experience, and instrument availability.

Operative Steps

The steps in a robotically-assisted radical hysterectomy are the same as in a radical hysterectomy performed with conventional laparoscopic equipment or an open incision. If SLN assessment is also being done, the lymphadenectomy should be performed first. If SLNs are not to be assessed, the lymphadenectomy may be done either before or after the radical hysterectomy. Regardless, both the radical hysterectomy and pelvic lymphadenectomy are begun by opening of the retroperitoneal space, generally by incising an avascular space in the anterior broad ligament or over the pelvic sidewall that is extended cranially and caudally parallel to the infundibulopelvic (IP) ligament (Fig. 17.5) [24].

Opening of the avascular spaces should continue, and this may be done mostly in a blunt fashion. The paravesical space is opened next; it is delineated by the obliterated umbilical artery medially, the pubic symphysis anteriorly, the cardinal ligament posteriorly, and the external iliac vessels laterally. This is followed by the pararectal space, which is defined by the ureter and posterior broad ligament medially, the internal iliac vessels laterally, and the cardinal ligament anteriorly [24]. If evaluating SLNs, it is important to remember that most are found in the internal or external

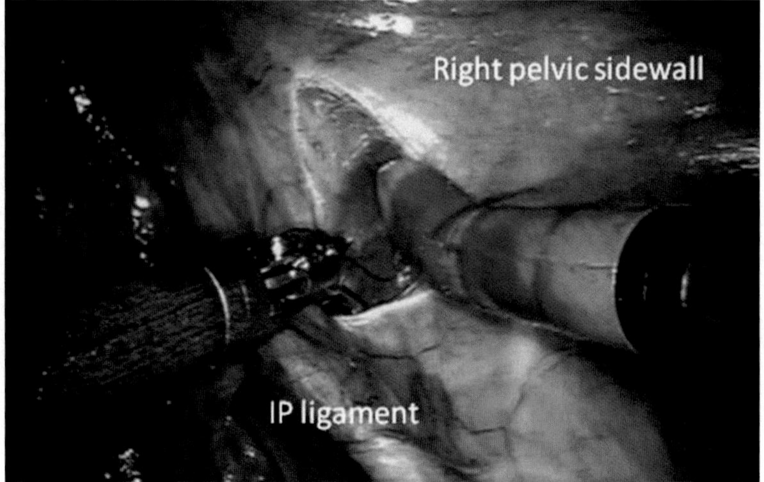

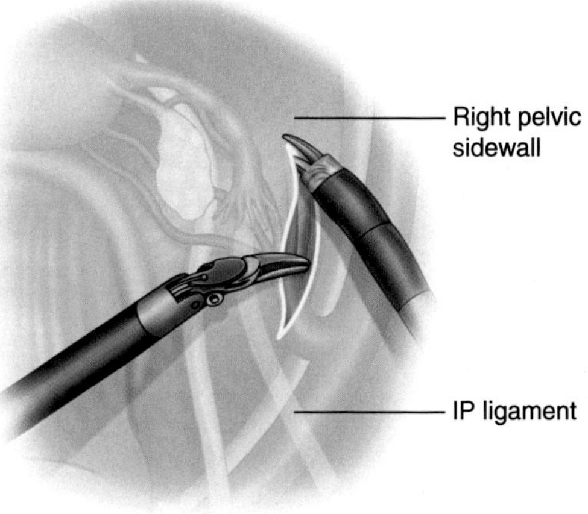

Fig. 17.5 The retroperitoneal space is opened by incising an avascular space over pelvic sidewall, extending it parallel to infundibulopelvic ligament

iliac nodal basin, with the majority lying in the interiliac region [16]. These areas are easily accessed with the paravesical and pararectal spaces open, and SLNs are identified and excised (Fig. 17.6).

After these spaces are opened and the SLNs removed, attention is turned to the IP ligament if an oophorectomy is planned. The IP ligament may be isolated by opening an avascular space in the posterior broad ligament. This skeletonization allows easy transection of the IP ligament; it should first be cauterized with a robotic bipolar instrument and then transected using the scissors and monopolar energy. If an oophorectomy is not planned, the IP ligament should be left intact and the utero-ovarian ligament and fallopian tube transected instead, in the same fashion [24].

The round ligament may be transected while opening the paravesical and pararectal spaces or transected prior to development of the vesicouterine space (i.e., the "bladder flap"). With elevation of the bladder and cranial retraction of the uterus, the vesicouterine space is easily developed with the use of monopolar cautery and blunt dissection (Fig. 17.7). A uterine manipulator or other instrument in the vagina will help to delineate the anterior fornix. The dissection may be carried as caudally as is necessary to achieve an adequate vaginal margin [24].

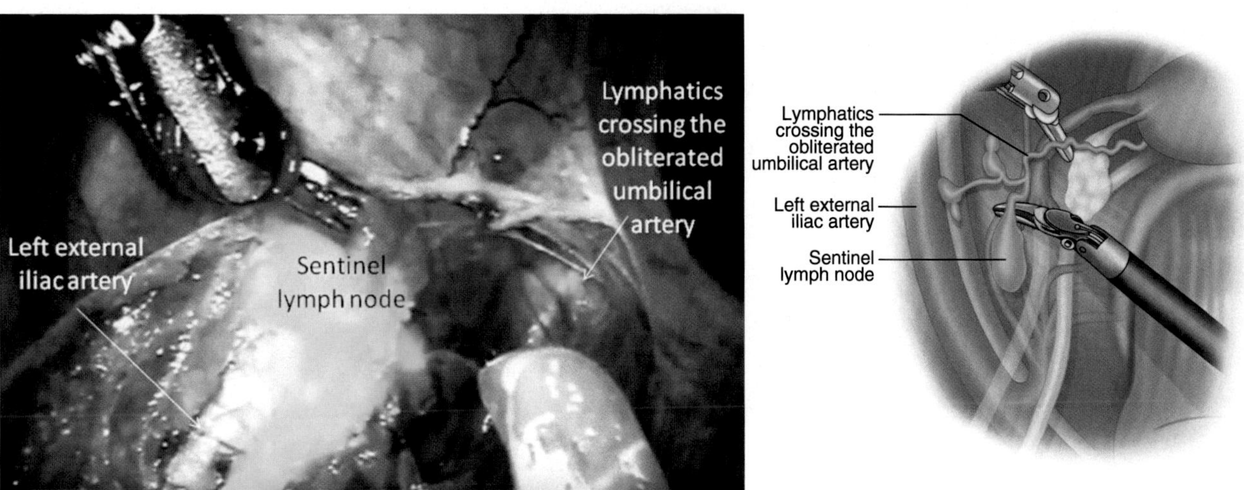

Fig. 17.6 A left external iliac sentinel lymph node identified with Firefly™ Fluorescence Imaging after cervical injection of indocyanine green. The lymphatic trunks cross over obliterated umbilical artery

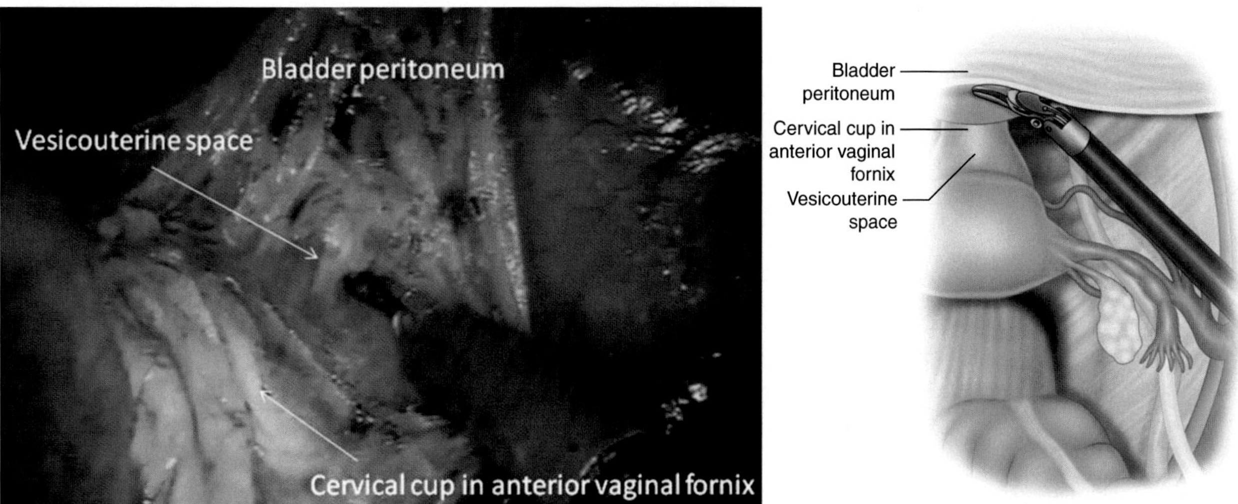

Fig. 17.7 The vesicouterine space is developed with both blunt dissection and monopolar cautery. The bladder peritoneum is tented up with robotic fourth arm

The uterine artery is identified next and traced back toward its origin from the internal iliac artery. Its relationship to the ureter is identified, and the two are separated. The uterine artery may then be transected lateral to the ureter, using bipolar and then monopolar cautery (Fig. 17.8) [24]. This is followed by cauterization and transection of the superficial uterine vein. The anterior portion of the cardinal ligament is carefully mobilized to "unroof" the ureter (Fig. 17.9), and incision of the cardinal ligament medial to the ureter is done after the ureter is rolled laterally (Fig. 17.10) [25].

The medial leaf of the broad ligament is incised to the desired transection point on the uterosacral ligament. The uterosacral ligament is then transected (Fig. 17.11). Anterior traction is placed on the uterus, and the posterior peritoneum is retracted toward the sacrum. The peritoneum is then incised, and the rectovaginal space is developed as caudally as is necessary to achieve an adequate vaginal margin; this is achieved using both blunt dissection and monopolar cautery (Fig. 17.12).

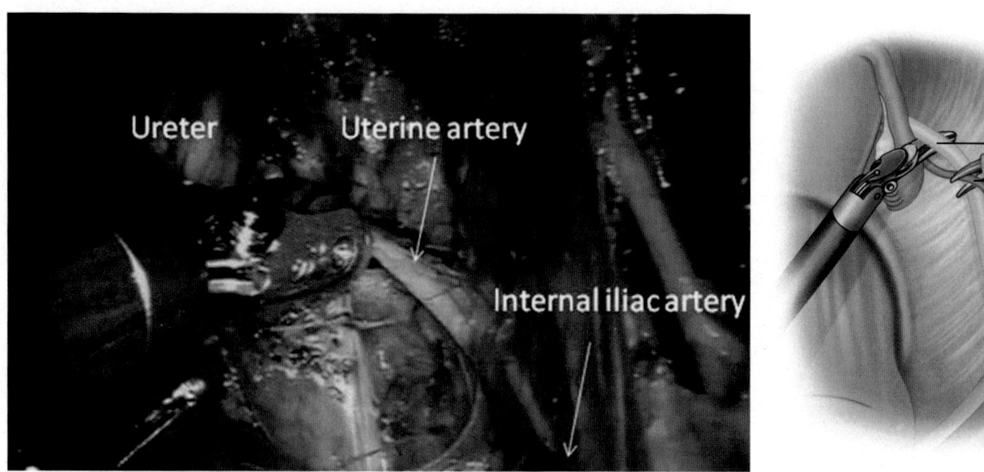

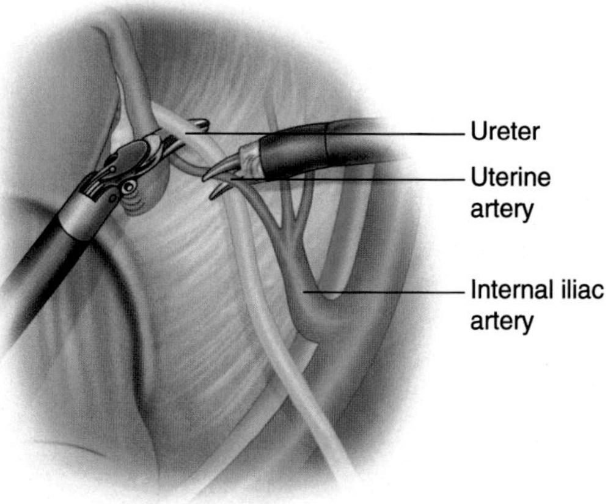

Fig. 17.8 The right uterine artery is cauterized and transected lateral to the ureter. The ureter (upper left corner) retracted medially by robotic fourth arm (lower left corner)

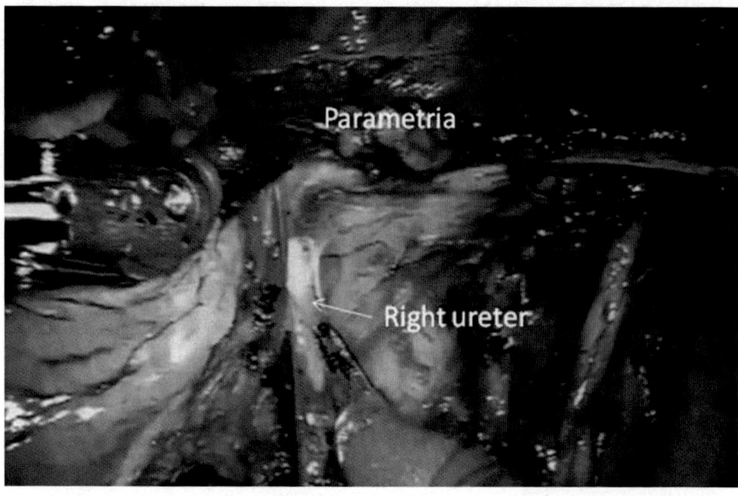

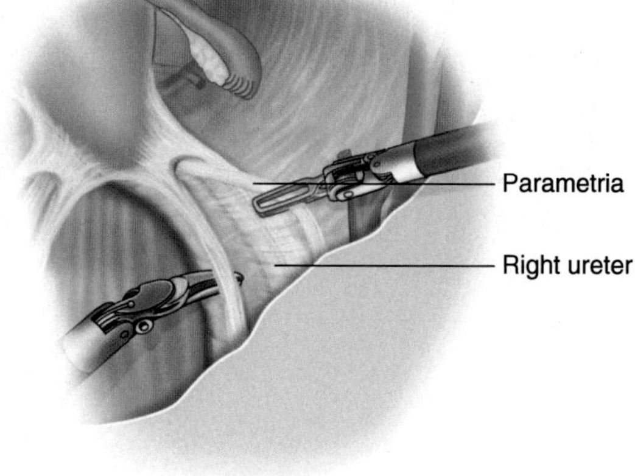

Fig. 17.9 The right parametria dissected from the right ureter

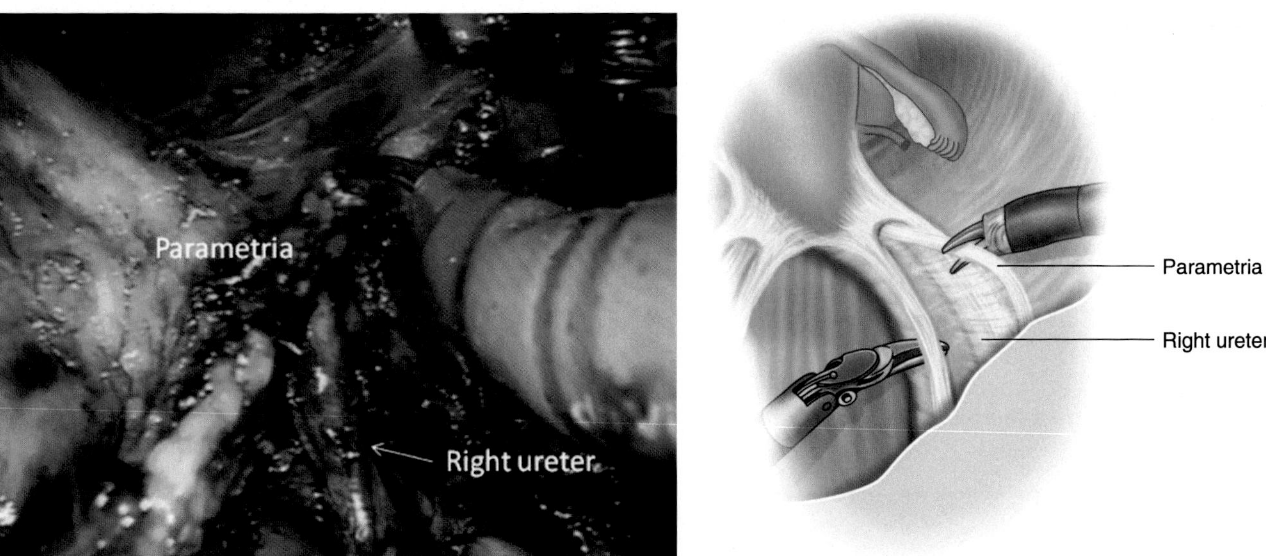

Fig. 17.10 The right parametria transected above the right ureter

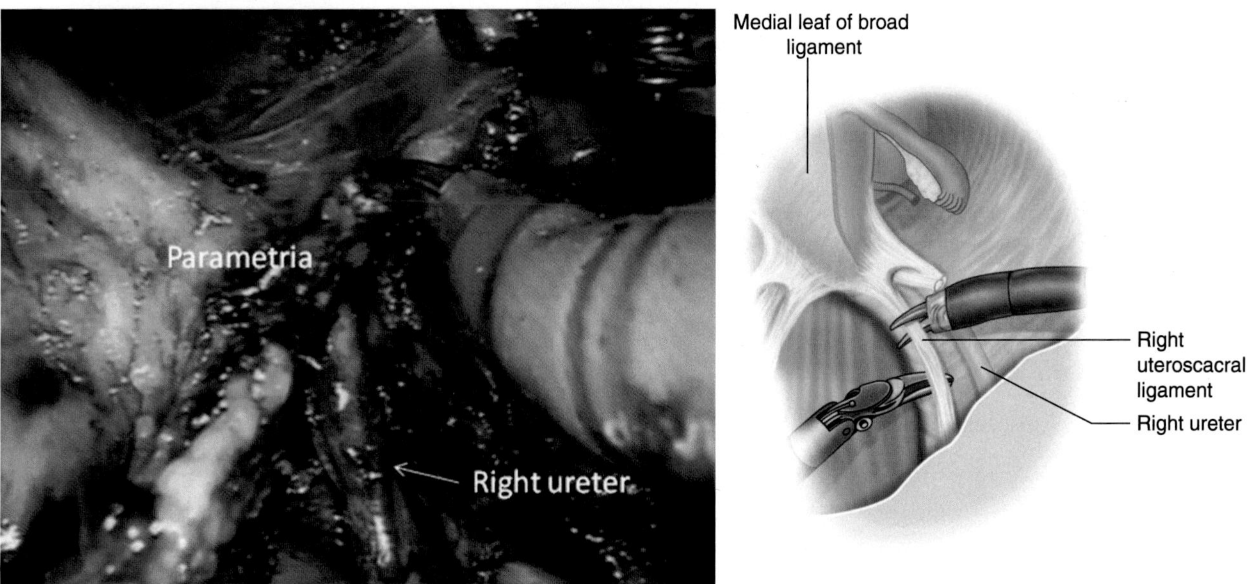

Fig. 17.11 The medial leaf of the broad ligament is incised; the right uterosacral ligament is transected. The right ureter mobilized from medial leaf of broad ligament

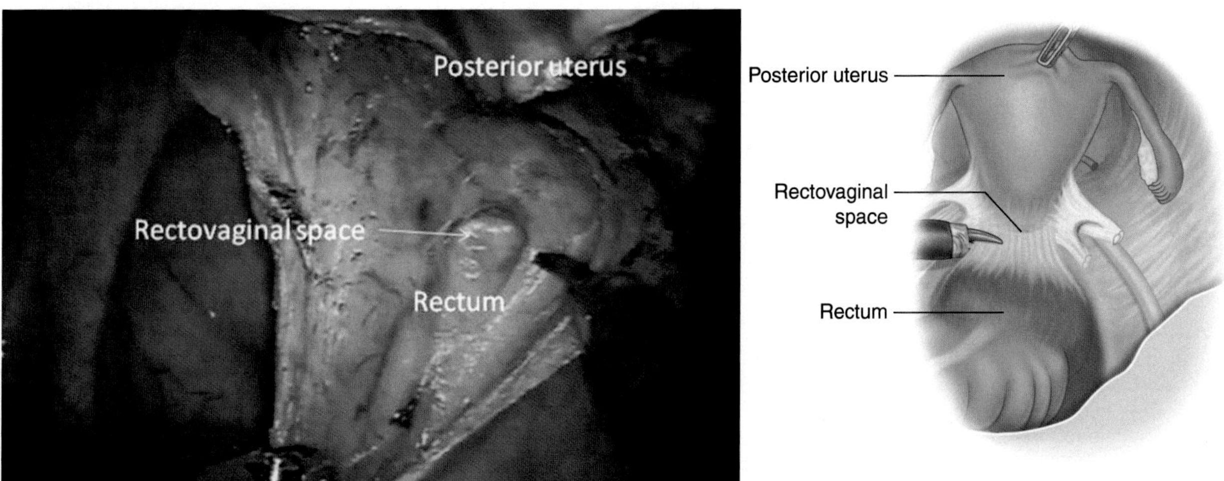

Fig. 17.12 Downward traction on posterior peritoneum facilitates development of rectovaginal space

After uterine arteries and uterosacral ligaments have been transected and the rectovaginal space developed, the colpotomy is made. If the uterine manipulator that is being used does not have a pneumo-occluder, or if a uterine manipulator is not being used, a pneumo-occluder should be placed prior to incising the vagina. The incision is then started at the desired point on the vagina using monopolar cautery and extended circumferentially (Fig. 17.13). The specimen is removed through the vagina and inspected, to ensure that adequate margins have been achieved.

The instruments in arms 1 and 3 may be replaced with robotic needle drivers at this time, and whichever suture the surgeon prefers may be passed through the accessory trocar. Frequently-used sutures include barbed suture, which can rapidly close the cuff in a running fashion, as no knots are required. Standard monofilament or braided sutures may also be used without much additional difficulty, given the ease of knot-tying afforded by the superior dexterity of the robotic system. Generally these non-barbed sutures are cut to approximately 15 inches, which prevent the excess suture from becoming cumbersome during closing of the vaginal cuff. The same principles of instrument knot-tying that are utilized during open surgery apply to the robotic instruments as well (Fig. 17.14) [24]. The vagina is closed, making sure to incorporate both peritoneum and vaginal

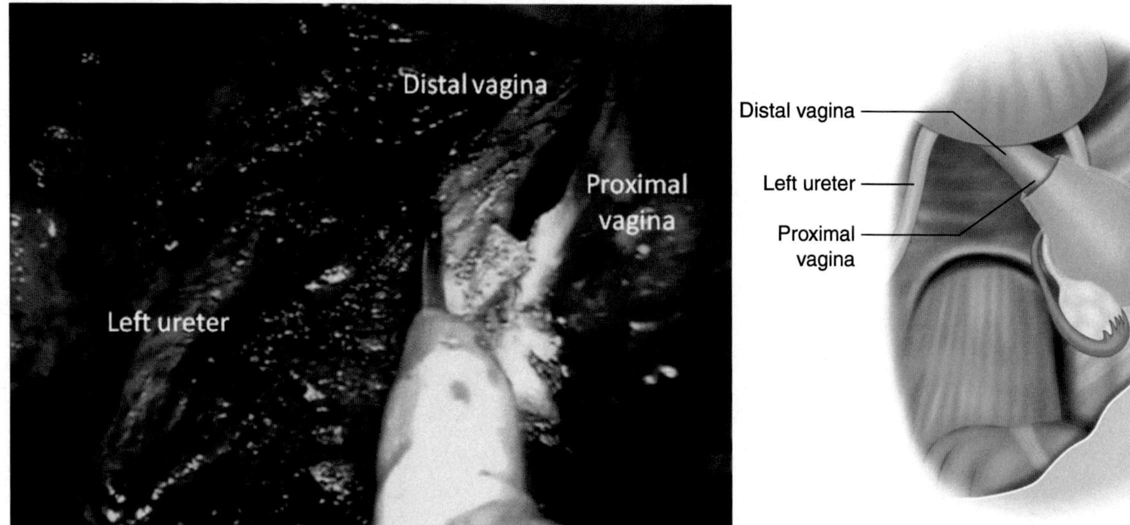

Fig. 17.13 Colpotomy is made circumferentially with monopolar cautery

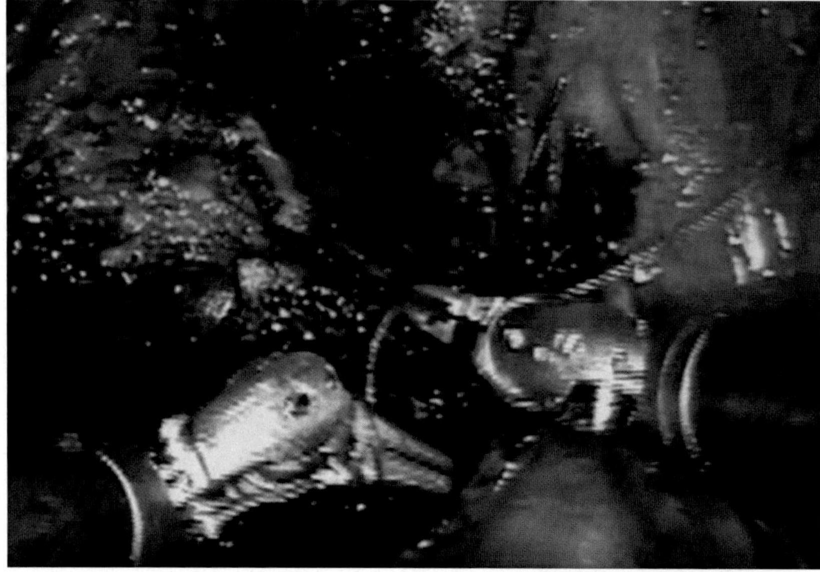

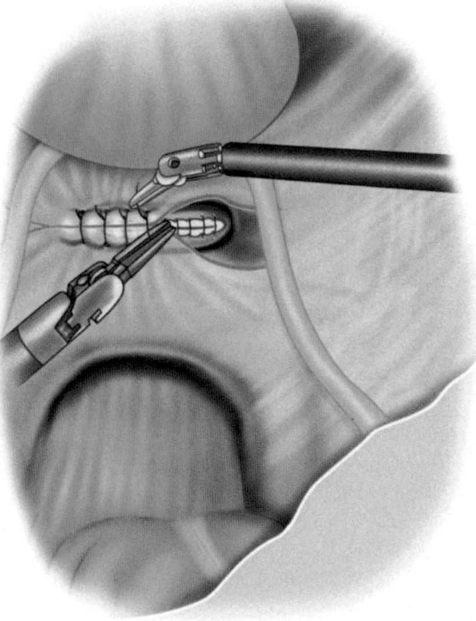

Fig. 17.14 If suture requires knot-tying, use same principles of instrument-tying as in open surgery

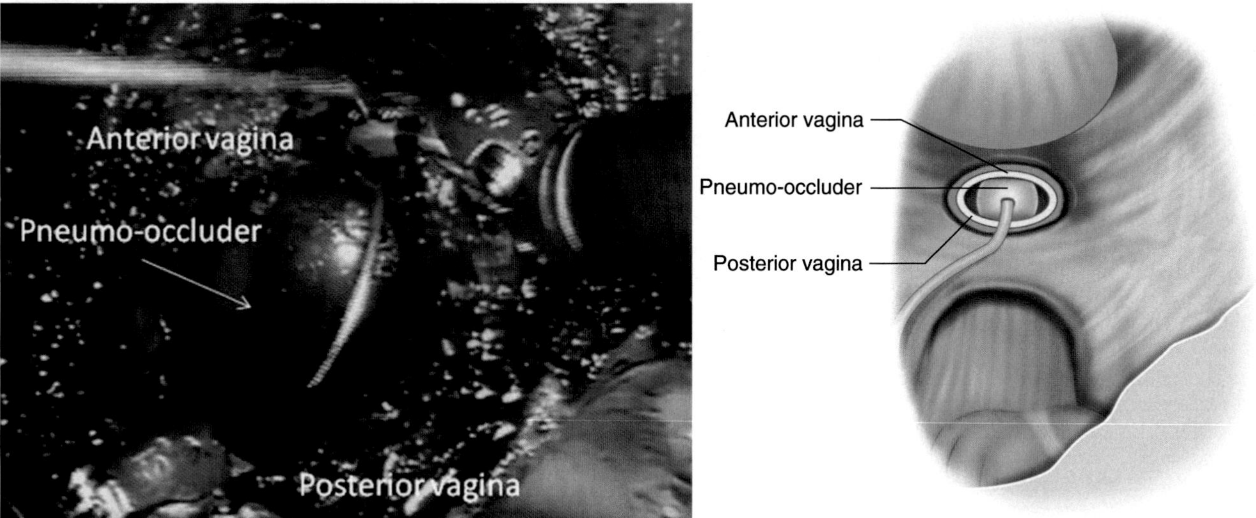

Fig. 17.15 The vaginal cuff is closed. Ensure that both peritoneum and vaginal mucosa are incorporated into the closure. A pneumo-occluder seen in the vagina

mucosa (Fig. 17.15). Hemostasis is then confirmed, the robot undocked, and trocars removed. The fascia must be closed for any port site larger than 1 cm, generally the camera port when using the da Vinci S® or Si®, and the accessory port. The risk of herniation is very low with the robotic 8 mm incisions, and, in general, these do not require fascial closure [26].

Conclusion

Radical hysterectomy performed with the robotic platform has been demonstrated to be a safe and feasible minimally invasive option in the management of early-stage cervical cancer, with or without SLN assessment. It continues to gain popularity among gynecologic oncologists due to the improved dexterity and superior visualization it provides to the surgeon and the improved perioperative outcomes for patients compared to laparotomy. The advantages of the robotic system make it ideal for use in more complicated dissections, and, as such, the need for extended lateral dissection is not in and of itself an indication for laparotomy.

The first randomized trial comparing minimally invasive surgery and laparotomy for radical hysterectomy in the management of early-stage cervical cancer was recently presented [27]. These preliminary data indicate worse progression-free survival with minimally invasive surgery, contradicting prior retrospective reports. The full report and analysis is awaited prior to drawing definitive conclusions.

References

1. Hoogendam JP, Verheijen RHM, Wegner I, Zweemer RP. Oncological outcome and long-term complications in robot-assisted radical surgery for early stage cervical cancer: an observational cohort study. BJOG. 2014;121:1538–45.
2. Sert B, Abeler V. Robotic radical hysterectomy in early-stage cervical carcinoma patients, comparing results with total laparoscopic radical hysterectomy cases. The future is now? Int J Med Robot Comput Assist Surg. 2007;3:224–8.
3. Boggess JF, Gehrig PA, Cantrell L, Shafer A, Ridgway M, Skinner EN, et al. A case-control study of robot-assisted type III radical hysterectomy with pelvic lymph node dissection compared with open radical hysterectomy. Am J Obstet Gynecol. 2008;199:357.e1–7.
4. Magrina J, Kho RM, Weaver AL, Montero RP, Magtibay PM. Robotic radical hysterectomy: comparison with laparoscopy and laparotomy. Gynecol Oncol. 2008;109:86–91.
5. Geisler JP, Orr CJ, Khurshid N, Phibbs G, Manahan KJ. Robotically assisted laparoscopic radical hysterectomy compared with open radical hysterectomy. Int J Gynecol Cancer. 2010;20:438–42.
6. Conrad LB, Ramirez PT, Burke W, Naumann RW, Ring KL, Munsell MF, et al. Role of minimally invasive surgery in gynecologic oncology: an updated survey of members of the Society of Gynecologic Oncology. Int J Gynecol Cancer. 2015;25:1121–7.
7. Soliman PT, Frumovitz M, Sun CC, dos Reis R, Schmeler KM, Nick AM, et al. Radical hysterectomy: a comparison of surgical approaches after adoption of robotic surgery in gynecologic oncology. Gynecol Oncol. 2011;123:333–6.
8. Estape R, Lambrou N, Diaz R, Estape E, Dunkin N, Rivera A. A case matched analysis of robotic radical hysterectomy with lymphadenectomy compared with laparoscopy and laparotomy. Gynecol Oncol. 2009;113:357–61.
9. Chen CH, Chiu LH, Chang CW, Yen YK, Huang YH, Liu WM. Comparing robotic surgery with conventional laparoscopy and laparotomy for cervical cancer management. Int J Gynecol Cancer. 2014;24:1105–11.

10. Cantrell LA, Mendivil A, Gehrig PA, Boggess JF. Survival outcomes for women undergoing type III robotic radical hysterectomy for cervical cancer: a 3-year experience. Gynecol Oncol. 2010;117:260–5.
11. Piver MS, Rutledge F, Smith JP. Five classes of extended hysterectomy for women with cervical cancer. Obstet Gynecol. 1974;44:265–72.
12. Querleu D, Morrow CP. Classification of radical hysterectomy. Lancet Oncol. 2008;9:297–303.
13. Lecuru F, Mathevet P, Querleu D, Leblanc E, Morice P, Darai E, et al. Bilateral negative sentinel nodes accurately predict absence of lymph node metastasis in early cervical cancer: results of the SENTICOL study. J Clin Oncol. 2011;29:1686–91.
14. Cormier B, Diaz JP, Shih K, Sampsom RM, Sonoda Y, Park KJ, et al. Establishing a sentinel lymph node mapping algorithm for the treatment of early cervical cancer. Gynecol Oncol. 2011;122: 275–80.
15. Altgassen C, Hermann H, Brandstadt A, Kohler C, Durst M, Schneider A. Multicenter validation study of the sentinel lymph node concept in cervical cancer: AGO study group. J Clin Oncol. 2008;26:2943–51.
16. Holman LL, Levenback CF, Frumovitz M. Sentinel lymph node evaluation in women with cervical cancer. J Minim Invasive Gynecol. 2014;21:540–5.
17. Wright JD, Herzog TJ, Neugut AI, Burke WM, Lu YS, Lewin SN, et al. Comparative effectiveness of minimally invasive and abdominal radical hysterectomy for cervical cancer. Gynecol Oncol. 2012;127:11–7.
18. Reynisson P, Persson J. Hospital costs for robot-assisted laparoscopic radical hysterectomy and pelvic lymphadenectomy. Gynecol Oncol. 2013;130:95–9.
19. Penner KR, Fleming ND, Barlavi L, Axtell AE, Lentz SE. Same-day discharge is feasible and safe in patients undergoing minimally invasive staging for gynecologic malignancies. Am J Obstet Gynecol. 2015;212:186.e1–8.
20. Smith B, Backes F. The role of sentinel lymph nodes in endometrial and cervical cancer. J Surg Oncol. 2015;112:753–60.
21. Buda A, Di Martino G, Vecchione F, Bussi B, Dell'Anna T, Palazzi S, et al. Optimizing strategies for sentinel lymph node mapping in early-stage cervical and endometrial cancer: comparison of real-time fluorescence with indocyanine green and methylene blue. Int J Gynecol Cancer. 2015;25(8):1513.
22. Abu-Rustum NR, Khoury-Collado F, Gemignani ML. Techniques of sentinel lymph node identification for early-stage cervical and uterine cancer. Gynecol Oncol. 2008;111:S44–50.
23. Ramirez PT, Frumovitz M, Dos Reis R, Milam MR, Bevers MW, Levenback CF, et al. Modified uterine manipulator and vaginal rings for total laparoscopic radical hysterectomy. Int J Gynecol Cancer. 2008;18:571–5.
24. Leitao MM Jr, Sert MB. Robot-assisted laparoscopic radical hysterectomy. In: Abu-Rustum NR, Barakat RR, Levine DA, editors. Atlas of procedures in gynecologic oncology. 3rd ed. Boca Raton, FL: CRC Press; 2013.
25. Andou M, Kanao H, Ota Y, Hada T. Laparoscopic radical hysterectomy. In: Abu-Rustum NR, Barakat RR, Levine DA, editors. Atlas of procedures in gynecologic oncology. 3rd ed. Boca Raton, FL: CRC Press; 2013.
26. Schiavone MB, Bielen MS, Gardner GJ, Zivanovic O, Jewell EL, Sonoda Y, et al. Herniation formation in women undergoing robotically assisted laparoscopy or laparotomy for endometrial cancer. Gynecol Oncol. 2016;140:383–6.
27. Ramirez PT, Frumovitz M, Pareja R, Lopez A, Vieira MA, Ribeiro R. Phase III randomized trial of laparoscopic or robotic versus abdominal radical hysterectomy in patients with early-stage cervical cancer: LACC trial. Society of Gynecologic Oncology Annual Meeting, 2018.

18 Robotically-Assisted Sacrocolpopexy

Steven Minaglia and Maurice K. Chung

Introduction

The presacral space lies in the true pelvis anterior to the sacrum. Within the presacral space lies the anterior longitudinal ligament (ALL), which covers a portion of the anterior sacrum. Fixation to the ALL of the pelvic floor and reproductive tract in women has been performed for several decades as a treatment of pelvic organ prolapse (POP) (Fig. 18.1) [1]. The specific area of interest for the pelvic reconstructive surgeon lies caudal to the bifurcation of the great vessels and medial to the right ureter and sigmoid colon.

Robotically-assisted sacrocolpopexy (RASC) has become a widely accepted surgical treatment of POP although open and laparoscopic approaches are still performed. A brief rationale for the development and implementation of this approach is as follows. A 2008 Cochrane review indicated that abdominal sacrocolpopexy was associated with a lower rate of recurrent vault prolapse and dyspareunia than the vaginal sacrospinous colpopexy. However sacrocolpopexy was shown to take longer and be more expensive [2]. Laparoscopic sacrocolpopexy compared to open sacrocolpopexy has been shown to take longer but is associated with less intraoperative blood loss, shorter hospital stay, and reduced postoperative ileus and small bowel obstruction [3]. The rationale for robotic assistance over "straight-stick" laparoscopic performance includes three-dimensional visualization of structures, the potential for enhanced surgeon comfort given console ergonomics and a seated position, and use of wristed instruments to facilitate fine dissection and suturing at multiple fixation points mundane to the sacrocolpopexy. A systematic review evaluating two randomized trials comparing RASC to laparoscopic sacrocolpopexy indicated increased cost and postoperative pain related to RASC [4]. A meta-analysis comparing the two procedures further included nonrandomized trials and showed RASC was associated with longer operative times and increased postoperative pain [5]. Both reviews found no differences in anatomical outcomes and quality of life [4, 5]. While use of the laparoscopic-only approach may be increasing for some surgeons due to enhanced skill and concern for costs and increased postoperative pain, the RASC will likely be performed in future years.

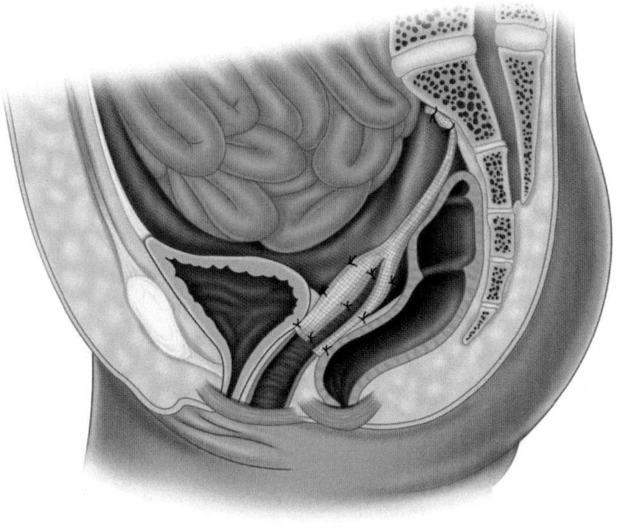

Fig. 18.1 Sacrocolpopexy

S. Minaglia, MD, MBA (✉)
Division of Urogynecology and Pelvic Reconstructive Surgery, Department of Obstetrics and Gynecology, John A. Burns School of Medicine, University of Hawaii, Kapi'olani Medical Center for Women and Children, Honolulu, HI, USA
e-mail: minaglia@hawaii.edu

M. K. Chung, MD, RPh
Midwest Regional Center of Excellence for Endometriosis, Pelvic Pain and Bladder Control, Lima, OH, USA

Y. Fong et al. (eds.), *The SAGES Atlas of Robotic Surgery*, https://doi.org/10.1007/978-3-319-91045-1_18

Indications for Surgery

Indications include repair of posthysterectomy vaginal vault or cervical prolapse, uterine prolapse, cystocele, rectocele, enterocele, and perineal descent. Fixation points of the graft ultimately depend on the defects being repaired. Historically, surgeons appeared to prefer the use of sacrocolpopexy to repair large anterior or apical defects. Additionally, patients with prolapse and a short vaginal length may benefit from the sacrocolpopexy as some transvaginal approaches have been associated with decreased vaginal length postoperatively [6]. Patients are often counseled about the need for concomitant vaginal repairs, especially when the surgeon aims to limit graft exposure to the vaginal canal and/or distal pelvic floor defects persist after sacrocolpopexy.

Robotic Surgical Approach Considerations

In general, patients who are candidates for open abdominal sacrocolpopexy are also candidates for RASC. Issues precluding RASC include contraindication to pneumoperitoneum, intolerance of steep Trendelenburg positioning, and difficult laparoscopic access among others.

Anesthesia

The standard approach for RASC utilizes general anesthesia. In a small retrospective study comparing combined spinal and general anesthesia to general anesthesia alone, patients in the combined group used less intravenous opioids during and after the procedure. Hospital stay did not differ in the study [7].

Patient Positioning

Robotically-Assisted Sacrocolpopexy

Patients are routinely positioned in the dorsal lithotomy position using Yellowfins stirrups (Allen Medical Systems Inc.; Acton, MA, USA) or similar. This allows access to the abdomen, pelvis, and vagina during the procedure. Arms are typically tucked next to the patient's abdomen bilaterally in order to facilitate surgeon and assistant access to the abdomen as well as to limit potential injury created by dynamic motions of robotic arms. Careful attention to positioning with appropriate application of padding must be made to avoid any nerve injury.

Gel or foam is commonly used to prevent the patient sliding during positioning. Trendelenburg positioning is required in order to move small bowel and portions of the sigmoid colon out of the pelvis. In general, the patient may be placed in steep Trendelenburg position until the presacral space and vaginal apex are accessible. The degree of Trendelenburg can then be reduced slowly until the degree is at a minimum and the operative site is still accessible (Fig. 18.2). Tilting the patient to the left often aids in moving the sigmoid colon away from the operative site. The deleterious consequences of prolonged surgery in Trendelenburg position are likely to decrease in frequency as surgeons become faster and more familiar with robotic technology and patient positioning for this procedure.

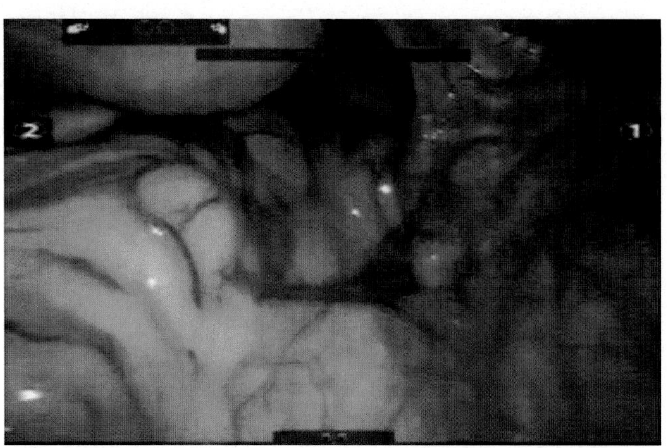

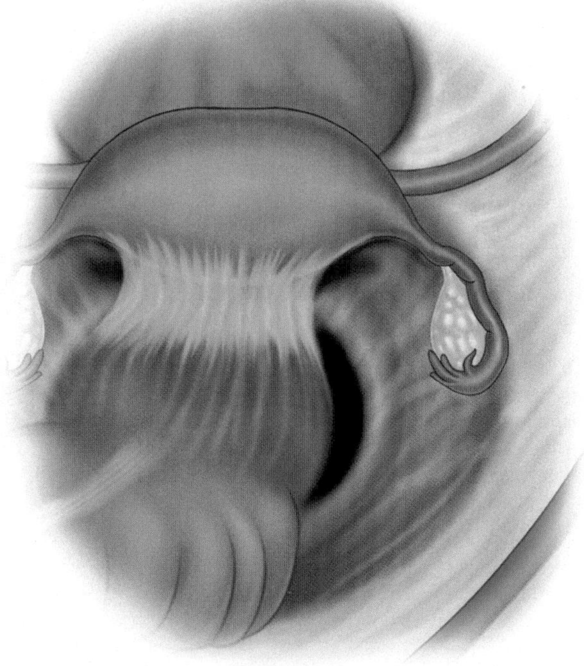

Fig. 18.2 View of the presacral space

A small retrospective study demonstrated a statistically significant decrease in mean total operative time of 75 minutes over a 4-year period during early adoption of the procedure [8].

Approach Options for RASC Combined with Hysterectomy

In the case of concomitant hysterectomy, whether total or supracervical, uterine manipulation to achieve views anterior and posterior to the uterus is important.

Optimally, the uterine manipulator should function in a way that the spaces anterior, posterior, and directly lateral to the uterus are easily visualized (Figs. 18.3, 18.4, 18.5, and 18.6). This fundamental principle is necessary for hysterectomy with concomitant pelvic floor repair to easily perform extirpation of the uterus, creation of the bladder flap, and amputation of the uterus above the cervix or creation of the vaginal cuff.

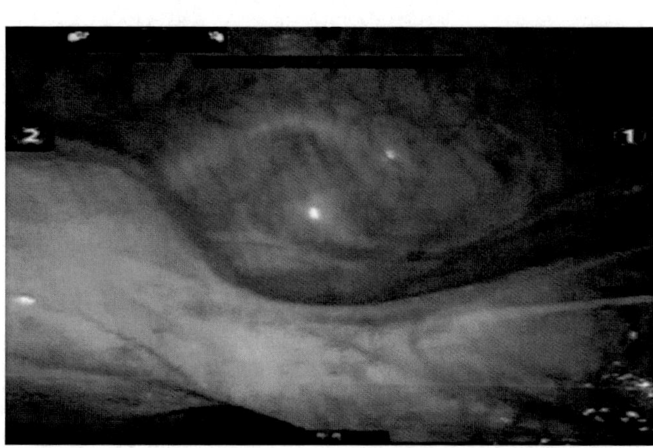

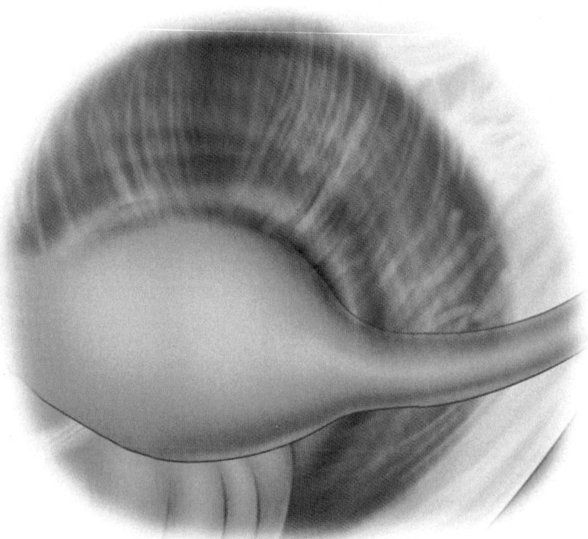

Fig. 18.3 Anterior, posterior, and lateral view of the uterus

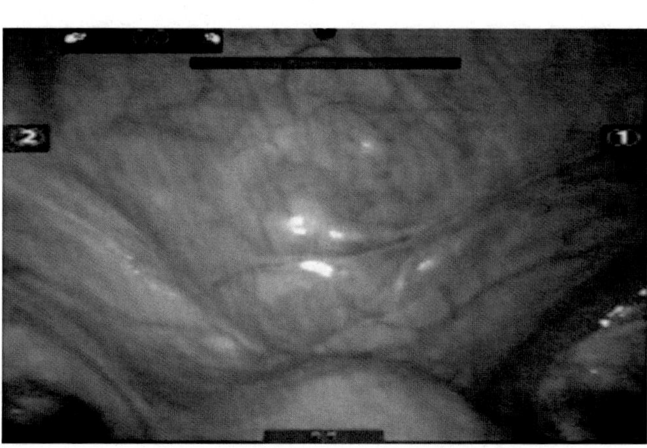

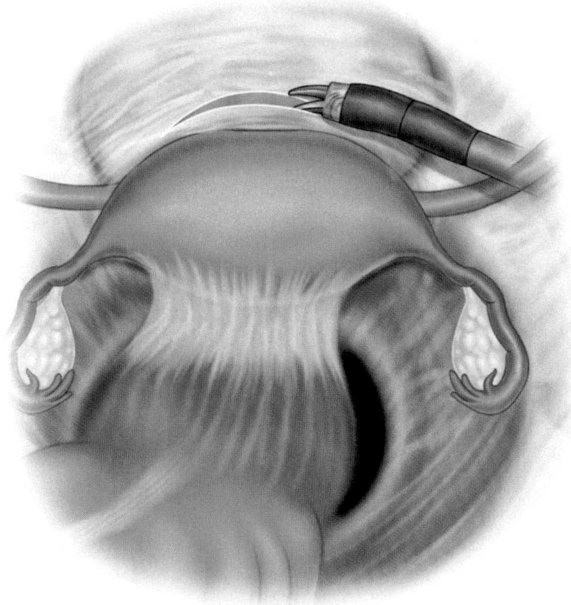

Fig. 18.4 Site of bladder flap creation

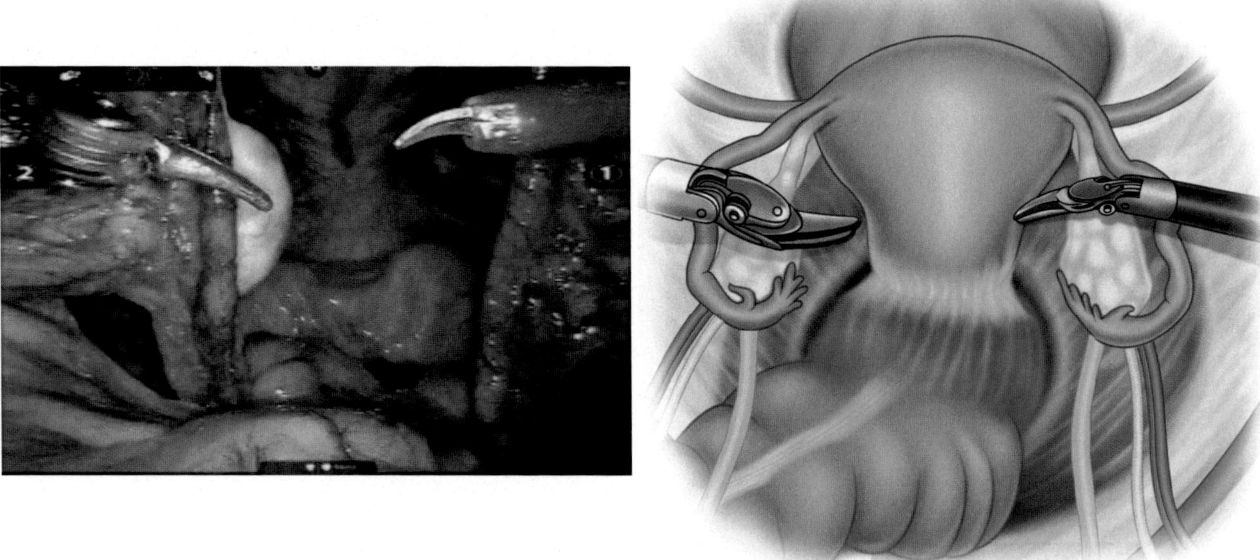

Fig. 18.5 Posterior view of uterus and cervix

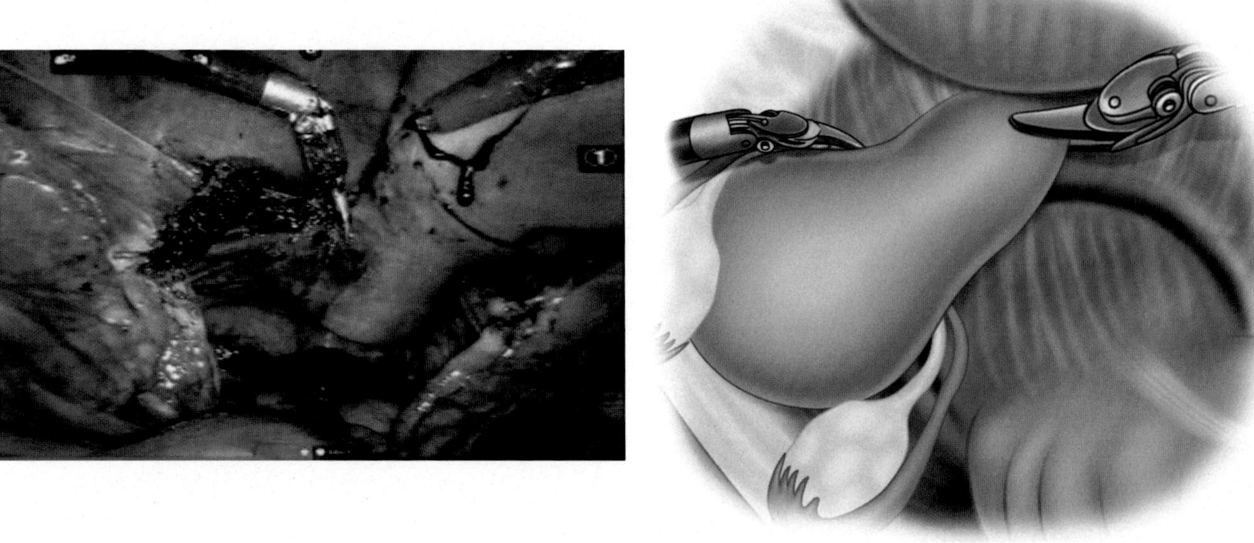

Fig. 18.6 Lateral view during hysterectomy

Approach Options for RASC without Hysterectomy

Vaginal manipulation is necessary to create spaces for graft fixation in the case of prior hysterectomy, whether total or supracervical. Concomitant trachelectomy (if indicated after prior supracervical hysterectomy) is beyond the scope of this chapter. There is a wide range of options that allow distension and elongation of the vaginal canal during the procedure: examples include sponges, gloved sponges, EEA sizers, vaginal cylinders, a gloved sponge stick, and Hoyte Sacro Tips (CooperSurgical Inc.; Trumbull, CT, USA).

Trocar Placement

Advanced preparation for abdominal and pelvic adhesions is necessary when attempting to complete a minimally invasive approach. Prior cesarean section and intestinal and/or gynecologic surgery may predispose the patient to the development of adhesions that may limit access to the pelvis. To begin, having a camera small enough to rotate among trocars as they are placed is necessary in order to gain different perspectives of adhesions and how they affect the conduct of the procedure. Laparoscopic dissection prior to docking the robot is often optimal during the early stages of the procedure due to the possible need for patient position changes. With rotation of the camera, graspers and dissectors may also be rotated in order to approach adhesions from different vectors. In general, trocar placement will occur as planned provided adhesions are removed in a manner to visualize the entire pelvis and presacral space.

Common trocar placement strategies are depicted in (Fig. 18.7a, b). The "W" configuration depicted in (Fig. 18.7b) was popularized with the introduction of robotic technology. This configuration allowed for roughly equal spacing between robotic arms, thus minimizing limitations on arm movement. Surgeons who performed laparoscopic sacrocolpopexy prior to the introduction of robotic technology likely utilized the trocar positions represented in (Fig. 18.7a) and merely continued using trocars in this configuration during robotic assistance. Placement of lower quadrant trocars likely developed for several reasons, including the need for standard length laparoscopic instruments to reach both the presacral space and distal pelvic floor fixation points and the need for the surgeon to avoid standing near the head of the operating table where bulky operating room equipment is commonly placed. Additionally, the lower quadrant trocars are mundane to several other gynecologic procedures.

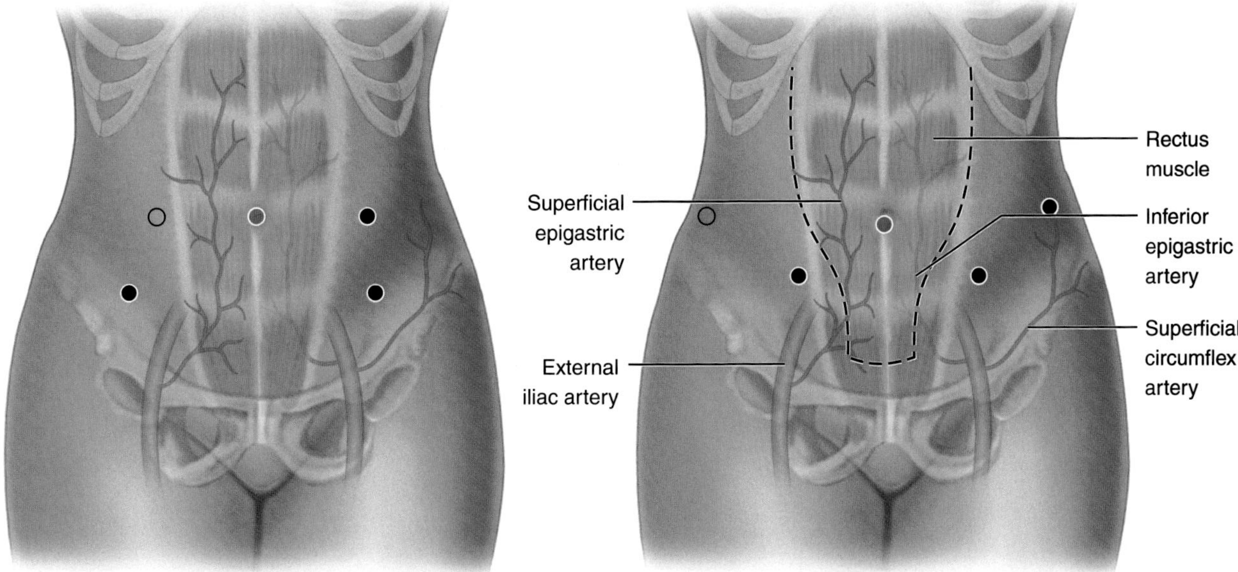

Fig. 18.7 (**a**) Trocar placement for laparoscopic sacrocolpopexy. (**b**) Trocar placement for RASC

Patient Cart Positioning

Placing the patient cart to the left of the patient (side docking) (Fig. 18.8) and placing it between the legs (Fig. 18.9) are two different strategies. Allowing easy access to the pelvis, whether for uterine manipulation, vaginal manipulation, and/or specimen removal, is the key rationale for placing the patient cart on the left side of the patient. A drawback of the side-docked patient cart is that all robotic arms emerge from the patient's left side, leaving limited space for dynamic motions. Given adequate yet modest vaginal access and the potential use of non-robotic instruments on the patient's left side, some surgeons still place the patient cart between the legs.

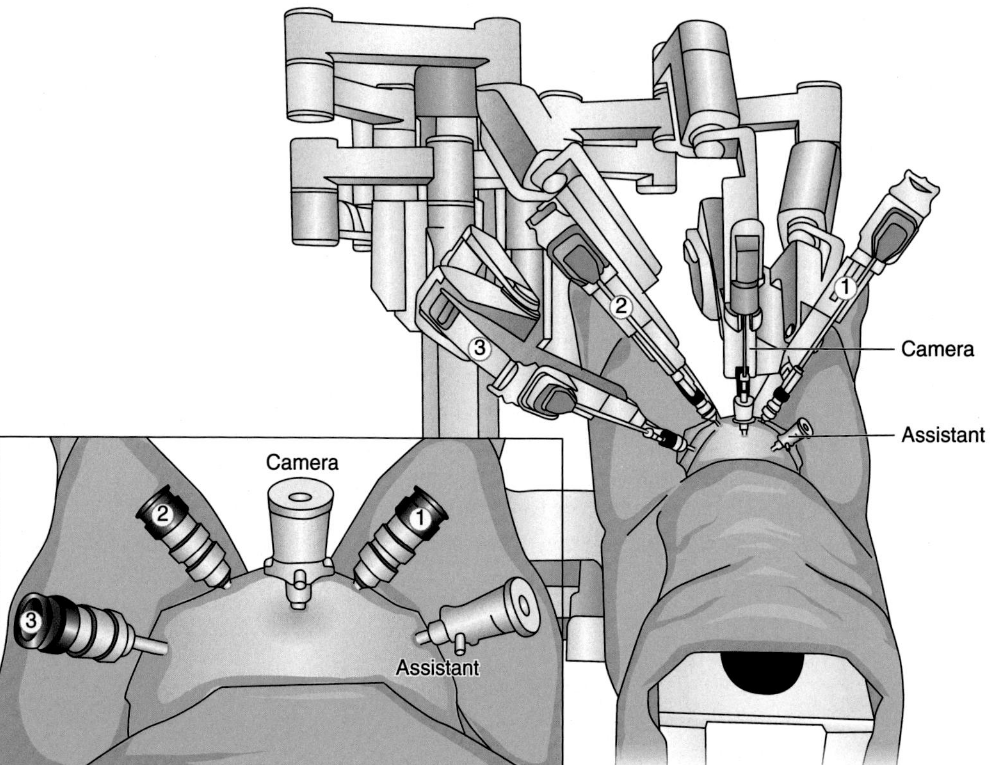

Fig. 18.8 Patient cart side docking to patient left

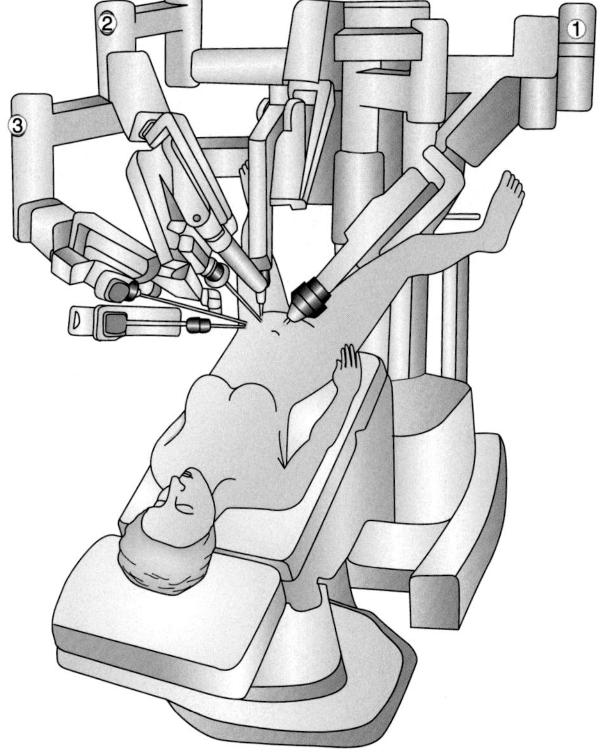

Fig. 18.9 Patient cart placed between the legs

Endoscopic Instrumentation

The da Vinci Surgical System (Intuitive Surgical Inc.; Sunnyvale, CA, USA) is the most widely used robotic surgical system for RASC and is used in all RASC surgical technique descriptions to follow. In general, the following instruments are used: monopolar scissors, PK dissecting forceps, large needle driver, and SutureCut needle driver (Intuitive Surgical, Inc., Sunnyvale, CA). A ProGrasp (Intuitive Surgical, Inc.) may be used with the robotic third arm in cases where additional retraction is needed. The assistant commonly uses a suction irrigator, needle driver, and assorted graspers. A cauterizing loop and Endo Catch bag are used in the case of supracervical hysterectomy.

RASC with Hysterectomy Steps

Various techniques of RASC have been described in the literature without any particular technique demonstrating superiority. Therefore, we present our technique as an option and attempt to outline its rationale using available evidence where appropriate.

A uterine manipulator is placed along with a Foley catheter to gravity after the patient is sterilely prepped and draped. The robot is docked after access to the pelvis is obtained as described above. The hysterectomy and possible bilateral salpingo-oophorectomy are performed before RASC. Complete steps to these procedures are described elsewhere in this text. Of note, the bladder flap is created and anterior vaginal wall exposed while the uterine manipulator is in place regardless of the type of hysterectomy planned. This step may be facilitated by counter traction created by the uterine manipulator. Further anterior dissection may be performed if needed after the hysterectomy with the aid of a vaginal manipulator.

In the case of supracervical hysterectomy, we amputate the cervix at the level of the internal os using a cauterizing endoloop. The cervix is then oversewn using absorbable suture. There is no general consensus on the importance of oversewing the cervical stump prior to RASC; case reports, however, appear to suggest that oversewing the cervical stump may reduce complications [9, 10]. In the case of a total hysterectomy, the vaginal cuff is closed prior to beginning RASC. In the case of a posthysterectomy vaginal vault prolapse, it is important to identify the cuff, assess for any cuff dehiscence, and close the cuff completely prior to mesh fixation (Figs. 18.10 and 18.11). We begin RASC as further described below after completing the total hysterectomy or oversewing the cervical stump after supracervical hysterectomy.

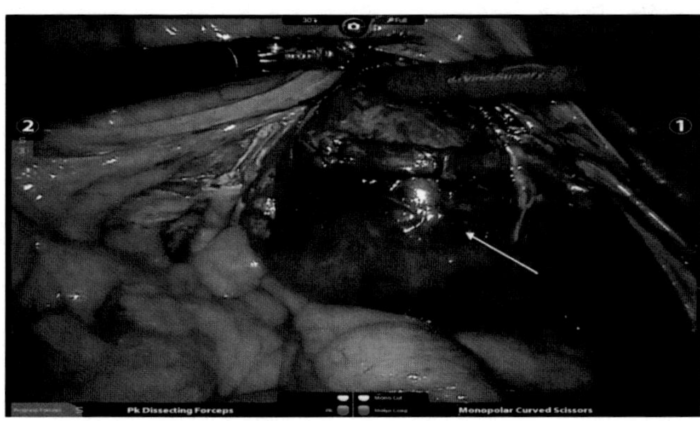

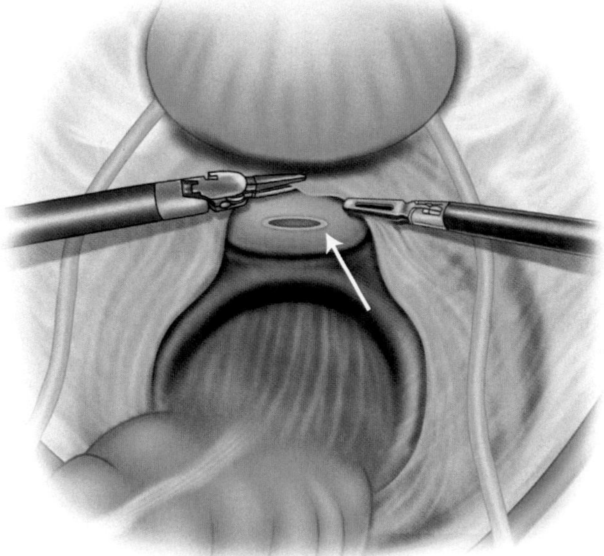

Fig. 18.10 Vaginal cuff dehiscence, white arrow

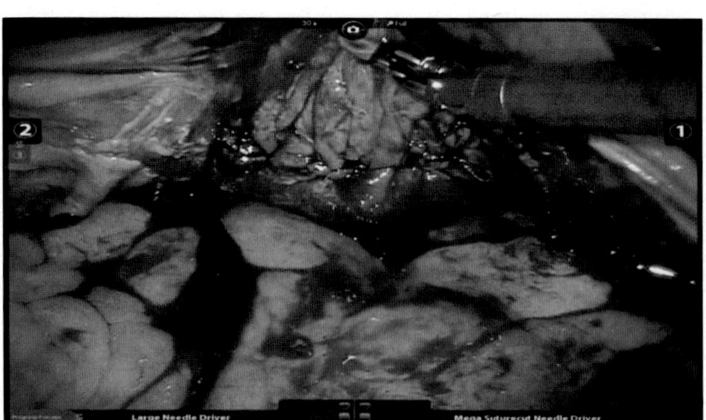

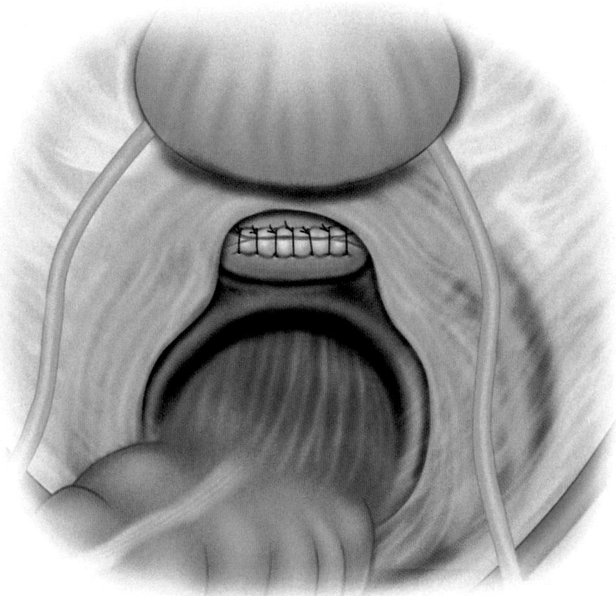

Fig. 18.11 Vaginal cuff closure

RASC without Hysterectomy Steps

Vaginal dissection is similar in cases of posthysterectomy vaginal vault prolapse, concomitant total hysterectomy, or concomitant supracervical hysterectomy with the exceptions noted above. Monopolar Endo Shears are placed in the first arm and bipolar Maryland graspers placed in the second arm. The surgeon has a few choices to retract the sigmoid colon. The robotic third arm may be used on the left side with an instrument such as the ProGrasp. Alternatively an endoscopic tissue grasper may be placed on the left side and locked on sigmoid epiploica for retraction. Lastly, the bedside assistant can retract the colon from the right-sided accessory trocar, and the left-sided accessory trocar can then be entirely deleted. In general, since peritoneal and bladder dissection are easily facilitated by the assistant from the right-sided accessory trocar, routine use of a left-sided accessory trocar is questionable. Routine assessment of the risks and benefits of all trocars is advised.

Vaginal Dissection

The peritoneum is incised starting at the vaginal apex. Anterior and posterior planes are created with blunt and/or sharp dissection for a length of approximately 4–6 cm. Use of electrocautery should be minimized. Careful measurements of the vagina, including the total vaginal length and location of the urethrovesical junction, must be taken at the outset of the procedure in order to determine the extent of the dissection. The length of the anterior dissection should not exceed the total vaginal length minus the urethral length. In order to limit mesh contact with the anterior rectum, the surgeon may choose to limit posterior dissection to the extent of the posterior cul-de-sac. A ruler may be used to determine exposed vaginal length if needed. Alternatively, the monopolar Endo Shears may be used as a reference. The distance between the tips of the monopolar Endo Shears and the end of the gray line is 5.4 cm. Using Pythagorean theorem, the distance from the apex to the distal margin of the dissection is just over 4 cm in the midline given the 30-degree orientation of the instrument when the tips are placed at the distal margin of the dissection (Fig. 18.12).

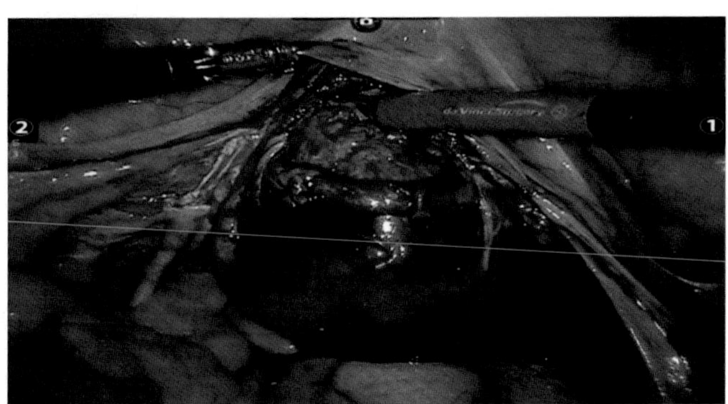

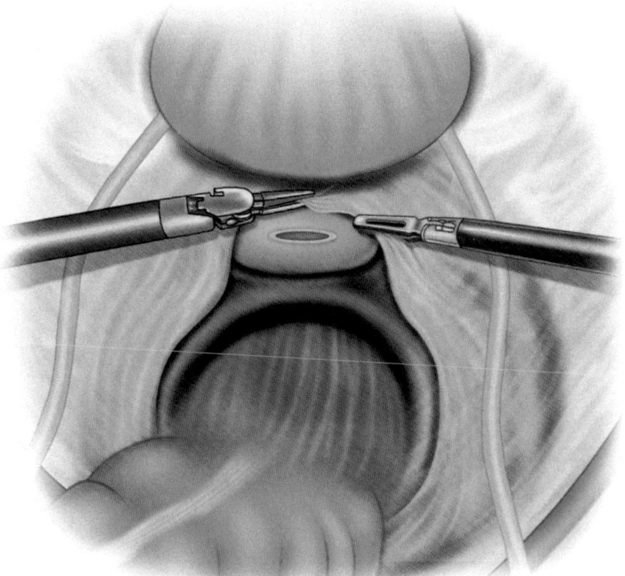

Fig. 18.12 Estimation of anterior dissection length

Sacral Promontory Dissection

Access to the presacral space is bounded on the left by the sigmoid colon and the right by the right ureter. Care must also be taken to avoid the common iliac vessels. The peritoneal incision is begun at the level of the sacral promontory and is carried all the way down to the posterior aspect of the cervix and/or vagina using Endo Shears (Fig. 18.13). Some authors advocate the use of two separate peritoneal incisions, one near the posterior cervix or vagina and the other near the sacral promontory, in order to avoid the extra time involved in peritoneal closure. In this situation, the mesh is tunneled beneath the intact peritoneum from the posterior cervix and/or vagina up to the presacral space.

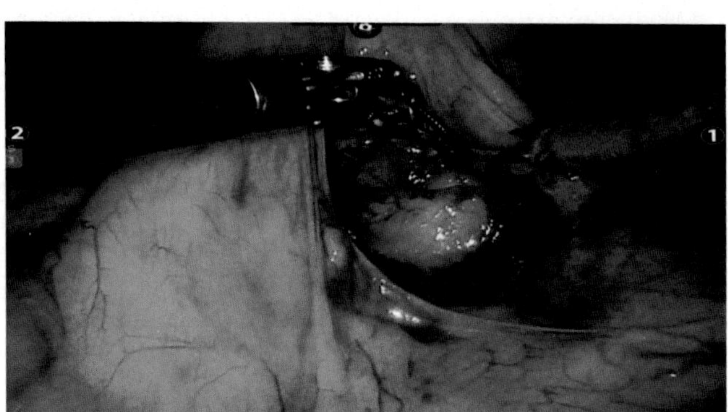

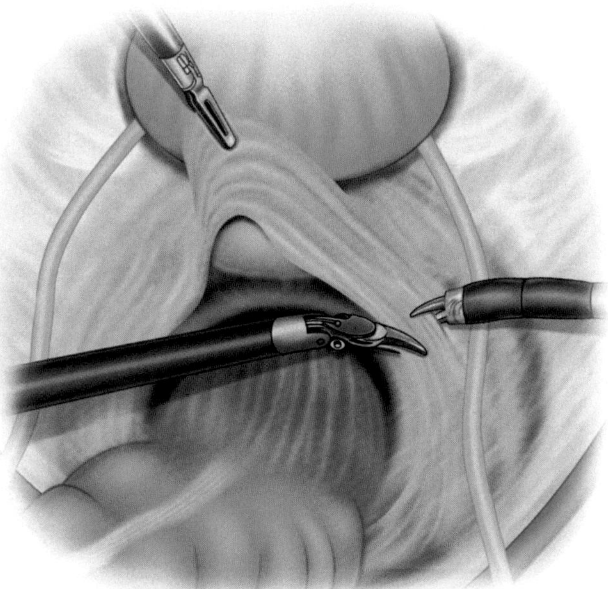

Fig. 18.13 Peritoneal dissection from the promontory

The anterior longitudinal ligament is then identified and carefully exposed. Avoidance of sacral vessels is critical during the suturing phase of the procedure. Vessels may be cauterized with bipolar energy when avascular portions of the ALL cannot be readily identified. Bleeding in this area can be life-threatening. Several methods to achieve hemostasis in this area include application of direct pressure, increased insufflation pressure, application of hemostatic agents, oversewing with suture, and application of thumbtacks. Conversion to laparotomy must be considered if hemostasis cannot be achieved endoscopically. It is strongly advised to endoscopically pack the presacral space and arrange for blood products immediately prior to undocking the robot and laparotomy.

Vaginal Mesh Attachment

Mesh type and configuration depend on surgeon preference and the pelvic floor defects to be repaired. In general the mesh should be lightweight and porous. Eleven out of 13 studies reported use of a macroporous monofilament polypropylene mesh in a recent systematic review and meta-analysis [11]. Mesh may be configured into a single rectangular piece or a "Y" shape. Some surgeons prefer to use Gore-Tex suture to attach the mesh to the vaginal walls and ALL; recent studies, however, have shown similar outcomes with the use of absorbable sutures [12, 13]. Partial thickness sutures are placed in the anterior and posterior vaginal walls and cervical stump, when present (Figs. 18.14 and 18.15).

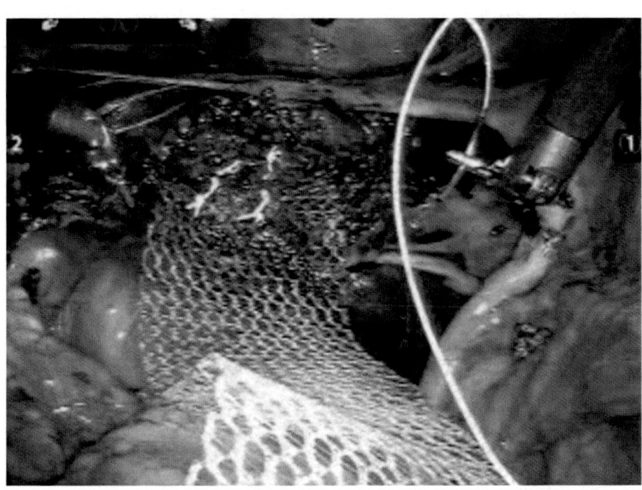

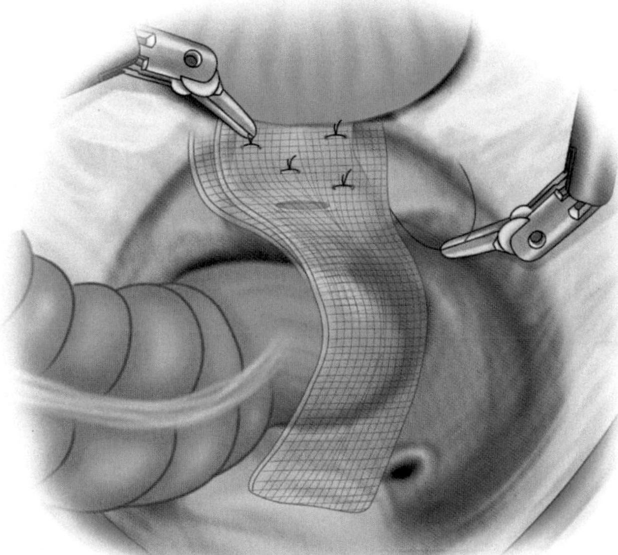

Fig. 18.14 Mesh attachment to the anterior vagina

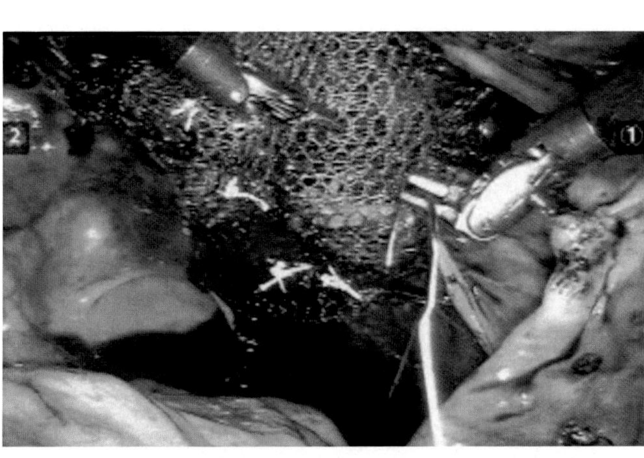

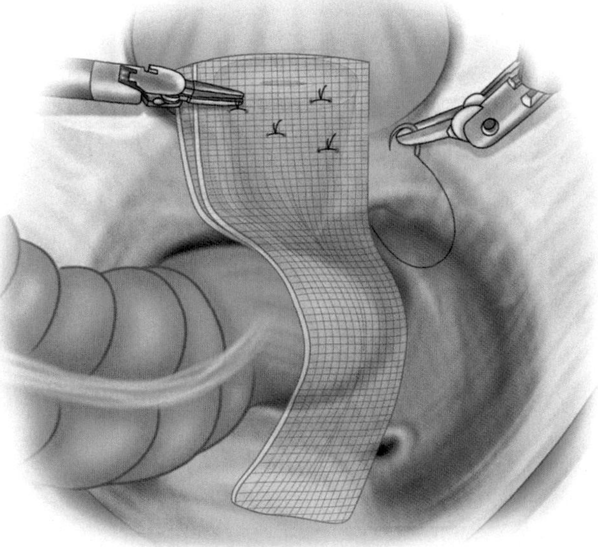

Fig. 18.15 Mesh attachment to the posterior vagina

Sacral Mesh Attachment

The mesh is either tunneled under the peritoneum or placed within the peritoneal incision prior to attachment to the ALL. Tensioning of the mesh is performed using a vaginal retractor held by the assistant. Maximal cephalad orientation of the vaginal apex is first demonstrated, followed by allowing the retractor to occupy the vagina without tension (Fig. 18.16). The mesh is then attached to the ALL using 2–3 interrupted Gore-Tex sutures (Fig. 18.17). Care must be taken to ensure the needle and suture pass through the ALL, and not deeper. The needle is ideally held parallel to the plane of the anterior sacrum as soon as the ligament is penetrated in order to avoid deeper structures such as bone or disc. Visualization is important given the lack of tactile cues. Anatomic studies reveal that the disc is most often located at the maximal anterior deflection of the promontory [13]. Case reports have indicated that sutures placed into the disc can lead to discitis and additional surgery [14]. The redundant mesh at the level of the promontory is removed in an elliptical fashion (Fig. 18.18). Care is taken to trim any corners that may oppose the great vessels, sigmoid colon, and/or the right ureter. A soft vaginal retractor is best removed at this stage while visualizing the mesh in case vaginal wall sutures were placed transmurally into the retractor.

Peritoneal Closure

The peritoneum is closed with absorbable suture in one or two lengths, taking care to extraperitonealize the mesh (Fig. 18.19).

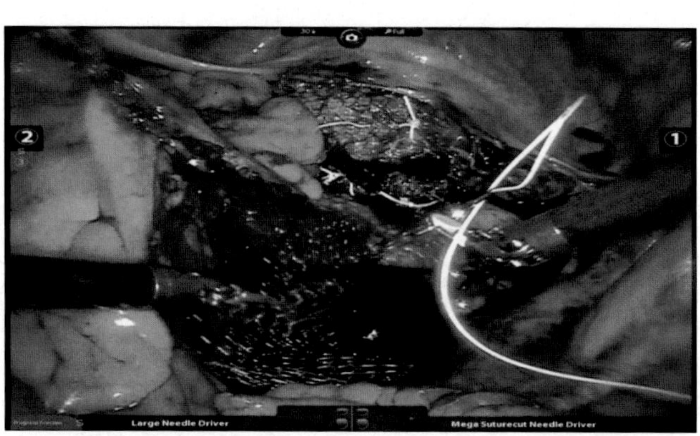

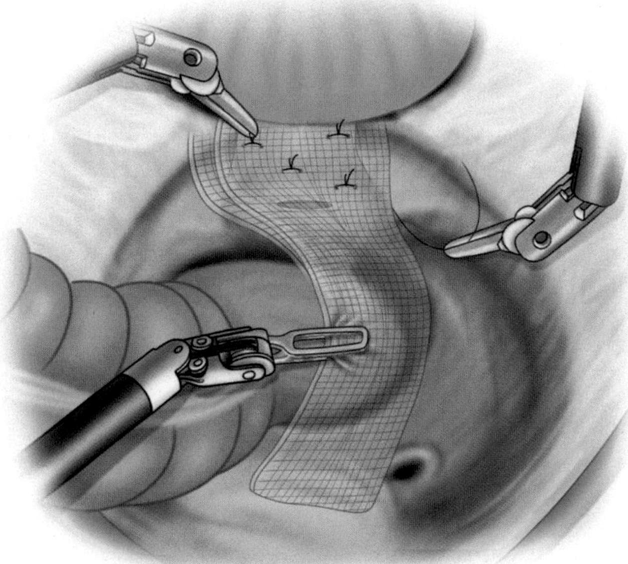

Fig. 18.16 Assessment of mesh tension

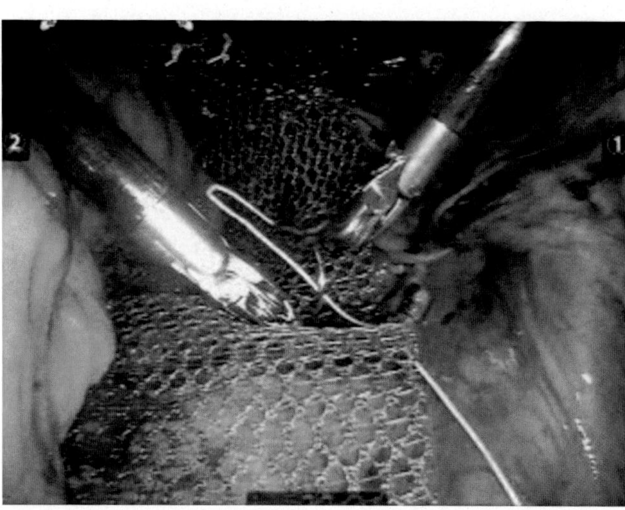

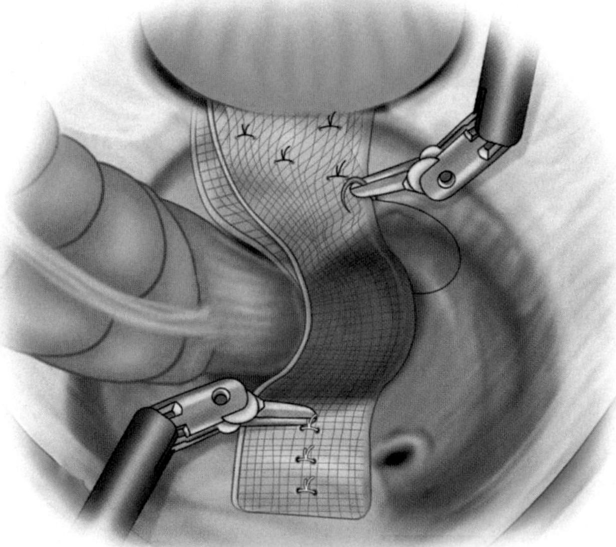

Fig. 18.17 Mesh attachment to the anterior longitudinal ligament

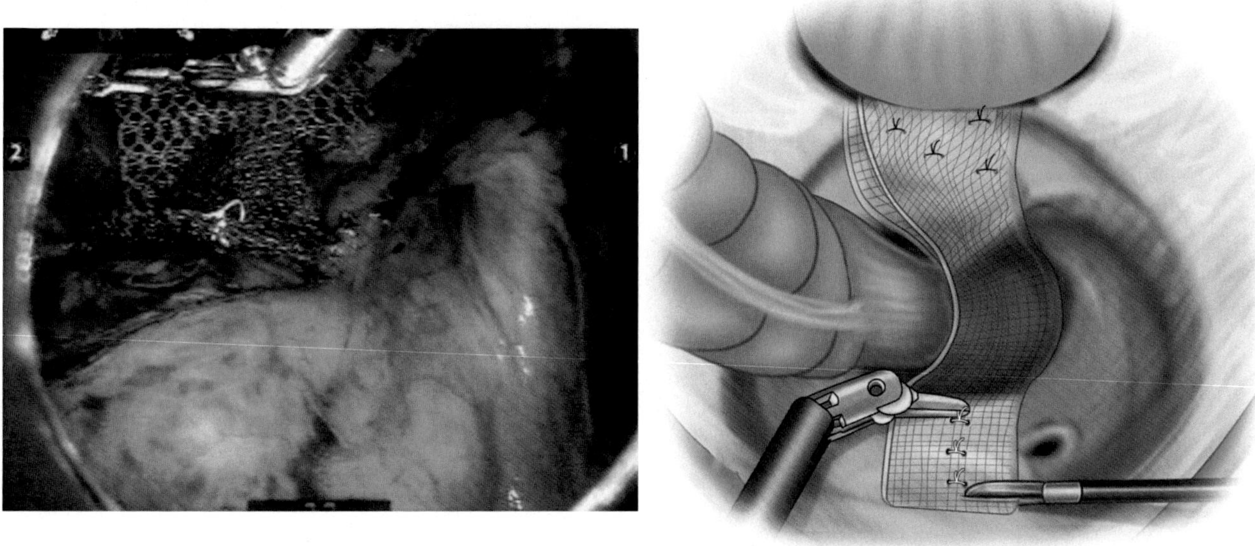

Fig. 18.18 Trimming excess mesh at the promontory

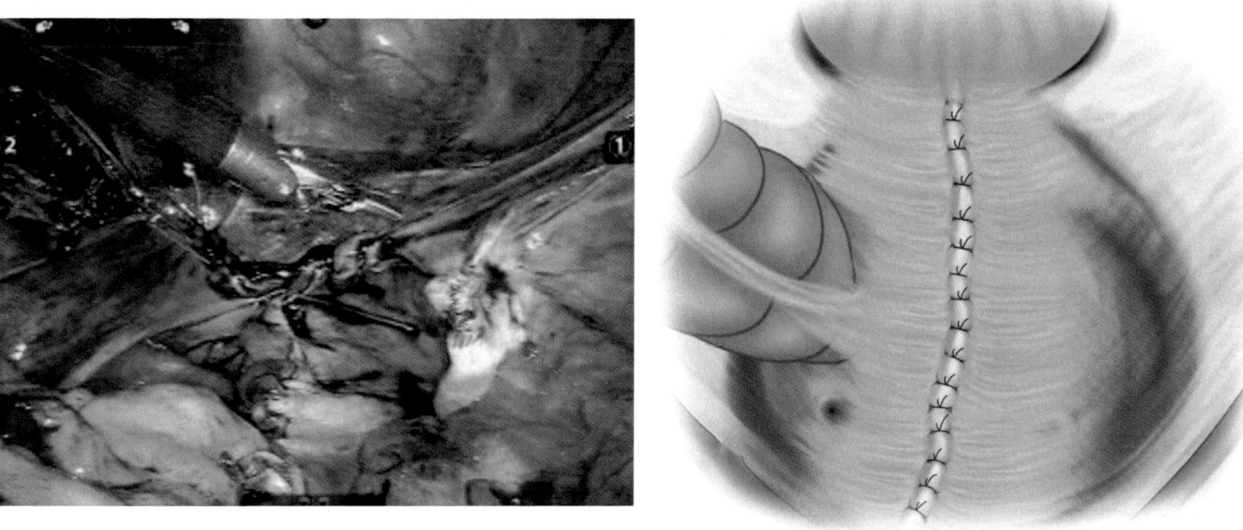

Fig. 18.19 Closure of the peritoneum over the mesh

Postoperative Care

Postoperatively, patients are extubated in the operating room and should be observed in a monitored setting. Once ambulatory, a voiding trial is typically instituted due to the high likelihood of concomitant repairs and/or anti-incontinence surgery. Patients are usually discharged once pain control is adequate and there are no signs of complications. This is typically on postoperative day 1 with a follow-up visit in 2 weeks.

References

1. Lane FE. Repair of posthysterectomy vaginal-vault prolapse. Obstet Gynecol. 1962;20:72–7.
2. Maher C, Baessler K, Glazener CM, Adams EJ, Hagen S. Surgical management of pelvic organ prolapse in women: a short version cochrane review. Neurourol Urodyn. 2008;27(1):3–12.
3. Campbell P, Cloney L, Jha S. Abdominal versus laparoscopic sacrocolpopexy: a systematic review and meta-analysis. Obstet Gynecol Surv. 2016;71(7):435–42.
4. Callewaert G, Bosteels J, Housmans S, Verguts J, Van Cleynenbreugel B, Van der Aa F, et al. Laparoscopic versus robotic-assisted sacrocolpopexy for pelvic organ prolapse: a systematic review. Gynecol Surg. 2016;13:115–23.
5. De Gouveia DSM, Claydon LS, Whitlow B, Dolcet Artahona MA. Robotic versus laparoscopic sacrocolpopexy for treatment of prolapse of the apical segment of the vagina: a systematic review and meta-analysis. Int Urogynecol J. 2016;27(3):355–66.
6. Tan JS, Lukacz ES, Menefee SA, Luber KM, Albo ME, Nager CW. Determinants of vaginal length. Am J Obstet Gynecol. 2006;195:1846–50.
7. Minaglia SM, Santiago TD, Lee JM, Kagihara J, Ruel M, Oyama I. Combined spinal and general anesthesia reduces intra- and postoperative opioid requirements in patients undergoing robotic-assisted laparoscopic sacrocolpopexy. Female Pelvic Med Reconstr Surg. 2012;18(5S):S179–80.
8. Minaglia SM, Santiago TD, Lee JM, et al. Changes in robotic-assisted laparoscopic sacrocolpopexy operative time: an analysis of technical factors. Female Pelvic Med Reconstr Surg. 2012;18(5S):S183.
9. Minaglia SM. Vaginal trachelectomy following laparoscopic supracervical hysterectomy and sacrocervicopexy. Female Pelvic Med Reconstr Surg. 2014;20(2):116–8.
10. Moulder JK, Cohen SL, Morse AN, Einarsson JI. Mesh extrusion through the internal cervical os: an unusual complication following laparoscopic sacrocervicopexy. Female Pelvic Med Reconstr Surg. 2013;19:309–11.
11. Hudson CO, Northington GM, Lyles RH, Karp DR. Outcomes of robotic sacrocolpopexy: a systematic review and meta-analysis. Female Pelvic Med Reconstr Surg. 2014;20:252–60.
12. Linder BJ, Anand M, Klingele CJ, Trabuco EC, Gebhart JB, Occhino JA. Outcomes of robotic sacrocolpopexy using only absorbable suture for mesh fixation. Female Pelvic Med Reconstr Surg. 2017;23:13–6.
13. Shepherd JP, Higdon HL 3rd, Stanford EJ, Mattox TF. Effect of suture selection on the rate of suture or mesh erosion and surgery failure in abdominal sacrocolpopexy. Female Pelvic Med Reconstr Surg. 2012;16:229–33.
14. Propst K, Tunitsky-Bitton E, Schimpf MO, Ridgeway B. Pyogenic spondylodiscitis associated with sacral colpopexy and rectopexy: report of two cases and evaluation of the literature. Int Urogynecol J. 2014;25:21–31.

Part IV

Gastrointestinal Procedures

Total Gastrectomy

19

Luke V. Selby and Vivian E. Strong

Introduction

Total gastrectomy is utilized with curative intent for gastric adenocarcinoma occurring in the proximal stomach, at the gastroesophageal junction, or for tumors, regardless of location, with diffuse histology. It is also the surgical technique for patients undergoing prophylactic gastrectomy with a diagnosis of hereditary diffuse gastric cancer [1]. Since the publication of the MacDonald trial [2] and the MAGIC trial [3], advanced gastric cancer has been treated in a multidisciplinary fashion, with patients undergoing either neoadjuvant or adjuvant chemotherapy. Unfortunately, studies have routinely shown that not all patients eligible for postoperative chemotherapy receive this therapy, often because of a prolonged recovery from their operation.

The first use of minimally invasive techniques for gastrectomy was reported in 1994 [4]; since then, minimally invasive techniques for gastrectomy have been widely adopted. Several randomized controlled trials have compared laparoscopic gastrectomy and open gastrectomy with encouraging results [5–10]. These trials have individually established oncologic equivalency between laparoscopic and open gastrectomies and found lower complication rates in the laparoscopic resections. A recent meta-analysis of these trials and several other high-quality retrospective series comparing laparoscopic and open distal gastrectomy found that the laparoscopic approach was associated with a shorter postoperative hospital stay and fewer postoperative complications [11]. Retrospective single-institution series have shown that patients who underwent laparoscopic gastrectomy were more likely to receive indicated adjuvant therapy than well-matched controls who underwent open gastrectomy [12], although longer-term follow-up is not yet available.

Robotic surgery for gastric cancer was first described in 2003 [13, 14] and first reported in the United States in 2007 [15]. A recent meta-analysis comparing robotic gastrectomy to both laparoscopic and open gastrectomy found that robotic surgery was associated with a shorter length of stay than open gastrectomy and lower intraoperative blood loss than laparoscopic surgery, but a longer operative time than either approach; morbidity and lymph node retrieval did not differ between the groups [16].

Clinical trials comparing robotic gastrectomy with open gastrectomy are currently ongoing, but none have published interim results, so it is not possible to make a direct comparison between robotic approaches and either open or laparoscopic gastrectomy. However, there are several advantages to the robotic approach when compared with laparoscopy. Both of these minimally invasive surgery (MIS) techniques are associated with decreased hospital length of stay and earlier return to activity, but robotic approaches have several benefits over laparoscopic surgery, all related to the robotic platform. Articulating hands provide improved dexterity and finer control than is available with laparoscopic instruments; visualization is much improved, owing to the three-dimensional camera available on robotic systems; imaging integration with the intraoperative view is much stronger; and surgeon comfort is far greater with the robotic platform.

Patient Selection

Patient selection, especially at the beginning of a surgeon's experience, is vitally important. Because robotic resections have a longer operative time than either laparoscopic or open resections [12], the surgeon should initially operate on patients without significant medical comorbidities, with small tumors, and with normal BMI and intestinal histology. Patients undergoing prophylactic total gastrectomy to

L. V. Selby, MD, MS
Department of Surgery, University of Colorado Health Sciences Center, Aurora, CO, USA
e-mail: luke.selby@ucdenver.edu

V. E. Strong, MD (✉)
Department of Surgery, Memorial Sloan Kettering Cancer Center, New York,, NY, USA

Y. Fong et al. (eds.), *The SAGES Atlas of Robotic Surgery*, https://doi.org/10.1007/978-3-319-91045-1_19

prevent hereditary diffuse gastric cancer associated with a mutation in *CHD1* are ideal candidates for a robotic approach. These patients, who have an approximately 80% lifetime risk of developing gastric adenocarcinoma [17], nearly always have foci of high-grade dysplasia or intramucosal carcinoma within the stomach, and as such do not require more than a D1 lymphadenectomy. The critical element of a prophylactic total gastrectomy is ensuring, via frozen section, that the proximal and distal margins are free of gastric mucosa.

As a surgeon's individual and institutional experience with robotic total gastrectomy increases, it is reasonable to expand indications for a robotic total gastrectomy to include patients with worse medical comorbidities, more advanced disease, and a higher BMI [18]. As with all potentially morbid surgical procedures, it is important to prospectively record patient characteristics and individual patient outcomes. Gastric cancer is rare in Western centers, so total gastrectomy, regardless of surgical approach, is a relatively infrequent procedure. Consistent prospective data collection will allow multiple institutions to pool their clinical outcomes and allow for analysis of procedure-specific and overall outcomes.

Relative contraindications to robotic gastrectomy may include patients with significant intraabdominal adhesions, diffuse histology, large tumor size or invasion into adjacent organs, and lack of institutional support. Just as with laparoscopic surgery, intraabdominal adhesions can prevent safe visualization of important structures and therefore the technical performance of the operation. In patients with diffuse histology, the proximal and distal extents of the tumor cannot be predicted preoperatively. For these tumors, haptic feedback is essential, as palpation is often important in determining the proximal and distal extent of tumor and the appropriate resection margin. Though the proximal and distal margins should be sent for frozen section to confirm normal esophageal and duodenal mucosa, the inability to confirm via palpation that the area of resection is grossly normal makes robotic resection of diffuse histology more difficult.

Institutional experience with, and support for, robotic operations is essential for the safe performance of robotic surgery at any anatomic location. Robotic surgery requires coordinated teamwork within the operating room, with all team members having familiarity not only with the procedure being performed but also with robotic surgery.

Robotic Setup and Patient Positioning

We have previously described patient positioning for laparoscopic gastrectomy [19]; positioning for robotic gastrectomy is similar (Fig. 19.1). The patient's arms can either be tucked or positioned on arm boards, with appropriate attention paid to padding the elbows, hands, and other pressure points. The patient is well secured to the table at the shoulders, hips, and knees. Robotic total gastrectomy requires the patient to be placed in steep reverse Trendelenburg position of at least 45°, so foot boards are commonly used to additionally secure the patient. Final patient positioning must be achieved prior to docking the robot, as any change in position cannot occur with the robotic arms in place.

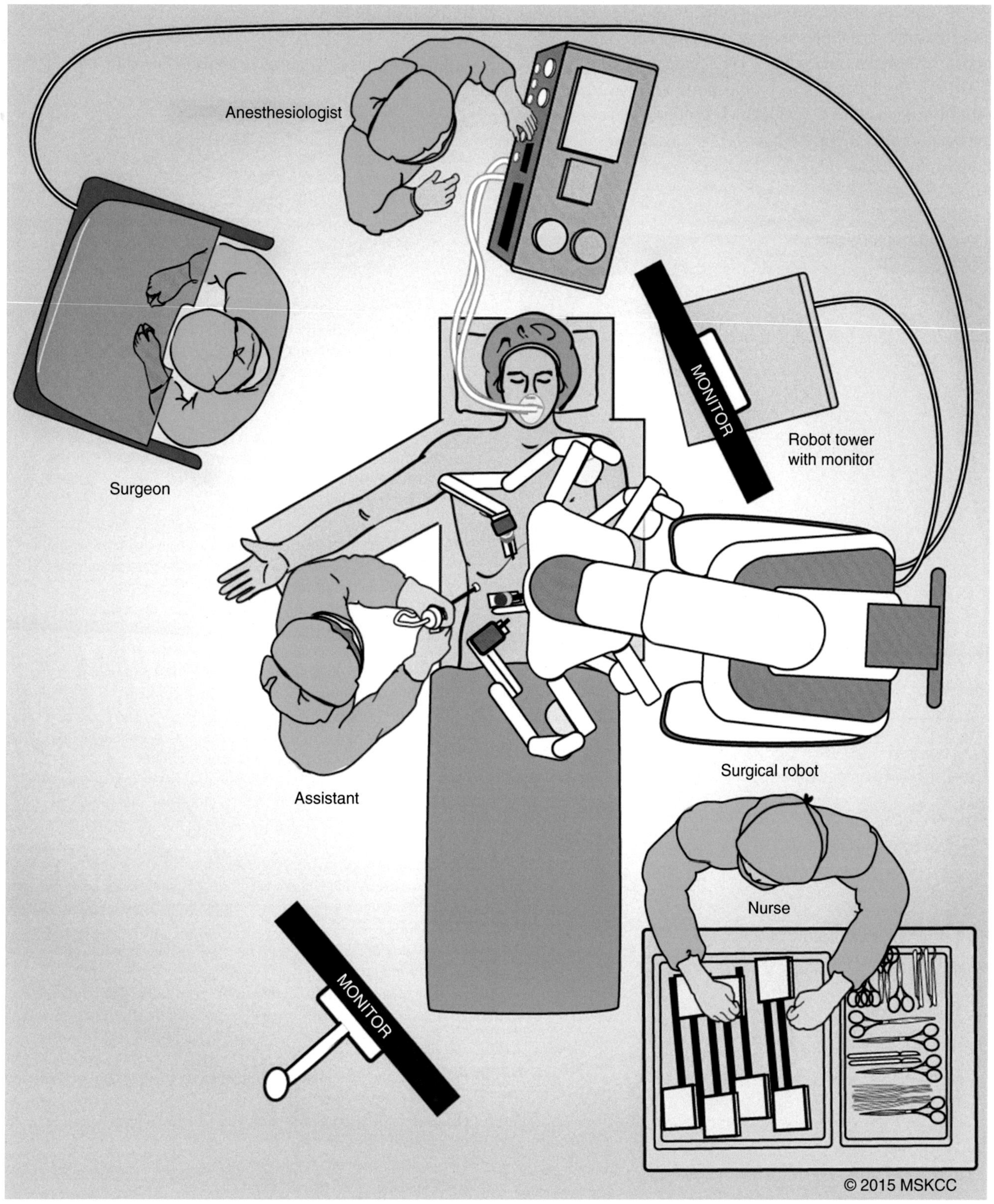

Fig. 19.1 Position for a patient undergoing robotic total gastrectomy. Of note, the operation is generally performed in steep reverse Trendelenburg position, and the patient must be positioned prior to docking the robot (©2016, Memorial Sloan Kettering Cancer Center; *reprinted with permission*)

Port placement for robotic gastrectomy (Fig. 19.2) follows the same principles as port placement for any laparoscopic or robotic procedure. The camera port is placed 15–20 cm from the stomach, and ports are placed at least 8 cm from each other. As with any procedure, there are variations in port placement; we have found great success with the setup in Fig. 19.2.

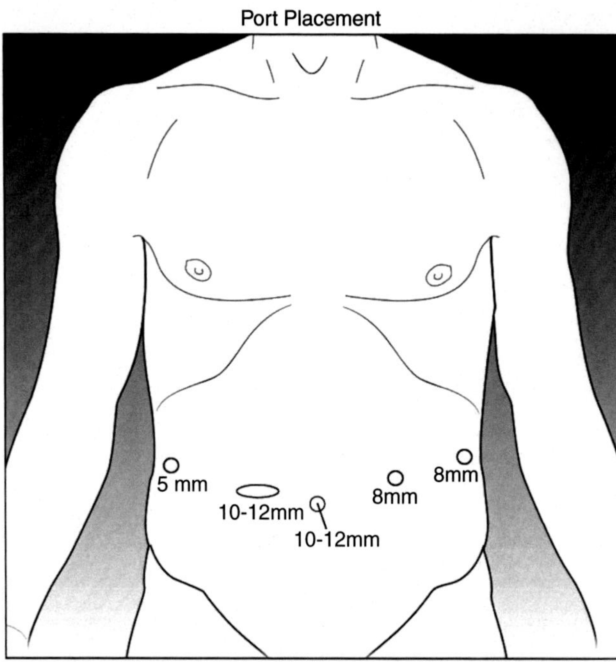

Fig. 19.2 Port placement for robotic total gastrectomy (©2016, Memorial Sloan Kettering Cancer Center; *reprinted with permission*)

Procedural Details

A summary of the key operative steps is found in Table 19.1.

Table 19.1 Key operative steps

1.	Explore the abdomen for intraabdominal adhesions that prevent the technical performance of robotic surgery or previously unidentified peritoneal tumor spread
2.	Identify the location of the tumor on the extraluminal surface or with the assistance of intraoperative endoscopy
3.	Position the patient and dock the robot
4.	Dissect the omentum from the transverse colon toward the splenic flexure to enter the lesser sac
5.	After grasping the posterior wall of the stomach, retract the stomach anteriorly and to the right to allow identification and ligation of the short gastric vessels
6.	Incise the peritoneum over the left crux and expose the posterolateral esophagus
7.	Retract the stomach to the left upper quadrant, and complete the omentectomy by carrying it toward the hepatic flexure. When the omentum is fully freed from the transverse colon, place it in the left upper quadrant
8.	Divide the attachments between the stomach and the pancreas
9.	Identify the right gastroepiploic vessels at the superior border of the pancreas near their origin from the gastroduodenal vessels, and divide them with a linear stapler
10.	Incise the gastrohepatic attachments near the pylorus to identify and ligate the right gastric artery
11.	While creating a window at the level of the pylorus, dissect the lymphatic tissues along the proper and common hepatic arteries so that they remain with the specimen
12.	Mobilize the posterior aspect of the pylorus and proximal duodenum, and divide the duodenum with a linear stapler with bioabsorbable staple line reinforcement
13.	Continue the dissection of lymphatic tissues toward the celiac axis and proximal splenic artery, and ligate the left gastric vein and artery, ensuring that all lymphatic tissue remains with the specimen
14.	Ensure that all gastrohepatic attachments at the esophageal hiatus are divided, and level 1 and 3 lymph nodes up to the right crux and esophagus remain with the specimen
15.	Complete the mobilization of the distal esophagus, and divide it with a linear stapler with bioabsorbable staple line reinforcement
16.	Transfer the robotic camera to the port in the right midaxillary line, remove the specimen in a specimen bag introduced via the umbilical port, and send margins of interest for frozen section analysis
17.	Divide the jejunum 30–40 cm distal to the ligament of Treitz with a linear stapler
18.	Create the jejunojejunostomy 60–70 cm downstream of the divided jejunum
19.	Create the esophagojejunostomy
20.	Close mesenteric defects and Petersen's space
21.	Ensure that all specimens are removed from the peritoneal cavity and hemostasis is complete

Conversion to Open

There should be a low threshold for conversion from a robotic approach to an open approach based on the clinical experience and judgment of the operation surgeon. During the preoperative timeout, the entire operative team discusses the protocol for converting the operative approach and should clarify roles during the conversion.

Procedural Setup

Pneumoperitoneum is established either near the umbilicus (where a 10–12-mm port will be placed), at another trocar site, or with a Veress needle in the left upper quadrant. If pneumoperitoneum is not established through the umbilicus, a 10–12-mm trocar is then placed either directly above or below the umbilicus (depending on the patient's habitus). Generally, the infraumbilical position is caudal enough for the omentectomy and construction of the jejunojejunal anastomosis and close enough to the esophageal hiatus for construction of the esophagojejunostomy. Following placement of the midline port, two 8-mm ports are placed in the left midclavicular line and left anterior axillary lines. On the right side of the abdomen, a 10–12-mm port is placed in the midclavicular line, and a 5-mm port is placed in the anterior axillary line (Fig. 19.2). A liver retractor is also frequently placed in the left upper quadrant via a small subxiphoid stab incision. This retractor facilitates significant retraction of the left lateral lobe of the liver and exposure of the esophageal hiatus.

Following satisfactory port setup, the abdomen is explored for adhesions, evidence of previously unrecognized peritoneal disease, and extraluminal identification of the tumor. If the tumor is not appreciable, especially in the case of tumors at the gastroesophageal junction, endoscopy should be utilized to confirm its location. The surgeon must ensure that a resection margin of 2–4 cm can be obtained with the transabdominal approach. Once these details are confirmed and the decision to proceed with robotic resection is made, the patient is placed in steep reverse Trendelenburg of approximately 45°, and the robot is docked. Arms 1 and 3 are placed in the left-sided ports, and arm 2 is placed in the 12-mm right-sided port. Initially a fenestrated bipolar grasper is placed in arm 2, arm 1 receives monopolar scissors or an energy sealant device, and grasping forceps are placed in arm 3.

Omentectomy

The first step of the procedure is the omentectomy, which is accomplished by retracting the greater omentum cephalad, identifying the transverse colon, and dividing the colon from the omentum by entering the avascular plane between the two and proceeding toward the splenic flexure. Once visualization of the posterior wall of the stomach confirms entrance to the lesser sac, the posterior wall is retracted by the bedside assistant anteriorly and to the right (Fig. 19.3). As omentectomy proceeds toward the splenic flexure, the short gastric vessels are identified and ligated under direct vision by the energy sealant device in arm 1. The left crux of the diaphragm is now identified, the peritoneum overlying it is incised, and the crural muscle fibers are identified. Gentle blunt dissection along the crus exposes the posterolateral esophagus. The posterior wall of the stomach is grasped and retracted toward the patient's left shoulder, and the omentectomy is completed by proceeding toward the hepatic flexure; when it is removed from its colonic attachments, it can be placed in the left upper quadrant for later removal.

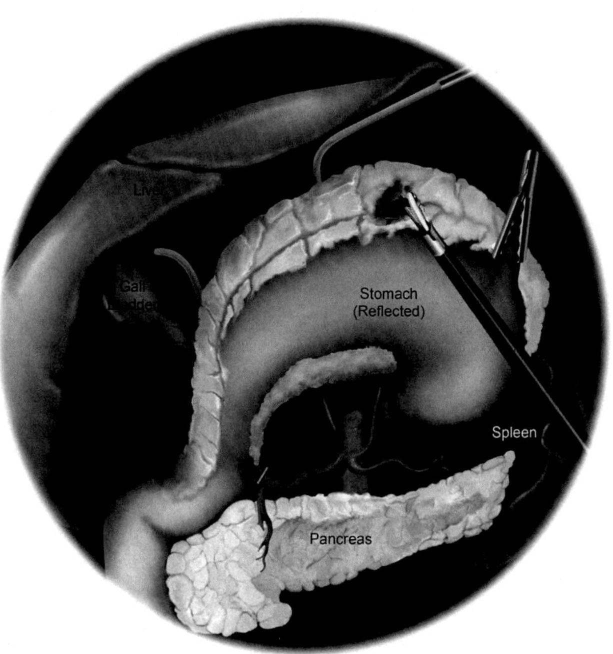

Fig. 19.3 Entering the lesser sac and visualizing the posterior wall of the stomach allow the omentectomy to proceed safely to the splenic flexure (©2016, Memorial Sloan Kettering Cancer Center; *reprinted with permission*)

Dissection of the Greater Curvature

Following omentectomy, attention is turned to dividing the stomach from its posterior attachments to the pancreas, using either the energy sealant device or sharp dissection. The right gastroepiploic vessels are identified at the superior border of the pancreas and dissected circumferentially at their origin from the gastroduodenal vessels. To divide them with a linear stapler, remove arm 2 of the robot from the 12-mm port in the right midclavicular line to allow the bedside assistant to use the stapler.

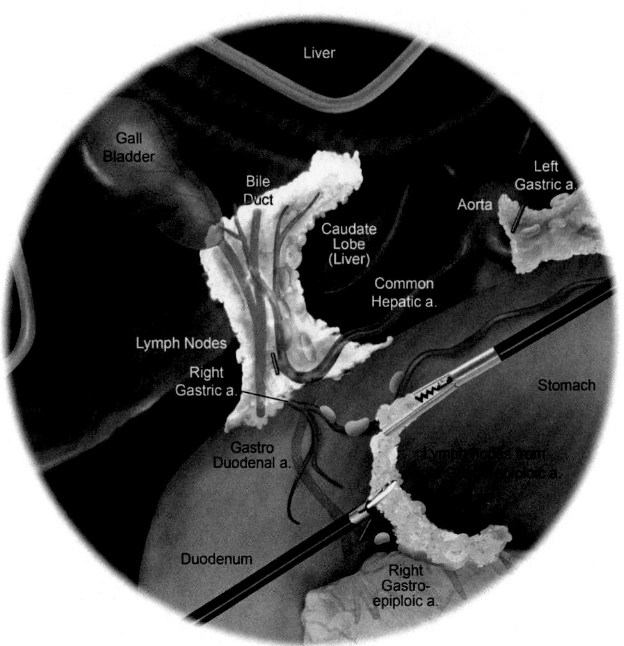

Fig. 19.4 View of the proximal duodenum during dissection of the lymph nodes from the right gastroepiploic artery (©2016, Memorial Sloan Kettering Cancer Center; *reprinted with permission*)

Division of the Proximal Duodenum

The gastrohepatic attachments are now divided using the energy sealant device in arm 1. The right gastric artery is ligated at its base, lymphatic tissues along the proper and common hepatic arteries are swept medially toward the stomach, and a window is created at the level of the pylorus (Fig. 19.4). Using a combination of blunt dissection and electrocautery, the posterior aspect of the pylorus and the proximal duodenum are gently elevated off of the retroperitoneum. A linear stapler with a bowel load and bioabsorbable reinforcement is introduced through the right-sided 12-mm port, and the proximal duodenum is divided just beyond the pylorus.

Lymphadenectomy

The stomach is now reflected into the left upper quadrant to allow for the D2 lymphadenectomy. This dissection was previously started along the proper hepatic artery and is now continued along the common hepatic artery toward the celiac axis and the proximal splenic artery. During this dissection, the left gastric artery and vein are identified at the celiac axis. Their surrounding lymphatic tissue is carefully swept up toward the specimen, and then the vessels are divided at their origin with surgical clips or a linear stapler.

Division of the Distal Esophagus

The gastrohepatic omentum is now further incised up to the level of the esophageal hiatus with the energy sealant device. Level 1 and 3 lymph nodes are dissected with the proximal stomach up to the right crux of the diaphragm. The peritoneal fat and any fat overlying the esophagus are opened, and the distal esophagus is circumferentially dissected. Finally, the distal esophagus is divided with a linear stapler.

Specimen Retrieval

Following division of the esophagus, the robotic camera is positioned in the right-sided 12-mm port, and a specimen bag is introduced into the peritoneum via the umbilical port. The umbilical incision is generally enlarged to remove the specimen in its bag. The proximal margin is marked with a stitch and routinely sent for frozen section margin analysis. We do not routinely send the distal margin for analysis unless the operation is a prophylactic total gastrectomy for hereditary diffuse gastric cancer, in which case frozen section must reveal normal esophageal mucosa at the proximal margin and normal duodenal mucosa at the distal margin. In distal gastrectomies with tumor located near the pylorus, the surgeon may choose to send frozen section analysis of the distal margin. While pathologists are examining the margins, the Roux-en-Y jejunojejunostomy is created.

Roux-En-Y Reconstruction

Unlike distal gastrectomies, all total gastrectomies are reconstructed with a Roux-en-Y esophagogastrectomy. The colon is elevated cephalad to identify the ligament of Treitz. A mobile piece of jejunum 30–40 cm downstream of the ligament of Treitz is identified, making sure it will reach to the esophageal hiatus and the divided end of the distal esophagus. The identified jejunum is then divided with a linear stapler. Using the linear stapler, the jejunojejunostomy is created another 60–70 cm downstream, and the common enterotomy of the end-to-side anastomosis is closed with running 2-0 silk.

The Roux limb is now prepared for the esophagojejunostomy. Though the esophagojejunostomy can be created with either linear or circular staples, we prefer the use of a transoral anvil (Orvil™, Covidien, New Haven, CT) (Fig. 19.5) [20]. This device has an anvil attached to a nasogastric tube and is introduced transorally by the anesthesiologist and passed distally until the tip of the nasogastric tube reaches the stapled end of the esophagus. A small esophagotomy is made with electrocautery to allow the tube to be pulled into the peritoneal cavity. The tubing is pulled out of the abdomen through the 12-mm port, pulling the anvil down the esophagus. The staple line of the Roux limb is removed with the energy sealant device, the other end of the circular stapler is placed into the proximal end of the Roux limb, and it is fired. Two intact donuts and visual inspection confirm a successful anastomosis, and the open end of the Roux limb is closed with a linear stapler. The donuts are sent to pathology for examination, as they represent the true final esophageal margin. Mesenteric defects from the jejunojejunostomy and Petersen's space are sutured closed with running 3-0 Vicryl suture [21]. Following this, the robot is undocked, the patient flattened out, the port sites are closed, and the procedure is completed.

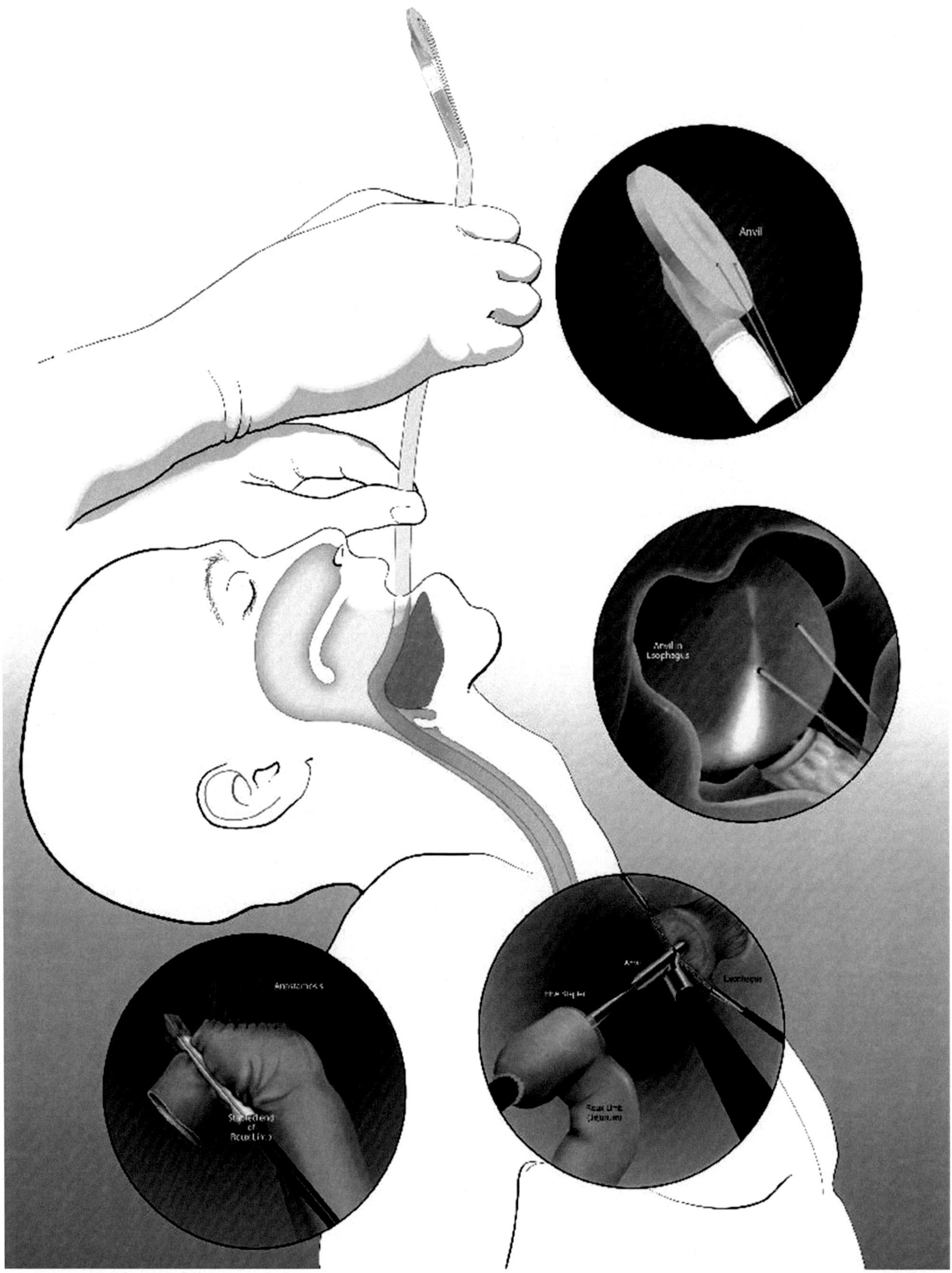

Fig. 19.5 Use of a transoral anvil for construction of the esophagojejunostomy during total gastrectomy (©2016, Memorial Sloan Kettering Cancer Center; *reprinted with permission*)

Postoperative Care and Complications

Postoperatively, neither nasojejunal drainage nor artificial nutrition is necessary [22, 23]. Patients with a normal clinical exam and normal vital signs are started on sips of clear liquids on their first postoperative day and advanced daily. In the postoperative patient with normal vital signs and a normal abdominal exam, early initiation of oral feeding is advantageous [23–25], and by the fourth postoperative day, patients may be consuming a postgastrectomy diet (multiple small meals daily). All patients lose weight postoperatively, but weight loss is rarely dangerous and seldom requires invasive intervention [22].

A leak of the esophagojejunal anastomosis is the most common major complication following total gastrectomy. Most leaks are diagnosed prior to discharge, and almost all are diagnosed within 3 weeks of operation [26]. Routine radiologic evaluation of the esophagojejunal anastomosis is not indicated, but changes in vital signs, tachycardia, or another clinical suspicion of an esophagojejunal leak warrants either a contrast-enhanced CT scan of the abdomen and pelvis or an esophagogram with water-soluble contrast.

Postoperative Outcomes

Several recent retrospective series have compared MIS total gastrectomy versus open gastrectomy [27–29]. Consistently, laparoscopic total gastrectomy, when compared with open total gastrectomy, is associated with decreased blood loss, less postoperative pain, faster return of bowel function, shorter hospital stay, lower postoperative morbidity, and longer operative times. No long-term follow-up data have been published comparing laparoscopic approaches with open approaches. One recent meta-analysis comparing robotic gastrectomy with laparoscopic and open gastrectomy found that robotic surgery was associated with a shorter length of stay than open gastrectomy and lower intraoperative blood loss than laparoscopic surgery but longer operative time than either of the other approaches; morbidity and lymph node retrieval did not differ between the groups [16].

Summary

Minimally invasive gastrectomy (either laparoscopic or robotic) is associated with improved short-term outcomes when compared with open total gastrectomy, but data on long-term cancer-specific outcomes do not yet exist. Robotic gastrectomy has several benefits over laparoscopic gastrectomy, including improved visualization, improved dexterity, and surgeon comfort. These advantages are associated with increased cost when compared with laparoscopic gastrectomy [30], and as yet no prospective data have established superiority of robotic surgery over laparoscopic surgery for gastric cancer. As robotic gastrectomy becomes more established, it is hoped that prospective data collection and well-designed studies will clarify the role of robotic surgery in the treatment of gastric cancer.

References

1. Strong VE, Gholami S, Shah MA, Tang LH, Janjigian YY, Schattner M, et al. Total gastrectomy for hereditary diffuse gastric cancer at a single center: postsurgical outcomes in 41 patients. Ann Surg. 2017;266(6):1006–12.
2. Macdonald JS, Smalley SR, Benedetti J, Hundahl SA, Estes NC, Stemmermann GN, et al. Chemoradiotherapy after surgery compared with surgery alone for adenocarcinoma of the stomach or gastroesophageal junction. N Engl J Med. 2001;345:725–30.
3. Cunningham D, Allum WH, Stenning SP, Thompson JN, Van de Velde CJ, Nicolson M, MAGIC Trial Participants, et al. Perioperative chemotherapy versus surgery alone for resectable gastroesophageal cancer. N Engl J Med. 2006;355:11–20.
4. Kitano S, Iso Y, Moriyama M, Sugimachi K. Laparoscopy-assisted Billroth I gastrectomy. Surg Laparosc Endosc. 1994;4:146–8.
5. Kim W, Kim HH, Han SU, Kim MC, Hyung WJ, Ryu SW, Korean Laparo-endoscopic Gastrointestinal Surgery Study (KLASS) Group, et al. Decreased morbidity of laparoscopic distal gastrectomy compared with open distal gastrectomy for stage I gastric cancer: short-term outcomes from a multicenter randomized controlled trial (KLASS-01). Ann Surg. 2016;263:28–35.
6. Kitano S, Shiraishi N, Fujii K, Yasuda K, Inomata M, Adachi Y. A randomized controlled trial comparing open vs laparoscopy-assisted distal gastrectomy for the treatment of early gastric cancer: an interim report. Surgery. 2002;131:S306–11.
7. Lee JH, Han HS, Lee JH. A prospective randomized study comparing open vs laparoscopy-assisted distal gastrectomy in early gastric cancer: early results. Surg Endosc. 2005;19:168–73.
8. Huscher CG, Mingoli A, Sgarzini G, Sansonetti A, Di Paola M, Recher A, Ponzano C. Laparoscopic versus open subtotal gastrectomy for distal gastric cancer: five-year results of a randomized prospective trial. Ann Surg. 2005;241:232–7.
9. Kim YW, Baik YH, Yun YH, Nam BH, Kim DH, Choi IJ, Bae JM. Improved quality of life outcomes after laparoscopy-assisted distal gastrectomy for early gastric cancer: results of a prospective randomized clinical trial. Ann Surg. 2008;248:721–7.
10. Kim HH, Hyung WJ, Cho GS, Kim MC, Han SU, Kim W, et al. Morbidity and mortality of laparoscopic gastrectomy versus open gastrectomy for gastric cancer: an interim report—a phase III multicenter, prospective, randomized trial (KLASS trial). Ann Surg. 2010;251:417–20.
11. Vinuela EF, Gonen M, Brennan MF, Coit DG, Strong VE. Laparoscopic versus open distal gastrectomy for gastric cancer: a meta-analysis of randomized controlled trials and high-quality nonrandomized studies. Ann Surg. 2012;255:446–56.
12. Kelly KJ, Selby L, Chou JF, Dukleska K, Capanu M, Coit DG, et al. Laparoscopic versus open gastrectomy for gastric adenocarcinoma in the west: a case-control study. Ann Surg Oncol. 2015;22:3590–6.
13. Hashizume M, Sugimachi K. Robot-assisted gastric surgery. Surg Clin North Am. 2003;83:1429–44.
14. Giulianotti PC, Coratti A, Angelini M, Sbrana F, Cecconi S, Balestracci T, Caravaglios G. Robotics in general surgery: personal experience in a large community hospital. Arch Surg. 2003;138:777–84.

15. Anderson C, Ellenhorn J, Hellan M, Pigazzi A. Pilot series of robot-assisted laparoscopic subtotal gastrectomy with extended lymphadenectomy for gastric cancer. Surg Endosc. 2007;21: 1662–6.
16. Marano A, Choi YY, Hyung WJ, Kim YM, Kim J, Noh SH. Robotic versus laparoscopic versus open gastrectomy: a meta-analysis. J Gastric Cancer. 2013;13:136–48.
17. Gaya DR, Stuart RC, Going JJ, Stanley AJ. Hereditary diffuse gastric cancer associated with E-cadherin mutation: penetrance after all. Eur J Gastroenterol Hepatol. 2008;20:1249–51.
18. Selby LV, DeMatteo RP, Tholey RM, Jarnagin WR, Garcia-Aguilar J, Strombom PD, et al. Evolving application of minimally invasive cancer operations at a tertiary cancer center. J Surg Oncol. 2017;115(4):365–70.
19. Kelly KJ, Strong VE. Minimally invasive total gastrectomy. In: Kim J, Garcia-Aguilar J, editors. Surgery for cancers of the gastrointestinal tract. New York: Springer; 2015. p. 87–97.
20. LaFemina J, Vinuela EF, Schattner MA, Gerdes H, Strong VE. Esophagojejunal reconstruction after total gastrectomy for gastric cancer using a transorally inserted anvil delivery system. Ann Surg Oncol. 2013;20:2975–83.
21. Kelly KJ, Allen PJ, Brennan MF, Gollub MJ, Coit DG, Strong VE. Internal hernia after gastrectomy for cancer with roux-Y reconstruction. Surgery. 2013;154:305–11.
22. Davis JL, Selby LV, Chou JF, Schattner M, Ilson DH, Capanu M, et al. Patterns and predictors of weight loss after gastrectomy for cancer. Ann Surg Oncol. 2016;23:1639–45.
23. Selby L, Rifkin M, Yoon S, Ariyan C, Strong V. Decreased length of stay and earlier oral feeding associated with standardized postoperative clinical care for total gastrectomies at a cancer center. Surgery. 2016;160(3):607–12.
24. Mortensen K, Nilsson M, Slim K, Schäfer M, Mariette C, Braga M, Enhanced Recovery After Surgery (ERAS®) Group, et al. Consensus guidelines for enhanced recovery after gastrectomy: enhanced recovery after surgery (ERAS®) society recommendations. Br J Surg. 2014;101:1209–29.
25. Lassen K, Kjaeve J, Fetveit T, Tranø G, Sigurdsson HK, Horn A, Revhaug A. Allowing normal food at will after major upper gastrointestinal surgery does not increase morbidity: a randomized multicenter trial. Ann Surg. 2008;247:721–9.
26. Selby LV, Vertosick EA, Sjoberg DD, Schattner MA, Janjigian YY, Brennan MF, et al. Morbidity after total gastrectomy: analysis of 238 patients. J Am Coll Surg. 2015;220:863–71.
27. Shim JH, Yoo HM, Oh SI, Nam MJ, Jeon HM, Park CH, Song KY. Various types of intracorporeal esophagojejunostomy after laparoscopic total gastrectomy for gastric cancer. Gastric Cancer. 2013;16:420–7.
28. Corcione F, Pirozzi F, Cuccurullo D, Angelini P, Cimmino V, Settembre A. Laparoscopic total gastrectomy in gastric cancer: our experience in 92 cases. Minim Invasive Ther Allied Technol. 2013;22:271–8.
29. Nagai E, Ohuchida K, Nakata K, Miyasaka Y, Maeyama R, Toma H, et al. Feasibility and safety of intracorporeal esophagojejunostomy after laparoscopic total gastrectomy: inverted T-shaped anastomosis using linear staplers. Surgery. 2013;153:732–8.
30. Park JY, Jo MJ, Nam BH, Kim Y, Eom BW, Yoon HM, et al. Surgical stress after robot-assisted distal gastrectomy and its economic implications. Br J Surg. 2012;99:1554–61.

Radical Distal Subtotal Gastrectomy and D2 Lymphadenectomy for Gastric Cancer

20

Yanghee Woo and Woo Jin Hyung

Introduction

Robotic radical subtotal distal gastrectomy with D2 lymphadenectomy is a safe, feasible, and oncologically sound minimally invasive option for curative resection of gastric cancer located in the antrum or distal half of the stomach [1]. Minimally invasive surgery (MIS) performed with curative intent for gastric cancer demonstrates improved patient outcome measures when compared to the traditional open radical gastrectomy including less pain and overall earlier recovery [2–7].

Since Drs. M. Hashizume from Japan and PC. Giulianotti from the United States published the first series of successful robotic gastrectomy for cancer in 2003 [8, 9], numerous case series, retrospective comparative studies, and a prospective trial comparing robotic and laparoscopic approaches to gastric cancer have advanced the field with Dr. WJ Hyung (South Korea) recommending procedural standardization in 2016 [10–17]. As the debate over the cost and benefits of emerging technologies continues, robotic surgery for the treatment of gastric cancer is increasingly becoming the approach of choice for many surgeons [18, 19].

Robotic radical gastrectomy not only offers the patient benefits of MIS comparative to laparoscopy, it provides the use of significantly more sophisticated and technologically advanced capabilities to the surgeons. Mastery of the robotic procedure requires expertise in the proper oncologic procedure as well as understanding of technological potential of the robotic surgery platform and can result in maximum benefit for both the patient and the surgeon during well-planned robotic radical subtotal distal gastrectomy with D2 lymphadenectomy.

Robotic Surgical Platform

The da Vinci® Surgical Systems (Si and Xi) (Intuitive Surgical; Sunnyvale, CA), currently the only robotic surgical systems approved by the Food and Drug Administration in the United States for complex abdominal operations, have been used to assist surgeons in performing gastric cancer operations since 2003. The da Vinci® Surgical Systems are equipped with several key features that are particularly beneficial during a totally robotic distal subtotal gastrectomy with lymphadenectomy. The advantages of the robotic system include control of four arms, steady 3D operative view, tremor-filtered precision, and EndoWrist® instruments.

Y. Woo, MD (✉)
Department of Surgery, City of Hope National Medical Center, Duarte, CA, USA
e-mail: ywoo@coh.org

W. J. Hyung
Robotic Surgery, Yonsei University Health System, Seoul, South Korea

Y. Fong et al. (eds.), *The SAGES Atlas of Robotic Surgery*, https://doi.org/10.1007/978-3-319-91045-1_20

The robotic surgical platform gives the surgeon access to four robotic arms at the console, allowing control of the camera and three additional instruments, providing almost complete control of the operative environment throughout the operation. Timely camera movements to obtain the surgeon's desired operative view and the necessary repositioning of the exposure arm for proper retraction can be achieved without delay and regardless of the assistant's skill level. Another distinct advantage, the 3D view of the operative field, provides depth perception superior to that of laparoscopic flat, two-dimensional images. This feature is especially useful during the retroperitoneal lymph node (LN) dissection around the celiac axis and its branches. Moreover, the robotic arms do not fatigue; steady and accurate movements are maintained through the duration of the operation. EndoWrist® capability of the robotic instruments such as the Maryland bipolar forceps significantly improves angled dissections around vessels. The Large Needle Driver and the Mega™ Suture Needle Driver are EndoWristed with 7 degrees of articulation, facilitating ease of intracorporeal suturing of the gastrojejunostomy and jejunojejunostomy, the oversewing of staple lines, or quicker and more precise control of bleeding vessels.

On the other hand, one of the notable limitations of robotic surgical systems is the lack of haptic sense. This limitation makes thorough and meticulous preoperative planning for a robotic gastrectomy and lymphadenectomy ever more important. This planning involves the careful review of the endoscopic findings, the endoscopic ultrasound (EUS), and the CT scan of the abdomen. The endoscopic localization of the tumor can aid in the determination of the proximal margin, the EUS will help guide the extent of lymph node dissection, and the CT scan may allow for identification of aberrant vascular anatomy, especially replaced left hepatic artery off of the left gastric artery, which can easily be divided during the hepatogastric ligament dissection.

Procedure Preparation

Operating Room Setup

Before starting the operation, the surgeon should ensure that the configuration of the operating room is optimized for the safety of the patient and the convenience of the members of the OR team of surgeons, anesthesiologists, scrub technologists, and circulating nurses. The optimal configuration of the robot, the surgeon console, the surgical cart, and the anesthesia cart, along with the proper placement of monitors, is described relative to the patient on the operating table. However, limitations of space and fixed structures in each operating room are likely to require flexibility and repositioning.

- The robot system is brought in directly cephalad (Si System) to the patient with the center of the robotic cart aligned with the patient's head or perpendicular to the OR table (Xi System), and the boom is rotated appropriately.
- The anesthesia cart and the anesthesiologist are positioned at either the left or right side of the patient's head for easy access to the patient's airway.
- Since the assist-port will be placed on the patient's left side, the patient-side assistants will need to stand or sit on the left side of the patient, with the main assistant monitor on the opposite side facing the assistant.
- The vision cart is usually placed at the foot of the operating table. If space does not allow for this configuration, the vision cart can be placed to the patient's upper right, close enough for all the connecting wires to reach without tension.
- The surgeon console should be placed in one corner or edge of the operating room, to provide the surgeon with a panoramic view of the patient and ready access to the patient.

Patient Setup, Trocar Placement, and Instrument Selection

After the patient is placed under general endotracheal anesthesia with two large-bore peripheral intravenous accesses and an arterial line for constant blood pressure monitoring, the patient's arms are tucked to the sides. Wide prepping of the abdomen from the nipple line to the suprapubic region is followed by draping in the standard sterile fashion. Once the patient is prepped and draped, the operation begins with the placement of the five required ports—four trocars for the robotic arms and one assist trocar (Fig. 20.1). A 10-mm, 12-mm, or 15-mm trocar can be used for the assistant, but 15 mm is preferred. The proper placement of the ports is essential to the ease of a successful operation. One reason is that despite the articulation of most of the instruments, the ultrasonic shears—a very useful instrument in the lymphadenectomy portion of the procedure—do not articulate, so proper port placement for the dissection using the ultrasonic shears is important. If another articulating instrument is used instead of the ultrasonic shears, such as the hot shears or vessel sealer, then the placement of the right-sided port can be more forgiving. Port placement also should account for the patient's abdominal wall girth and the intra-abdominal anatomy, because the distance between the ports and the placement of the ports determine the reach and direction of the robotic instruments:

- For patients who have a large dome, the surgeon should consider moving the right ports to a more medial location so that the instruments on these two robotic arms can easily reach the left-side extent of the dissection.
- The right-sided midclavicular robotic port site should be at the level of the first portion of the duodenum.

First, insert the camera port approximately 16–20 cm inferior to the xiphoid process (usually, just infraumbilical or just supraumbilical), and place the patient in the reverse Trendelenburg position (approximately 15–30°) prior to placing the remaining trocars. Before docking the robot, an exploration of the intraperitoneal surfaces should be performed to evaluate for the presence of metastatic disease. After confirming the absence of distant disease, the robotic surgical cart is aligned with the operating table and brought in to be docked over the patient.

The camera is inserted first, using the infraumbilical port. The selected instruments should then be inserted into the abdominal cavity under direct visualization. The preferred instruments include curved bipolar Maryland forceps on the first arm and ultrasonic shears or a monopolar device and the Cadiere forceps, interchangeably, on the second and third arms.

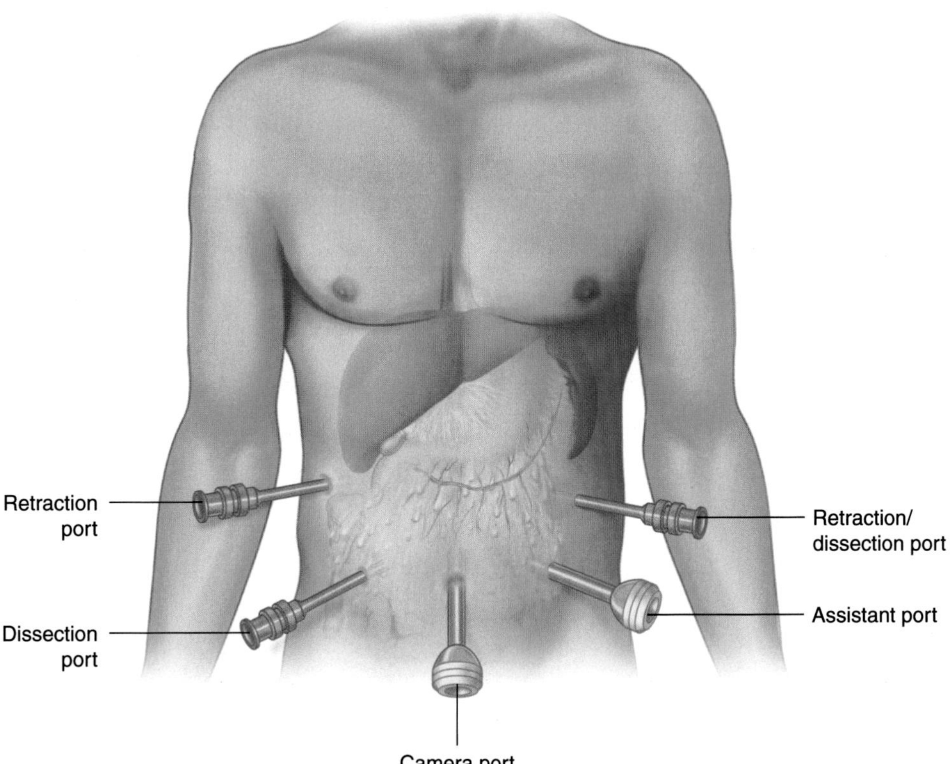

Fig. 20.1 Once the patient is prepped and draped, the operation begins with the placement of the five ports. Four trocars will be used for the robotic arms and one trocar for the assistant

Preparation of the Operative Field

Exposure is paramount to the successful completion of a totally robotic distal subtotal gastrectomy with D2 lymphadenectomy. It is required to prevent open conversion, an unnecessary increase in operative time, and surgeon frustration. Three key maneuvers to optimize exposure prior to the start of the main portion of the procedure and to facilitate accurate resection are complete gastric decompression, self-sustaining liver retraction, and proper placement of the robotic trocars (as described above).

Gastric decompression is recommended to increase the operative domain and permit easy manipulation of the stomach during the operation. The most common methods of gastric decompression are either the insertion of an orogastric/nasogastric tube or percutaneous needle aspiration/suction using a long, 18- to 20-gauge spinal needle.

Self-sustaining **liver retraction** helps expose the hepatoduodenal and hepatogastric ligaments and provides easy access to the lesser curvature of the stomach, the celiac axis, and the esophageal crux; such access is very useful throughout the operation, especially during lymph node dissection of stations 7, 8a, 9, 11p, and 12a. Before beginning the dissection, the left lobe of the liver can easily be retracted using any of several described techniques [20–22], including the suture-gauze liver suspension method.

Surgical Procedure Overview

Procedure of Robotic Distal Subtotal Gastrectomy and D2 Lymph Node Dissection

The procedure of radical distal subtotal gastrectomy involving the en bloc dissection of the N2-level lymph nodes as described by the Japanese Gastric Cancer Association can be performed using a directional method with major named vessels as key landmarks of lymph node stations (Fig. 20.2) [23, 24].

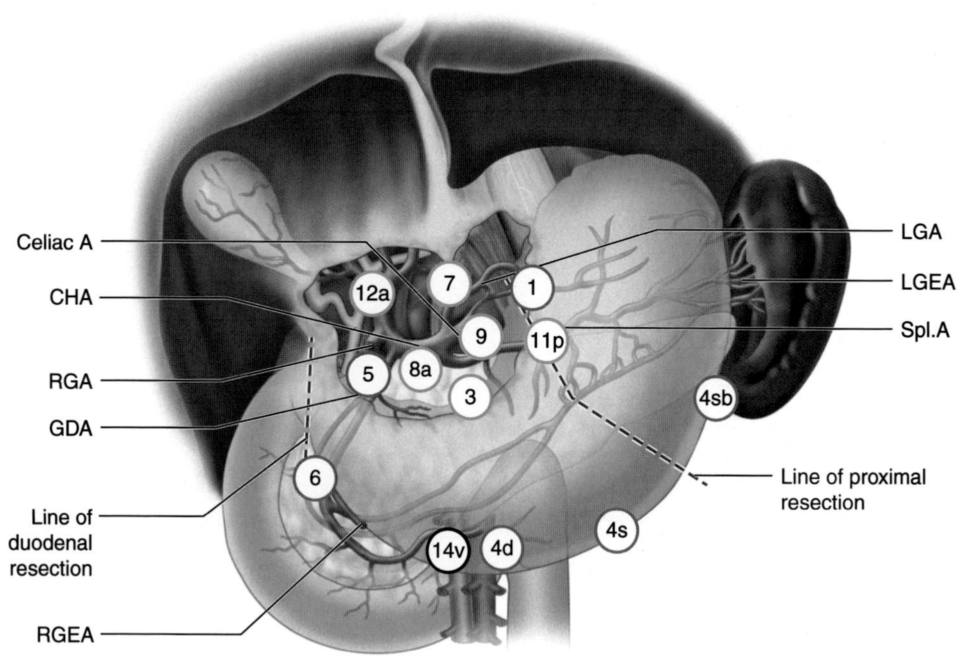

Fig. 20.2 Dissection of the lymph nodes using a directional method with major named vessels as key landmarks of lymph node stations. *CHA* common hepatic artery, *GDA* gastroduodenal artery, *LGA* left gastric artery, *LGEA* left gastroepiploic artery, *PHA* proper hepatic artery, *RGA* right gastric artery, *RGEA* right gastroepiploic artery

Left-Sided Greater Curvature Dissection (Lymph Node Stations 4d and 4 S)

The dissection begins with a partial omentectomy starting 5 cm away from the proximal edge of the greater curvature of the antrum, left laterally toward the left gastroepiploic vessels. If total omentectomy is required, the dissection of the greater omentum is more easily performed at the end of the dissection, prior to the reconstruction. The optimum exposure is achieved using the right lateral robotic arm (Cadiere forceps). Grasp the soft tissues on the edge of the greater curvature of the stomach about 8 cm proximal to the pylorus using the Cadiere forceps and pulling superiorly and slightly anteriorly. This creates a draping of the omentum, separates the stomach from the colon, and provides the initial exposure to enter the lesser sac (Fig. 20.3a).

- Begin the dissection using the ultrasonic shears in the left dissection arm approximately 6 cm away from the edge of the greater curvature in the omental draping. Divide the gastrocolic ligament to enter the lesser sac. Once the posterior wall of the stomach is visible, be sure to divide the filmy layer separating the instruments from the posterior wall of the stomach. (Take care not to enter the colonic mesentery or injure the colon or the duodenum.)
- Remember to use the Cadiere to improve the surgical exposure and view by grasping more proximal areas of the edge of the stomach along the greater curvature and moving the operative field toward the liver.
- As the dissection nears the lower pole of the spleen, the left gastroepiploic vessels arising from the splenic vessels can be identified. Once identified, clear the vessels from the surrounding soft tissue, ligate them with Hem-o-lok® clips (Teleflex; Wayne, PA), and divide the vessels leaving one Hem-o-lok® clip on the patient side (Fig. 20.3b).
- Then, identify the first set of short gastric vessels. Using it as an anatomic landmark, divide the soft tissue until the edge of the greater curvature of the stomach is reached. Clear the soft tissue off the greater curvature of the stomach until the proximal resection margin is reached.
- This allows for en bloc retrieval of lymph node station 4 s.

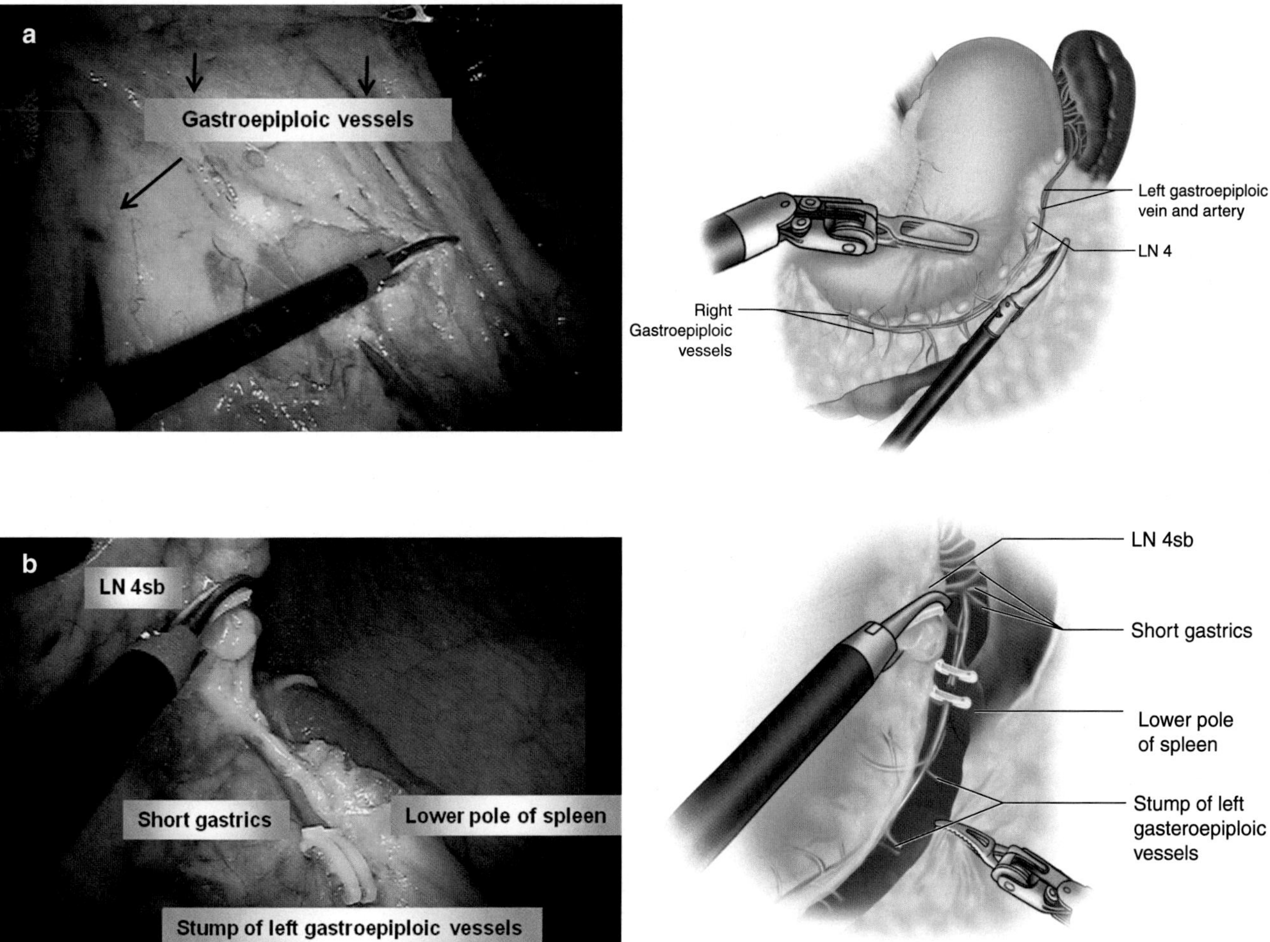

Fig. 20.3 Left-sided greater curvature dissection. (**a**) Initial exposure. (**b**) Dividing the gastroepiploic vessels until the identification of the left gastroepiploic artery and vein. LN station #4d

Distal Stomach Dissection

Start the right-sided greater curvature dissection by repositioning the Cadiere exposure arm and grasping the greater curvature of the stomach at the level of the cut edge of the gastrocolic ligament. Divide the gastrocolic ligament distally toward the head of the pancreas (HOP). Before pursuing the identification of the right gastroepiploic vessels, divide the duodenocolic ligament to separate the right colon from the duodenum until the first portion of the duodenum, about 2 cm distal to the pylorus.

Return to dissect the anterior and inferior portion of the head and neck of the pancreas, and remove the soft tissues containing lymph node station #6. The borders of station #6 are defined by the right gastroepiploic vein (RGEV), the anterior superior pancreaticoduodenal vein (ASPDV), and the middle colic vein (MCV) (Fig. 20.4).

- Reposition the third arm by grasping the posterior stomach near the pylorus and retracting upward toward the liver.
- Dissect free the posterior pylorus from the HOP, and identify the anterior surface of the gastroduodenal artery.
- Proceed carefully and dissect the soft tissue off the HOP, and identify the RGEV and ASPDV. Include the soft tissue around the RGEV and superior to the ASPDV in the specimen retrieval.
- Identify the RGEV and clear the vessel as it joins the ASPDV. (This dissection is facilitated by the exposure arm grasping the inferoposterior edge of the pylorus.) Isolate, ligate, and divide the RGEV at its base as it drains into the MCV.
- This allows for the retraction of the divided RGEV and exposure of the right gastroepiploic artery, which is usually located more posteriorly as it branches from the gastroduodenal artery (GDA). Ligate and divide the right gastroepiploic artery at this point.
- Continue the dissection along the anterior surface of the GDA, and detach its attachments to the posterior duodenum until the common hepatic artery (CHA) is identified.

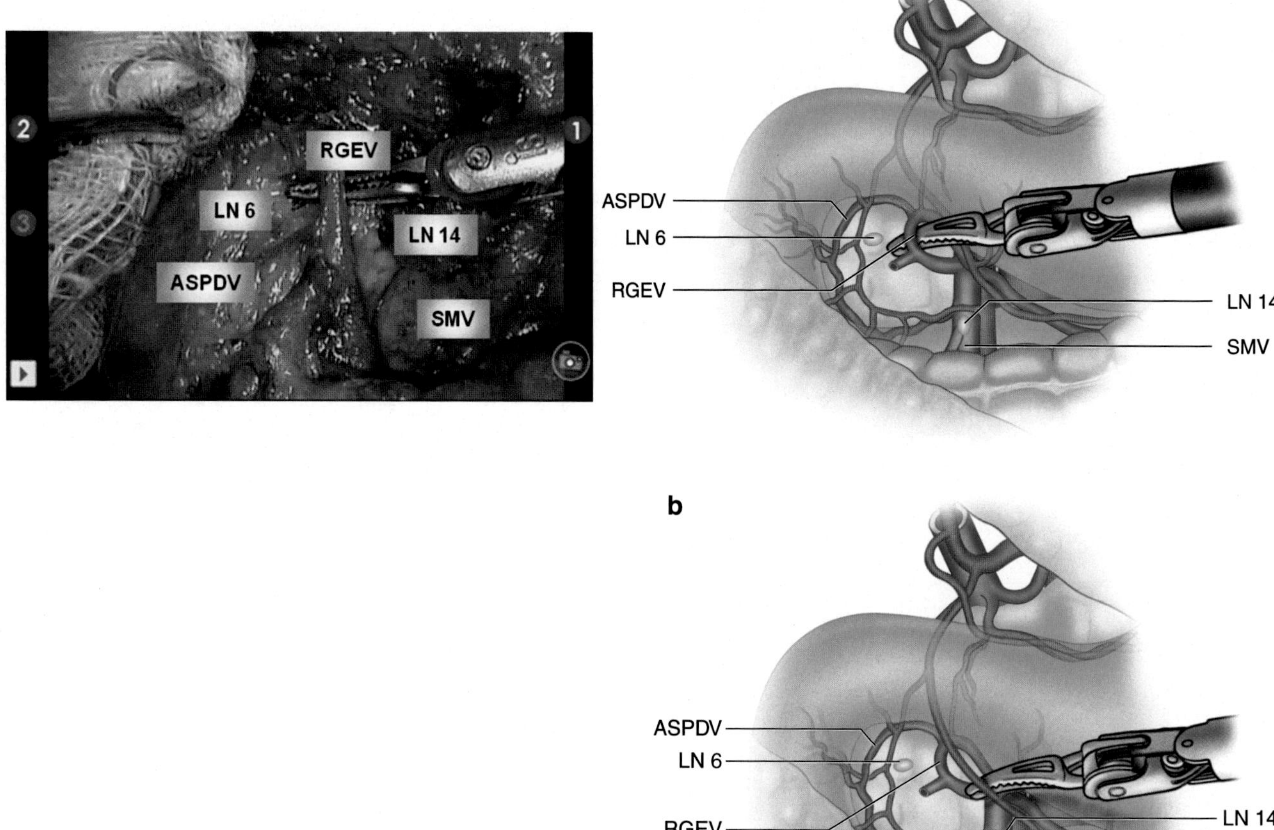

Fig. 20.4 (**a, b**) Right-sided greater curvature dissection, with removal of LN station #6. *ASPDV* anterior superior pancreaticoduodenal vein, LN station #6; *RGEV* right gastroepiploic vein, *SMV* superior mesenteric artery

Placing a 4 × 4-inch gauze anterior to the GDA and posterior to the area of the duodenum to be divided can protect the proper hepatic artery as it branches into the GDA. The gauze can be identified during the supraduodenal dissection.

- Clear the duodenal attachments to the hepatoduodenal ligament approximately 2 cm distal to the pylorus, using caution not to injure the proper hepatic artery. Once the duodenum is cleared, an Endo linear stapler or the robotic stapler can be used to transect it at this point.

Lesser Curvature Dissection (Lymph Node Dissection 12a, 8a, 7, 9, 11p, 1, and 3)

Hepatoduodenal ligament dissection requires that the liver is retracted to expose this area. To create the necessary additional exposure, pull the stomach to the patient's left. This move identifies the soft tissue that is encasing the right gastric artery as it is attached to the proper hepatic artery.

- Follow the dissection that was performed along the anterior GDA until the proper hepatic artery (PHA) is identified. Then, as the soft tissue along the anterior proper hepatic artery is being dissected, the right gastric artery can be identified at its base, isolated, ligated, and divided for retrieval of the lymph node station #5 (Fig. 20.5a)
- Continue the meticulous and precise dissection along the anterior and left lateral side of the PHA until the anterolateral border of the portal vein (PV) is identified (Fig. 20.5b). To improve the exposure, gentle downward retraction of the common hepatic artery (CHA) can be provided by the assistant.
- Clear the soft tissue in this area and dissect the soft tissues distally until CHA is identified. Continue to clear the soft tissue along the CHA to retrieve the 8a lymph node station.

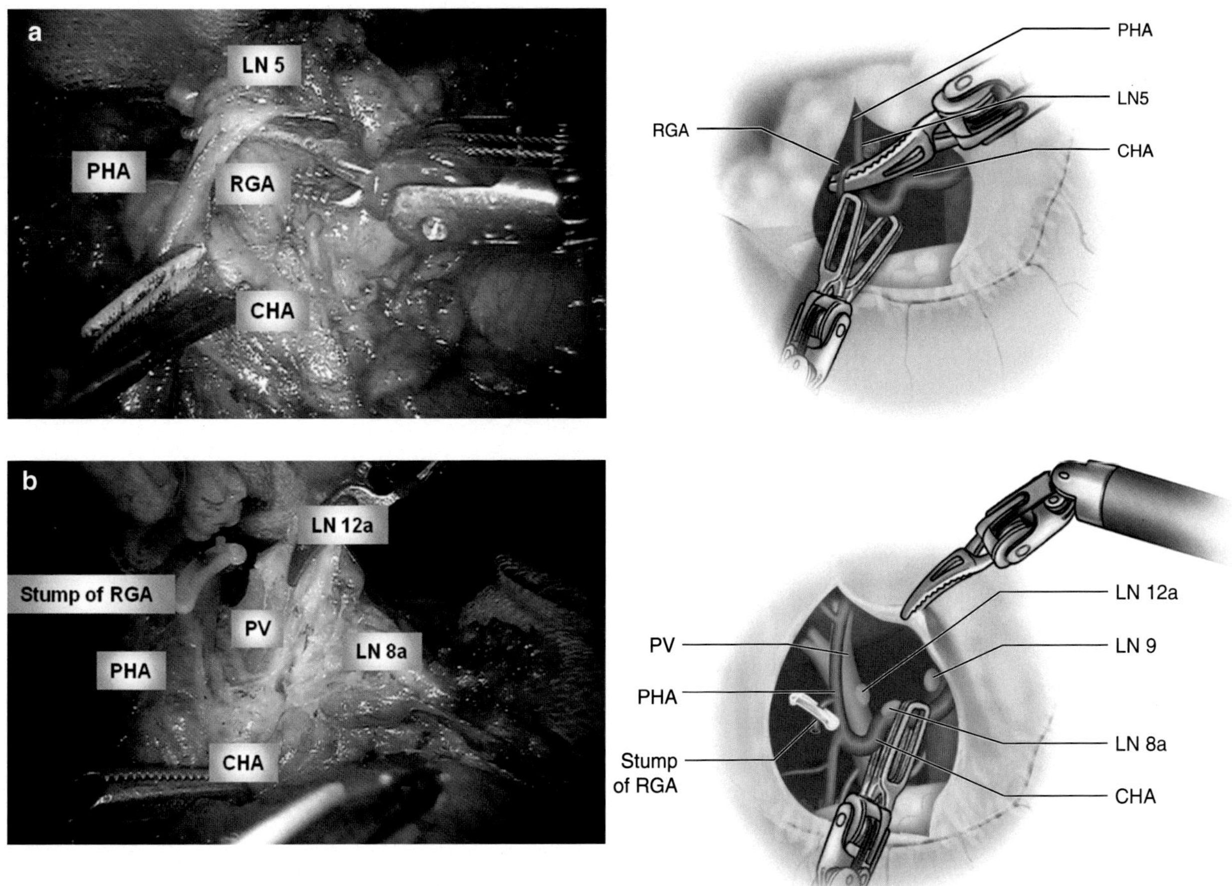

Fig. 20.5 Lesser curvature dissection. (**a**) Retrieval of LN station #5 along the right gastric artery. (**b**) Dissection of soft tissue (LN station #12a) anteromedial to the proper hepatic artery (PHA) and identifying the anterolateral border of the portal vein (PV)

Suprapancreatic and Celiac Axis Dissection

Continued skeletonization of the CHA toward the celiac axis will help to identify the left gastric vein as it drains toward the portal vein. Isolate the left gastric vein, ligate with Hem-o-lok® clips, and divide it. (*Caution:* Occasionally, the left gastric vein drains into the splenic vein and can course anterior to the splenic artery.) This allows for the stomach to be retracted more left laterally as its attachments to the celiac axis help isolate the left gastric artery. Retrieve the soft tissues around the celiac artery, which contain lymph node station #9 (Fig. 20.6).

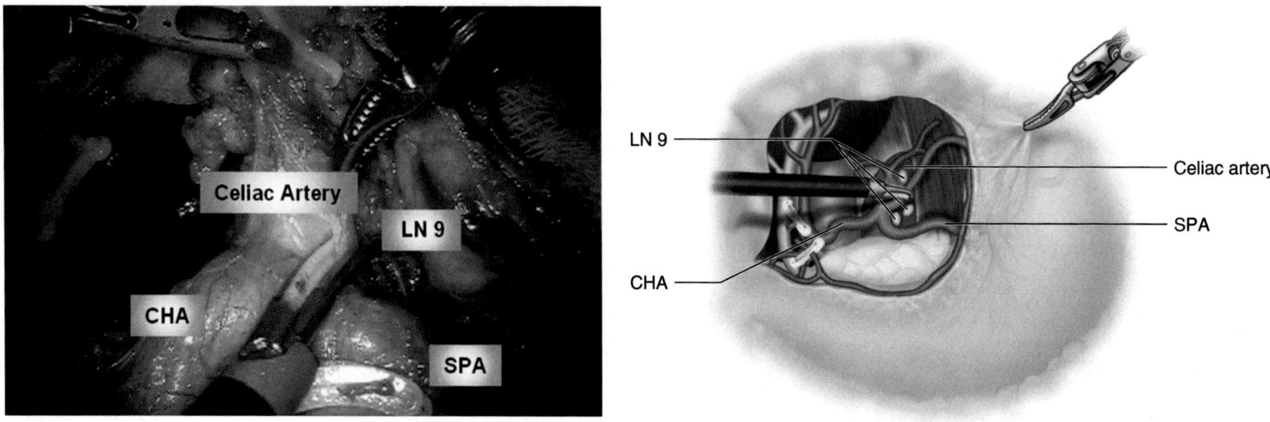

Fig. 20.6 Celiac artery dissection for LN station #9. *SPA* splenic artery

Left Gastric and Splenic Artery Dissections

The soft tissues surrounding the left gastric artery (LGA) are retrieved as lymph node station #7, and the tissues along the splenic artery are retrieved as station #11p (Fig. 20.7).

- To improve access to the origin of the LGA from the celiac axis, divide the retroperitoneal attachments along the lesser curvature of the stomach, along the right diaphragmatic crux.
- Using the Cadiere grasper (robot arm #3), grasp the soft tissues along the lesser curvature of the stomach to straighten out the LGA perpendicular to the celiac axis.
- Clear the soft tissues surrounding the root of the LGA, ligate the LGA with clips or a vascular stapler, and divide the LGA at its root.

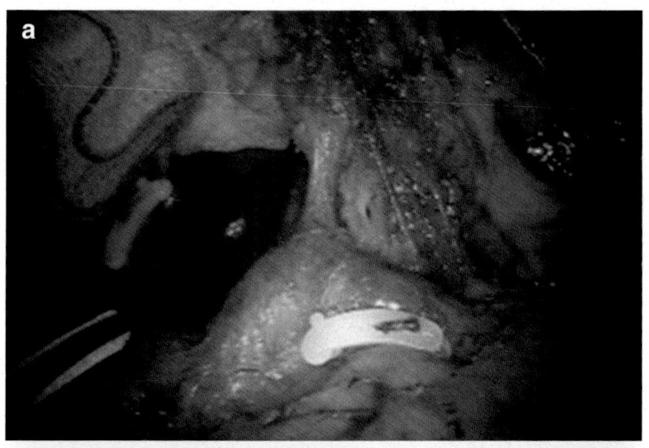

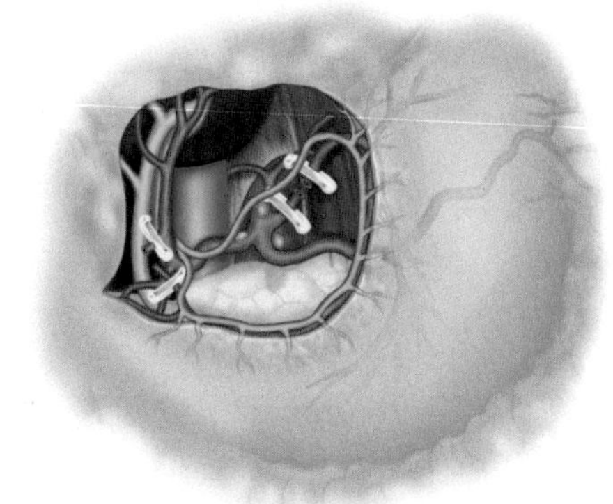

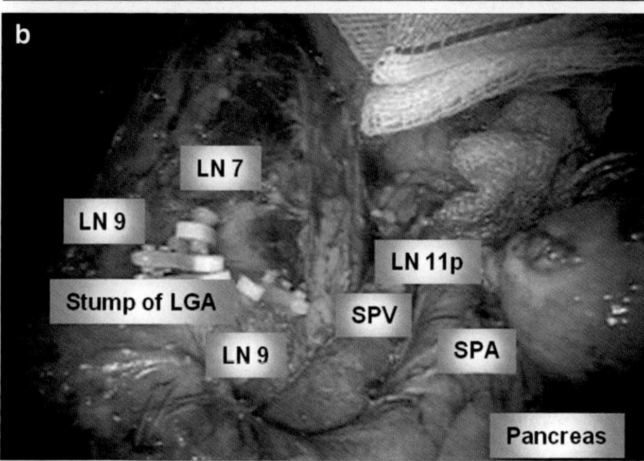

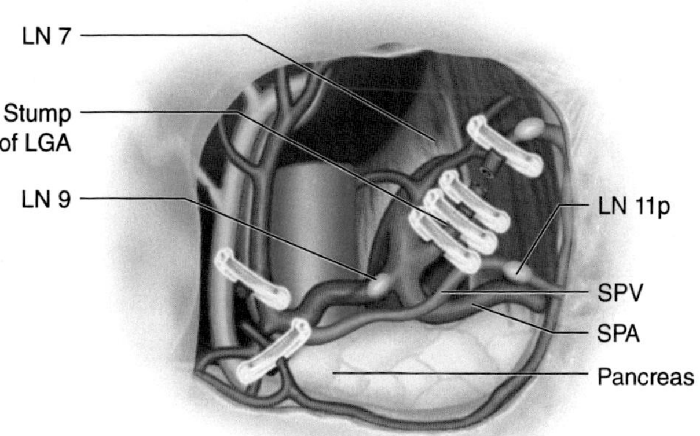

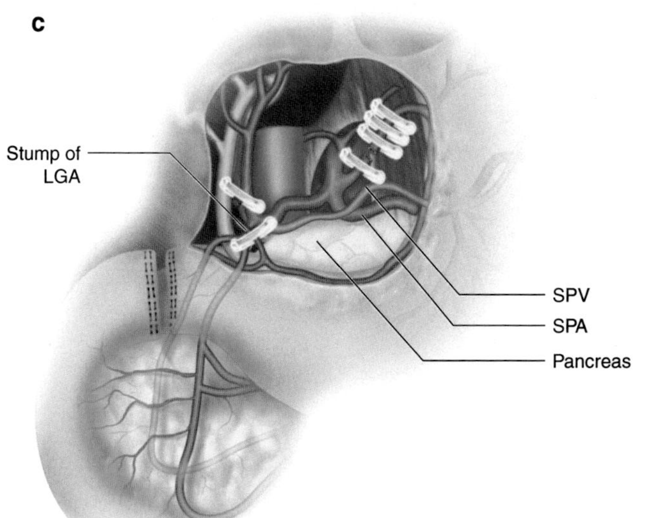

Fig. 20.7 (**a–c**) Dissection of the left gastric artery (LGA) as it branches from the celiac artery and soft tissue (LN station #11p) along the proximal half of splenic artery (SpA). *SPV* splenic vein

- The dissection around the LGA along the celiac axis can be facilitated by starting the dissection along the splenic artery and clearing the attachments for a couple of centimeters.
- Once the LGA has been divided, continue the skeletonization, and retrieve the soft tissues off the anterior surface of the splenic artery until approximately half of the distance of the splenic artery has been cleared. This completes the dissection of lymph node station #11p.

Proximal Lesser Curvature Dissection and Proximal Resection

- To complete the D2 lymphadenectomy, lymph node stations #1 and #3 along the proximal lesser curvature of the stomach are dissected. This dissection requires the removal of the soft tissues along the intra-abdominal esophagus, the right cardia, and the lesser curvature of the stomach until the proximal resection margin (Fig. 20.8).
- Anterior and posterior vagus nerves should also be identified during this portion of the procedure and divided.
- Divide any remaining posterior attachments to prepare for proximal gastric resection. Confirm the proximal resection line from the greater curvature to the lesser curvature, and divide using a stapler (either Endo-GIA™ or robotic).

This completes the procedure of robotic D2 lymphadenectomy for distal subtotal gastrectomy.

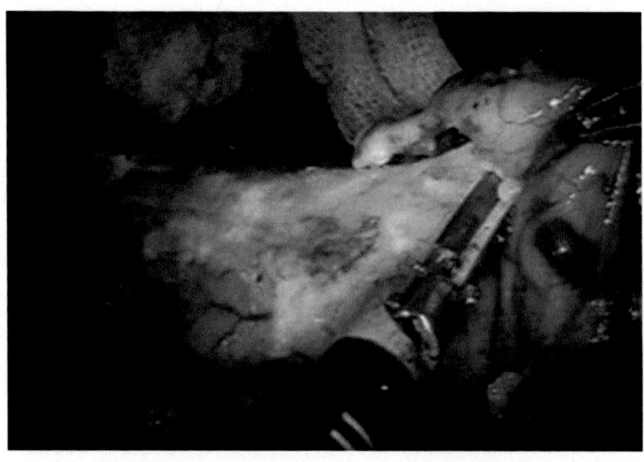

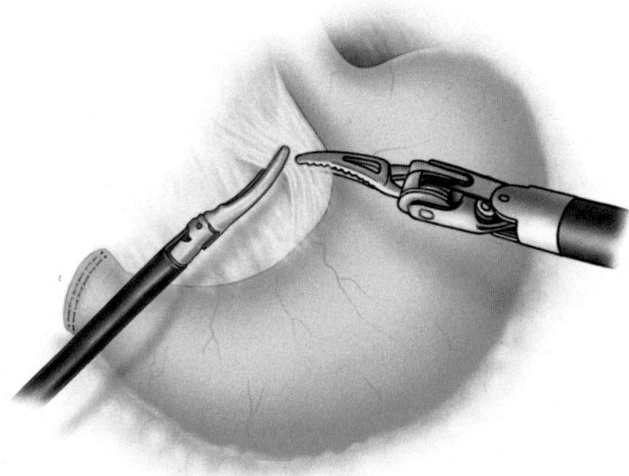

Fig. 20.8 Proximal lesser curvature dissection. Clearance of the LN stations #1 and #3

Methods of Reconstruction

For the gastrojejunal reconstruction, either a loop gastrojejunostomy or a Roux-en-Y gastrojejunostomy can be performed completely robotically, either using staplers or by robotic suturing. Each approach has advantages and disadvantages, and the selection of the gastrointestinal reconstruction technique after robotic gastric cancer surgery will be guided by the extent of stomach resection and the surgeon's preference. Usually, stapled anastomoses are quicker, but they may require expertise at the bedside for assistance [12, 25, 26]. Robot-assisted sutured anastomosis is another option and can easily be performed using the robotic needle drivers [27].

Figure 20.9 illustrates the steps in a side-to-side, completely stapled loop gastrojejunostomy. In general, some of the many methods described for laparoscopic reconstruction can be adapted to a robotic operation. Moreover, with the recent addition of robotic staplers, the anastomoses can be performed using the robotic instruments.

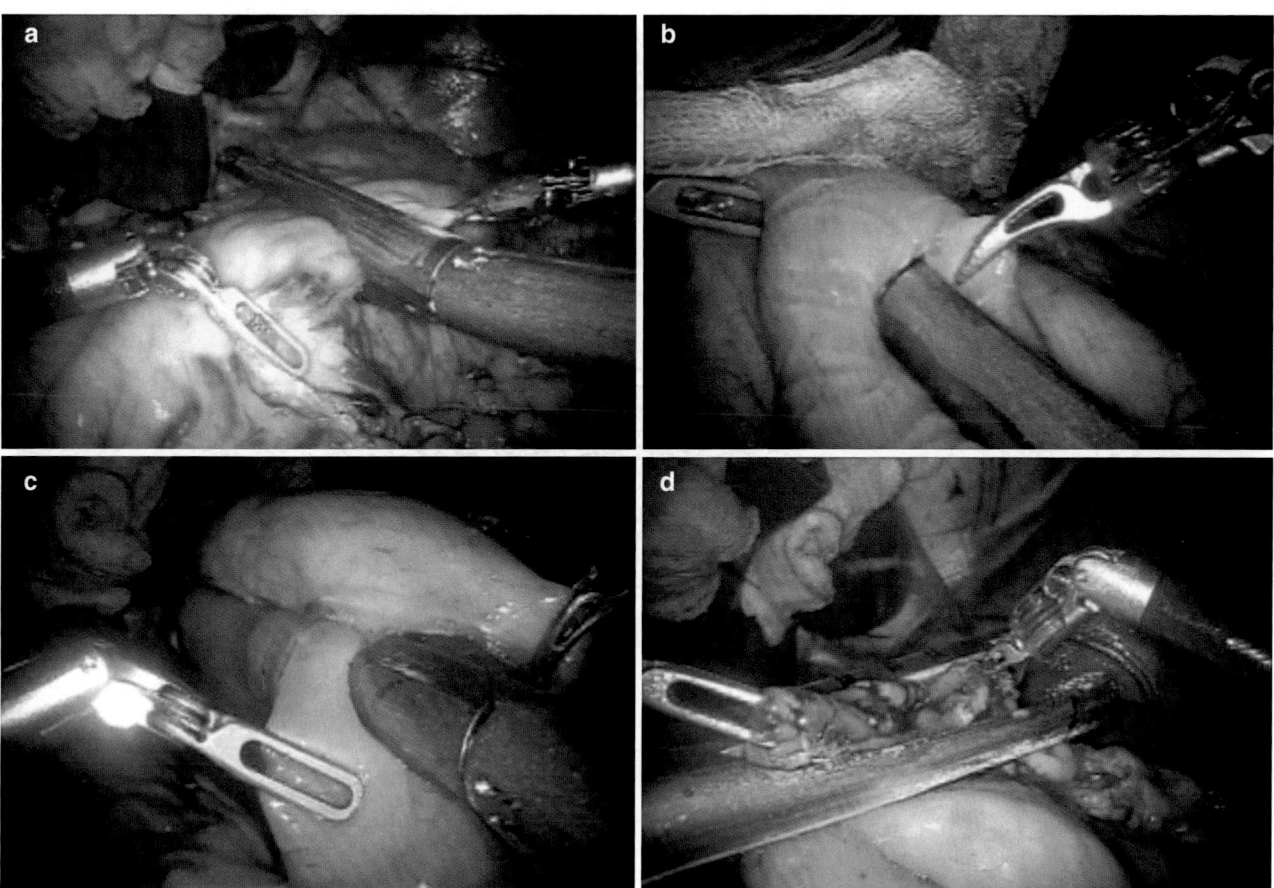

Fig. 20.9 A side-to-side, completely stapled loop gastrojejunostomy. (**a**) Proximal resection of the stomach. (**b**) Intracorporeal intubation of the two mouths of the stapler in the gastrostomy (previously made 50 cm proximal to the staple along the greater curvature) and the jejunostomy. (**c**) Stapling of the gastrojejunostomy, using a 60-mm linear stapler. (**d**) Closure of the common enterotomy

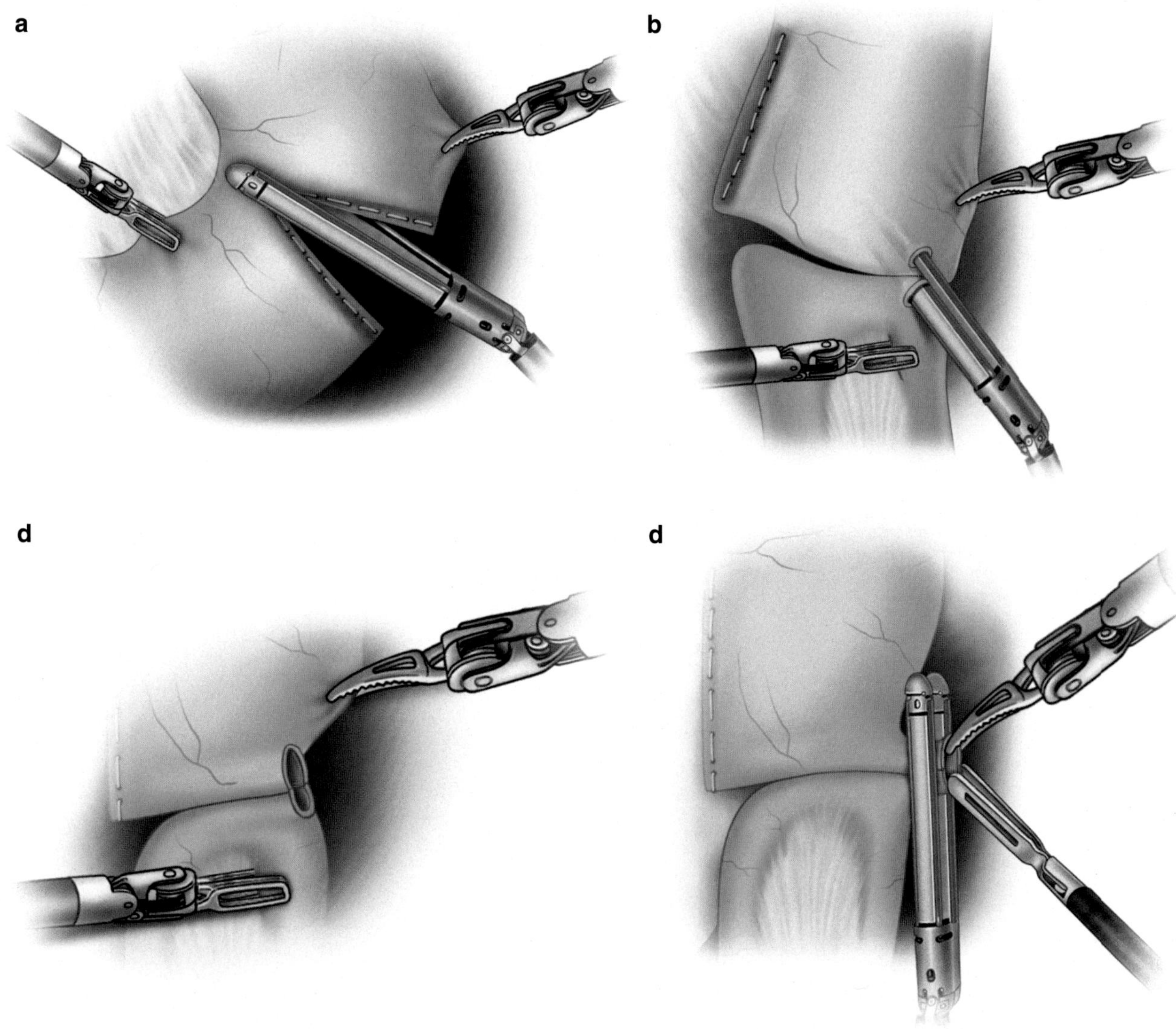

Fig. 20.9 (continued)

Postoperative Management

Postoperative management of patients who have undergone robotic gastrectomy can follow an enhanced recovery program after surgery. The patients are kept NPO on maintenance fluids for the first 24 h. They are monitored for nausea, pain, urinary output (with a Foley catheter), and infection. Patient-controlled analgesia and deep vein thrombosis prophylaxis are provided. In the absence of complications, the expected hospital course is as follows:

- POD1: Start water intake, remove Foley catheter, and encourage out of bed.
- POD 2: Advance to clear liquid diet.
- POD 3 and 4: Advance to regular diet with postgastrectomy restriction and small portions.

The median length of hospital stay is usually 5 days if there are no complications.

Potential Complications

The most common complications for robotic gastrectomy for gastric cancer are wound infections, intraluminal bleeding, and anastomotic leakage [28–30]. The morbidity is higher with D2 lymphadenectomy than for D1 lymphadenectomy. There are also several other possible complications:

- Intra-abdominal fluid collections or abscesses
- Intraluminal and intra-abdominal bleeding
- Pancreatitis, pancreatic leak, or pancreatic fistula
- Anastomotic leak or stricture
- Gastroparesis or ileus
- Obstruction

Conclusions

Robotic surgery is an oncologically sound minimally invasive surgical option for patients who require distal subtotal gastrectomy with D2 lymphadenectomy. [31] Surgeons have successfully applied robotic gastrectomy for early and advanced stage diseases and in elderly and obese gastric cancer patients [32, 33]. It provides surgeons the opportunity not only to more easily adopt minimally invasive surgery to benefit our gastric cancer patients but also to identify the utility of integrating novel technology in improving the outcome of our cancer patients. The optimum application of currently available technology such as near-infrared imaging and multi-input console view are still being investigated as the robotic surgical technology with the potential for automation is being explored and developed [34–37].

References

1. Woo Y, Hyung WJ, Pak KH, Inaba K, Obama K, Choi SH, et al. Robotic gastrectomy as an oncologically sound alternative to laparoscopic resections for the treatment of early-stage gastric cancers. Arch Surg. 2011;146:1086–92.
2. Huscher CG, Mingoli A, Sgarzini G, Sansonetti A, Di Paola M, Recher A, et al. Laparoscopic versus open subtotal gastrectomy for distal gastric cancer: five-year results of a randomized prospective trial. Ann Surg. 2005;241:232–7.
3. Kim HH, Hyung WJ, Cho GS, Kim MC, Han SU, Kim W, et al. Morbidity and mortality of laparoscopic gastrectomy versus open gastrectomy for gastric cancer: an interim report–a phase III multicenter, prospective, randomized trial (KLASS trial). Ann Surg. 2010;51:417–20.
4. Kitano S, Shiraishi N, Uyama I, Sugihara K, Tanigawa N, Japanese Laparoscopic Surgery Study Group. A multicenter study on oncologic outcome of laparoscopic gastrectomy for early cancer in Japan. Ann Surg. 2007;245:68–72.
5. Huang KH, Lan YT, Fang WL, Chen JH, Lo SS, Hsieh MC, et al. Initial experience of robotic gastrectomy and comparison with open and laparoscopic gastrectomy for gastric cancer. J Gastrointest Surg. 2012;16:1303–10.
6. Caruso S, Patriti A, Marrelli D, Ceccarelli G, Ceribelli C, Roviello F, et al. Open vs. robot-assisted laparoscopic gastric resection with D2 lymph node dissection for adenocarcinoma: a case-control study. Int J Med Robot. 2011;7:452–8.
7. Pernazza G, Gentile E, Felicioni L, Tumbiolo S, Giulianotti PC. Improved early survival after robotic gastrectomy in advanced gastric cancer. Surg Laparosc Endosc Percutan Tech. 2006;16:286.
8. Giulianotti PC, Coratti A, Angelini M, Sbrana F, Cecconi S, Balestracci T, et al. Robotics in general surgery: personal experience in a large community hospital. Arch Surg. 2003;138(8):777–84.
9. Hashizume M, Sugimachi K. Robot-assisted gastric surgery. Surg Clin North Am. 2003;83:1429–44.
10. Buchs NC, Bucher P, Pugin F, Morel P. Robot-assisted gastrectomy for cancer. Minerva Gastroenterol Dietol. 2011;57:33–42.
11. Song J, Oh SJ, Kang WH, Hyung WJ, Choi SH, Noh SH. Robot-assisted gastrectomy with lymph node dissection for gastric cancer: lessons learned from an initial 100 consecutive procedures. Ann Surg. 2009;249:927–32.
12. Hyung WJ, Woo Y, Noh SH. Robotic surgery for gastric cancer: a technical review. J Robot Surg. 2011;5:241–9.
13. D'Annibale A, Pende V, Pernazza G, Monsellato I, Mazzocchi P, Lucandri G, et al. Full robotic gastrectomy with extended (D2) lymphadenectomy for gastric cancer: surgical technique and preliminary results. J Surg Res. 2011;166:e113–20.
14. Song J, Kang WH, Oh SJ, Hyung WJ, Choi SH, Noh SH. Role of robotic gastrectomy using da Vinci system compared with laparoscopic gastrectomy: initial experience of 20 consecutive cases. Surg Endosc. 2009;23:1204–11.
15. Patriti A, Ceccarelli G, Bellochi R, Bartoli A, Spaziani A, Di Zitti L, et al. Robot-assisted laparoscopic total and partial gastric resection with D2 lymph node dissection for adenocarcinoma. Surg Endosc. 2008;22:2753–60.

16. Anderson C, Ellenhorn J, Hellan M, Pigazzi A. Pilot series of robot-assisted laparoscopic subtotal gastrectomy with extended lymphadenectomy for gastric cancer. Surg Endosc. 2007;21:1662–6.
17. Kim YM, Son T, Kim HI, Noh SH, Hyung WJ. Robotic D2 lymph node dissection during distal subtotal gastrectomy for gastric cancer: toward procedural standardization. Ann Surg Oncol. 2016;23(8):2409–10.
18. Park SS, Kim MC, Park MS, Hyung WJ. Rapid adaptation of robotic gastrectomy for gastric cancer by experienced laparoscopic surgeons. Surg Endosc. 2012;26(1):60–7.
19. Marano A, Choi YY, Hyung WJ, Kim YM, Kim J, Noh SH. Robotic versus laparoscopic versus open gastrectomy: a meta-analysis. J Gastric Cancer. 2013;13(3):136–48.
20. Woo Y, Hyung WJ, Kim HI, Obama K, Son T, Noh SH. Minimizing hepatic trauma with a novel liver retraction method: a simple liver suspension using gauze suture. Surg Endosc. 2011;25:3939–45.
21. Shabbir A, Lee JH, Lee MS, Park do J, Kim HH. Combined suture retraction of the falciform ligament and the left lobe of the liver during laparoscopic total gastrectomy. Surg Endosc. 2010;24:3237–40.
22. Yoshikawa K, Shimada M, Higashijima J, Nakao T, Nishi M, Takasu C, et al. Combined liver mobilization and retraction: a novel technique to obtain the optimal surgical field during laparoscopic total gastrectomy. Asian J Endosc Surg. 2016;9(2):111–5.
23. Japanese Gastric Cancer Association. Japanese classification of gastric carcinoma: 3rd English edition. Gastric Cancer. 2011;14:101–12.
24. Japanese Gastric Cancer Association. Japanese gastric cancer treatment guidelines 2010 (ver. 3). Gastric Cancer. 2011;14:113–23.
25. Kim MC, Heo GU, Jung GJ. Robotic gastrectomy for gastric cancer: surgical techniques and clinical merits. Surg Endosc. 2010;24:610–5.
26. Lee HH, Hur H, Jung H, Jeon HM, Park CH, Song KY. Robot-assisted distal gastrectomy for gastric cancer: initial experience. Am J Surg. 2011;201:841–5.
27. Hur H, Kim JY, Cho YK, Han SU. Technical feasibility of robot-sewn anastomosis in robotic surgery for gastric cancer. J Laparoendosc Adv Surg Tech A. 2010;20:693–7.
28. Eom BW, Yoon HM, Ryu KW, Lee JH, Cho SJ, Lee JY, et al. Comparison of surgical performance and short-term clinical outcomes between laparoscopic and robotic surgery in distal gastric cancer. Eur J Surg Oncol. 2012;38:57–63.
29. Kim HI, Han SU, Yang HK, Kim YW, Lee HJ, Ryu KW, et al. Multicenter prospective comparative study of robotic versus laparoscopic gastrectomy for gastric adenocarcinoma. Ann Surg. 2016;263(1):103–9.
30. Yang SY, Roh KH, Kim YN, Cho M, Lim SH, Son T, et al. Surgical outcomes after open, laparoscopic, and robotic gastrectomy for gastric cancer. Ann Surg Oncol. 2017;24(7):1770–7.
31. Okumura N, Son T, Kim YM, Kim HI, An JY, Noh SH, et al. Robotic gastrectomy for elderly gastric cancer patients: comparisons with robotic gastrectomy in younger patients and laparoscopic gastrectomy in the elderly. Gastric Cancer. 2016;19(4):1125–34.
32. Kwon IG, Cho I, Guner A, Kim HI, Noh SH, Hyung WJ. Minimally invasive surgery as a treatment option for gastric cancer in the elderly: comparison with open surgery for patients 80 years and older. Surg Endosc. 2015;29(8):2321–30.
33. Lee J, Kim YM, Woo Y, Obama K, Noh SH, Hyung WJ. Robotic distal subtotal gastrectomy with D2 lymphadenectomy for gastric cancer patients with high body mass index: comparison with conventional laparoscopic distal subtotal gastrectomy with D2 lymphadenectomy. Surg Endosc. 2015;29(11):3251–60.
34. Woo Y, Choi GH, Min BS, Hyung WJ. Novel application of simultaneous multi-image display during complex robotic abdominal procedures. BMC Surg. 2014;14:13.
35. Kim YM, Baek SE, Lim JS, Hyung WJ. Clinical application of image-enhanced minimally invasive robotic surgery for gastric cancer: a prospective observational study. J Gastrointest Surg. 2013;17(2):304–12.
36. Kim H, Lee SK, Kim YM, Lee EH, Lim SJ, Kim SH, et al. Fluorescent iodized emulsion for pre- and intraoperative sentinel lymph node imaging: validation in a preclinical model. Radiology. 2015;275(1):196–204.
37. Son T, Kwon IG, Hyung WJ. Minimally invasive surgery for gastric cancer treatment: current status and future perspectives. Gut Liver. 2014;8(3):229–36.

Multiport and Single-Site Robotic Cholecystectomy

21

Eric Kubat, Dan Eisenberg, and Sherry M. Wren

This chapter reviews the fundamentals and technology, robotic setup, general operative technique, and adoption considerations for robotically-assisted multiport and single-site cholecystectomy. Basic fundamental knowledge of the robotic system, the procedure setup, and instrumentation is critical prior to performing robotically-assisted cholecystectomy. A graduated training program that includes online education, simulation, direct observation, bedside assistance, and case proctoring is important for the implementation of a safe and effective robotically-assisted cholecystectomy.

Robotic cholecystectomy has been shown to be safe and effective. Since its introduction in 1997, it has become the most commonly performed robotic operation in general surgery. Although lacking haptic feedback, the three-dimensional, high-definition visualization, wristed instruments, and improved ergonomics offer a theoretical technical advantage for the operating surgeon.

With growing interest in single-incision procedures, a single-site robotic platform was specifically developed to mitigate the technical difficulties inherent to single-incision laparoscopic surgery. As a consequence, this procedure is associated with a short learning curve and favorable operative outcomes.

A basic fundamental knowledge of the robotic system, room setup, and instruments, along with simulation training and case proctoring, is important to successfully establish a safe and effective robotic cholecystectomy program. This chapter reviews the setup and technique of multiport and single-site robotic cholecystectomy.

E. Kubat, MD · D. Eisenberg, MD · S. M. Wren, MD (✉)
Department of General Surgery, Stanford University School of Medicine, VA Palo Alto Health Care System, Palo Alto, CA, USA
e-mail: ekubat@stanford.edu

Fundamentals and Technology

The first robotically-assisted cholecystectomy was performed in 1997. Using a computerized interface, Belgian surgeons were able to safely remove the gallbladder of an elderly woman using three-dimensional visualization and wristed, articulating instruments [1]. The added benefit of improved visualization, wristed articulation, and enhanced instrument precision created an appealing alternative to standard laparoscopic cholecystectomy, but these benefits came at the expense of tactile or haptic feedback. The widespread use of the surgical robotic platform increased exponentially, and its use expanded into other surgical procedures [2]. Currently, Intuitive Surgical (Sunnyvale, CA) is the sole producer of commercially available robotic surgical systems for general surgery that have been cleared by the US Food and Drug Administration (FDA), but other robotic surgery companies are developing competing platforms. As of early 2016, the da Vinci Si® and da Vinci Xi® are the most recent iterations of the system.

The efficacy and feasibility of robot-assisted multiport cholecystectomy have been established [3]. The surgeon may experience improved ergonomics, enhanced visualization, and improved precision through maximal instrument degrees of freedom and the elimination of tremor [4]. No published evidence has yet demonstrated the superiority of robotic multiport cholecystectomy over standard multiport cholecystectomy. Possible increased operative time, cost, and the loss of tactile feedback all need to be considered carefully when choosing this operative approach, especially during the early learning curve. Cosmetic benefit is postulated only for single-site robotic cholecystectomy; robotic multiport cholecystectomy uses the equivalent number of trocars as standard laparoscopy.

Importantly, the robotic multiport cholecystectomy is often used as an introductory operation that allows the surgeon to become familiar with and gain experience with the robotic platform prior to undertaking more complex robotically-assisted surgical procedures.

Y. Fong et al. (eds.), *The SAGES Atlas of Robotic Surgery*, https://doi.org/10.1007/978-3-319-91045-1_21

The robotic platform for laparoscopic single-incision surgery was first introduced for use with the da Vinci® robotic surgical system in 2010 (Intuitive Surgical, Sunnyvale, CA). The da Vinci Single-Site® platform was designed specifically to mitigate the challenges presented by laparoscopic single-site surgery and is the only commercially available robotic single-incision platform available at the present time. Laparoscopic single-site surgery presents significant visual and ergonomic challenges for the surgeon. Loss of triangulation of camera and instruments relative to target anatomy results in disorientation of the anatomy, difficult visualization, and instrument collisions (both intracorporeal and extracorporeal), thus increasing the level of difficulty of even simple laparoscopic tasks. The robotic single-site platform includes a multichannel port that provides access to the abdominal cavity for an 8-mm 3D high-definition laparoscope, two 5-mm curved robotic instruments, and a 5-mm assistant instrument.

The robotic instruments used in this platform are semirigid and are introduced through specifically designed curved cannulae (Fig. 21.1). The curved cannulae cross at the remote center fulcrum at the level of the abdominal wall, and the introduced semirigid instruments follow the course of the cannulae. Thus, they reestablish triangulation with respect to the camera at the target anatomy, with minimal collisions of the robotic arms.

Operating at the console, the surgeon does not experience additional ergonomic strain. In addition, the control of the robotic arms can be programmed such that the robotic right arm (left instrument on the monitor) is controlled by the surgeon's left hand. This effectively compensates for the crossed intra-abdominal instruments, and the surgeon's hand movements at the console correctly correspond to the movement of the instruments and the image on the screen [5]. Thus, the da Vinci Single-Site® platform restores intuitive control of the instruments and avoids the need to cross hands, which captures the feel of multiport laparoscopic surgery. Complex surgical tasks can be performed with significantly greater facility using this robotic single-site platform, compared with conventional single-site laparoscopy [6].

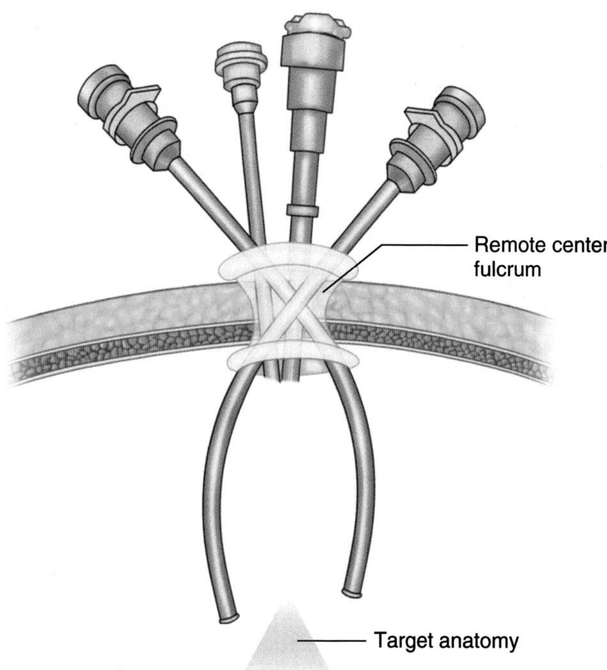

Fig. 21.1 Orientation of the da Vinci Single-Site® port and cannulae (Intuitive Surgical, Sunnyvale, CA). The curved cannulae cross at the remote center fulcrum at the level of the abdominal wall, and the flexible instruments follow the curved course of the cannulae

Preoperative Considerations

Operative indications for robotic multiport and single-incision cholecystectomy are similar to those for standard laparoscopic cholecystectomy. The indications have remained unchanged since the original NIH Consensus Development Conference Statement on Gallstones and Laparoscopic Cholecystectomy [7]. The most frequent indication for cholecystectomy is symptomatic cholelithiasis, but common indications also include biliary dyskinesia, acute and chronic cholecystitis, and complications related to choledocholithiasis. Relative contraindications to robotically-assisted multiport cholecystectomy are similar to those for standard laparoscopic cholecystectomy. These include untreated coagulopathy, a lack of equipment, a lack of surgeon expertise, dense upper abdominal adhesions, advanced cirrhosis or liver failure, and known or suspected gallbladder cancer [8].

Robotic Multiport Cholecystectomy

Room Setup

- Room setup (Fig. 21.2) will be dependent upon the robotic platform to be used. Described here are the setups for a da Vinci Si® and Xi® system. The Xi system is less dependent on the physical position of the robot and does not require the center column to be in alignment with the camera port.
- The operating room (OR) table should be positioned so that the Si® robot can be positioned over the patient's right shoulder and the anesthesiologist can still maintain access to the patient's airway and intravenous access. The Xi® system is usually positioned to the patient's left or right side with the rotation of the robot boom determining the final arm positions.

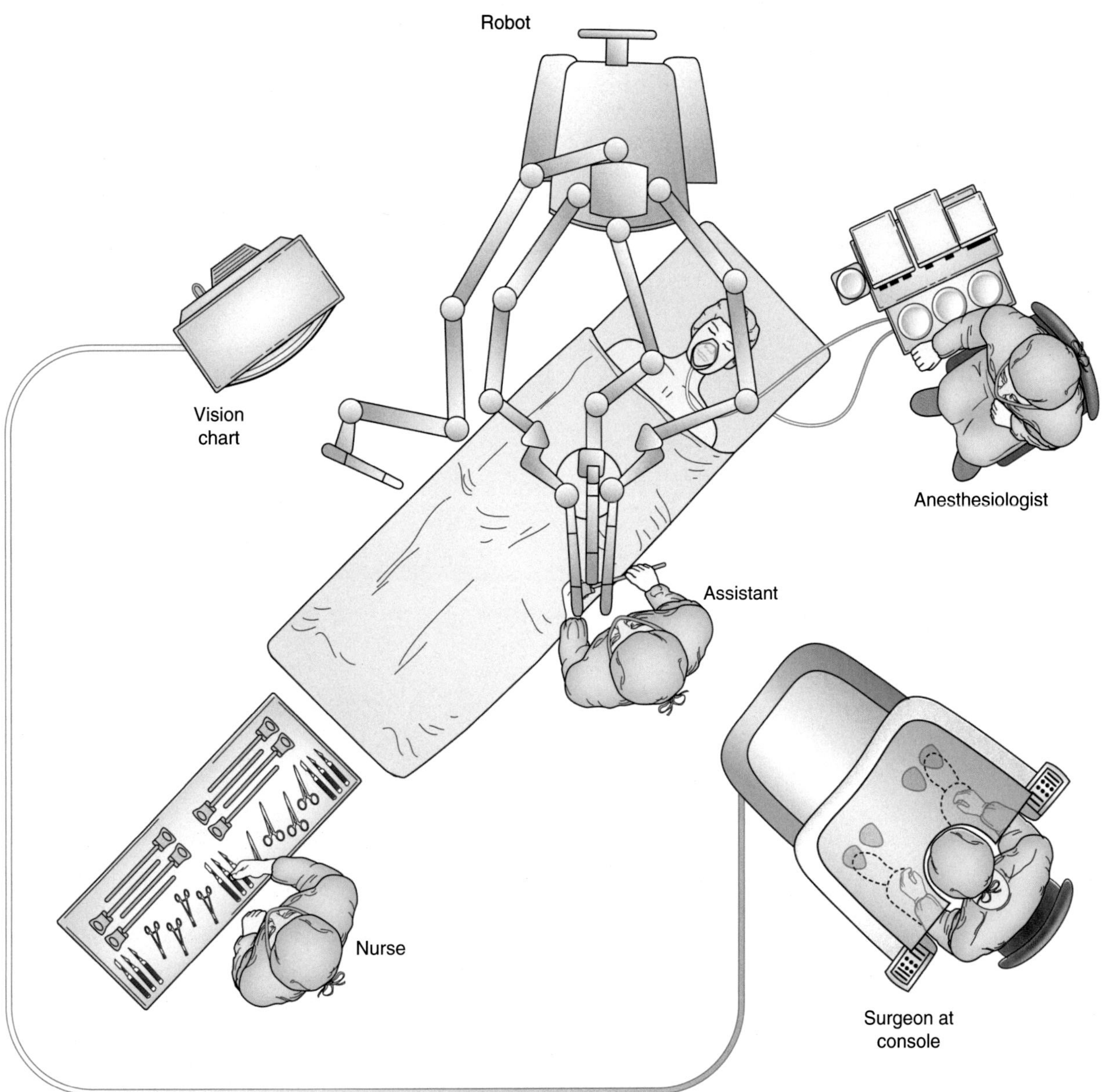

Fig. 21.2 Operative room setup for robotic cholecystectomy

- The vision tower should be positioned so that the bedside assistant has a direct line of view to the monitor. The instrument table is positioned near the patient's feet and the vision tower, to the patient's right. The bedside assistant can then position himself or herself to the patient's left, opposite the vision cart.
- The surgeon console is usually positioned to the patient's left side, with a direct line of vision to the bedside assistant.

Patient Preparation

- Supine with the right arm secured at the side. The left arm can be secured at the side or remained out.
- Reverse Trendelenburg (10–15°) with slight left table tilt.
- Sequential compression devices applied to the lower extremities.
- Standard surgical preparation of the abdomen.
- Other possibilities include urinary catheter, orogastric or nasogastric decompression, and a footboard to prevent sliding.

Port Placement

- Three to four trocars are used for Si® multiport cholecystectomy (Fig. 21.3). The 8-mm or 12-mm camera port is inserted at the umbilicus. The remaining 8-mm trocars are inserted as follows: left upper quadrant trocar (at the left midclavicular line, just inferior to the level of the falciform ligament), right upper quadrant trocar (at the right midclavicular line, 5–10 cm below the costal margin), and right upper quadrant trocar (8–10 cm lateral and inferior). If needed, an additional assistant's trocar can be inserted left of and lateral to the umbilicus, along the midclavicular line. The setup for the Xi® system is straightforward. An 8-mm trocar is placed at the umbilicus, and three additional 8-mm trocars are placed parallel to the umbilical trocar, usually two in the right lower quadrant and one in the left lower quadrant. The distance between the trocars should be 8–10 cm apart. An assistant's trocar may be placed laterally in the left lower quadrant (Fig. 21.4) if necessary.

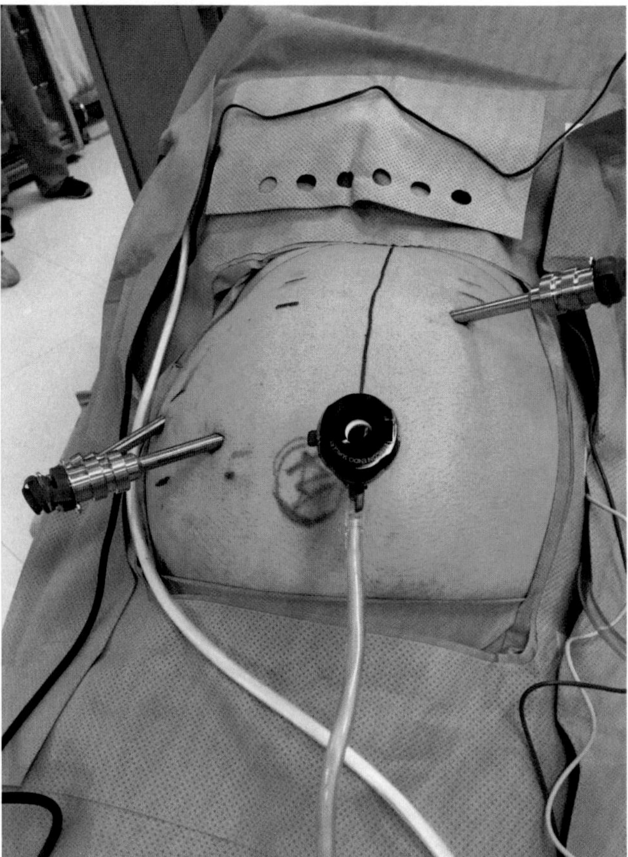

Fig. 21.3 Robotic multiport cholecystectomy trocar placement using the da Vinci Single-Si® system. The robotic camera trocar is inserted at the umbilicus. Robotic instrument trocars are then inserted in the left upper quadrant and the right upper quadrant. Note the distance from the target anatomy to account for instrument length

- In general, trocars are inserted further from the target anatomy than in standard laparoscopy because of the robotic instrument length and the need to position the robotic arms.
- Position the remote center of the cannula at the level of the peritoneum (*black band*).
- Trocars should all be placed 8–10 cm apart to avoid robotic instrument arm collisions.
- We frequently establish pneumoperitoneum to 15 mmHg via the Veress needle inserted near Palmer's point. After insufflation, direct insertion of a trocar is then performed, and the remaining robotic trocars are inserted under direct laparoscopic visualization. Hasson and direct insertion techniques may be used to gain access to the peritoneal cavity with equivalent safety [9].

Docking

- If using the Si® system, clear a path for the patient cart to approach the patient over the right shoulder (at 45°). The Xi® robot may be brought in from the patient's left or right using the targeting mechanism. Remove all lights and equipment from the intended patient cart path.
- Lower the table, and position the instrument arms to avoid collisions with the patient and equipment.
- Align the patient cart with the anatomy or according to the robot system prompts, and position the camera arm appropriately.
- Using port and arm clutch maneuvers, the Si® camera arm is attached to the umbilical trocar, instrument arm 1 is attached to the left upper quadrant trocar, instrument arm 2 is attached to the right upper quadrant trocar, and instrument arm 3 (optional) is attached to the lateral right upper quadrant trocar (Fig. 21.5). If using the Xi® system, the endoscopic camera is inserted into the umbilical trocar and attached to arm 3. Arms 1 and 2 are attached to the right lower quadrant trocars and arm 4 to the left lower quadrant trocar. The camera can also be moved to other arms/trocars on the Xi® system and the instrument arms varied accordingly.
- Instrument arms should be spaced far enough apart to avoid collisions.
- Alternatively, a 5-mm laparoscopic instrument can be utilized through a 5-mm right upper quadrant trocar in place of instrument arm 3 (or arm 1 with the Xi® system).
- With the Si® system, we use three instrument arms and use a laparoscopic instrument and port in place of instrument arm 3 only if we have additional bedside assistants to aid with retraction. If the Xi® system is used, we typically use all four arms.
- Once the system is docked, the OR table cannot be moved. Xi® innovations allow for coordinated OR table movement even when the robot is docked.

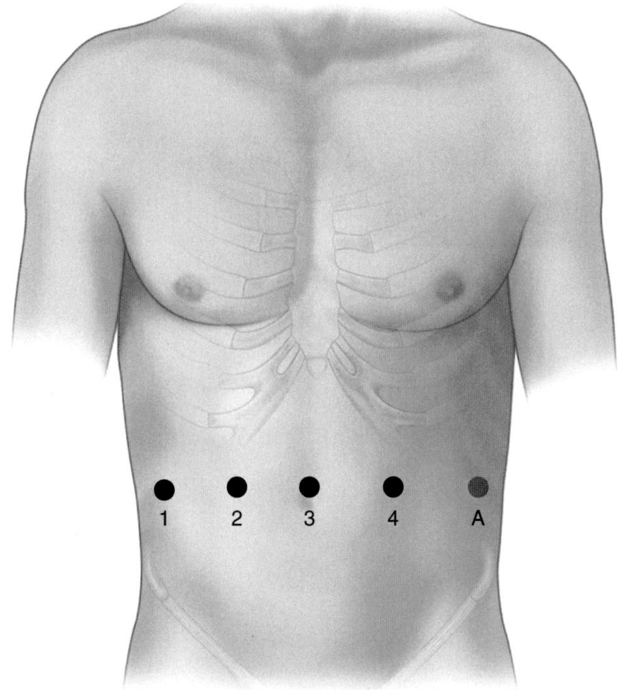

Fig. 21.4 Da Vinci Xi® robotic multiport cholecystectomy trocar placement. The trocars are inserted in parallel. They are placed at least 8 cm apart from each other. The robotic camera is usually inserted into arm 3. If an assistant trocar is used, it is usually placed in the left lower abdomen (A)

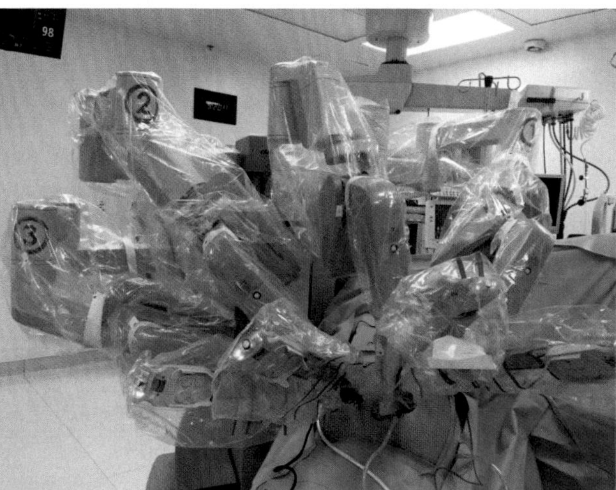

Fig. 21.5 Docked camera and instrument arms for robotic multiport cholecystectomy using the da Vinci Si® system

Instruments

- Once pneumoperitoneum is established, trocar placement is verified, and instrument arms are connected, the instruments are chosen:
  - Monopolar instruments
    Monopolar cautery with hook tip
    Monopolar cautery spatula
    Monopolar curved scissors
  - Retraction and dissection
    Cadiere forceps
    Maryland bipolar forceps
    Double-fenestrated grasper
    Grasping forceps
  - Ligation
    Medium-large clip appliers
    Scissors
  - Suction/irrigation
    EndoWrist® suction/irrigation (Intuitive Surgical)
- We regularly start the procedure using the Si® system with monopolar cautery with hook tip (instrument 1), Maryland bipolar forceps (instrument 2), and grasping forceps (instrument 3). Once we are ready to clip the cystic duct or artery, we exchange the hook electrocautery for the medium-large clip applier. Similarly with the Xi® system, we utilize two grasping forceps or Maryland bipolar forceps attached to arms 1 and 2. A hook electrocautery is attached to arm 4.

Operative Steps

- A standard cholecystectomy dissection is performed to achieve the critical view of safety [10]:
  - Initial exposure of the gallbladder
  - Wide dissection of Calot's triangle and achievement of the critical view of safety (Figs. 21.6, 21.7, 21.8, 21.9, and 21.10)
  - Intraoperative cholangiography or near-infrared cholangiography (optional)
  - Ligation and division of the cystic duct and artery
  - Gallbladder bed dissection
- To remove the gallbladder, an endoscopic retrieval bag is inserted through any trocar (upsized if needed), and the specimen is collected.
- Once the specimen is secured, the robotic instruments are removed and the arms are undocked. The trocars are removed under direct vision and the specimen is retrieved.
- The fascia is closed at the port sites if the trocar is 10 mm or larger.
- Intraoperative cholangiography can be performed either via traditional cholangiography techniques or via the integrated FireFly™ near-infrared fluorescence cholangiography (Fig. 21.10). It is best to decide preoperatively whether FireFly™ will be used, so the correct camera can be chosen and medication given before surgery.
  - Select the Firefly™-equipped (8- or 10-mm) camera and calibrate for fluorescence.
  - Inject 1.5–2 mL (3.5–5 mg) of reconstituted indocyanine green (ICG) intravenously at least 45 min prior to planned imaging of the biliary anatomy. (We do this in the anesthesia holding area.)
  - The robotic camera should be changed to near-infrared fluorescence mode (FireFly™) to image the cystic and common bile duct anatomy.

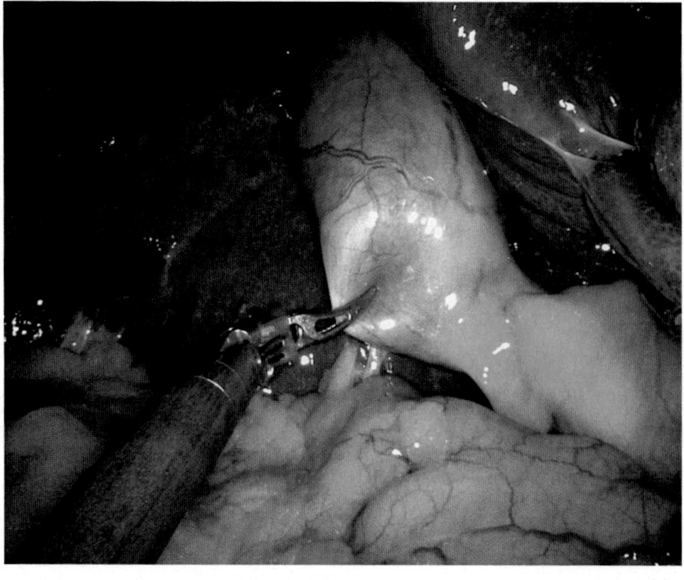

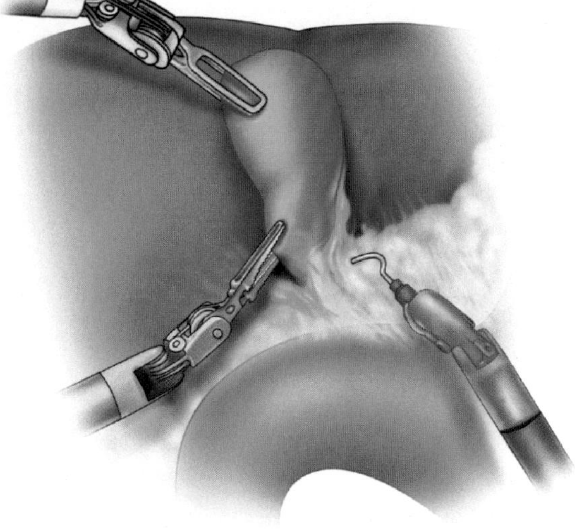

Fig. 21.6 Initial exposure of the gallbladder

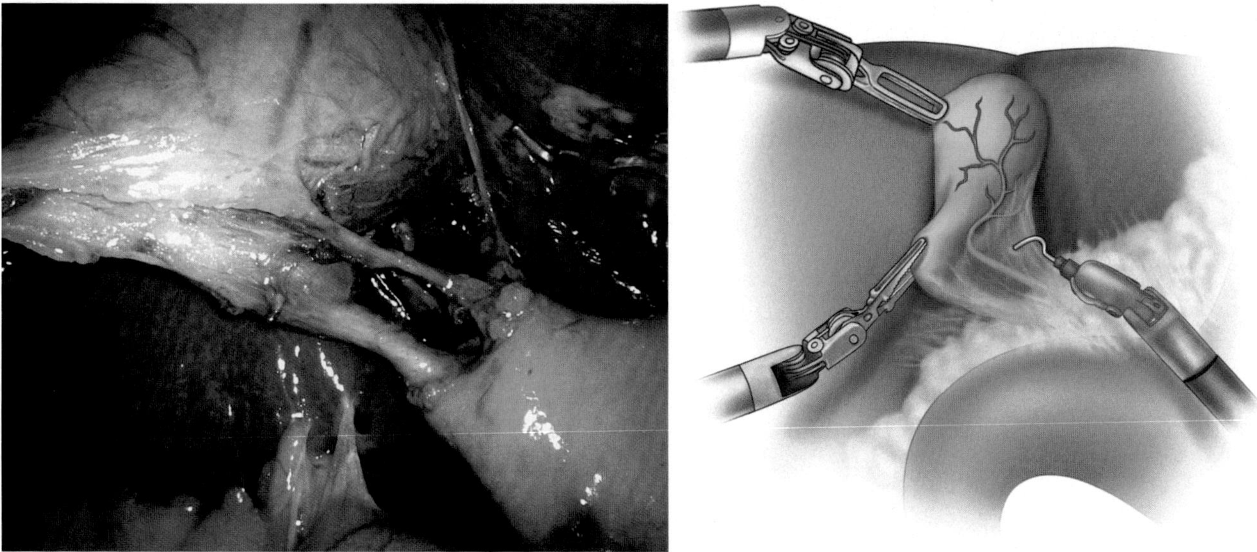

Fig. 21.7 Wide dissection of Calot's triangle and achievement of the critical view of safety

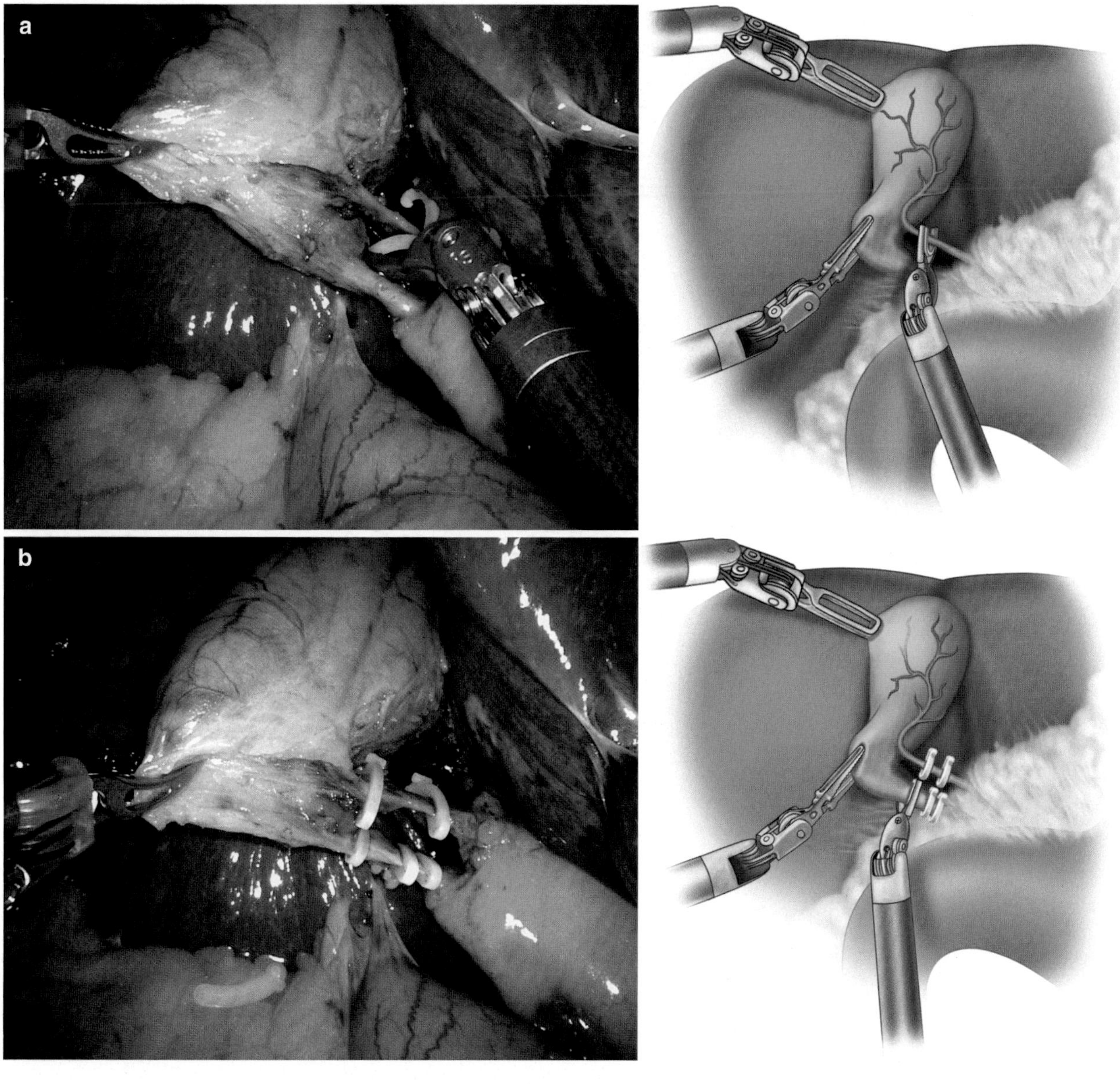

Fig. 21.8 Ligation (**a**) and division (**b**) of the cystic duct and artery

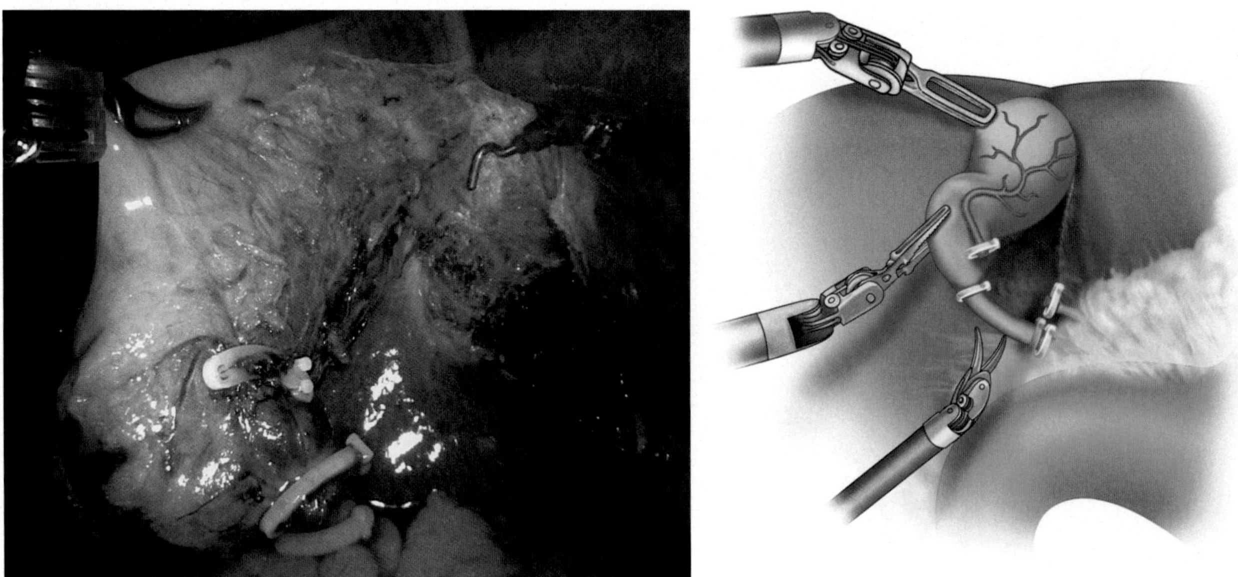

Fig. 21.9 Gallbladder dissection of the cystic plate

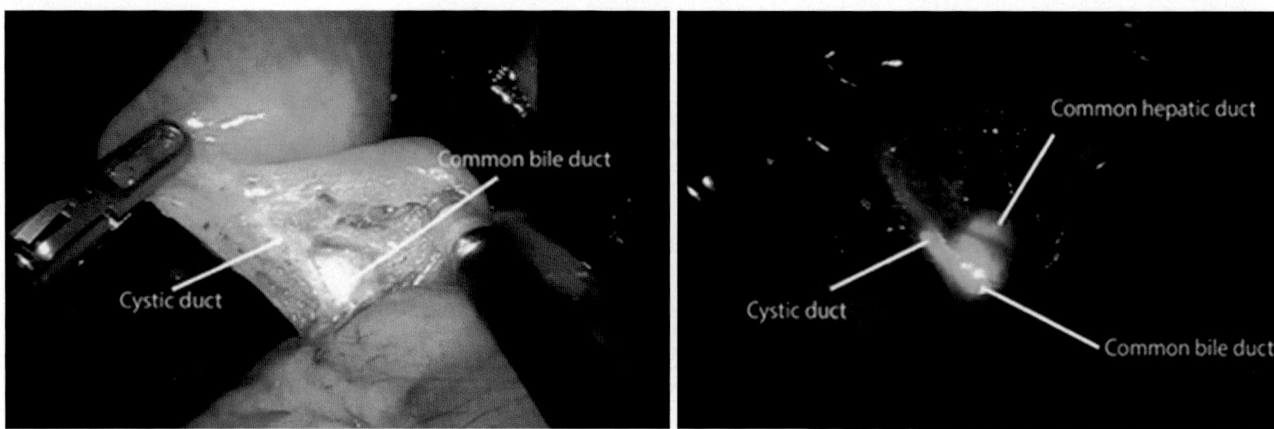

Fig. 21.10 Near-infrared fluorescence cholangiography. On the left is the normal-appearing biliary anatomy. To the right is the biliary anatomy following intravenous indocyanine green (ICG) injection and visualization via a Firefly™-equipped near-infrared fluorescence endoscopic camera

Robotic Single-Site Cholecystectomy

At the present time, single-site cholecystectomy is available only with the Si® model, but additional platforms are being developed for the Xi® with expansion of the application of the Sp single-port system (cleared by the FDA in 2014), which includes an articulating 3D HD camera and three fully articulating instruments through a single 25-mm cannula.

Room Setup

- The OR table should be positioned so that the robot can be positioned over the patient's right shoulder, and the anesthesiologist can still maintain access to the patient's airway and intravenous access.
- The vision tower should be positioned so that the bedside assistant has a direct line of view to the monitor. The instrument table is positioned near the patient's feet and the vision tower, to the patient's right. The bedside assistant can then position himself or herself to the patient's left, opposite the vision cart.
- The surgeon console is usually positioned to the patient's left side with a direct line of vision to the bedside assistant.

Patient Preparation

- Patient placed supine on bed, arms tucked (left arm may remain out) and secured safely.
- Reverse Trendelenburg (10–15°) with slight left table tilt.
- Sequential compression devices and standard surgical preparation of the abdomen.
- After induction of anesthesia, the surgeon can determine the need for a urinary catheter, orogastric or nasogastric tube, and antibiotic prophylaxis.

Port Placement and Docking

- A Single-Site® silicone port (Fig. 21.11) is inserted at the umbilicus. This port contains insertion sites for an 8-mm trocar (robotic endoscope), two 5-mm curved trocars (instruments), and a 5-mm assistant trocar.
- To insert the Single-Site® port, a transumbilical incision 2–2.5 cm in length is performed and carried down to the midline fascia; it may be necessary to transect the umbilical stalk.
- Enter through the fascia carefully, and use a finger to check for and sweep away any underlying intra-abdominal adhesions. Then extend the fascial incision to

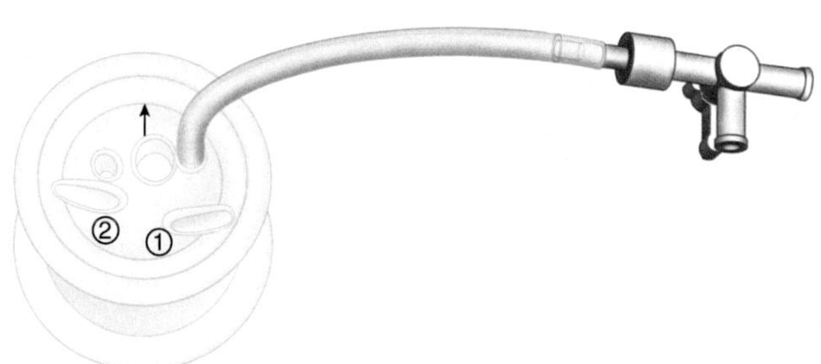

Fig. 21.11 Single-Site® silicone port. This contains insertion sites for an 8-mm port for the robotic endoscope, two 5-mm curved ports (1 and 2), and a 5-mm assistant port. Pneumoperitoneum is maintained via the attached insufflation tubing

2.5 cm. Creating a larger fascial incision may result in slipping of the port into or out of the abdomen and will create difficulty in maintaining a pneumatic seal.

- Inspect the silicone port; clamp using an atraumatic clamp just below the lower rim, being sure not to clamp the insufflation barb.
- Dip the port in saline or water to facilitate ease of port placement. (*Never* use a water-soluble lubricant like KY Jelly or Surgilube.)
- Using a small retractor, gently place the port into the abdomen (Fig. 21.12); carefully remove the retractor and clamp without withdrawing the port.
- Align the pre-marked arrow on the top of the port by rotating the port within the incision to target the gallbladder location.
- Attach the insufflation tubing to the insufflation port with a three-way stopcock and insufflate to 12–15 mm Hg. After insufflation, check to ensure that the port is in good position and flush against the abdominal wall.

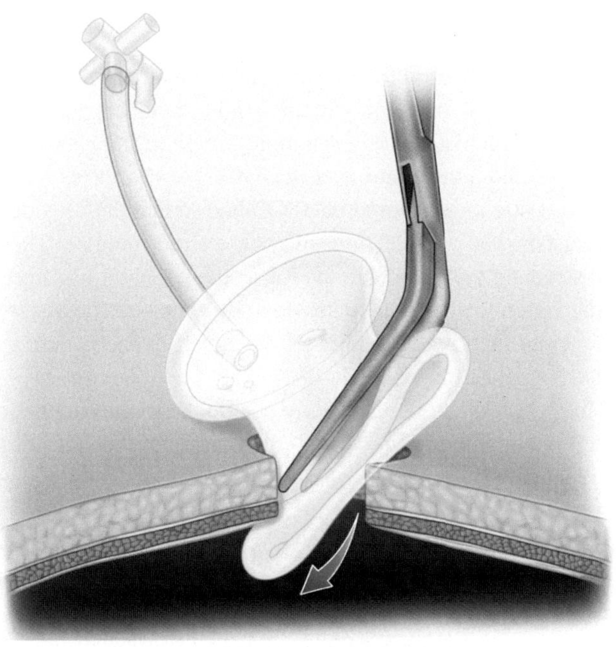

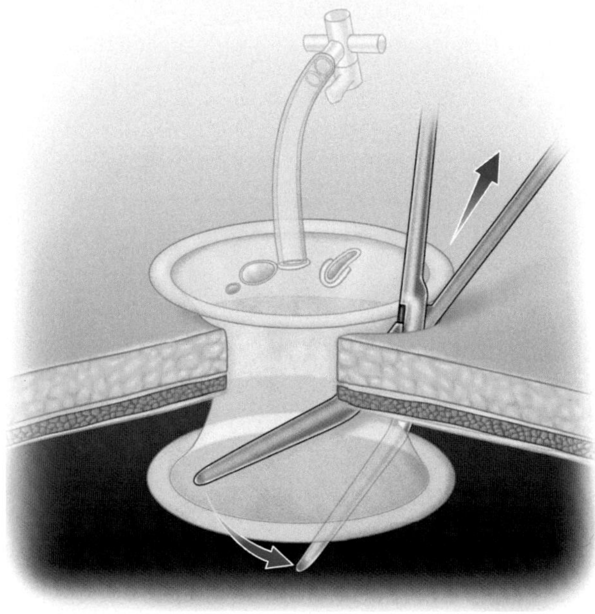

Fig. 21.12 Insertion of the robotic Single-Site® port. An atraumatic clamp is used to guide the lower portion of the port beneath the fascia. Saline or water may facilitate insertion

- Place an 8-mm camera trocar and the 5-mm assistant trocar into the designated trocar sites.
- Using a 0-degree or 30-degree down robotic endoscope, inspect the anatomy and readjust the position of the table appropriately.
- Grasp the gallbladder with a laparoscopic grasper through the 5-mm assistant trocar, and check for mobility and whether an adequate anatomic view has been achieved; adjust the table if necessary to achieve the best view. (Avoid excessive reverse Trendelenburg, which will create difficulty by bringing the operative anatomy too close to the instruments.) Remove the assistant trocar (to be replaced after docking; see below).
- The robot should be arranged so that the camera arm is aligned with the center column, and instrument arms 1 and 2 have straight setup joints (Fig. 21.13). Instrument arm 3 is not used for this procedure and should be secured out of the way.
- Clear a path for the patient cart to approach the patient over the right shoulder (at 45°). Remove all lights and equipment from the intended patient cart path.
- Bring the camera arm in alignment with the camera trocar and target anatomy, and dock.
- After lubricating the two curved cannulae with water or saline, first dock instrument arm 2, followed by instrument arm 1. Care must be taken to follow the trocar with the camera at all times, to avoid unintended visceral injury. Use of the dock assist device can help facilitate arm docking.
- Replace the 5-mm assistant trocar and have the bedside assistant grasp the gallbladder fundus and retract superiorly.
- Once the gallbladder is retracted, the camera must then be positioned to visualize the target anatomy.

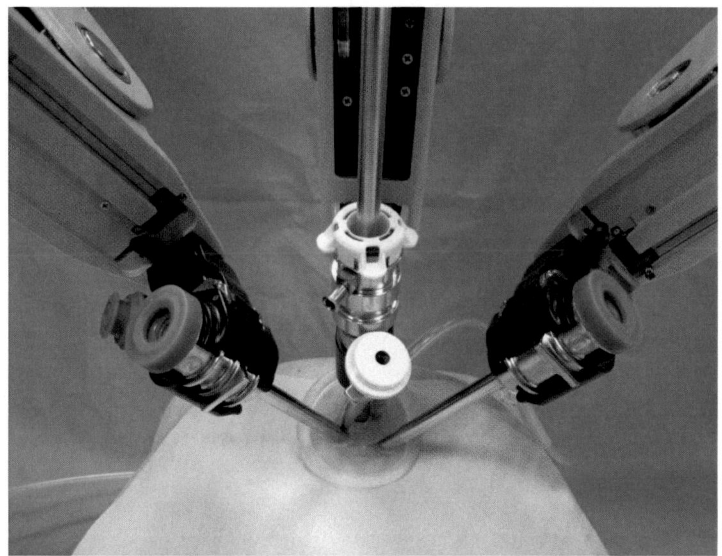
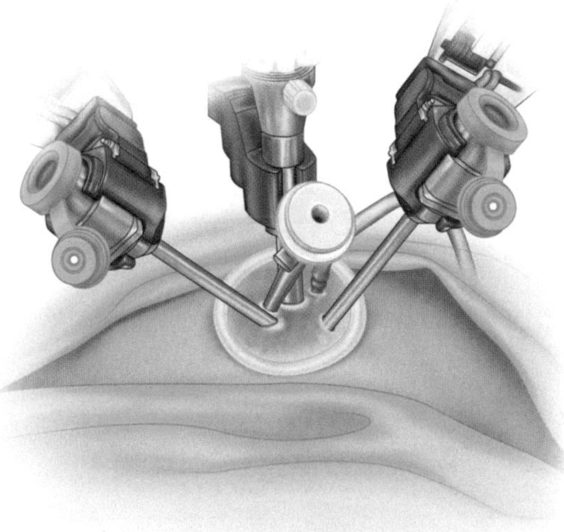

Fig. 21.13 Appearance of robot docked to trocars in a Single-Site® port

Instruments

- Instrument choices are specific to the Single-Site® platform. They consist of non-wristed, flexible-shaft instruments that fit through the curved cannulae.
- Examples include:
  - Monopolar cautery hook
  - Maryland dissector
  - Curved scissors
  - Cadiere forceps
  - Crocodile forceps
  - Hem-o-lok® clip applier
  - Suction irrigator
- To begin, a grasping instrument (Cadiere or crocodile forceps) is attached to instrument arm 1, and a monopolar cautery hook or Maryland grasper is attached to instrument arm 2. The robotic interface will then automatically set arm 1 to be the screen left instrument, even though it is on the patient's left, and arm 2 to screen right, so that movements are intuitive (Fig. 21.14).

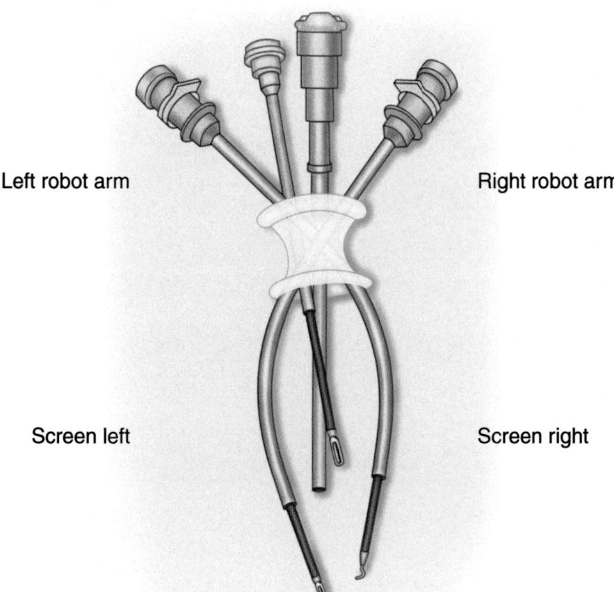

Fig. 21.14 Robotic single-site port with inserted curved cannulae and nonrigid instruments. The right robot arm controls the instrument on the left of the screen and vice versa, but the robotic interface can then be set, so the surgeon's left hand controls the right robot arm and thus the intuitive left side of the screen

Operative Steps

- A standard cholecystectomy dissection is performed to achieve the critical view of safety [10].
- A Hem-o-lok® clip applier is inserted and clips are used to ligate the duct and artery. Curved scissors are then used to transect (Fig. 21.15).
- The gallbladder is then removed from the liver bed by a standard approach, and the area is inspected to ensure hemostasis. The assistant port is replaced with a 10-mm port to allow the introduction of an endoscopic retrieval bag.
- The gallbladder is placed in the endoscopic retrieval bag, and the operative field is inspected. A suction irrigator can be replaced through either curved cannula.
- The robotic instrument arms are then undocked. The curved trocars are removed under direct vision.
- After removing the camera, the silicone port, the remaining trocars, and the gallbladder specimen are removed.
- The umbilical fascia defect is closed with interrupted 0-Vicryl suture, the umbilicus is tacked down to the fascia if necessary, and the skin closed with absorbable subcuticular suture.

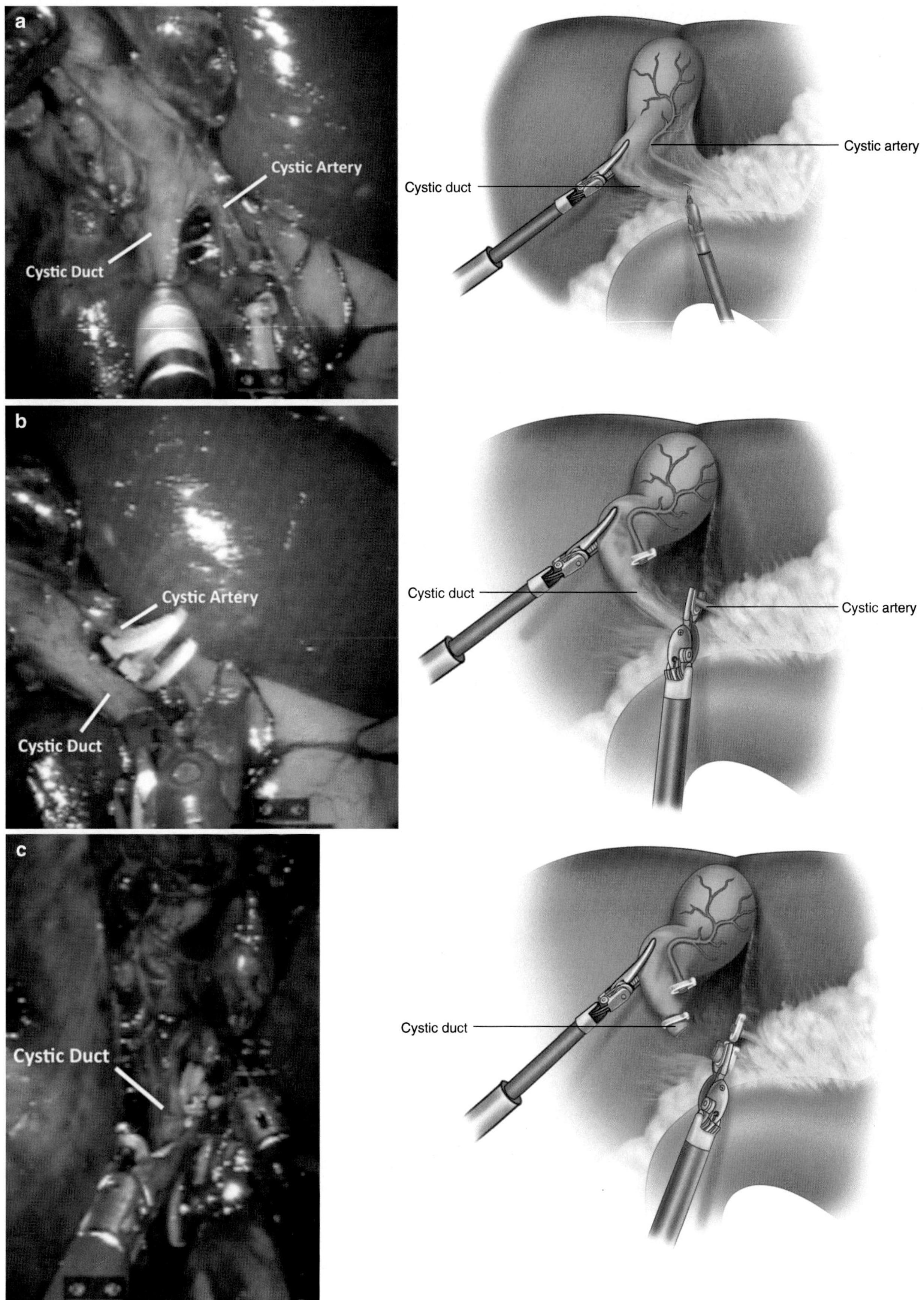

Fig. 21.15 Cholecystectomy performed using the da Vinci Single-Site® system. (**a**) Identification of the cystic duct and cystic artery. (**b**, **c**) Plastic clips are applied and the cystic duct and artery are ligated

Procedure-Specific Complications

The establishment of abdominal access and safe facilitation of trocar placement is paramount to the application of minimally invasive surgery, including robotic multiport cholecystectomy. If not performed carefully, serious visceral and vascular injury can occur. There is no difference in the safety of open versus closed-entry technique to establish abdominal access [9]. The choice of entry should be directed by the surgeon's training and skill and patient characteristics. We commonly employ a closed-entry technique using either a Veress needle inserted in the left upper quadrant or an optical trocar inserted at the umbilicus. A high index of suspicion and immediate recognition of access injuries is crucial to treat any associated complications.

Common bile duct injuries are serious complications that may arise in minimally invasive cholecystectomy. The current accepted rate of major bile duct injury during cholecystectomy is 0.1–0.6%. Surgeon experience, patient age, male sex, and the degree of inflammation all affect the identification of biliary anatomy [8]. Misidentification of the biliary duct is the most common reason for major bile duct injury, and we believe obtaining a "critical view of safety" is just as important in robotically-assisted multiport cholecystectomy as it is in standard laparoscopic cholecystectomy. The critical view of safety has three requirements [10]:

1. The triangle of Calot is cleared of fat and fibrous tissue.
2. The lowest portion of the gallbladder must be separated from the cystic plate.
3. Only two structures should be seen entering the gallbladder.

Once these three requirements are met, the "critical view of safety" has been obtained.

Intraoperative cholangiography can aid in identifying biliary anatomy and help to improve injury recognition, using either standard cholangiography techniques or ICG near-infrared cholangiography. Using the integrated near-infrared endoscopic visualization system in either robotic multiport or single-site cholecystectomy, real-time visualization of the biliary anatomy can occur. To do so, ICG (3.5–5 mg reconstituted), which is excreted in bile, is injected 45 minutes prior to planned imaging. In robotic single-site cholecystectomy, ICG near-infrared fluorescent cholangiography is especially useful and can be incorporated into the surgeon's armamentarium. Standard cholangiography can be technically difficult in the setting of single-site surgery, and the integrated near-infrared technique allows visualization of the biliary anatomy without additional access sites. Near-infrared cholangiography is well documented in single-site cholecystectomy [11, 12]. We exercise caution in interpreting near-infrared cholangiography anatomy in obese patients and those with significant inflammation, as biliary anatomy often can be difficult to discern.

Avoiding equipment malfunction is also important to a successful operation. During trocar placement, it is important to place trocars 8–10 cm apart to avoid external instrument and robotic arm collisions. Identifying the "sweet spot" of the robotic camera arm and positioning the arms to allow for maximal arm movement will decrease the need to reposition the robotic arms during the operation. One should also keep the robotic instrumentation within the visual field at all times. Instruments are followed from insertion at the trocar site to the position in the operative field. Failure to do so may result in inadvertent visceral injury.

Lastly, care should be exercised in closure of trocar sites and transumbilical incisions. Hernia rates range from 2% to more than 15%, depending on patient factors such as obesity, age, and medical conditions. Meticulous attention should be given to fascial closure to prevent future incisional hernias.

Postoperative Care

Similar to standard laparoscopy, robotic multiport cholecystectomy can generally be performed as an outpatient or short-stay (<24 h) procedure. Typical postoperative care instructions are given. These include removal of dressings, bathing instructions, and routine weight-lifting restrictions. Return precautions include fever, jaundice, worsening abdominal pain, abdominal distension, persistent nausea or vomiting, and problems with bowel or bladder function. The patient is usually seen 1–2 weeks postoperatively in the outpatient setting and can be followed based on the surgeons' standard practice.

Costs, Adoption, and Training

Intuitive Surgical (Sunnyvale, CA) is currently the only provider of surgical robotic systems. The initial or fixed cost for the platform ranges from $1 million to $2.5 million per unit [13]. The yearly costs for additional consumables and yearly maintenance for the platform can be greater than $125,000 [14]. The financial burden that is associated with implementation of the robot is real, but the true financial burden is a topic of debate. In healthcare systems that have already obtained the robotic platform and have the robotic infrastructure in place, cost-containment strategies involving minimizing instrument use and OR time utilization create a favorable financial picture for robotically-assisted cholecystectomy [14, 15].

Other approaches to single-site robotic surgery are in development. The SPIDER (Single-Port Instrument Delivery Extended Research) device (TransEnterix, Research Triangle Park, NC) has been designed to improve the laparoscopic single-site surgical environment with re-approximation of triangulated instruments and camera. It has been shown to be safe and intuitive in single-port cholecystectomy [16]. As a consequence, a robotically-assisted device employing the SPIDER system with the surgeon at the bedside, the SurgiBot™, was developed with the potential of an additional future platform for robotic single-site surgery [17]. No data is yet available for its implementation in human surgery.

The learning curve for robotic multiport cholecystectomy is relatively short; proficiency may be reached in 20–30 cases [3]. The time to complete the procedure is dependent upon setup of the robotic instrumentation, operative time, and wound closure. Setup time in both multiport and single-site approaches improves with familiarity with the instrumentation and docking; the operative time similarly also decreases [18–20]. Robotic multiport cholecystectomy is a common general-surgery procedure that can provide the basic robot platform training as a step toward completing more complex robotic procedures.

The ability of the robotic platform to overcome the technical limitations of laparoscopic single-site surgery is reflected in a short learning curve for the single-site cholecystectomy. However, insertion of additional laparoscopic trocars, reported in fewer than 10% of single-site robotic cholecystectomies, can be used to avoid conversion to multiport laparoscopy or open surgery [20, 21].

Training in robotic cholecystectomy may be provided through industry-sponsored training, direct observation, and case proctoring. Surgical residency training programs have begun integrating robotic surgical training into their curriculum, and the robotic multiport cholecystectomy is a useful procedure to introduce residents to the robotic platform.

References

1. Himpens J, Leman G, Cadiere GB. Telesurgical laparoscopic cholecystectomy. Surg Endosc. 1998;12:1091.
2. Hughes-Hallett A, Mayer EK, Marcus HJ, Cundy TP, Pratt PJ, Parston G, et al. Quantifying innovation in surgery. Ann Surg. 2014;260:205–11.
3. Vidovszky TJ, Smith W, Ghosh J, Ali MR. Robotic cholecystectomy: learning curve, advantages, and limitations. J Surg Res. 2006;136:172–8.
4. Miller DW, Schlinkert RT, Schlinkert DK. Robot-assisted laparoscopic cholecystectomy: initial Mayo Clinic Scottsdale experience. Mayo Clin Proc. 2004;79:1132–6.
5. Wren SM, Curet MJ. Single-port robotic cholecystectomy: results from a first human use clinical study of the new da Vinci single-site surgical platform. Arch Surg. 2011;146:1122–7.
6. Eisenberg D, Vidovszky TJ, Lau J, Guiroy B, Rivas H. Comparison of robotic and laparoendoscopic single-site surgery systems in a suturing and knot tying task. Surg Endosc. 2013;27:3182–6.
7. NIH releases consensus statement on gallstones, bile duct stones and laparoscopic cholecystectomy. Am Fam Physician. 1992;46:1571–4.
8. SAGES. Guidelines for the clinical application of laparoscopic biliary tract surgery. 2010. http://www.sages.org/publications/guidelines/guidelines-for-the-clinical-application-of-laparoscopic-biliary-tract-surgery. Accessed 4 Nov 4 2015. 2013 Jun 24:1–30.
9. Ahmad G, O'Flynn H, Duffy JMN, Phillips K, Watson A. Laparoscopic entry techniques. Cochrane Database Syst Rev. 2012;2:CD006583.
10. Strasberg SM, Brunt LM. Rationale and use of the critical view of safety in laparoscopic cholecystectomy. J Am Coll Surg. 2010;211:132–8.
11. Ishizawa T, Kaneko J, Inoue Y, Takemura N, Seyama Y, Aoki T, et al. Application of fluorescent cholangiography to single-incision laparoscopic cholecystectomy. Surg Endosc. 2011;25:2631–6.
12. Spinoglio G, Priora F, Bianchi PP, Lucido FS, Licciardello A, Maglione V, et al. Real-time near-infrared (NIR) fluorescent cholangiography in single-site robotic cholecystectomy (SSRC): a single-institutional prospective study. Surg Endosc. 2012;27:2156–62.
13. Barbash GI, Glied SA. New technology and health care costs--the case of robot-assisted surgery. N Engl J Med. 2010;363:701–4.
14. Rosemurgy A, Ryan C, Klein R, Sukharamwala P, Wood T, Ross S. Does the cost of robotic cholecystectomy translate to a financial burden? Surg Endosc. 2015;29:2115–20.
15. Bedeir K, Mann A, Youssef Y. Robotic single-site versus laparoscopic cholecystectomy: which is cheaper? A cost report and analysis. Surg Endosc. 2016;30(1):267–72.
16. Pryor AD, Tushar JR, DiBernardo LR. Single-port cholecystectomy with the TransEnterix SPIDER: simple and safe. Surg Endosc. 2010;24:917–23.
17. Wiyandini JR. A framework to determine the potential for success of new medical robotic products: assessment by Cooper Scoring Model and TOPSIS analysis. 2014. http://purl.utwente.nl/essays/65837. Accessed 4 Nov 2015.
18. Nelson EC, Gottlieb AH, Müller H-G, Smith W, Ali MR, Vidovszky TJ. Robotic cholecystectomy and resident education: the UC Davis experience. Int J Med Robotics Comput Assist Surg. 2013;10:218–22.
19. Spinoglio G, Lenti LM, Maglione V, Lucido FS, Priora F, Bianchi PP, et al. Single-site robotic cholecystectomy (SSRC) versus single-incision laparoscopic cholecystectomy (SILC): comparison of learning curves. First European experience. Surg Endosc. 2011;26:1648–55.
20. Ayloo S, Choudhury N. Single-site robotic cholecystectomy. JSLS. 2014;18:e2014.00266. https://doi.org/10.4293/JSLS.2014.00266.
21. Konstantinidis KM, Hirides P, Hirides S, Chrysocheris P, Georgiou M. Cholecystectomy using a novel single-site(®) robotic platform: early experience from 45 consecutive cases. Surg Endosc. 2012;26:2687–94.

Colectomy

22

Kurt Melstrom

Introduction

A colectomy, removing a section of the colon, is based on the blood supply that feeds that segment. Colectomies, therefore, are broadly grouped into right-sided colectomies (right hemicolectomy, transverse colectomy) and left-sided colectomies (left hemicolectomy, sigmoidectomy). Colectomies are traditionally performed through an open, midline incision, but the open procedure results in a long incision that leads to a long recovery. Robotic colon surgery is a new technique that allows the surgeon to perform surgery through smaller incisions, with a magnified view and improved dexterity. This chapter describes the standard approach to a right colectomy and a left colectomy. Patient positioning, port placement, and the key steps of the operation are all highlighted.

Background

Since its introduction to colon surgery in the early 2000s, the robotic approach has been gaining in use and popularity. The potential advantages of general robotic surgery have been well advertised. These include a three-dimensional view of the operative field, improved magnification, and motion scaling. Other advantages include more independence from surgical assistants. The surgeon controls the camera, and it remains stable when not being moved. The robot also has a third arm for retraction, which helps the operating surgeon provide his or her own traction without instruction.

Perhaps the greatest advantage is the multiple degrees of freedom of the instruments, which allow for better handling as compared to straight laparoscopic instruments. Because of these reasons, the robot has been adapted to operations in narrow and tight cavities where precision is needed, such as the pelvis. Consequently, colorectal surgeons have utilized the robot most often for rectal surgery and low anterior resections. A colon resection, on the other hand, is not performed in a small space but encompasses a rather large working space. In addition, suturing is limited in colon surgery. Therefore the use of robotics has not been as widely adopted for colon surgery as for rectal surgery, but with the introduction of the da Vinci Xi® robotic system (Intuitive Surgical, Sunnyvale, CA), operating in multiple abdominal quadrants has been simplified, and more and more surgeons are adopting robotics for all colon and rectal surgery.

This chapter presents the step-by-step techniques of a standardized robotic right colon resection [1]. The description of a robotic left/sigmoid colon resection will follow [2]. Conventional preoperative and postoperative considerations will be highlighted. Finally, outcomes from the multitude of small robotic colectomy trials are discussed.

Indications

The indications for robotic colon surgery should parallel those of laparoscopic surgery. The most common indication is carcinoma of the right, left, or sigmoid colon. Although diverticulitis was once thought to be a contraindication for minimally invasive surgery, such surgery is now commonplace. Inflammatory bowel disease is another common colorectal disease that can be operated on with the robot.

Patients who have had multiple abdominal operations are most likely not a great match for robotics. Certainly, a diagnostic laparoscopy can be performed to start, but multiple abdominal wall and intraloop adhesions will render a robotic approach infeasible. Obesity is not a contraindication, but the working space is greatly reduced. This is especially true in men with a large amount of intraabdominal adiposity. It is probably not wise to proceed with a robotic surgery if the pedicles cannot be properly exposed. Finally, there is currently no role for robotics in an emergent setting, save for repair of a colonoscopic perforation in a prepped patient.

K. Melstrom, MD
City of Hope National Medical Center, Duarte, CA, USA
e-mail: kmelstrom@coh.org

Y. Fong et al. (eds.), *The SAGES Atlas of Robotic Surgery*, https://doi.org/10.1007/978-3-319-91045-1_22

Preoperative Preparation

There are no specific variations in the preoperative process for robotic versus laparoscopic or open surgery. The only exception would be full disclosure to the patient about the robotic technique and its potential advantages and disadvantages. A full oncologic work-up is standard, including colonoscopy, carcinoembryonic antigen (CEA) level, and CT scan of the chest, abdomen, and pelvis. A general preoperative clearance is also necessary, with a cardiac work-up when indicated. For small lesions, it is vital that the tumor is marked preoperatively with tattooing via colonoscope. Any variation or abnormality in the colonoscopy report should prompt the surgeon to perform another colonoscopy personally to confirm the findings. Enhanced recovery after surgery (ERAS) guidelines should be utilized. When coupled with robotic surgery, the length of stay is significantly reduced. Bowel preparations are optional, but preoperative antibiotics and deep vein thrombosis prophylaxis are a must.

Robotic Right Colectomy

Patient and Robot Positioning

The patient should be placed in a low lithotomy position with the arms tucked at the patient's side. There is no contraindication to keeping the patient supine, but this position helps to keep the patient from moving and allows the surgeon to operate between the legs on the rare occasion when that is needed. It is important that all pressure points are properly padded. The patient should have some form of immobilization. This could be foam padding on the table, inflatable bean bags, shoulder harnesses, or a chest strap. Special precautions should be taken with obese patients, as they tend to move more during surgery. The robot should come in from the right side, either straight on or from the patient's right shoulder (Fig. 22.1). Variations in the robot placement depend on the robotic model, operating room setup, and surgeon preference.

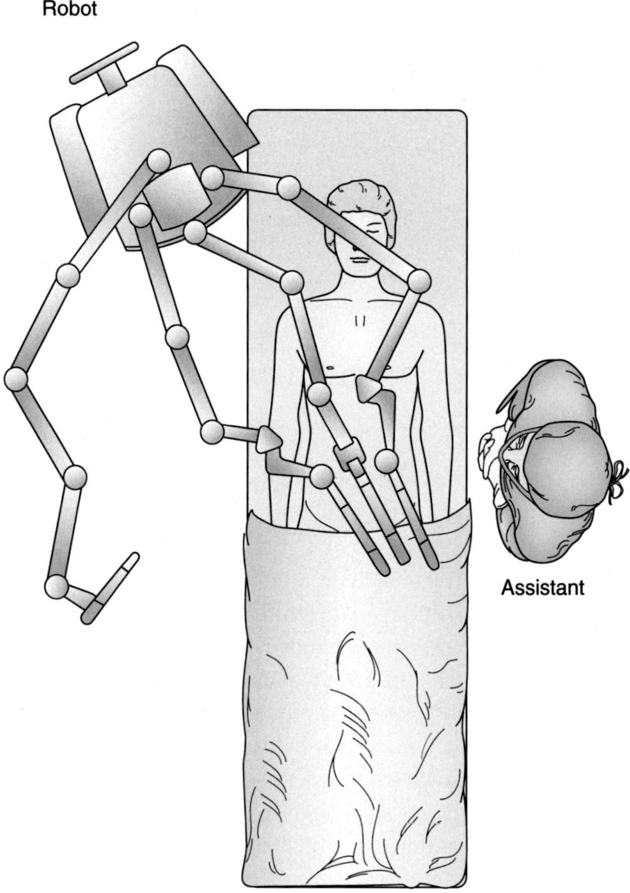

Fig. 22.1 Right colectomy docking setup. The robot should be docked over the right shoulder of the patient at a 45-degree angle

Port Placement and Instruments

Pneumoperitoneum is established via the Veress needle or the Hasson technique, at any of the proposed port sites, Palmer's point, or at the umbilicus. There are many variations to port placement. These should follow standard laparoscopic trocar placement with some exceptions. Specimen extraction through a Pfannenstiel incision would require a suprapubic port. The standard port placement for a robotic right colon surgery with intracorporeal anastomosis with da Vinci® Si model (Intuitive Surgical, Sunnyvale, CA) is shown in Fig. 22.2a. Robotic 8-mm

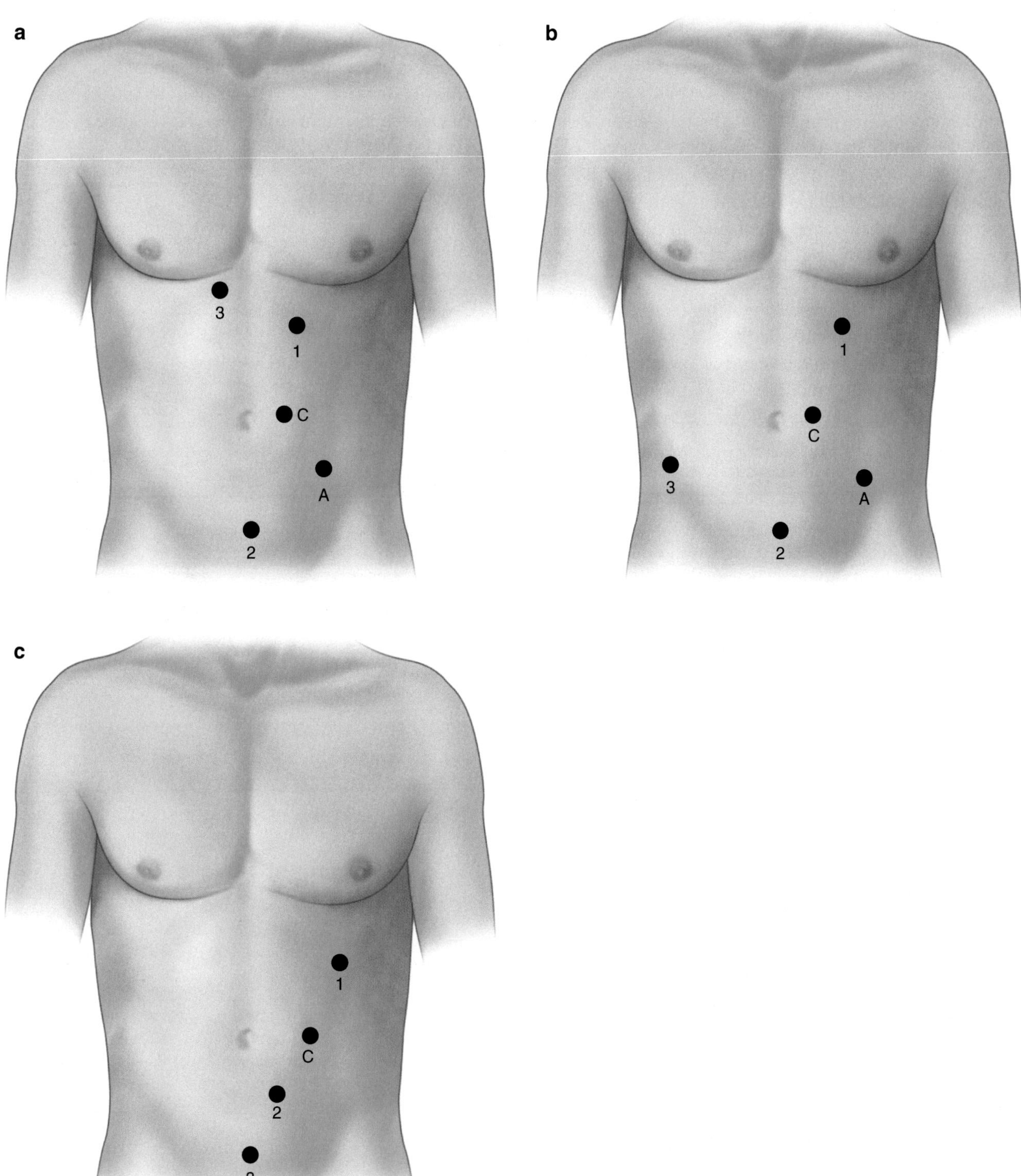

Fig. 22.2 Right colectomy port placement. Trocars: 1, arm 1; 2, arm 2; 3, arm 3; C, camera; A, assistant. (**a**) Standard port placement for a right colectomy. (**b**) Alternative port placement with arm 3 directly over the ascending colon. (**c**) Port placement when using the da Vinci Xi® system (Intuitive Surgical, Sunnyvale, CA)

trocars are used throughout. A 12-mm trocar should be used for trocar 1 to allow the use of the robotic stapler. Trocar 3 is the retraction arm and can be placed just to the right of the subxiphoid space. An alternative would be to place it in the right mid-abdomen (Fig. 22.2b). There should be an average of 6–8 cm between ports to avoid arm clashing. The assistant port should be a standard 10-mm trocar to allow the easy passage of needles if suturing. The da Vinci Xi® robotic system has a different setup. The ports should be placed in a straight line starting at the suprapubic port and travelling cranially toward the left midclavicular line (Fig. 22.2c). Finally, a single-port setup is an option through the umbilicus. A single-site port is placed, and the camera and two arms are used in the single-site port [3]. This placement requires crossing of instruments and switching the hand controls for arms 1 and 2. The left arm will be controlled with the right hand and vice versa.

Trocar 1 should be for the right hand. It should be a monopolar instrument, generally the hook or scissors. This will be replaced later with the vessel sealer and the stapler. Trocar 2 is for the left hand. It should be a bipolar instrument, either the Maryland dissector, fenestrated bipolar, or PK dissecting instrument. Trocar 3 is for retraction and can be the Cadiere or small grasping retractor. The camera can be 0-degree or 30-degree. The assistant should use a bowel grasper for retraction and the suction irrigator when necessary. The table will need to be tilted toward the patient's left side and should be in Trendelenburg position, allowing the small bowel to fall into the left upper quadrant. For the da Vinci Xi® system, the setup should be lower abdominal, and the target should be the ascending colon or hepatic flexure.

Ileocolic Pedicle Isolation and Ligation

The procedure begins by ensuring that all omentum and small bowel are out of the way and then identifying the ileocolic pedicle. Gentle retraction near the ligament of Treves will tent the pedicle. Dissection should then be performed just beneath the pedicle to open the space into the retroperitoneum. Early identification of the duodenum is key; it is mobilized away from the pedicle. A rent should be made in the mesentery above the pedicle, and it should be cleaned of all overlying fat (Fig. 22.3). The pedicle should then be divided close to its origin with either the vessel sealer or the white load stapler.

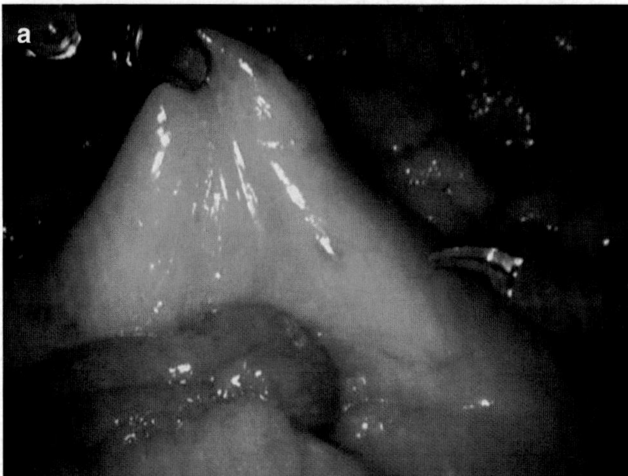

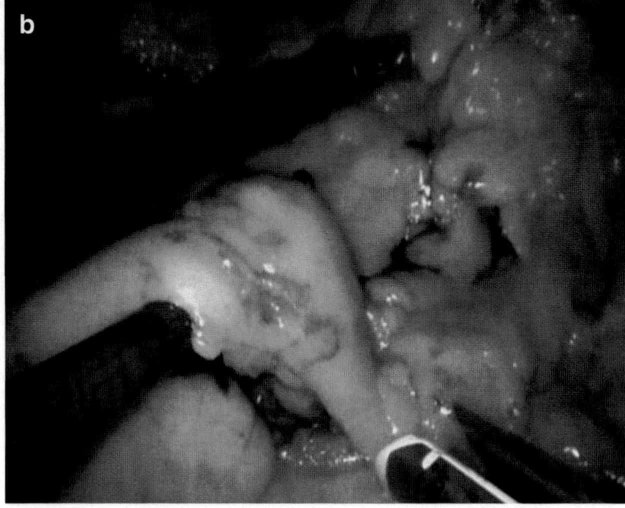

Fig. 22.3 Ileocolic pedicle. (**a**) The mesentery is tented upward, revealing the ileocolic pedicle coursing from the superior mesenteric artery. (**b**) The ileocolic pedicle has been isolated and mobilized away from the underlying duodenum. It is now ready for ligation

Mobilization of the Right Colon

Retraction is then placed on the cut pedicle, and medial-to-lateral mobilization of the right colon is performed. It is helpful to use the elbows or wrists of the vessel sealer and arm 2 to accomplish this gentile, blunt mobilization, which should be taken to the right abdominal wall laterally, inferiorly beyond the cecum, superiorly as far as possible, and medially just to the start of the pancreatic head. The cecum is then retracted medially, and the already dissected space usually can be seen as a purple discoloration. This should be incised to mobilize the cecum. The dissection is then carried out superiorly along the lateral attachments of the right colon. This dissection is made much easier by a full mobilization medially first. Once the hepatic flexure is reached, the mobilization is complete.

Hepatic Flexure Mobilization

The hepatic flexure is mobilized by first grasping the omentum with the third arm. The assistant can then retract the colon inferiorly by grasping an epiploic appendage. The omentum can then be removed from the transverse colon, allowing visualization of the gastrocolic ligaments. Again, the prior mobilization might be readily identified through the attachments. The ligament should be taken down, advancing laterally until the colon is completely mobile. Visualization of the duodenum usually indicates a sufficient mobilization.

Specimen Resection

The next step is to divide the mesentery. The cut ileocolic pedicle is grasped and retracted medially and superiorly. The ileal mesentery is then divided just medial to the pedicle to a proposed terminal ileum resection site approximately 5–10 cm from the ileocecal valve. The colonic mesentery is then divided, staying medial and travelling superiorly to the distal transverse colon, taking care to identify and ligate a variable right colon artery and the right branch of the middle colic artery. For tumors in the hepatic flexure and distal transverse colon, an extended right colectomy is necessary, with a larger mobilization of the transverse colon and division of the entire middle colic artery. For an extracorporeal anastomosis, the robotic portion of the operation is terminated at this point. For an intracorporeal anastomosis, both resection sites—the terminal ileum and transverse colon—are then divided with the robotic stapler (Fig. 22.4). The specimen can then be tucked away above the liver or in the pelvis for later extraction. The potential advantage of the intracorporeal technique is that it requires less mobilization of the transverse colon, as the extracorporeal technique requires the transverse colon to reach outside the body.

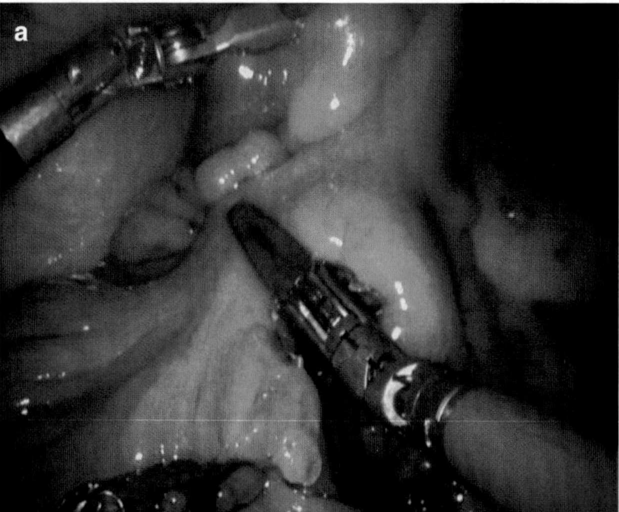

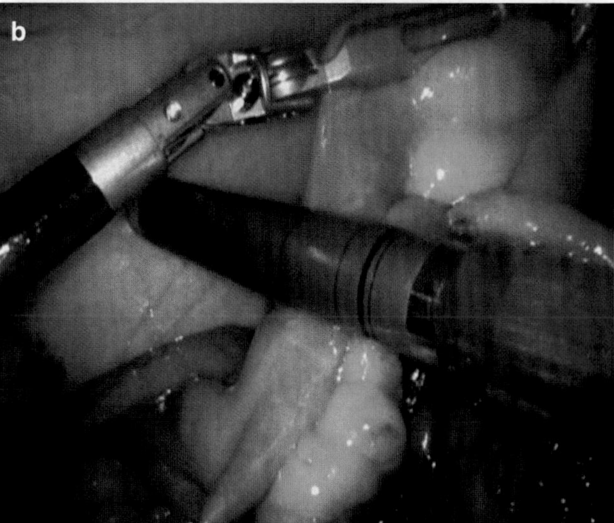

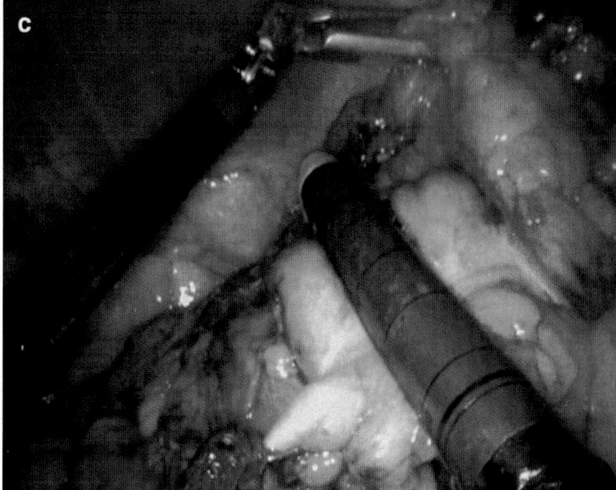

Fig. 22.4 Right colon resection. (**a**) The terminal ileal mesentery is divided with the vessel sealer. (**b**) The terminal ileum is divided with a stapler about 10 cm from the ileocecal valve. (**c**) The transverse colon is divided with a stapler

Anastomosis

Extracorporeal Anastomosis

The robot is undocked. A 6- to 8-cm incision is made around the umbilicus, a wound protector is placed, and the colon is brought outside the body. This step is made easier by mobilizing as much colon as possible and dividing the mesentery while in the body. Identification is also made easier by placing a grasper on the appendix and delivering it through the incision. The proposed resection sites are identified and cleaned of any fat. The bowel loops are paired, and enterotomies are made in the terminal ileum and transverse colon. A linear stapler is placed in each limb and firing is performed. The anastomosis is completed, and the specimen is resected with a second transverse firing of the stapler (Fig. 22.5). The anastomosis can be examined for completeness and hemostasis; it is then placed back in the abdomen, and the incision is closed.

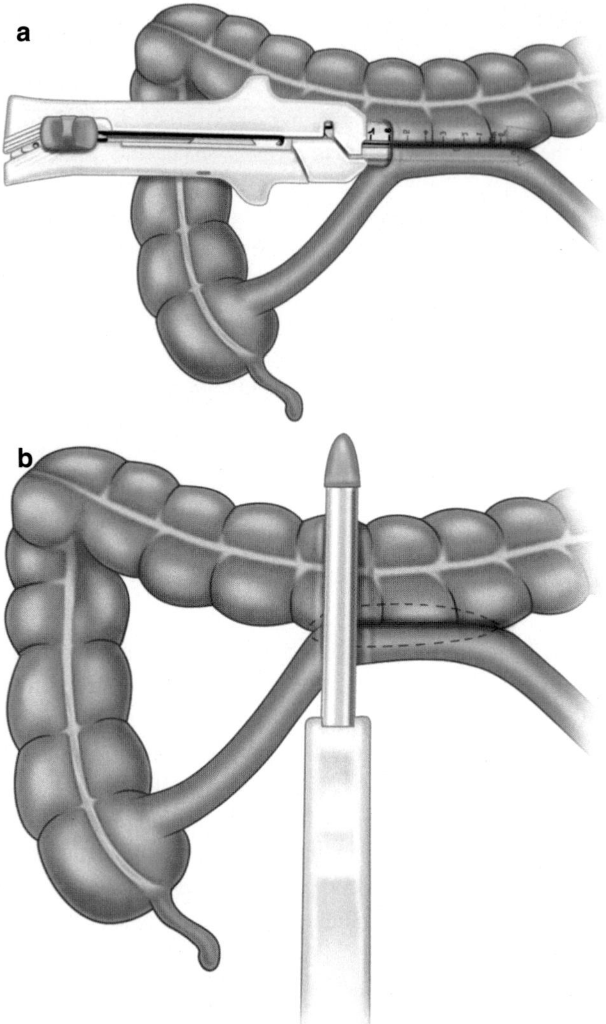

Fig. 22.5 Extracorporeal anastomosis. (**a**) Enterotomies are made in the terminal ileum and the transverse colon, and a gastrointestinal stapler is inserted in each limb and fired. (**b**) The anastomosis is completed, and the specimen is resected simultaneously with a transverse firing of the gastrointestinal stapler across the first staple line, excluding the original enterotomies

Intracorporeal Anastomosis

A side-to-side anastomosis is completed. The anastomosis can either be isoperistaltic, with stapled ends on both sides of the anastomosis, or it can be antiperistaltic, with the stapled ends on the same side. This choice is based on the surgeon's preference and how the bowel lines up. In either case, the two limbs of bowel should be approximated with a stay stitch distally. This is then retracted into the air by the third arm. Two small enterotomies are made in each limb of the bowel, and two firings of the robotic stapler are used to create the anastomosis. The common channel defect is then closed with robotic suturing in two layers (Fig. 22.6). It can also be stapled closed by placing stay stitches on each end of the opening. These ends are retracted into the air, and the robotic stapler is fired below, making sure that each corner has been appropriately resected and stapled closed.

For an intracorporeal anastomosis, any of the port sites can then be expanded for removal of the specimen. The suprapubic port site is a popular option because of its good cosmetic results and lower hernia rate. A 6-cm Pfannenstiel incision is made and a wound protector placed. The specimen is then removed and passed off the field. The incision is then closed in layers.

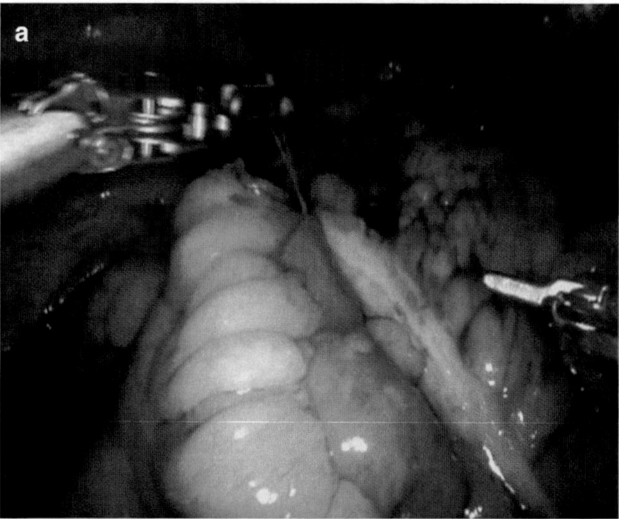

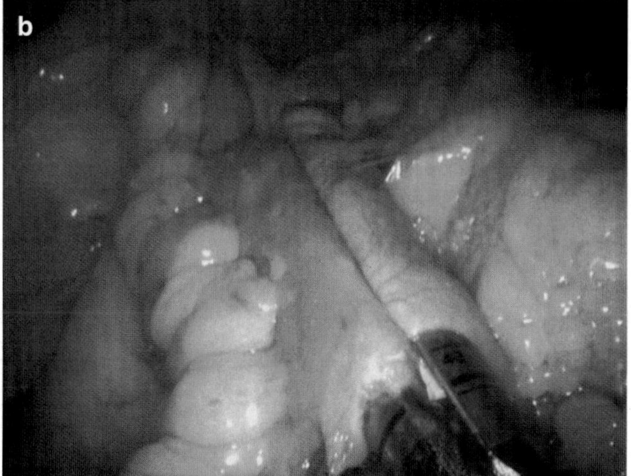

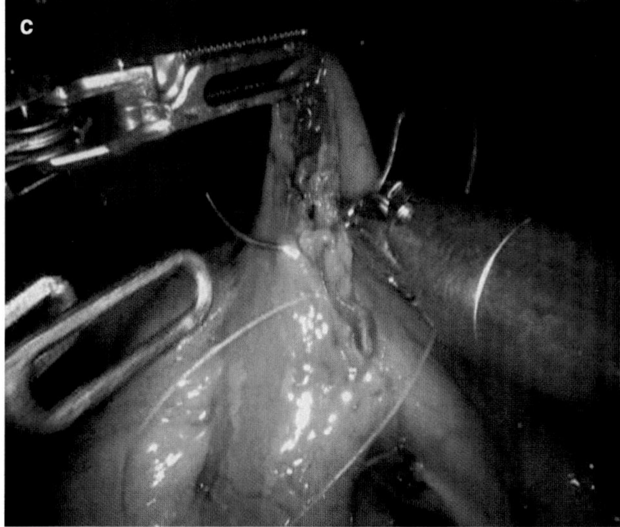

Fig. 22.6 Intracorporeal anastomosis. (**a**) A stay stitch is placed distally to line up the terminal ileum and transverse colon for anastomosis. (**b**) The stapler is placed in two enterotomies and fired to anastomose each limb of the bowel together. (**c**) The common channel defect is then closed in two layers in a running fashion

Robotic Left Colectomy and Sigmoidectomy

Patient and Robot Positioning

A robotic sigmoid colon resection is performed in much the same way as the more practiced robotic low anterior resection. A left colectomy for a descending colon tumor or splenic flexure tumor is adapted from these techniques with further mobilization of the transverse colon. The largest hindrance to performing these surgeries totally robotically is the splenic flexure takedown. As this is occurring in another quadrant of the abdomen, the surgical field needs to be altered. This can be addressed in four ways: (1) perform a hybrid approach by taking down the splenic flexure first or last laparoscopically; (2) double dock the robot on the left shoulder first and then the left leg; (3) single dock the robot and move arm 3 from the left of the robot to the right side; and (4) single dock the robot and do not move any arms. The fourth technique has been greatly facilitated by the use of the da Vinci Xi® robot and its *flex* joints.

The patient again should be placed in a low lithotomy position. The arms should be tucked and the patient appropriately secured. It is important to have the patient's buttocks as close to the edge of the bed as possible, as the transanal stapler will be used later and the patient will often slide cephalad. The robot will be docked along the patient's left side. It can come straight in from the left or be angled at 45 degrees, coming in from the patient's left leg (Fig. 22.7).

Port Placement and Instruments

As with a right colon resection, port placement depends on surgeon preference and the model of the robot. The standard setup for a single dock without changing arms is shown in Fig. 22.8a. This setup is ideal for the hybrid approach or if minimal splenic flexure work is needed. The camera is placed supraumbilically. Trocars 1 and 2 are placed in the lower quadrants on either side. Trocar 3 can be placed extremely lateral in the anterior axillary line on the left, offset from trocar 2.

Figure 22.8b shows a single-docking procedure. Arm 3 will be to the left of the robot, pointed down for the pelvis. It will be switched to the right of the robot and pointed upward for the splenic flexure. A final technique to single dock is seen in Fig. 22.8c. The splenic flexure mobilization is performed with arm 3 on trocar 4. The pelvic dissection requires arm 2 to move to trocar 4 and arm 3 to move to trocar 3.

If using the double-docking technique, the robot should first be docked from the left, about 15 degrees from the left shoulder. Figure 22.8d shows this configuration with arm 3 in trocar 3.1. The second dock is from the left leg and requires arm 3 on trocar 3.2. A similar double dock is shown in Fig. 22.8e, but arm 2 is changed instead of arm 3.

Finally, when using the da Vinci Xi® robot, the port placement again starts in a straight line, as seen in Fig. 22.8f. The line should start in the right lower quadrant and progress toward the left upper quadrant in a line connecting the right

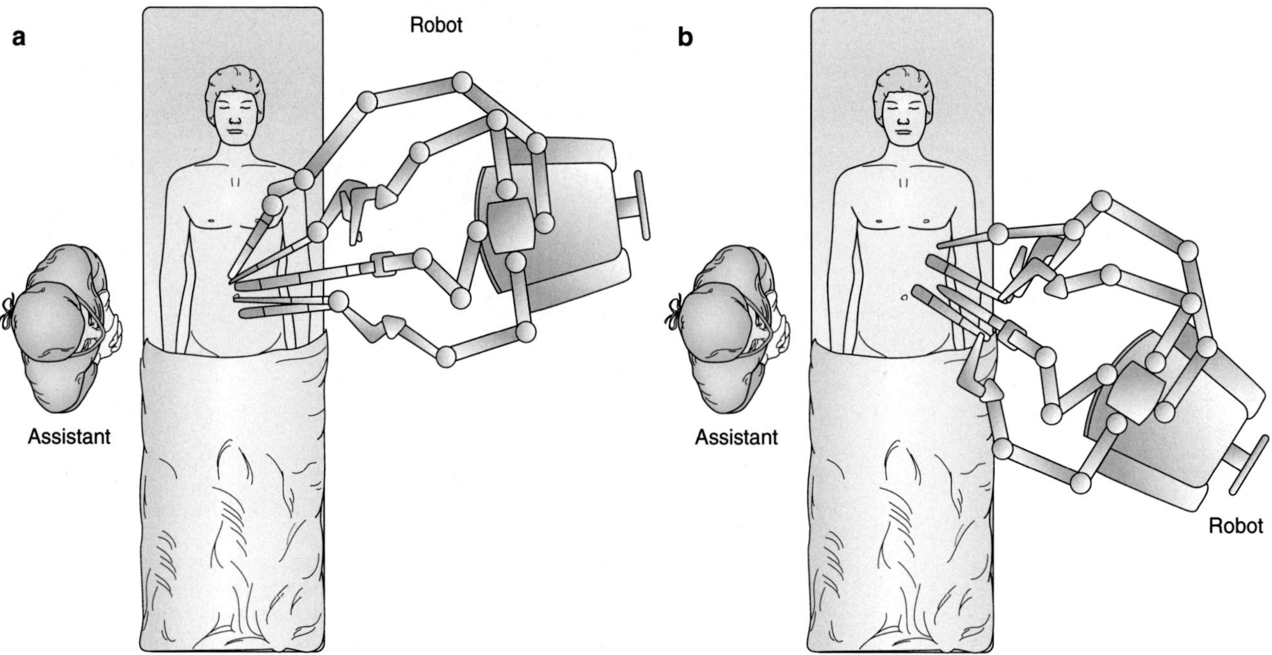

Fig. 22.7 Left colectomy docking setup. (**a**) The robot can be docked straight in from the left or at a 15-degree angle from the left shoulder. (**b**) The more popular docking method is from the patient's left leg at a 45-degree angle

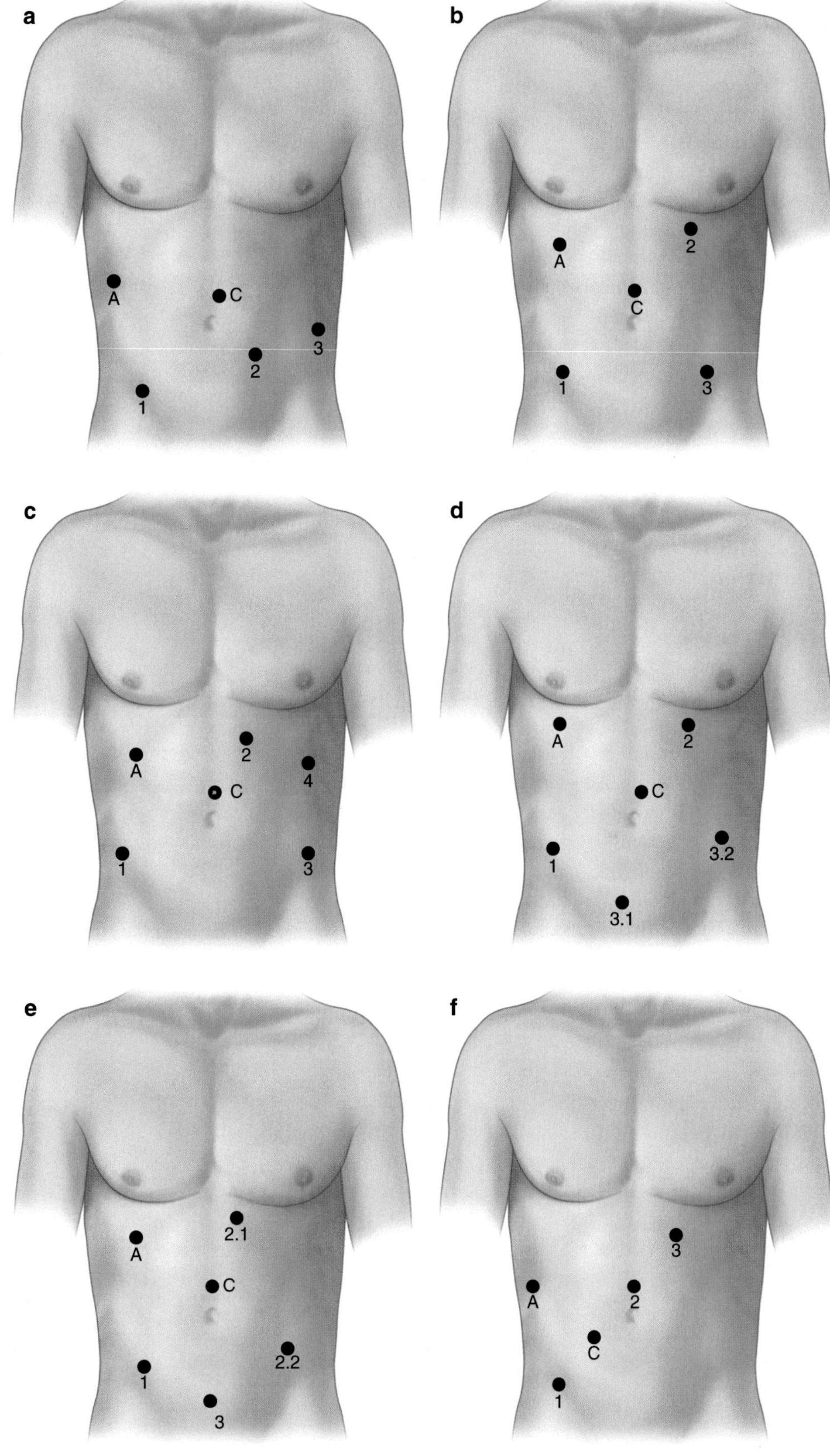

Fig. 22.8 Left colectomy port placement. Trocars: 1, arm 1; 2, arm 2; 3, arm 3; 4, extra port for arms 2 and 3; C, camera; A, assistant. (**a**) Single-docking method where arms do not move. (**b**) Single-docking method where arm 3 is brought on either side of the robot to reach the splenic flexure and the pelvis. (**c**) Single-docking method where both arms 2 and 3 are moved to approach each quadrant separately. (**d**) Double-docking method where arm 3 is moved. (**e**) Double-docking method where arm 2 is moved. (**f**) Standard port setup for the da Vinci Xi® model

femoral head to the left midclavicular line. It should intersect the midline with a supraumbilical camera port. Trocars should be the standard 8-mm robotic trocars except for the right lower quadrant trocar, which should be 12 cm to accommodate the stapler. One or two 5-mm assistant ports should be placed in the right mid to upper quadrant for retraction and suctioning.

Trocar 1 is the right hand and should be a monopolar instrument of the surgeon's choosing. Trocar 2 is for the left hand and should be a bipolar/retracting instrument. Finally, arm 3 is for retraction. Once all ports have been placed, the patient should be rotated to the right and placed in Trendelenburg position. The robot may then be docked. A hybrid option at this stage would be to take down the splenic flexure prior to any robotic work. The da Vinci Xi® system should be set to lower abdominal, with the target being the sigmoid colon.

Inferior Mesenteric Artery Isolation and Ligation

The omentum and bowel are retracted out of the field of view. The sigmoid colon is retracted out of the pelvis and toward the left sidewall. Often the natural attachments of the sigmoid colon will aid with retraction and should not be taken down immediately. The inferior mesenteric artery (IMA) pedicle is tented up, and a plane is developed underneath the pedicle just superior to the sacral promontory. The plane is then developed laterally until the left ureter is displayed and mobilized away to avoid any possible injury. The bare area superior to the IMA is incised, and the pedicle is isolated and cleaned of the overlying fat. The pedicle is then divided close to its origin with a stapler or vessel sealer (Fig. 22.9). The inferior mesenteric vein is identified at its origin, coming out underneath the duodenum. When extreme colon length is needed, as in a proctectomy, the vein should be divided here, but for a sigmoid resection, the vein usually can be ligated closer to the colon, when dividing the mesentery. For a true descending colon or splenic flexure tumor, the entire IMA does not need to be divided; instead, the left colic artery can be isolated, branching off the main IMA trunk, and ligated separately, leaving the sigmoidal blood supply intact.

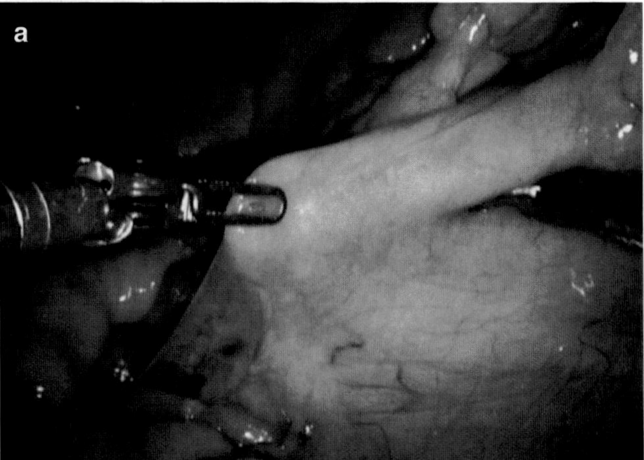

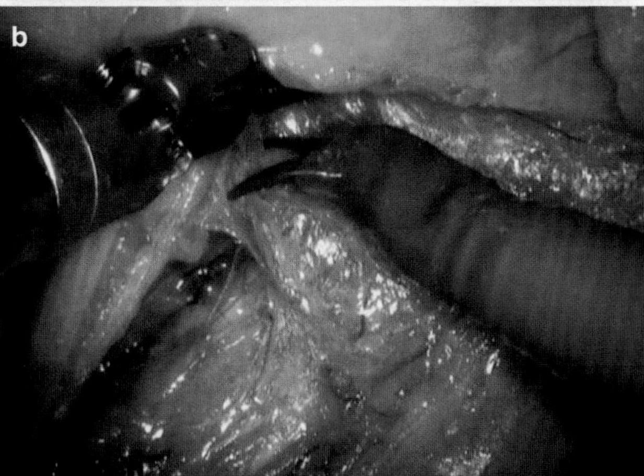

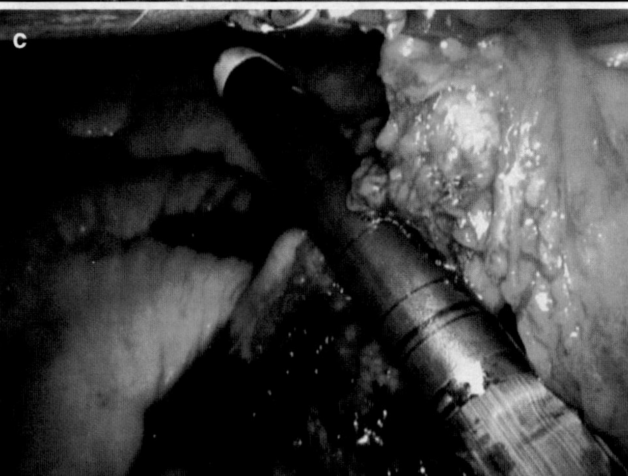

Fig. 22.9 Inferior mesenteric artery (IMA) isolation and ligation. (**a**) The mesentery is retracted superiorly, revealing the IMA pedicle inserting into its origin with the aorta. (**b**) Mobilization of the IMA off of the retroperitoneum. Note that the ureter has been identified and kept with the retroperitoneum. (**c**) Fully mobilized IMA pedicle ready for ligation with a vascular stapler

Mobilization of the Descending and Sigmoid Colon

A medial-to-lateral mobilization of the sigmoid and descending colon is the next step. Gentle, blunt separation with the elbows of the instruments will help to find the correct plane. This plane should be developed laterally to the abdominal sidewall, inferiorly to the start of the mesorectum, and superiorly to the border of the pancreas. The lateral-to-medial mobilization follows. If a complete mobilization was performed medially, only a thin layer of attachments should need to be incised. This is an important step, as it is very easy to mobilize underneath the retroperitoneum and kidney if the planes are not distinct. The mobilization should be taken as high on the splenic flexure as possible. The distal resection margin is often found at the rectosigmoid junction, requiring a partial mobilization of the mesorectum. This mobilization should be started in the posterior plane and then developed laterally for a small distance.

Splenic Flexure Mobilization

A sigmoid colectomy sometimes requires a full splenic flexure mobilization. A descending colon tumor usually will require a full mobilization to obtain clean margins and provide a tension-free anastomosis. At this point, the robot might need to be fully redocked. An alternative is to switch arms 1 and 3 [4]. Finally, the da Vinci Xi® system should be able to reach the splenic flexure with some minor alteration of the *flex* joints. Dissection is started medially, along the transverse colon. The omentum is retracted cephalad and the colon is retracted caudad. The two layers of the omentum should be incised off the transverse colon until entrance into the lesser sac has been accomplished. This is readily identified by the back of the stomach. The omentum and attachments are then sequentially divided, travelling laterally until the splenic flexure and the previous dissection are areas reached.

Distal Resection and Extraction

The proximal resection site should be identified. The mesentery must be split at this level, to allow it to reach outside the body. The entire mesentery can be divided up to the resection site and viability tested with the Firefly™ technology if desired. The distal resection margin is then identified, and the vessel sealer is used to clean off the entire mesentery. The distal margin is then stapled (Fig. 22.10). A retractor is placed on the end of the colon. If the tumor is in the splenic flexure or in the proximal descending colon, the resection should take place outside the abdomen instead.

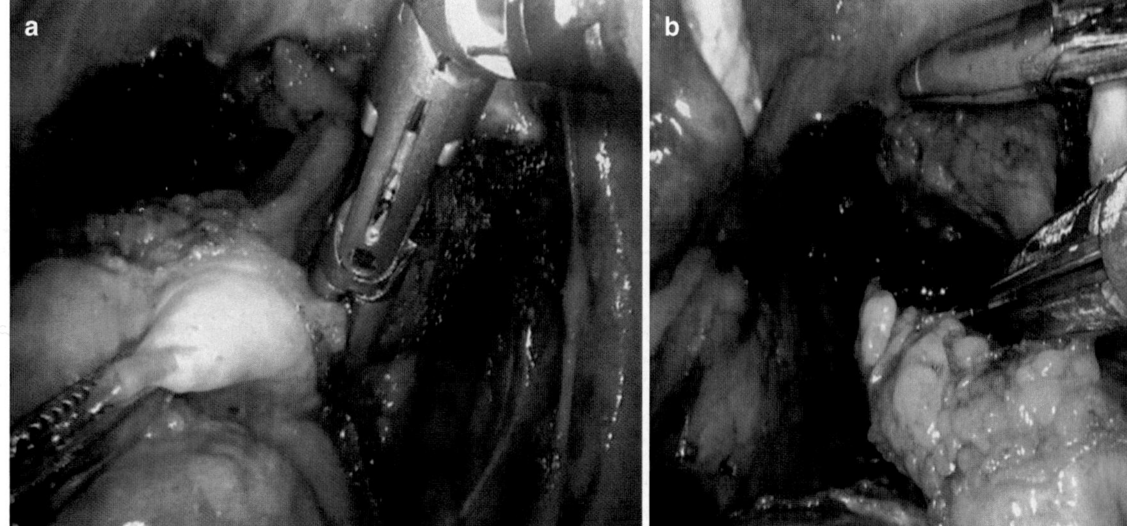

Fig. 22.10 Division of the distal colon. (**a**) The mesentery at the distal transection site is ligated with the vessel sealer. (**b**) The distal colon is then transected with the robotic stapler

Anastomosis

Descending Colon Anastomosis

The robot is undocked, and either the left lower quadrant port site or the umbilical port site is expanded to a 6- to 8-cm incision. A wound protector is placed, and the colon is extracorporealized. The specimen is then resected with appropriate margins. As is often the case with these surgeries, the bowel may not lay quite right when the staplers are used, so a hand-sewn anastomosis is often a better choice. The incisions are then closed in standard fashion.

Colorectal Anastomosis

The left lower quadrant port site is expanded and a wound protector is placed. The divided colon is extracorporealized and the proximal resection site identified. The specimen is resected at this point, and the circular stapler anvil is secured to the bowel with a purse-string stitch. This is placed back into the abdomen, and the incision site is closed partially, or a cap can be placed. The anastomosis is then completed laparoscopically with transanal placement of the circular stapler (Fig. 22.11). A leak test is performed and the pelvis is irrigated. The incisions are then closed.

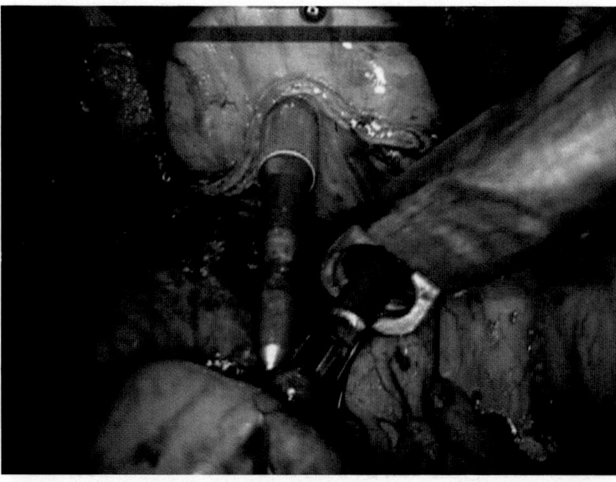

Fig. 22.11 Anastomosis. The circular stapler is placed transanally and the spike is deployed. Note the ideal placement of the spike just above the rectal stump staple line. The proximal colon is seen at the bottom of the picture with the anvil sutured in place. The anvil is ready to be paired with the spike to complete the anastomosis

Postoperative Course

Patients should be placed on an ERAS pathway with early ambulation and oral intake. Incisional pain should be significantly less than in an open operation, so the use of narcotics should be limited. Postoperative antibiotics are not necessary, but thrombosis prophylaxis should be continued.

Outcomes

As more surgeons have adopted robotic surgery into their colorectal practices, the long-term and short-term outcomes are starting to be reported. Most of the literature for robotic colorectal surgery focuses on rectal surgery and proctectomy, but there is a growing body of literature for robotic colectomies. Right colectomies are more frequently reported as stand-alone studies. Sigmoid and left colectomies are often lumped into rectal surgery papers, and several large national database studies mix right, left, and sigmoid colectomies together. The first comparison of laparoscopic versus robotic right colectomy was a retrospective review from 2010 [5]. Forty robotic cases were compared with 135 laparoscopic cases. The robot took significantly longer (158 vs. 118 min) and cost more to perform ($15,000 vs. $12,000). This review was followed by the only randomized controlled trial on the subject, a study from South Korea in 2012 [6]. There were 35 patients in each randomized group comparing robotic right colectomy versus laparoscopic right colectomy. As with the earlier study, operative time was significantly longer in the robot group (195 vs. 130 min), and the costs were also higher ($9000 vs. $6000). All the remaining variables were equivalent.

Lim et al. compared robotic versus laparoscopic sigmoid colectomies in 2013 [7]. There were 34 robotic sigmoidectomies, compared with 146 laparoscopic procedures. The robotic cases were shorter (217 vs. 252 min), and the robot group had minimally but significantly shorter stays and quicker return of bowel function. Three-year overall survival and disease-free survival were unchanged.

A 2013 study looked at the National Inpatient Database and compared 2423 laparoscopic colectomies with 160 robotic ones [8]. Robot surgeries had a lower conversion rate, 6 versus 10%. Morbidity and mortality were similar among the groups. As before, the robotic surgeries had a greater cost, $20,000 versus $16,000. Finally a meta-analysis from 2015 reviewed 14 major studies of robotic versus laparoscopic colectomies from the past decade [9]. The surgeries were approximately equally mixed between right colectomies and sigmoidectomies. Longer operative times were seen with robotic procedures. Conversion rates were lower when using robotic technologies, but much of the data is confounded with previous abdominal surgery and technique selection in those patients. Finally, short-term complications and return of bowel function were better when using robotic surgery.

In conclusion, the evidence to date shows that robotic surgery is more expensive than laparoscopic surgery and operative time is increased, especially for right colectomies. There is growing evidence of modest reductions, however, in conversions, length of stay, and return of bowel function when robotic surgery is performed.

Conclusions

Robotic colon surgery is an exciting and expanding field. The surgeon uses his or her basic principles from open and laparoscopic surgery and adapts them to the robot, so the standard approaches described here do not need to be followed to the letter. Medial-to-lateral or lateral-to-medial mobilizations are both feasible. Intracorporeal or extracorporeal anastomoses are both commonly performed. Finally, there are a myriad of port placement techniques and extraction sites. As more and more studies are published, the operative times have diminished, but they still remain longer than times for open or laparoscopic surgery. In addition, the costs with robotic surgery have always been higher than with the laparoscopic counterparts. Isolated studies have found improvements in complications, conversions, length of stay, and return of bowel function for robotic surgery. It is uncertain whether these modest improvements will be enough to make up for the increased cost of robotic surgery, but it does remain an exciting field that aids the surgeon's ability to enhance his or her own skills and technique.

References

1. Witkiewicz W, Zawadzki M, Rzaca M, Obuszko Z, Czarnecki R, Turek J, et al. Robot-assisted right colectomy: surgical technique and review of the literature. Wideochir Inne Tech Maloinwazyjne. 2013;8:253–7.
2. Luca F, Cenciarelli S, Valvo M, Pozzi S, Faso FL, Ravizza D, et al. Full robotic left colon and rectal cancer resection: technique and early outcome. Ann Surg Oncol. 2009;16:1274–8.
3. Ostrowitz MB, Eschete D, Zemon H, DeNoto G. Robotic-assisted single-incision right colectomy: early experience. Int J Med Robot. 2009;5:465–70.
4. Obias V, Sanchez C, Nam A, Montenegro G, Makhoul R. Totally robotic single-position 'flip' arm technique for splenic flexure mobilizations and low anterior resections. Int J Med Robot. 2011;7:123–6.
5. deSouza AL, Prasad LM, Park JJ, Marecik SJ, Blumetti J, Abcarian H. Robotic assistance in right hemicolectomy: is there a role? Dis Colon Rectum. 2010;53:1000–6.
6. Park JS, Choi GS, Park SY, Kim HJ, Ryuk JP. Randomized clinical trial of robot-assisted versus standard laparoscopic right colectomy. Br J Surg. 2012;99:1219–26.
7. Lim DR, Min BS, Kim MS, Alasari S, Kim G, Hur H, et al. Robotic versus laparoscopic anterior resection of sigmoid colon cancer: comparative study of long-term oncologic outcomes. Surg Endosc. 2013;27:1379–85.
8. Tyler JA, Fox JP, Desai MM, Perry WB, Glasgow SC. Outcomes and costs associated with robotic colectomy in the minimally invasive era. Dis Colon Rectum. 2013;56:458–66.
9. Chang YS, Wang JX, Chang DW. A meta-analysis of robotic versus laparoscopic colectomy. J Surg Res. 2015;195:465–74.

Robotic Total Colectomy

23

Patricio B. Lynn, Manuel Maya, and Julio Garcia-Aguilar

Robotic surgery is a relatively new technique that has become the preferred minimally invasive approach for colorectal procedures at Memorial Sloan Kettering Cancer Center.

The advantages of robotic surgical systems include a stable, surgeon-controlled camera platform, three-dimensional imaging combined with tenfold magnification, a third arm for fixed retraction, better ergonomics, and articulated instruments that provide superior dexterity (7 degrees of freedom, 90 degrees of articulation, fine-motion scaling, tremor reduction), allowing for complex and precise dissection and suturing [1, 2].

The usage of robotic assistance in colorectal surgery in the United States is still extremely low, ranging from 1 to 6% of all minimally invasive colectomies, but it is growing steadily [3–5]. In a recent retrospective review of the National Inpatient Sample Database comparing open versus laparoscopic and robotic approaches in total colectomies, only 2.6% of the cases were robotic. Notably, robotic surgery was associated with a significantly lower conversion rate, compared with laparoscopic approachcs [6].

Minimally invasive total abdominal colectomy is a significant technical challenge because it involves the abdomen's four quadrants. This operation is even more challenging when performed using a robot, as it may require not only changing the patient's position on the operating table to take full advantage of gravity but also moving the robotic platform from side to side relative to the operating table to allow access to the four quadrants of the abdominal cavity. Dual docking and moving the robotic platform from side to side is no longer necessary with the newest da Vinci Xi® platform (Intuitive Surgical, Sunnyvale, CA).

This chapter describes our technique for total abdominal colectomy in a step-by-step fashion.

Indications

Some surgeons will use minimally invasive approaches for an emergent or urgent total abdominal colectomy, but we limit the application of the robotic approach to elective cases. Several indications are the most common:

- Synchronous colon tumors
- Inflammatory bowel disease refractory to medical treatment
- Colonic inertia
- Familial adenomatous polyposis with few or no rectal polyps (in select circumstances)

Technique

Initial Considerations

We use the following technique in the treatment of patients with cancer. It follows the principles of total mesocolic excision, with sharp dissection between the embryological planes and central vascular ligation of the pedicles. The enhanced visualization and precise EndoWrist®-enabled movements of the robot allow a safe and appropriate mesocolic excision.

The da Vinci Xi® system in use at our institution, with a dual console, enables an integrated teaching and supervising

P. B. Lynn, MD
Department of Surgery, New York University School of Medicine, New York, NY, USA

Colorectal Service, Department of Surgery, Memorial Sloan Kettering Cancer Center, New York, NY, USA
e-mail: patricio.lynn@nyumc.org

M. Maya, MD
Instituto de Investigaciones Médicas Alfredo Lanari, Universidad de Buenos Aires, Buenos Aires, Argentina

Hospital Alemán de Buenos Aires, Buenos Aires, Argentina

J. Garcia-Aguilar, MD, PhD (✉)
Colorectal Service, Department of Surgery, Memorial Sloan Kettering Cancer Center, New York, NY, USA
e-mail: garciaaj@mskcc.org

Y. Fong et al. (eds.), *The SAGES Atlas of Robotic Surgery*, https://doi.org/10.1007/978-3-319-91045-1_23

environment without compromising operative and patient outcomes. For this procedure, rather than using a single-docking technique, we use a dual-docking approach with the robotic platform positioned between the patient's legs (Fig. 23.1). The enhanced reach of the robotic arms makes it possible to perform a two-step approach, first treating the right colon and then redocking and finalizing the operation by mobilizing the left colon and rectum without moving the platform to the other side of the table.

This technique could also be used with the da Vinci Si® platform, but not without moving the robot to the other side of the table during the procedure.

Patient Position and Docking

The patient is placed in a modified lithotomy position with both arms secured alongside the body and padded at pressure points to prevent injuries. A foam mattress is placed directly under the patient, and a foam pad is secured over the patient's chest to prevent sliding. The robot is placed between the patient's legs, and the arms are rotated 90° to the right (facing the right side of the patient). It is our practice to start the operation from the right side so that the left side of the operation will be done last, finishing with the rectal sectioning.

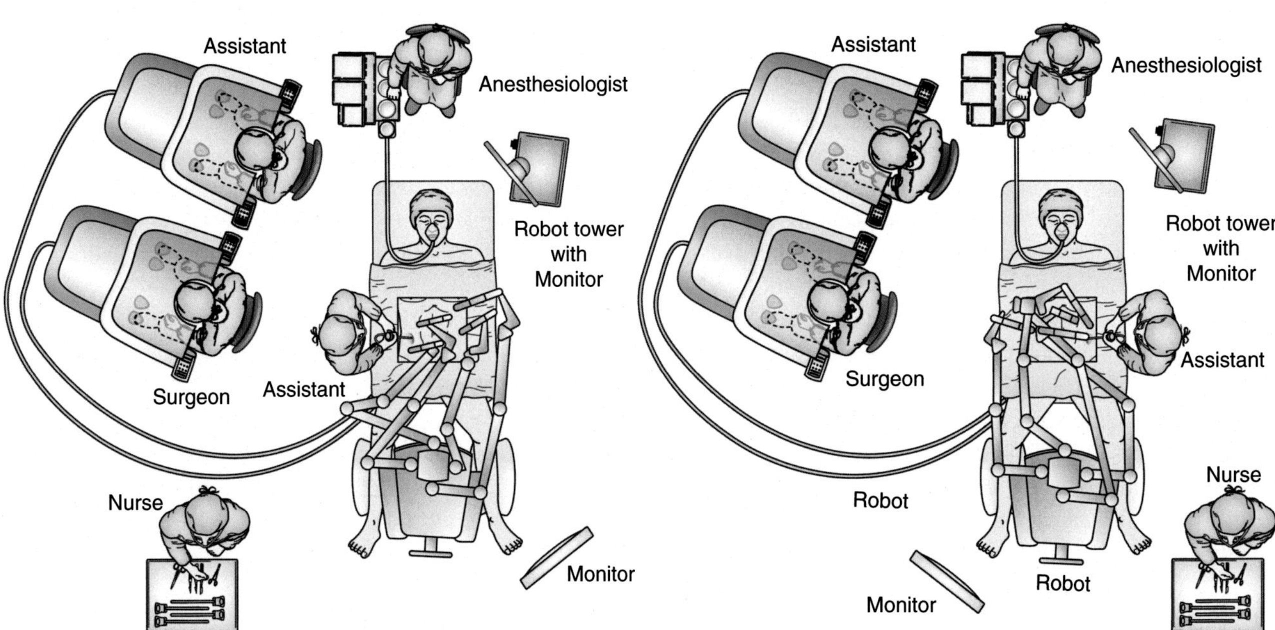

Fig. 23.1 Robot docking. Docking for right colon dissection (*left*). Docking for left colon/rectal dissection (*right*)

Port Placement

Trocar placement is illustrated in Fig. 23.2. Eight-millimetre robotic trocars are placed in the right and left upper quadrants and in the left lower quadrant. In the right lower quadrant, a 12-mm trocar is placed for the robotic or laparoscopic stapler. An additional 8-mm trocar for the camera is placed midline 2–3 cm superior to the umbilicus. Two 5-mm auxiliary trocars are placed in each flank for suction/retraction with a laparoscopic grasper. We have found that this disposition allows the performance of total colon mobilization with the use of the four robotic arms.

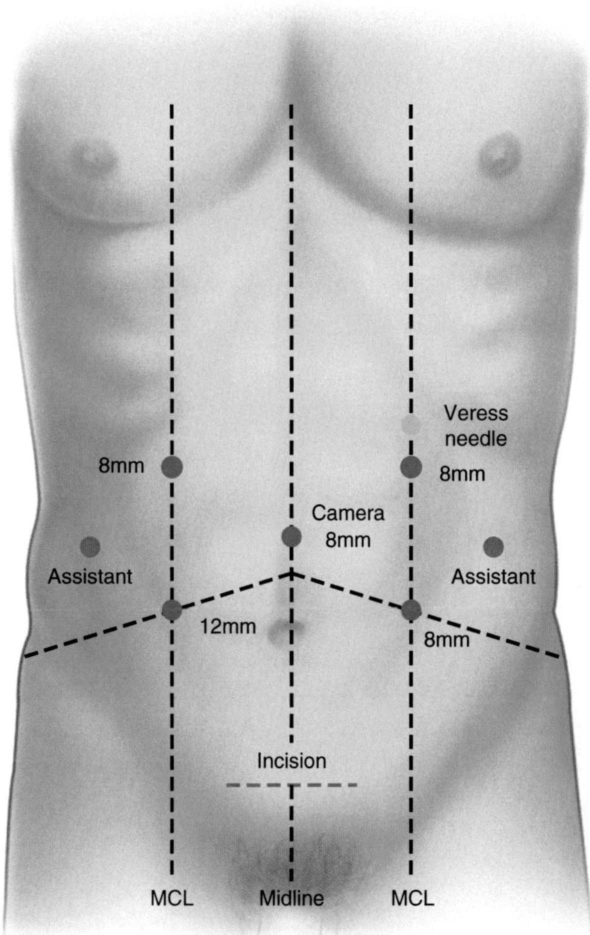

Fig. 23.2 Trocar positioning. MCL—midclavicular line

Operative Technique

Pneumoperitoneum is induced by placing a Veress needle in the left upper quadrant 5 cm below the costal border. An 8-mm camera port is inserted through the midline supra-umbilical incision, and an exploration of the abdominal cavity is undertaken to detect adhesions and assess resectability. The remaining trocars are placed under direct vision.

Before robot docking, patient is rotated left 15° and placed in Trendelenburg position (30º), laparoscopic inspection of the abdomen is completed with the robotic camera. Any adhesions are excised, the greater omentum is retracted cephalad (exposing the transverse colon), and small bowel loops are placed in the upper left quadrant to expose the right colon and mesocolon.

Robot docking is then performed (see Fig. 23.1a), aiming the target to the right colon. The cecum is retracted laterally and anteriorly, stretching the right mesocolon and exposing the ileocolic pedicle. The peritoneum is incised below the ileocolic vessels, identifying the avascular plane between the right mesocolon and the retroperitoneum (Fig. 23.3). Dissection continues along this plane laterally and cephalad. Using the vessel sealer device, ileocolic vessels are carefully dissected and transected up to the point of fusion with the superior mesenteric vein (SMV). In most cases we do not think it necessary to dissect the artery from the vein before sectioning, but doing so may facilitate the sectioning of these vessels in some selected cases.

Once the ileocolic pedicle has been transected, dissection continues over the SMV in a cephalad direction, identifying the second and third portion of the duodenum, the pancreatic head, and the middle colic vessels, which are then dissected and ligated (Fig. 23.4). The right colon has a high incidence of vasculature variation, and a right colic vessel that requires sectioning may be present in up to 20% of cases.

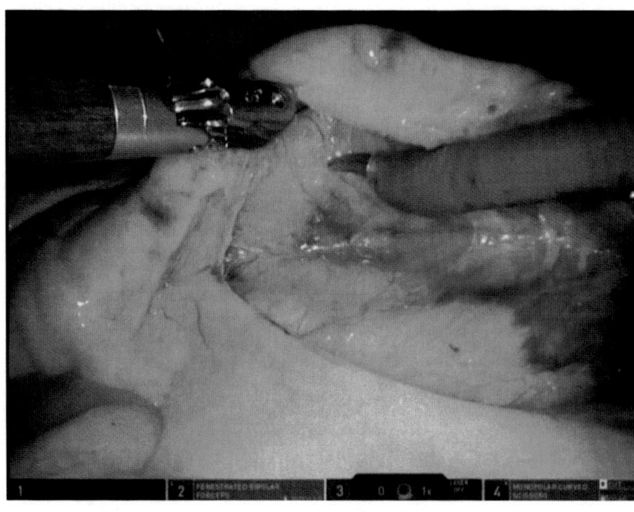

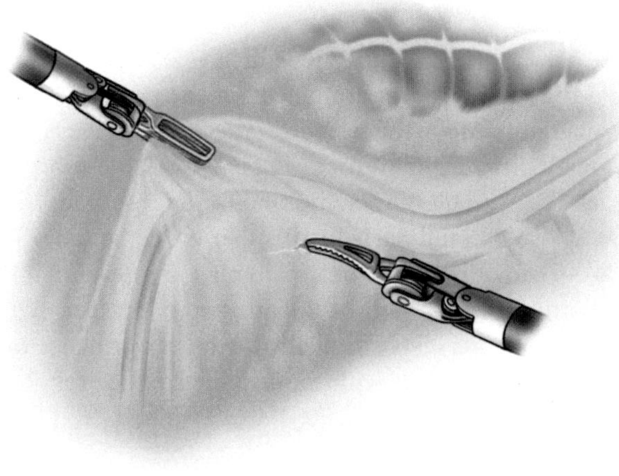

Fig. 23.3 Dissection below the ileocolic pedicle

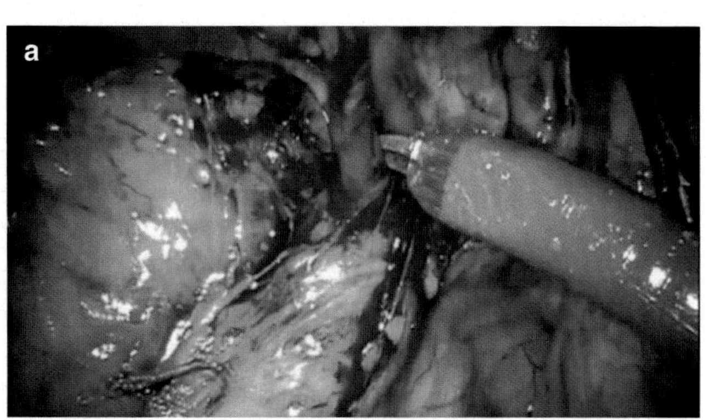

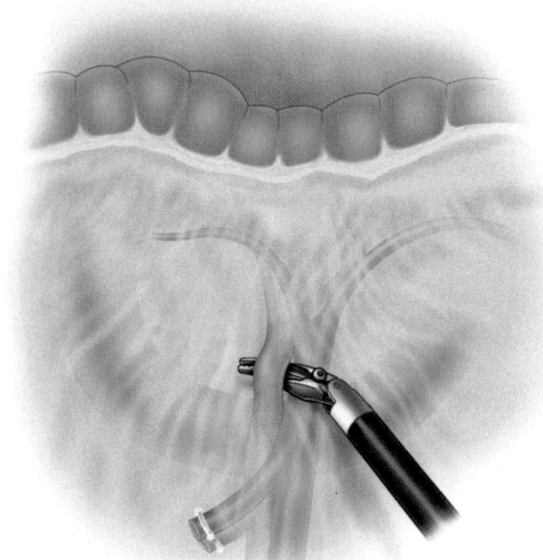

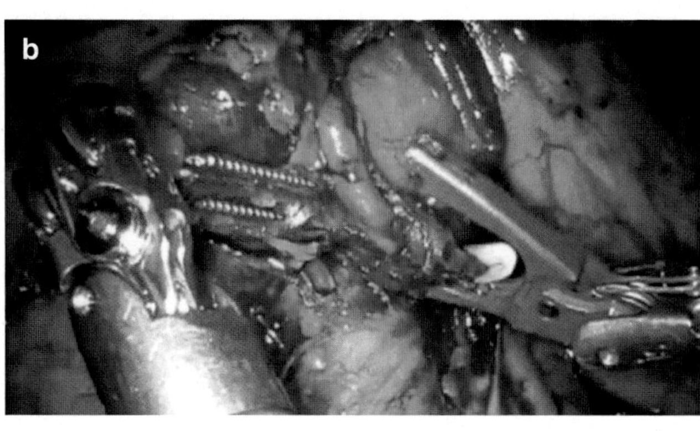

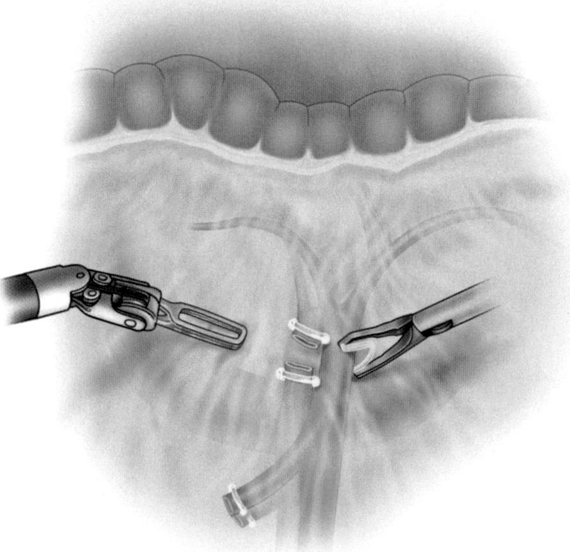

Fig. 23.4 Middle colic vessels: the vein (*top*) and artery (*bottom*)

Dissection below the mesocolon continues until the transverse colon (superiorly) and right colon (laterally) are exposed. The right transverse colon is then detached from the greater omentum. Lateral attachments are removed in a cranial-caudal fashion to the cecum and the last 15 cm of the ileum (Fig. 23.5). Finally, the mesentery of the distal ileum is sectioned with the vessel sealer device.

At this point the robot is redocked and oriented to the left flank. The arms are rotated 180° from right to left (see Fig. 23.1b). The patient is tilted right 15° and into the Trendelenburg position (30°), as above. For left colon mobilization, we prefer a medial-to-lateral approach and systematically start dissecting the inferior mesenteric vein (IMV), which is easily identifiable because of its proximity to the ligament of Treitz (Fig. 23.6). Lifting the vessel, the plane between the retroperitoneum (Gerota's fascia) and the mesocolon is encountered. The vessel is dissected and sectioned with the bipolar sealing device.

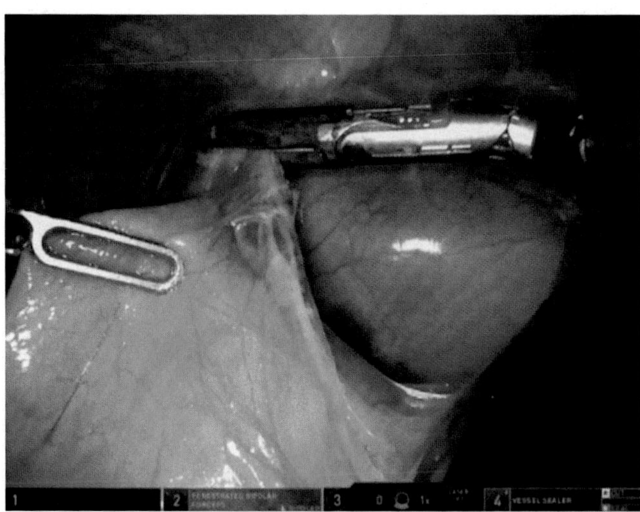

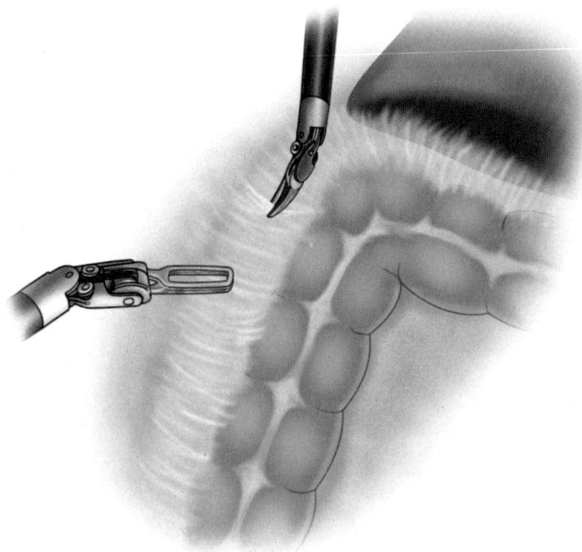

Fig. 23.5 Takedown of the right colon lateral attachments

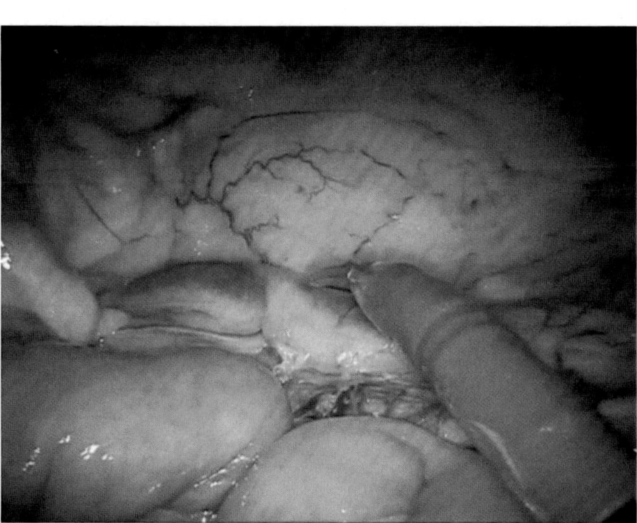

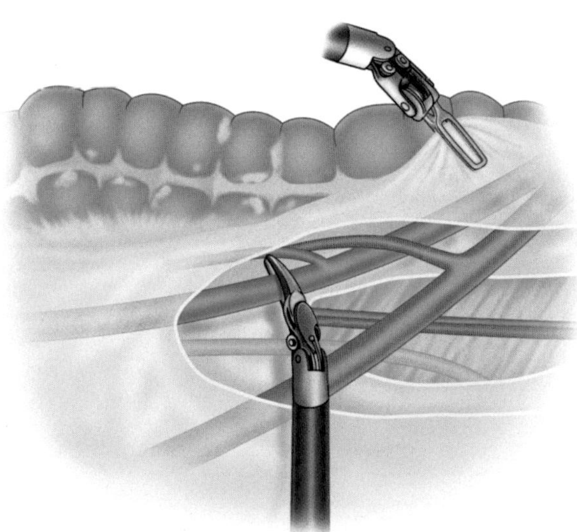

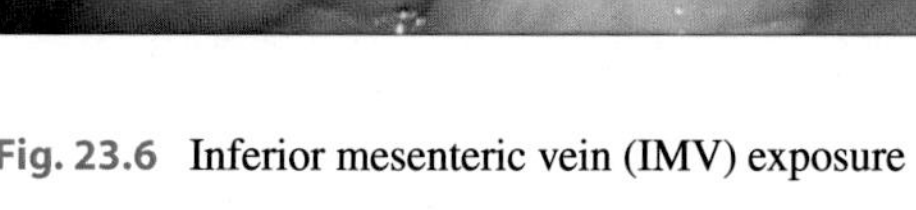

Fig. 23.6 Inferior mesenteric vein (IMV) exposure

Dissection continues in the previously identified plane, separating the mesocolon from the retroperitoneum laterally to the point where the left colon is visualized from below. Cephalad, the inferior border of the pancreas, is identified in the retroperitoneum, and the dissection is carried over the pancreas until the lesser sac is entered (Fig. 23.7). Following the anterior surface of the pancreas toward its tail and the hilum of the spleen, the left side of the transverse mesocolon is completely mobilized.

Splenic flexure mobilization is then undertaken. If the omentum is to be removed with the specimen, the lesser sac is entered by dividing the greater omentum outside of the gastroepiploic arcade. The rest of the left side of the omentum is then divided toward the hilum of the spleen. If the omentum is to be preserved, the greater omentum is completely detached from the transverse colon, starting at the mid transverse colon and finishing at the splenic flexure. Once completed, the splenic flexure is released, first taking down the lateral attachments to the abdominal wall and then continuing that plane from left to right and cephalad to caudal.

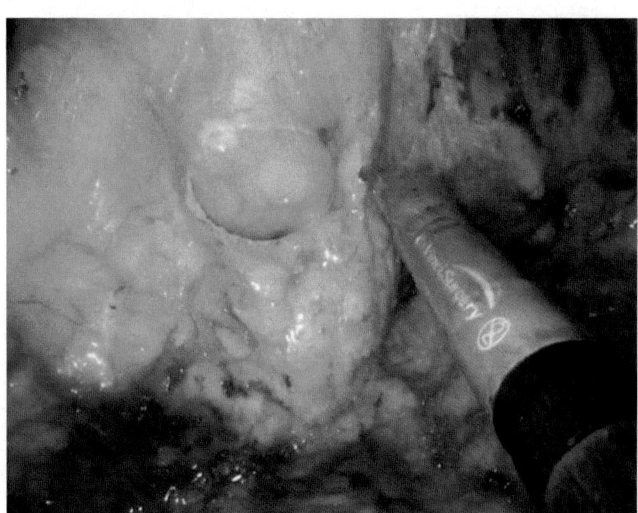

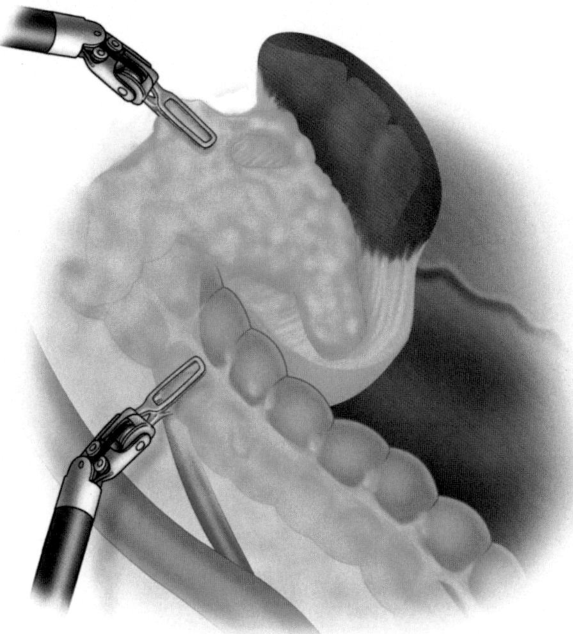

Fig. 23.7 Lesser sac opening

Dissection subsequently focuses inferiorly, continuing blunt dissection between the mesocolon and Gerota's fascia. The inferior mesenteric artery (IMA) is identified, emerging anteriorly from the abdominal aorta. The avascular plane between the IMA and the bifurcation of the aorta is identified, and the avascular plane between the sigmoid colon mesentery and the retroperitoneal structures is developed. Dissection progresses along this plane laterally until the attachments of the left sigmoid colon to the lateral abdominal wall are reached. During this dissection, it is essential to identify the left ureter and left gonadal vessels for preservation (Fig. 23.8).

Once completely dissected, the IMA can be divided between special clips, using the bipolar sealer device or a vascular stapler. This sectioning of the artery is performed 2 cm from its origin in order not to damage the autonomic nerves along the aorta (Fig. 23.9). Once the IMA is sectioned, the mesentery of the entire left colon can be separated from the retroperitoneum using blunt dissection. The remaining attachments of the descending and sigmoid colon to the abdominal wall along the left gutter are sectioned up to the splenic flexure, completing this stage of the procedure.

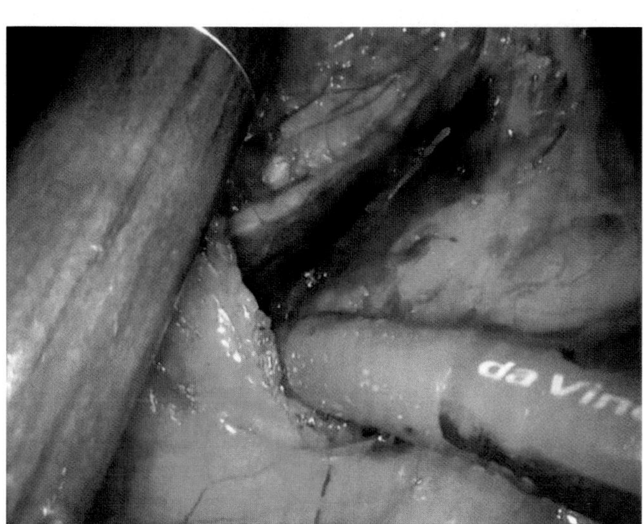

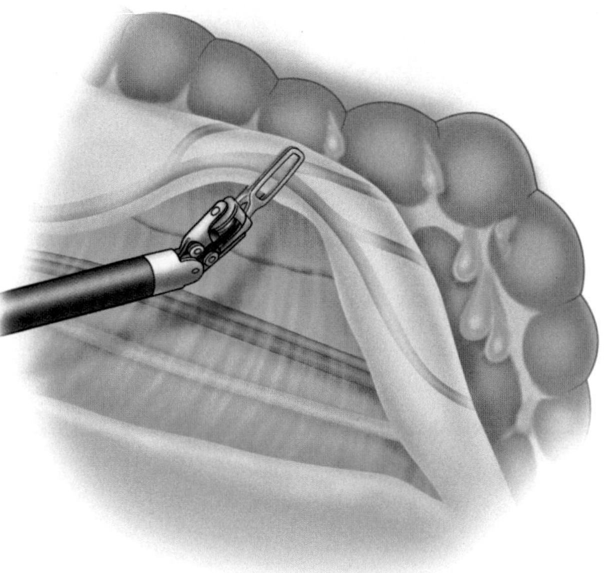

Fig. 23.8 Left ureter identification

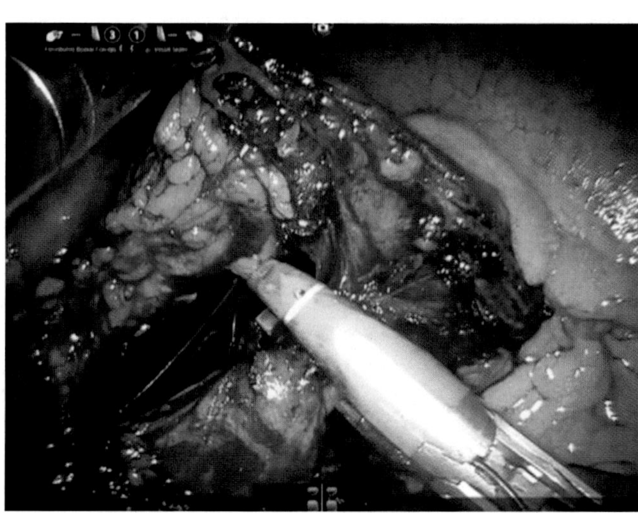

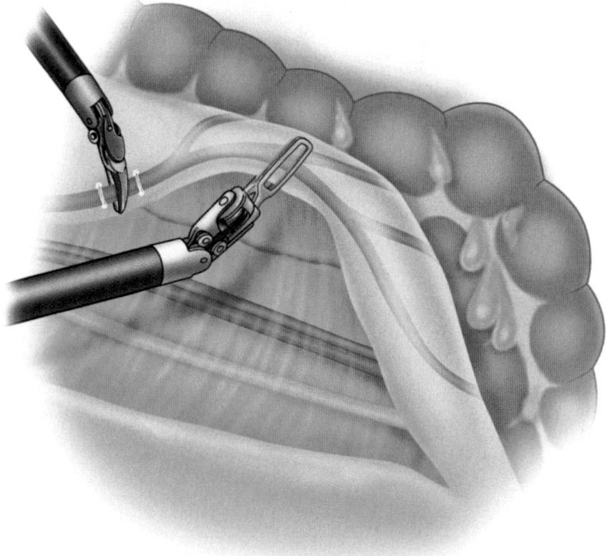

Fig. 23.9 Sectioning of the inferior mesenteric artery (IMA)

The rectal dissection is undertaken at this point. Following the dissection along the IMA and superior rectal pedicle, the mesorectal plane is entered at the level of the promontory (Fig. 23.10). The dissection continues, and the superior rectum is dissected free of the mesorectum with the vessel sealer device and transected with an endoscopic stapler (Fig. 23.11).

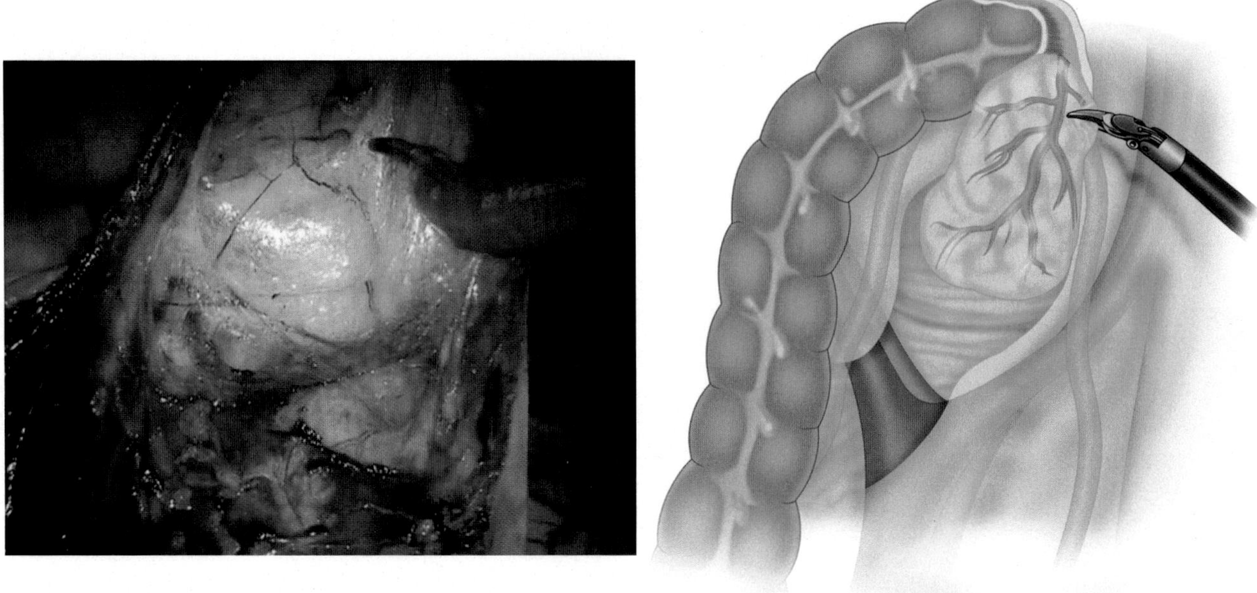

Fig. 23.10 Rectal dissection along the areolar space between the mesorectal and presacral fascias at the "holy plane"

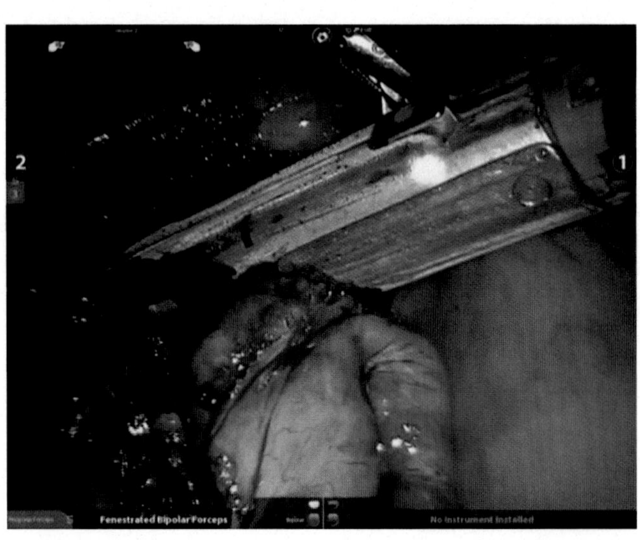

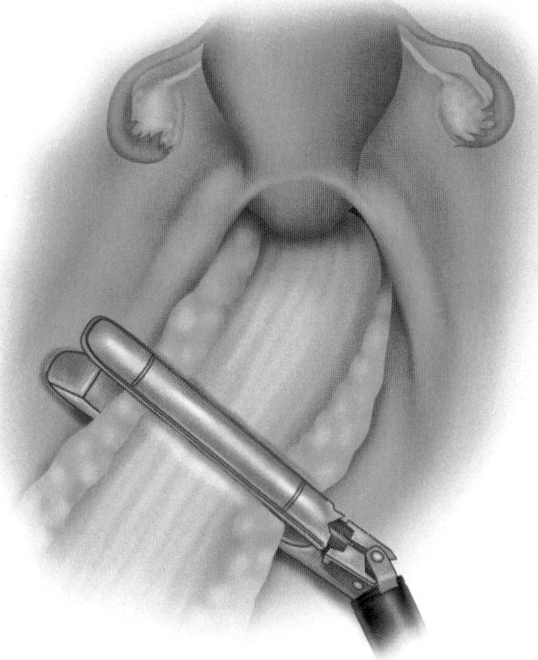

Fig. 23.11 Rectal transection

The robot is undocked and the proximal rectum is grasped with laparoscopic forceps. A 3- to 4-cm Pfannenstiel incision is performed, a wound protector is placed, and the specimen is extracted through the wound, starting with the sectioned rectum. Once the distal ileum is reached, the bowel is clamped and sectioned, and the surgical specimen is delivered. An anvil from the circular stapler is then inserted in the remaining distal ileum to perform an ileorectal anastomosis, preferably in a latero-terminal fashion. The distal ileum with the anvil is reinserted, the wound is closed, and the pneumoperitoneum is reinitiated. The robot is redocked, and stapled ileorectal anastomosis is performed after checking the small bowel for twisting. Hemostasis is secured, and a pelvic drain is placed posterior to the anastomosis and extracted through the left lower quadrant trocar site. At this point, the robot is undocked, the pneumoperitoneum is resolved, and the abdominal wound is closed.

Conclusions

The use of a robot to perform a total colectomy allows a precise dissection of the embryological planes. This operation also can be performed in an inverse order, starting with the left colon and finishing on the right side; this approach has the advantage that the most technically demanding part of the operation is performed first.

A single-docking technique has been described for this operation [7]. The time benefit gained by avoiding the redocking process must be carefully counterbalanced with the limitations of exposure inherent in such an approach. It is our belief that exposure is critical to the optimal performance of a total mesocolic excision and cannot be achieved with single docking without changing the patient decubitus. Having said that, a single-docking approach could be safely implemented for cases in which malignancy is not suspected.

References

1. Ballantyne GH, Moll F. The da Vinci telerobotic surgical system: the virtual operative field and telepresence surgery. Surg Clin North Am. 2003;83:1293–304. vii
2. Intuitive Surgical Inc. EndoWrist instruments. http://www.intuitivesurgical.com/products/instruments. Accessed 7 Jan 2017.
3. Tyler JA, Fox JP, Desai MM, Perry WB, Glasgow SC. Outcomes and costs associated with robotic colectomy in the minimally invasive era. Dis Colon Rectum. 2013;56:458–66.
4. Wormer BA, Dacey KT, Williams KB, Bradley JF 3rd, Walters AL, Augenstein VA, et al. The first nationwide evaluation of robotic general surgery: a regionalized, small but safe start. Surg Endosc. 2014;28:767–76.
5. Davis BR, Yoo AC, Moore M, Gunnarsson C. Robotic-assisted versus laparoscopic colectomy: cost and clinical outcomes. JSLS. 2014;18:211–24.
6. Moghadamyeghaneh Z, Hanna MH, Carmichael JC, Pigazzi A, Stamos MJ, Mills S. Comparison of open, laparoscopic, and robotic approaches for total abdominal colectomy. Surg Endosc. 2016;30:2792–8.
7. Harnsberger CR, Cajas-Monson LC, Oh SY, Ramamoorthy S. Robotic-assisted total abdominal colectomy. In: Ross H, Lee SW, Champagne BJ, Pigazzi A, Rivadeneira DE, editors. Robotic approaches to colorectal surgery. Cham: Springer International Publishing Switzerland; 2015. p. 149–55.

Robotic Low Anterior Resection

24

John V. Gahagan and Alessio Pigazzi

Introduction

With an estimated 39,220 new diagnoses in 2016, rectal cancer continues to be a common disease within the United States [1]. Treatment of rectal cancer involves a multidisciplinary approach that often includes surgery, chemotherapy, and radiotherapy.

Increased screening and the use of chemoradiotherapy have improved survival in rectal cancer. Despite these advances, surgical resection remains the mainstay of treatment. Low anterior resection (LAR) with a total mesorectal excision (TME) was first introduced by R.J. Heald in 1979 [2], and this technique has become the standard of care for surgical resection of rectal cancer [3]. An LAR with TME involves total resection of the tumor and surrounding mesorectal envelope and lymph nodes as a complete unit contained within the visceral fascia while preserving the underlying autonomic nerves.

The surgical management of rectal cancer can be technically challenging because of the anatomic constraints of the pelvis and the various nearby vital structures. The development of laparoscopy gave surgeons a new tool to better operate within the pelvis, providing easier maneuverability and visualization. Laparoscopy, however, is not without its own limitations, including limited range of motion and two-dimensional imaging. The advent of robotically-assisted surgery provided surgeons with the benefits of laparoscopy as well as improved ergonomics, improved range of motion and precision, and three-dimensional imaging. These added features make the surgical robot perfectly suited for use within the pelvis and on the rectum. Although the design of the first-generation da Vinci® system (Intuitive Surgical; Sunnyvale, CA) was not ideal for totally robotic rectal surgery, the newer da Vinci® models offer longer instruments and greater degrees of movement. These advancements allow for access to multiple areas of the abdomen and pelvis without repositioning the robot or performing an initial laparoscopic mobilization.

This chapter describes the technique of a robotic LAR with TME, with colon and splenic flexure mobilization. Described in addition to the totally robotic approach is the hybrid approach, in which the splenic flexure mobilization is performed laparoscopically and the TME is performed robotically.

Preoperative Planning

The rectum, the most distal portion of the large intestine, is identified where the taeniae coli splay near the sacral promontory, typically within 15 cm from the anal verge. The robotic approach to an LAR is most advantageous for tumors of the mid-rectum (5–10 cm from the anal verge) and low rectum (0–5 cm from the anal verge); the benefits of the robot are less apparent for more proximal tumors. A robotic approach is contraindicated for patients with hemodynamic instability or severe cardiac or pulmonary disease, which may make them unable to tolerate pneumoperitoneum. These comorbidities would also preclude a laparoscopic approach and necessitate an open approach.

A multidisciplinary approach to the management of rectal cancer allows patients to be evaluated for neoadjuvant and adjuvant therapy and undergo these treatments in a timely fashion. This team effort requires good communication between the medical oncology, radiation oncology, and surgical oncology teams [4]. The patient should also have a preoperative consultation with an ostomy nurse for ostomy education and skin marking, in case placement of an ostomy should become necessary during the operation [5].

All patients with rectal cancer should undergo a complete work-up prior to any treatment. The specifics of this work-up may vary, but several components are critical:

- Complete history and physical to assess for comorbid conditions and ability to tolerate an operation.
- Family history to evaluate for inherited cancer syndromes, with subsequent genetic counseling as necessary.

J. V. Gahagan, MD · A. Pigazzi, MD, PhD (✉)
Division of Colon and Rectal Surgery, Department of Surgery, University of California, Irvine, Orange, CA, USA
e-mail: gahaganj@uci.edu

Y. Fong et al. (eds.), *The SAGES Atlas of Robotic Surgery*, https://doi.org/10.1007/978-3-319-91045-1_24

- Laboratory studies: CEA, blood cell count, chemistry panel, and hepatic panel.
- Digital rectal exam and proctoscopy performed by the surgeon to confirm the location of the tumor.
- A full colonoscopy to evaluate for possible synchronous lesions.
- Pelvic imaging with endorectal ultrasound or high-resolution MRI to evaluate the depth of invasion and lymph node status.
- Metastatic disease work-up: CT imaging of the chest, abdomen, and pelvis. The role of PET imaging for rectal cancer has not yet been clearly defined.

In our practice, we routinely use a mechanical bowel preparation with a polyethylene glycol solution prior to rectal resections.

Operative Technique

The technique described here is for use with the da Vinci® S or Si models, but it can be adapted for the Xi model or future systems or models. Using this technique, the entire procedure can be performed without repositioning the robotic system. The first-generation da Vinci® Surgical System has more limited capabilities and therefore requires the hybrid approach described below.

Positioning and Preparation

The patient is placed in a modified lithotomy position using adjustable stirrups. The hips are flexed and slightly abducted such that the ipsilateral shoulders, hips, knees, and feet should form a straight line. To allow room for robot docking and for an assistant surgeon, both arms should be tucked. The patient should be securely strapped to the table to prevent shifting during movement of the table. All boney prominences must be well padded to avoid pressure injuries. Routine placement of ureteral stents is unnecessary and is not recommended. A nasogastric or orogastric tube should be placed for gastric decompression, and a Foley catheter should be placed for urinary bladder decompression. The assistant surgeon and the scrub technician both work from the patient's right side. The robot cart is docked from the patient's left side to allow for more neutral positioning of the lower extremities and to maintain access to the perineum during the operation (Fig. 24.1). The rectum is irrigated with 1–2 L of a dilute betadine solution to complete the bowel preparation. Prior to the start of the procedure, antibiotics that cover intestinal flora should be administered.

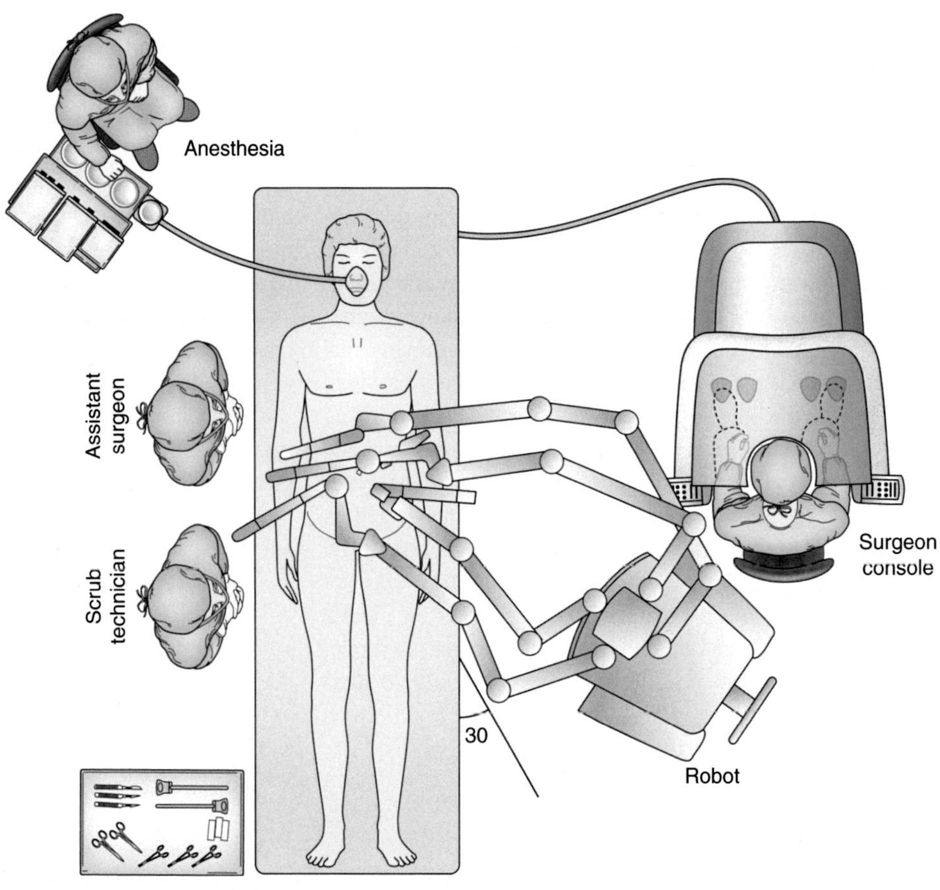

Fig. 24.1 Operating room configuration

Port Placement

A small incision is made at Palmer's point in the left upper quadrant, through which a Veress needle is placed to establish pneumoperitoneum (15 mm Hg). Next, the camera port (C, 12 mm trocar) is placed halfway between the xiphoid process and the pubic symphysis in the midline or slightly to the right (Fig. 24.2). This position will allow visualization of the left abdomen and the pelvis. The entire abdomen should be inspected for previously unknown metastatic disease or iatrogenic trocar/Veress needle injury. The additional trocars are then placed under direct visualization: four robotic (8 mm) ports and a 12 mm assistant port. The first robotic port (R1) is placed in the right lower quadrant at least 8 cm away from the camera, along a line that connects the camera to the anterior superior iliac spine, typically where this line crosses the midclavicular line. The second robotic port (R2) is placed in the left lower quadrant, as a mirror image of R1. An additional left lower quadrant port (R3) is placed approximately 8 cm lateral to R2 and superior to the anterior superior iliac spine. This port will be used during the TME. A fourth robotic port (R4) is placed in the epigastrium, approximately 5 cm inferior to the xiphoid and to the left of the falciform. This port will be used during the initial mobilization. This port configuration allows for triangulation by using R1, R2, and R4 during the mobilization and then using R1, R2, and R3 during the TME.

The assistant port (A, 12 mm), which can be used for retraction, suction, or stapling, is then placed in the right upper quadrant, approximately 8–10 cm cephalad to the right lower quadrant robotic port, along the midclavicular line. If necessary, a second assistant port can provide additional retraction; it can be placed in the right upper quadrant, approximately 5 cm cephalad to the first assistant port.

Robot Docking

The robotic cart is docked on the patient's left side, at an angle of 30° from the table, with arms projecting toward the patient's head. For the mobilization portion, a 30°-angled camera is used, and robotic arms R1 and R4 are docked. The left lower quadrant robotic arms will not be used until the pelvic portion of the operation. A monopolar curved scissors or a robotic vessel sealer is used in the R1 port (under right hand control), and a fenestrated bipolar grasper is docked in the R4 port (under left hand control). The assistant uses a grasper or suction to assist with retraction as necessary.

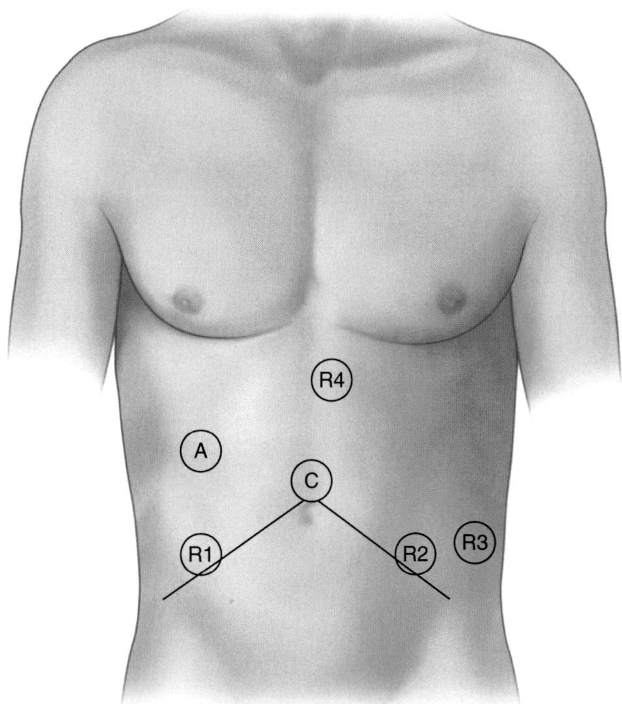

Fig. 24.2 Port placement

Mobilization

A medial-to-lateral mobilization of the left colon is started by first identifying the inferior mesenteric vein (IMV). The IMV is reliably found near the ligament of Treitz. As the assistant retracts the small bowel toward the right upper quadrant, the ligament of Treitz and attachments between the transverse mesocolon and proximal jejunum are sharply divided. Then the peritoneum surrounding the IMV is incised with monopolar scissors. Using blunt dissection, a space is developed between the mesocolon and Gerota's fascia toward the abdominal wall, skeletonizing the IMV. The IMV is then divided with a linear stapler, clips, or an energy-sealing device, through the assistant port. Early division of the IMV helps prevent traction injuries and bleeding complications.

The IMV is then traced distally toward the pelvis, as it travels with the left colic artery. The left colic artery will then lead to the origin of the inferior mesenteric artery (IMA). The origin of the IMA, the left colic artery, and the distal IMA form a T-shaped structure. The IMA is skeletonized. The left ureter and gonadal vessels should be identified and always remain posterior to the dissection plane to be avoided. The IMA is then divided at its origin using a linear stapler, clips, or an energy-sealing device (Fig. 24.3).

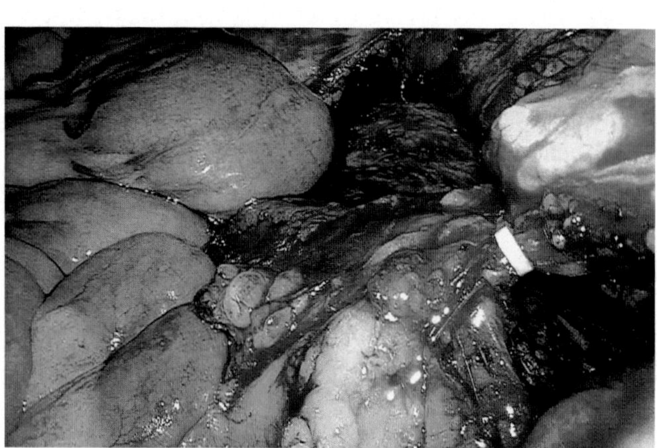

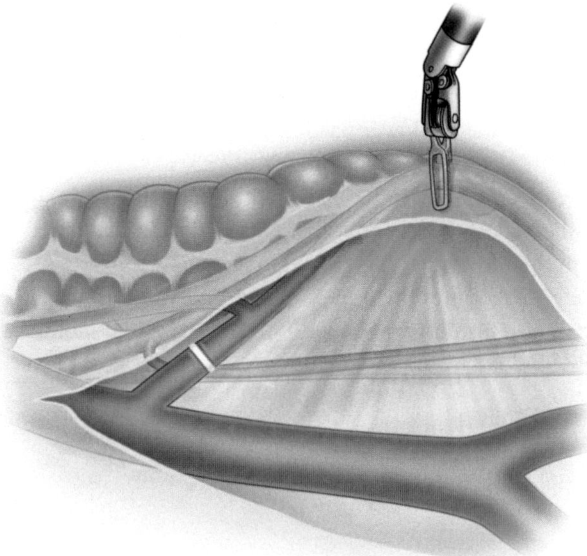

Fig. 24.3 Identification and clipping of the inferior mesenteric artery (IMA)

The medial-to-lateral mobilization is continued with blunt dissection in the avascular plane between the mesocolon and the retroperitoneum, until the white line of Toldt is reached. The assistant retracts the colon medially to provide countertraction. The white line of Toldt is then sharply incised, starting distally and moving proximally toward the splenic flexure. The dissection is continued toward the splenic flexure, which is then mobilized by dividing the splenocolic, phrenocolic, and gastrocolic ligaments.

Total Mesorectal Excision

After mobilization of the left colon and splenic flexure, the robotic arms are repositioned to facilitate dissection within the pelvis, but the robotic cart itself is not moved. The R1 port is unchanged and will continue to control the monopolar scissors. The robotic arm with the fenestrated grasper docked in R4 is moved to the R2 port. An additional fenestrated grasper is docked in the R3 port. The left hand can control the R2 and R3 arms interchangeably, although the R2 arm will be used primarily, and the R3 arm will provide exposure. The additional robotic arm in the R3 position gives the surgeon the ability to self-expose the pelvis, providing greater control of the rectal dissection. The camera is exchanged for a 0° endoscope, which will provide a better perspective in the pelvis.

The rectosigmoid mesentery is retracted superiorly and anteriorly, and the IMA is traced toward the pelvis. To perform a TME, the avascular plane between the fascia propria of the rectum and the parietal fascia ("holy plane") is identified and entered posterior to the rectum (Fig. 24.4). This plane will have very fine areolar tissue that can be divided sharply. It is important to avoid grasping the mesorectum, as it may tear and give rise to substantial bleeding. It is also important to have visualization of the ureters to prevent inadvertent injury. Keeping dissection within the avascular plane will help avoid damage to the ureters, which lie laterally, as well as the hypogastric nerves, which lie posteriorly. Dissection within this plane continues distally toward the coccyx. Once there has been sufficient posterior dissection, the anterior surface of the rectum is dissected first by incising the peritoneal reflection. The anterior dissection will likewise be performed in the avascular plane; it is continued distally until an adequate margin is achieved. The lateral stalks of the rectum can be divided with the fenestrated graspers and bipolar energy. In general, rectal cancer requires a 2 cm distal margin, but for very distal tumors, a 1 cm distal margin may be acceptable. Very distal tumors may require an intersphincteric resection or an abdominoperineal resection.

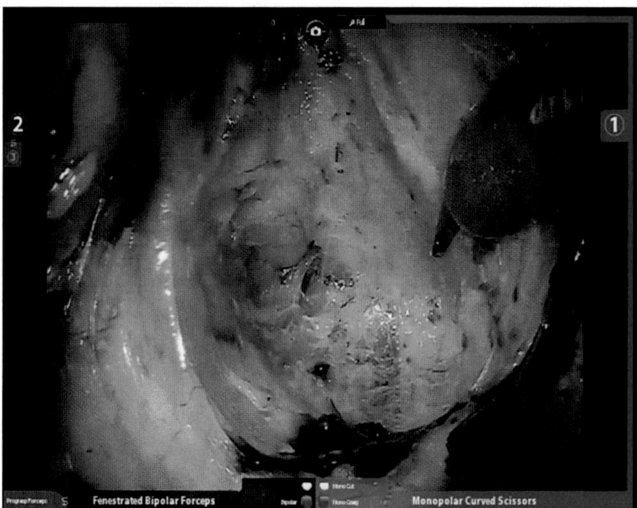

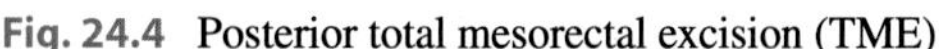

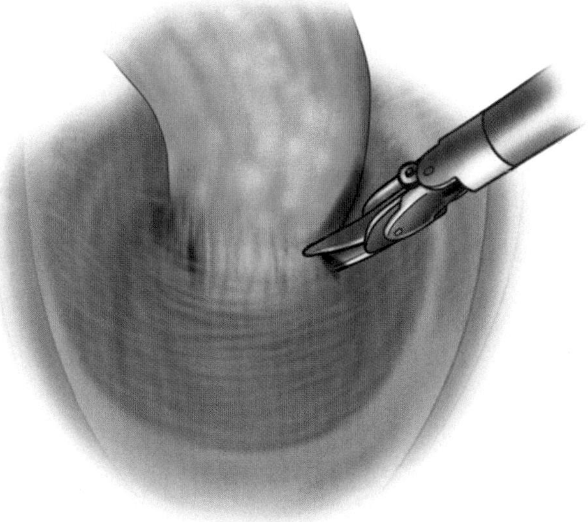

Fig. 24.4 Posterior total mesorectal excision (TME)

Specimen Extraction and Colorectal Anastomosis

To divide the rectum, the assistant will use a reticulating stapler through the assistant port (A). Alternatively, a robotic stapler can be used through the right lower quadrant port (R1) (Fig. 24.5). Complete division of the rectum may require multiple staple cartridges. After division of the rectum, the robot is undocked to allow for extraction of the specimen. The trocars are left in place to facilitate the subsequent anastomosis. The rectum is brought through a 4–5 cm Pfannenstiel incision with a wound protector. The proximal colon is divided sharply using Metzenbaum scissors, being careful not to spill stool into the abdomen. Prior to sending the specimen to pathology, it should be examined on a separate back table with separate instruments to ensure resection of the tumor with adequate margins. The anvil of an end-to-end circular stapler is inserted through the proximal colon and secured with a purse-string suture. The colon is then returned to the abdomen. The Pfannenstiel incision is closed, and the pneumoperitoneum is reestablished. Using an end-to-end circular stapler and laparoscopic instruments, the colorectal anastomosis is then constructed in the typical fashion. The proximal and distal tissue “donuts” from the end-to-end stapler are evaluated to ensure that both form complete circles, and they are then sent to pathology. The anastomosis should be inspected for integrity. This evaluation can be accomplished by direct visualization with a flexible sigmoidoscopy and with a “bubble test” (air insufflation through the sigmoidoscope with the anastomosis under irrigation and the proximal intestine occluded). If the anastomosis shows a leak or if there is concern about sufficient vascular supply, it should be reinforced or reconstructed with a new anastomosis [6]. Residual fluid or blood in the pelvis is then suctioned, and hemostasis should be confirmed.

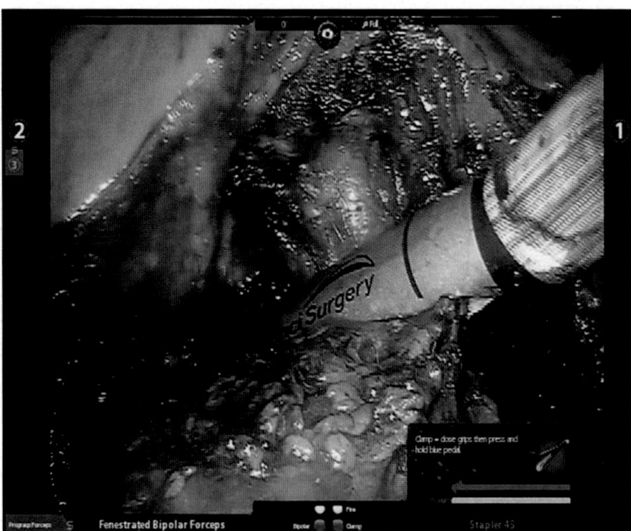

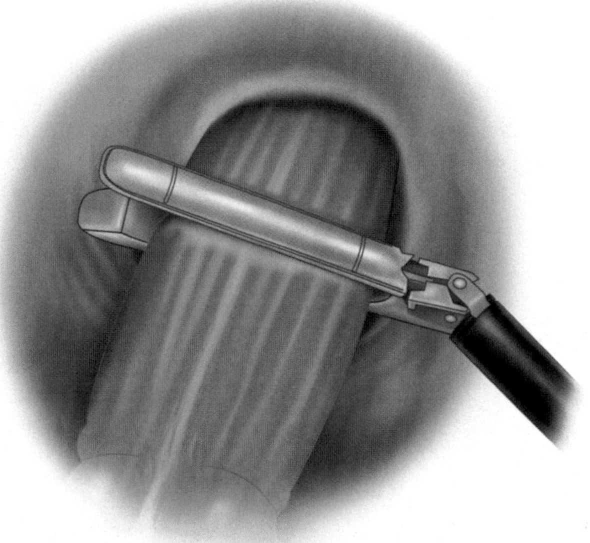

Fig. 24.5 Transection of the distal rectum using a robotic stapler

Ileostomy Construction and Drain Placement

An ileostomy is not considered mandatory. The decision to construct an ostomy is based on patient characteristics and surgeon preference. It can be considered for high-risk anastomoses, such as those in a male pelvis, malnutrition, or a low colorectal or colo-anal anastomosis [7]. If the patient did not have preoperative site marking and a stoma is desired, the ostomy can be placed at the right lower quadrant robotic trocar site. A loop of small intestine approximately 50 cm proximal to the ileocecal valve is identified and brought through a circular skin incision at the desired stoma site. The ostomy is then matured in the usual Brooke fashion after the other incisions are closed.

Laparoscopic-Robotic Hybrid Approach

Depending on surgeon preference, the mobilization portion of this operation can be performed laparoscopically for a hybrid laparoscopic-robotic approach [8]. There is no evidence to show that either a fully robotic or hybrid approach is better, and the choice of technique should be made based on surgeon comfort and skill.

In the hybrid approach, the surgeon uses the R1 port and the right upper quadrant assistant port as working ports, with the camera in the central abdomen (C) port. The mobilization is performed using the technique described above, starting with the identification of the IMV. Once the mobilization is complete, the robot is docked, and the rectal portion is completed as described above.

Transanal Specimen Extraction

The specimen can be extracted through a variety of incisions, and a transanal approach can be used as an alternative to a Pfannenstiel or lower midline incision [9]. To extract the specimen through the anus, the colonic mobilization and rectal dissection are performed as described above. The robotic cart remains docked to perform the extraction. The portion of the intestine to be resected is ligated with 1–0 suture 1 cm distal to the proximal resection margin and 1 cm proximal to the distal margin. The suture can be inserted through the assistant port and passed to the robotic arms. The colon (proximal to the suture) and rectum (distal to the suture) are then ligated using monopolar curved scissors. The specimen is then place into a collection bag, which is inserted and retrieved through the anus. A purse-string suture is then placed on the open proximal colon and another on the open distal rectum. The anvil of the EEA™ stapler (Medtronic; Minneapolis, MN) is then inserted through the anus, placed within the proximal colon, and secured with the purse-string suture. The stapler is then inserted through the anus. The spike is deployed and then encircled by the purse string. The end-to-end anastomosis is constructed in the usual fashion with subsequent integrity testing.

Postoperative Management

All patients who undergo a robotic LAR should follow a clinical pathway during the perioperative period. Clinical pathways after colorectal surgery have shortened hospital length of stay with lower morbidity compared with standard care [10]. The clinical pathway employed at our institution emphasizes early and frequent mobility, venous thromboembolism (VTE) prophylaxis, early removal of gastric tubes and Foley catheters, and early feeding. Patients are encouraged to ambulate starting on postoperative day 0 and work with a physical therapist to optimize mobility. Sequential compression devices are started in the preoperative holding area and are continued throughout the hospital stay. Chemical VTE prophylaxis should be started within 24 h of the operation. Nasogastric or orogastric tubes are removed prior to the end of the operation and are avoided in the postoperative period unless absolutely necessary. Foley catheters are typically removed on postoperative day 3. Patients are offered ice chips or clear liquids on postoperative day 1 and quickly advanced to a regular diet unless they develop nausea, vomiting, pain, or abdominal distension. Incentive spirometry is encouraged to help prevent atelectasis and pneumonia. Patients who received an ostomy should have a follow-up visit from the ostomy nurse prior to discharge to provide additional education and assist with ostomy care. In general, patients will be ready for discharge on postoperative day 4 or 5, with a scheduled return clinic visit within 1–2 weeks.

Complications and Limitations

The robotic approach to rectal surgery carries unique potential complications. Unlike laparoscopic surgery, the robot allows the surgeon to control multiple instruments simultaneously. Although this feature provides the surgeon with more control within the operative field, robotic arms outside the vision of the camera can cause inadvertent injuries that may not be recognized immediately. Constant awareness of all the robotic arms is critically important during robotic rectal surgery, as there are many vital structures within a small space. The robot facilitates a very precise dissection by providing delicate control of the instruments, but it lacks haptic feedback. Robotic surgery within the pelvis and on the rectum requires gentle, fluid movements. Therefore, the surgeon must utilize the three-dimensional visualization of the robot to assess how much tension, stretch, and pressure are being applied. Overly aggressive movements of the robotic arms can result in unintentional tissue injury and should be avoided. LAR is associated with a multitude of other complications, including anastomotic leak, sexual dysfunction, bladder dysfunction, pelvic abscess, or LAR syndrome, but these complications are common to all operative approaches and are not unique to the robotic approach.

Outcomes

A robotic LAR with TME was first described by Pigazzi et al. in 2006 as a hybrid approach [8]. The results showed that there were no significant differences in the short-term outcomes (such as operative time, blood loss, length of stay, node harvest, or margin status) between the laparoscopic arm and the robotic arm, concluding that a robotic LAR with TME was feasible. A few years later, in 2009 and 2010, four groups reported a fully robotic technique that eliminated the need for an initial laparoscopic mobilization [11–14]. Together, these reports demonstrated the safety and feasibility of a totally robotic approach to LAR. Because of the complexity of the robotic system and the need for setup and docking, the ability to use the robotic system requires the operating room staff to become familiar with the instruments, setup, and workflow. The surgeon must also become proficient with the robotic technology and the new surgical technique. It appears that the learning curve for robotic rectal resection requires approximately 20–25 cases for a surgeon to achieve an acceptable level of competency [15, 16].

In a comparison between robotic and laparoscopic LAR for rectal cancer, using the National Cancer Database, the outcomes appeared equivalent between the two groups. The robotic group had a significantly lower rate of conversion to open surgery than the laparoscopic group. Evaluation of lymph node harvest, margin status, 30-day mortality, readmission, and length of stay were no different between the two groups [17]. A single-center, randomized trial by Baik et al. comparing robotic versus laparoscopic LAR demonstrated comparable perioperative outcomes between the two approaches [18].

Preliminary data from the RObotic versus LAparoscopic Resection for Rectal Cancer (ROLARR) trial was presented at the 2015 Annual Scientific Meeting of the American Society of Colon and Rectal Surgeons. The ROLARR trial was a multi-institutional, international randomized control trial that compared robotic and laparoscopic rectal cancer surgery. Overall, the outcomes appeared equivalent between the two groups. Intraoperative and 30-day morbidity and 30-day mortality were similar in both groups. Circumferential radial margin (CRM) positivity was also similar in both groups, with an overall CRM positivity of 5.7%. On subgroup analysis, the robotic approach seemed to be most beneficial for male and obese patients.

References

1. Cancer.org. Key statistics for colorectal cancer. Atlanta, GA: American Cancer Society; 2016. http://www.cancer.org/cancer/colonandrectumcancer/detailedguide/colorectal-cancer-key-statistics. Accessed 9 Nov 2016
2. Heald RJ. A new approach to rectal cancer. Br J Hosp Med. 1979;22:277–81.
3. Kapiteijn E, van de Velde CJH. The role of total mesorectal excision in the management of rectal cancer. Surg Clin North Am. 2002;82:995–1007.
4. Obias VJ, Reynolds HL. Multidisciplinary teams in the management of rectal cancer. Clin Colon Rectal Surg. 2007;20:143–7.
5. American Society of Colon and Rectal Surgeons Committee Members; Wound Ostomy Continence Nurses Society Committee Members. ASCRS and WOCN joint position statement on the value of preoperative stoma marking for patients undergoing fecal ostomy surgery. J Wound Ostomy Continence Nurs. 2007;34:627–8.
6. Ricciardi R, Roberts PL, Marcello PW, Hall JF, Read TE, Schoetz DJ. Anastomotic leak testing after colorectal resection: what are the data? Arch Surg. 2009;144:407–11. discussion 411–2
7. Hanna MH, Vinci A, Pigazzi A. Diverting ileostomy in colorectal surgery: when is it necessary? Langenbeck's Arch Surg. 2015;400:145–52.
8. Pigazzi A, Ellenhorn JDI, Ballantyne GH, Paz IB. Robotic-assisted laparoscopic low anterior resection with total mesorectal excision for rectal cancer. Surg Endosc. 2006;20:1521–5.
9. Choi G-S, Park IJ, Kang BM, Lim KH, Jun S-H. A novel approach of robotic-assisted anterior resection with transanal or transvaginal retrieval of the specimen for colorectal cancer. Surg Endosc. 2009;23:2831–5.
10. Gouvas N, Tan E, Windsor A, Xynos E, Tekkis PP. Fast-track vs standard care in colorectal surgery: a meta-analysis update. Int J Color Dis. 2009;24:1119–31.
11. Hellan M, Stein H, Pigazzi A. Totally robotic low anterior resection with total mesorectal excision and splenic flexure mobilization. Surg Endosc. 2009;23:447–51.
12. Choi DJ, Kim SH, Lee PJM, Kim J, Woo SU. Single-stage totally robotic dissection for rectal cancer surgery: technique and short-term outcome in 50 consecutive patients. Dis Colon Rectum. 2009;52:1824–30.
13. Luca F, Cenciarelli S, Valvo M, Pozzi S, Faso FL, Ravizza D, et al. Full robotic left colon and rectal cancer resection: technique and early outcome. Ann Surg Oncol. 2009;16:1274–8.
14. Park YA, Kim JM, Kim SA, Min BS, Kim NK, Sohn SK, et al. Totally robotic surgery for rectal cancer: from splenic flexure to pelvic floor in one setup. Surg Endosc. 2010;24:715–20.
15. Bokhari MB, Patel CB, Ramos-Valadez DI, Ragupathi M, Haas EM. Learning curve for robotic-assisted laparoscopic colorectal surgery. Surg Endosc. 2011;25:855–60.
16. Pigazzi A, Luca F, Patriti A, Valvo M, Ceccarelli G, Casciola L, et al. Multicentric study on robotic tumor-specific mesorectal excision for the treatment of rectal cancer. Ann Surg Oncol. 2010;17:1614–20.
17. Speicher PJ, Englum BR, Ganapathi AM, Nussbaum DP, Mantyh CR, Migaly J. Robotic low anterior resection for rectal cancer: a national perspective on short-term oncologic outcomes. Ann Surg. 2015;262:1040–5.
18. Baik SH, Kwon HY, Kim JS, Hur H, Sohn SK, Cho CH, et al. Robotic versus laparoscopic low anterior resection of rectal cancer: short-term outcome of a prospective comparative study. Ann Surg Oncol. 2009;16:1480–7.

25 Transanal Excision

Sam Atallah and Elisabeth C. McLemore

The transanal excision technique has evolved significantly over the past 30 years. In 1983, Gerhard Buess introduced a disruptive technique into colorectal surgery, transanal endoscopic microsurgery (TEM) [1, 2]. Compared with transanal excision (TAE), TEM was associated with a superior quality of resection, demonstrated by higher rates of negative margins and lower rates of local recurrence [3–10].

Transanal minimally invasive surgery (TAMIS) was pioneered in 2009 [10] as a feasible alternative to TEM and transanal endoscopic operation (TEO) for local excision of rectal neoplasia. TAMIS utilizes disposable transanal access platforms to perform excision of rectal lesions using laparoscopic instrumentation. The TAMIS technique is associated with high-quality local excision and early results similar to the results of TEM [11–23].

Despite the advantages of TAMIS, it has some limitations when compared with TEM and TEO. The TAMIS technique requires both a surgeon and an operator to drive the laparoscopic camera. Similar to single-port abdominal surgery, there can be a great deal of instrument and camera collision with the inline reduced intraluminal working space. Similar to TEM, the closure of the local excision defect can be difficult, even with the TAMIS approach. For these reasons, surgeons have turned to robotic systems that can overcome the limitations of standard TAMIS. Specifically, the da Vinci® Robotic Surgical System (Intuitive Surgical; Sunnyvale, CA) has been deployed to perform transanal endoluminal surgical resection. This approach has been referred to as robotic TAMIS or robotic transanal surgery (RTS).

RTS was initially evaluated in the cadaveric model and found to be feasible [24]. This approach was also shown to be feasible using a bedside engineered glove port for transanal access [25, 26]. Subsequently, RTS has been successfully performed for local excision of a rectal neoplasm in the clinical setting [27]. A few centers have reported encouraging clinical results from their early experience using various transanal access ports [28–32]. RTS has also been used for applications beyond transanal local excision, such as transanal repair of complex rectourethral fistulae and transanal total mesorectal excision (taTME) [32].

Patient Selection

The indications for RTS are the same as for transanal endoscopic surgery (TEM, TEO, TAMIS) [33]. Though most segments of the rectum can be reached with RTS, this approach is most suited for lesions located in the mid-rectum (5–10 cm from the anal verge). The majority of transanal endoluminal surgical resection is performed for benign rectal neoplasms (Table 25.1) [33–41]. In addition, local excision and close clinical surveillance can be used to manage well-selected, histologically favorable T1 adenocarcinomas with the following characteristics:

- Mobile rectal mass
- Tumor ≤4 cm in diameter

Table 25.1 Transanal endoscopic surgery indications [33–41]

More common indications	Less common indications
Rectal adenoma	Anovaginal septal masses
Rectal carcinoid/ neuroendocrine tumors	Rectal advancement flaps for high rectovaginal fistulas or rectourethral fistulas
Rectal GIST (Gastrointestinal Stromal Tumors)	Low pelvic anastomotic bleeding or leak
	Rectal invasive adenocarcinoma

S. Atallah, MD
Professor of Surgery, University of Central Florida—College of Medicine, Orlando, FL, USA

Department of Colorectal Surgery, Florida Hospital, Orlando, FL, USA

Colorectal Surgery, Oviedo Medical Center, Orlando, FL, USA
e-mail: atallah@post.harvard.edu

E. C. McLemore, MD (✉)
Department of Surgery, Southern California Permanente Medical Group, Los Angeles, CA, USA
e-mail: elisabeth.c.mclemore@kp.org

Y. Fong et al. (eds.), *The SAGES Atlas of Robotic Surgery*, https://doi.org/10.1007/978-3-319-91045-1_25

- Well-differentiated to moderate differentiation
- Absence of vascular invasion
- Absence of lymphatic invasion
- Absence of tumor budding
- Thickness less than submucosal level 3 (sm3)

RTS should not be considered as an equivalent alternative to standard oncologic resection for local excision of higher-risk, locally advanced rectal tumors [34–41].

Preoperative Work-Up

A complete colonoscopy is recommended prior to undergoing surgery for a newly diagnosed rectal neoplasm, in order to complete colon and rectal cancer screening and prevention and manage any potential synchronous lesions. In cases of sporadic adenoma, the likelihood of a synchronous adenoma ranges from 30 to 40% [42, 43]. If the rectal mass is larger than 3 cm, the authors recommend performing the clinical work-up and staging for an invasive rectal neoplasm prior to undergoing transanal endoluminal surgical resection, as the risk of underlying occult malignancy increases with advanced adenoma size [44, 45]. In addition, clinical staging can be difficult to interpret after endoscopic or surgical resection performed for invasive rectal neoplasms; rectal neoplasms with associated enlarged mesorectal lymph nodes may be over- or under-staged after resection.

Clinical staging for rectal cancer includes pathologic findings of invasive adenocarcinoma on biopsy, carcinoembryonic antigen (CEA), complete colonoscopy, and local and systemic clinical staging. Local evaluation of the tumor thickness and assessment of the mesorectal lymph nodes are typically performed using ultrasound and/or MRI. Systemic clinical staging includes cross-sectional CT imaging of the chest, abdomen, and pelvis. Patients with stage IV disease or locally advanced lesions are not considered candidates for RTS unless the objective is palliation.

Patients with histologically favorable, early-stage malignancy (uTis or uT1uN0M0 cancer) are considered candidates for RTS but should be approached with caution, as the lymph node positivity rate for sessile T1 rectal neoplasms can range from 12 to 25% [45, 46]. Advanced training or experience with malignant polyps, Haggitt and Kikuchi classification systems, minimally invasive abdominal perineal resection, and low anterior resection is recommended for all surgeons who plan to perform RTS. Tumor characteristics favoring local endoluminal resection for T1 rectal neoplasms are those listed above in "Patient Selection" [34–41, 47]. Unfavorable lesions or locally advanced rectal neoplasms should be evaluated by a multidisciplinary tumor board [48, 49]. Published outcomes are listed in Table 25.2.

Operative Preparations

A full preoperative oral, mechanical bowel preparation is recommended for all patients to minimize stool contamination and obstruction of the operative field of view. Most rectal lesions can be removed using RTS with the patient in the lithotomy position, but the lateral approach has been described for low-lying lateral lesions and a prone-jackknife split-leg position for anterior lesions. A directional 30°-angled lens is preferred for most robotic transanal approaches.

The operating room should be fitted with standard laparoscopic equipment, including light source, video monitor, and CO_2 insufflator, as well as the da Vinci® Robotic System. The da Vinci® Si system is most often used, but use of the S and Xi Surgical Systems has also been described in RTS cases. General anesthesia with muscle paralysis is recommended to avoid collapse of the rectal wall, which often occurs with diaphragmatic excursion. Where available, a valveless trocar system should be used, because it significantly decreases smoke accumulation and bellowing (collapse of the rectal wall), thereby maintaining a less obstructed view of the surgical field [50].

Table 25.2 Preclinical and clinical outcomes: robotic transanal surgery for endoluminal local excision

Study	Year	Platform	Model	*N*	Size (cm)	Distance from AV (cm)	Operative time (min)	Margins
Atallah et al. [24]	2011	TAMIS-GP	Cadaver	2	n/a	n/a	35	n/a
Atallah et al. [27]	2012	TAMIS-GP	Human	1	3	7	105	1 Neg
Hompes et al. [25]	2012	Glove	Cadaver	2	n/a	n/a	--	n/a
Bardakcioglu [29]	2012	TAMIS-GP	Human	1	--	8	--	1 Neg
Buchs et al. [28]	2013	Glove	Human	3	3.2	10.2	110	3 Neg
Atallah [31]	2013	TAMIS-GP	Human	1	3.4	4	87	1 Neg
Gómez Ruiz et al. [55]	2014	Custom port	Cadaver	4	n/a	--	--	n/a
Hompes et al. [30]	2014	Glove	Human	16	5.3	8	108	13 Neg

AV anal verge, *GP* GelPoint path transanal access platform, *N* number of lesions resected, *TAMIS* transanal minimally invasive surgery

Figure 25.1 illustrates a setup for RTS with the patient in the modified lithotomy position, and the robotic cart docked parallel to the operating table. This configuration is one approach to RTS for endoluminal resection of rectal neoplasia. Alternate approaches for RTS are also feasible, including the lateral approach described by Buchs et al. [28] (Fig. 25.2) and the

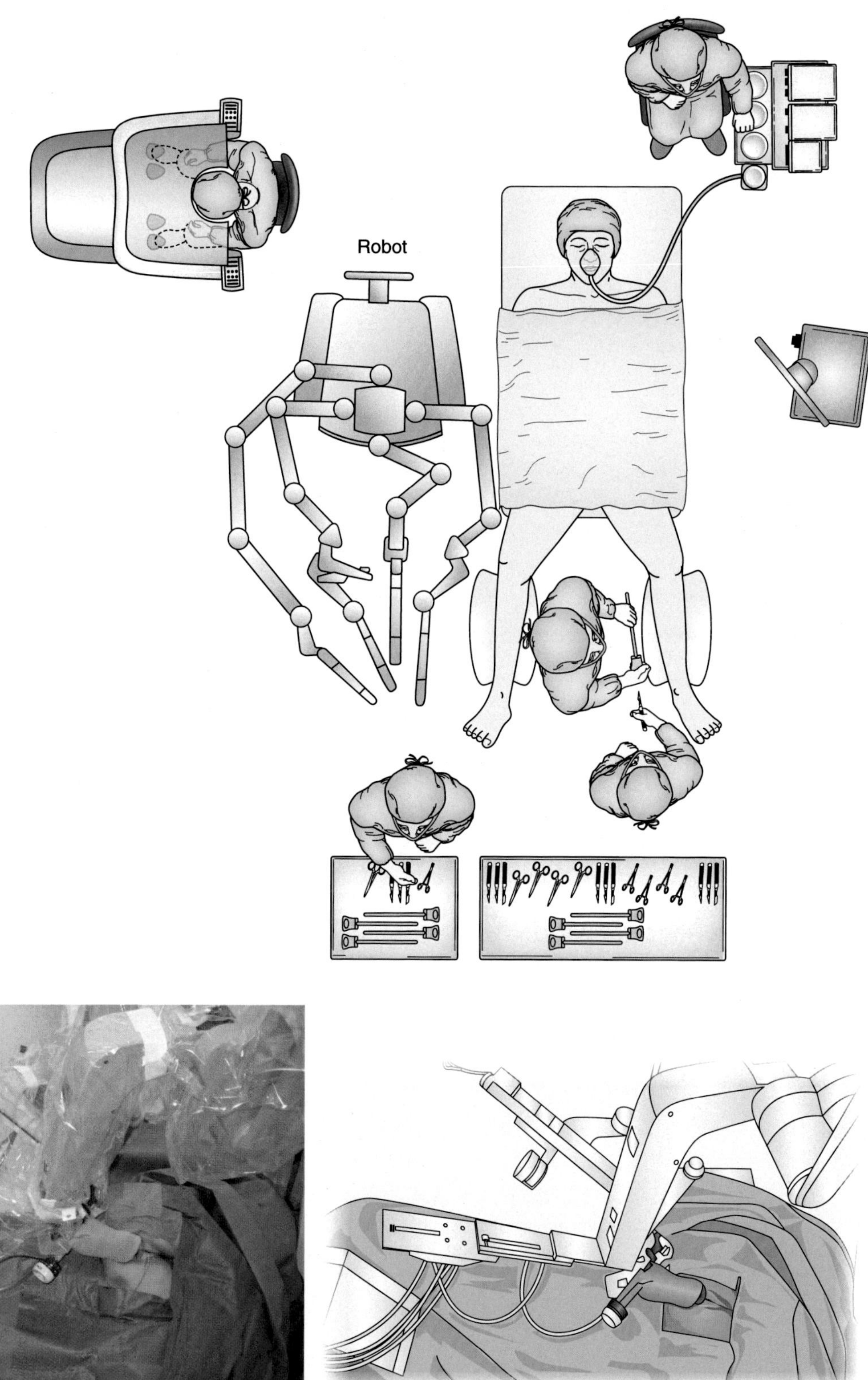

Fig. 25.1 The setup for robotic transanal surgery (RTS). The robotic cart is docked over the left (or right) shoulder, with the patient positioned in a modified lithotomy position in Allen stirrups. A bedside assistant operates a suction irrigator device to assist with smoke evacuation. The robotic arms are configured using either an 8 or 15 mm lens with 8 mm working arms

Fig. 25.2 RTS using a glove port and the lateral approach. Photo courtesy of Nicolas Buchs and Frederic Ris

prone-jackknife patient position demonstrated to be feasible by Hompes et al. (Fig. 25.3). Both of these variations in position and robotic cart docking utilize a glove-port technique, discussed below.

Parenteral antibiotics are administered 30 min prior to incision. The patient is then prepped and draped in the usual fashion. The abdomen should also be prepped, in case the lesion cannot be excised locally or abdominal access becomes necessary.

Robotic Transanal Surgery Using a Transanal Access Device

The most commonly used transanal access device for RTS is the GelPOINT path (Applied Medical; Rancho Santa Margarita, CA), which has been designed specifically for transanal access for TAMIS (Fig. 25.4). The device consists of a malleable cylindrical sleeve, which helps protect against injury to the sphincter mechanism. The sleeve is

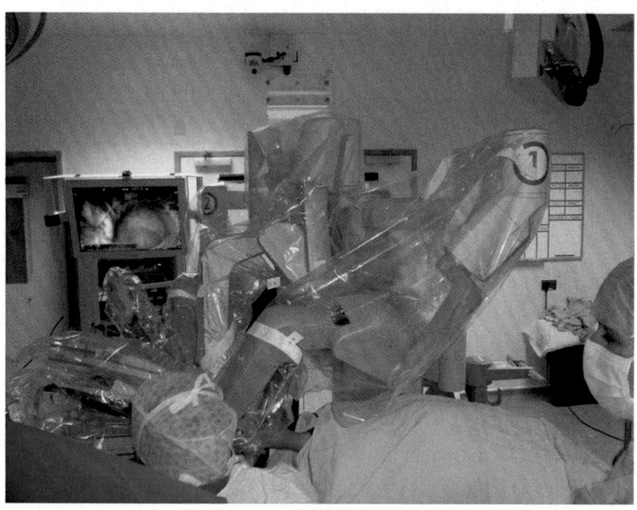

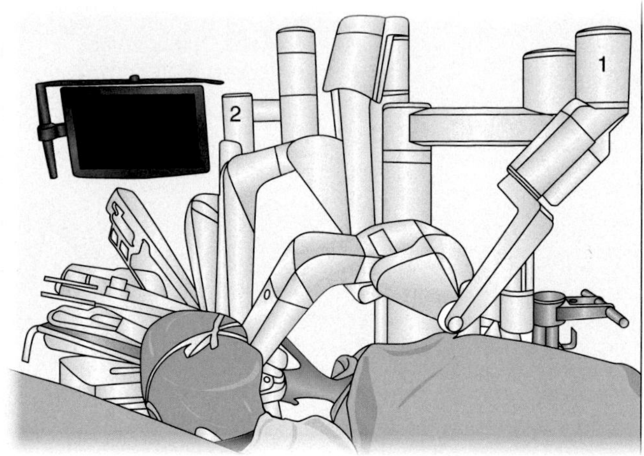

Fig. 25.3 RTS using a glove port and the prone-jackknife approach. Photo courtesy of Roel Hompes

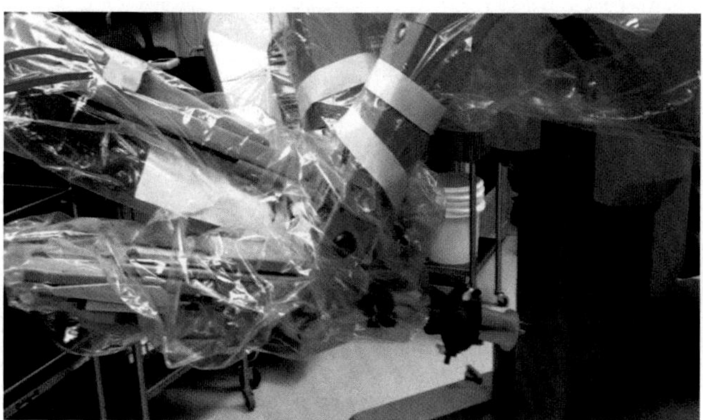

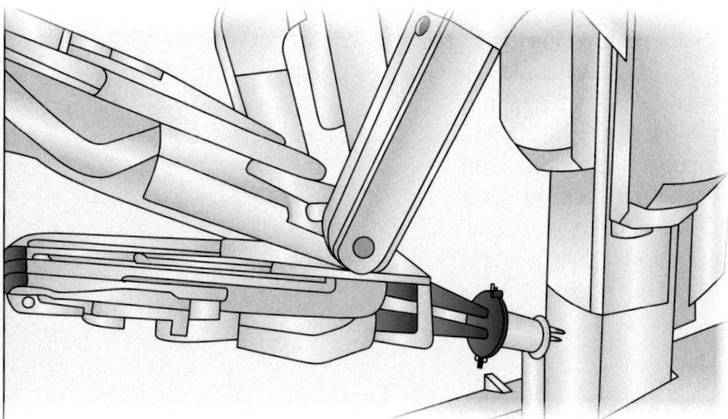

Fig. 25.4 The transanal access port (GelPOINT Path, Applied Medical), designed for transanal minimally invasive surgery (TAMIS), is most commonly used for RTS and is shown docked with the da Vinci® Si system using 5 mm instruments and an 8 mm 30° camera lens with a commonly used configuration

lubricated with petroleum jelly and introduced into the anal canal using an obturator provided by the manufacturer. Once seated above the anorectal ring, the sleeve can be sutured to the skin with 2–0 silk stay sutures if necessary. Typically, the TAMIS platform is used in combination with either a standard CO_2 insufflator or by using a valveless trocar system such as the AirSeal® insufflation system (CONMED; Utica, NY), which diminishes smoke accumulation and bellowing of the rectum, thereby improving surgical field visibility. All da Vinci® platforms have been used to perform RTS, including the da Vinci® Xi system (Fig. 25.5).

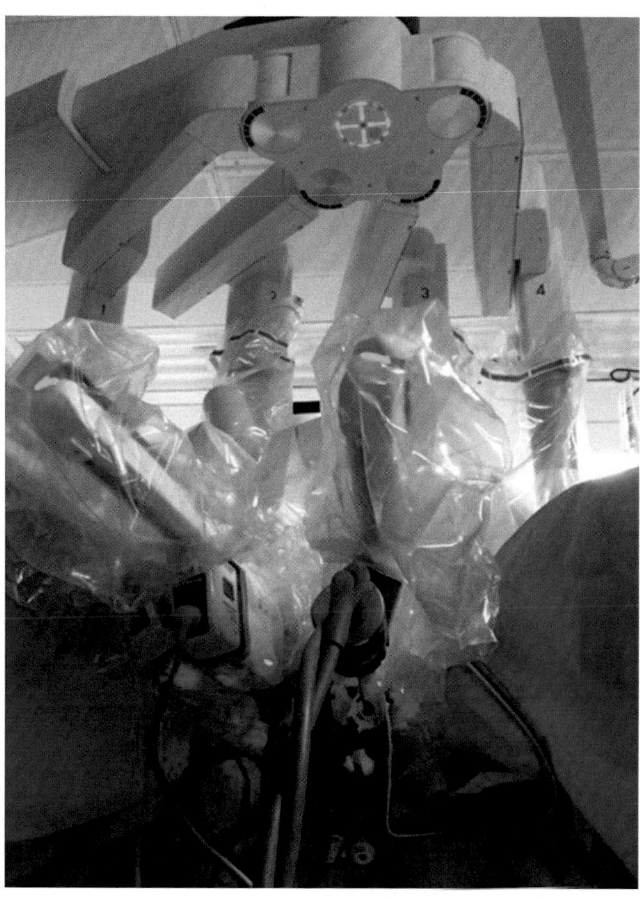

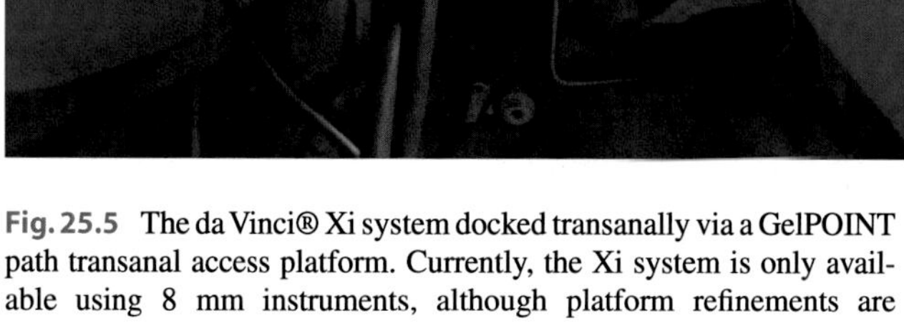

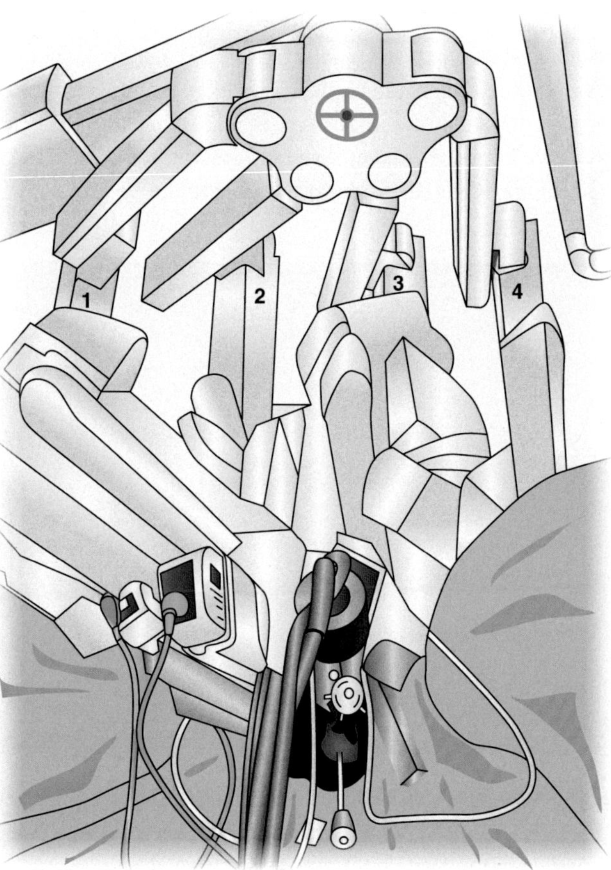

Fig. 25.5 The da Vinci® Xi system docked transanally via a GelPOINT path transanal access platform. Currently, the Xi system is only available using 8 mm instruments, although platform refinements are expected with 5 mm instruments, which are advantageous for operating within the confines of a narrow rectal lumen

Robotic Transanal Surgery Using the Glove Port

Alternatively, a glove port can be used, as described by R. Hompes et al. [25, 30]. Using a glove port, an 8.5 mm robotic 30° camera lens is introduced via trocar through the "thumb" of the glove in the "thumbs-up" camera position (Fig. 25.6). This arrangement can avoid excessive strain on the glove material, thus minimizing the risk of glove perforation from excessive torque. Though a variety of 8 and 5 mm wristed instruments can be used for RTS, Maryland bipolar forceps and monopolar hook cautery most typically are used, and no more than two robotic working arms are used with any type of RTS. For suture closure of defects, a robotic needle driver and forceps can be used in conjunction with a self-locking absorbable suture.

Robotic Transanal Surgery Using a Custom Rigid Port

A custom-made port developed by Dr. Marcos Gómez Ruiz combines a rigid steel platform that secures to the operating table with a mechanical arm and which uses the 80 mm, reusable GelPOINT gelatinous cap for an interface (Fig. 25.7). The steps require dilation of the anus with the aid of an obturator and then introduction of the rigid platform, which is secured into position using a Martin arm attached to the operating table rail. Finally, the disposable cap is placed onto the rigid, reusable platform. The robot is then docked along the patient's left at 45° to the vertical access of the operating table.

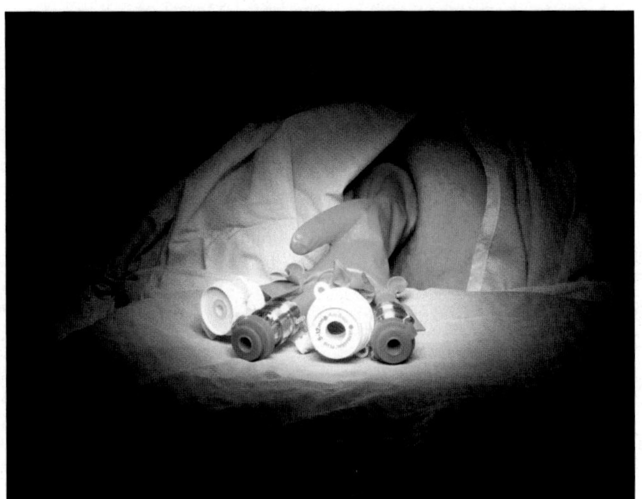

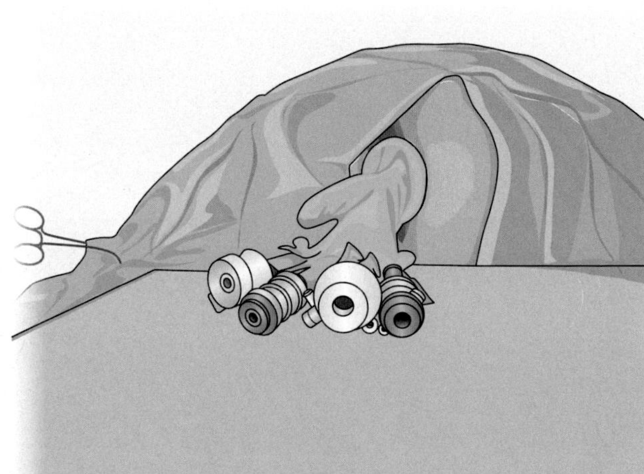

Fig. 25.6 The glove port for RTS. With the patient positioned in prone-jackknife and the thumb of the glove facing upward, the robotic cart is docked, and arm collision is minimized (Photo courtesy of Roel Hompes)

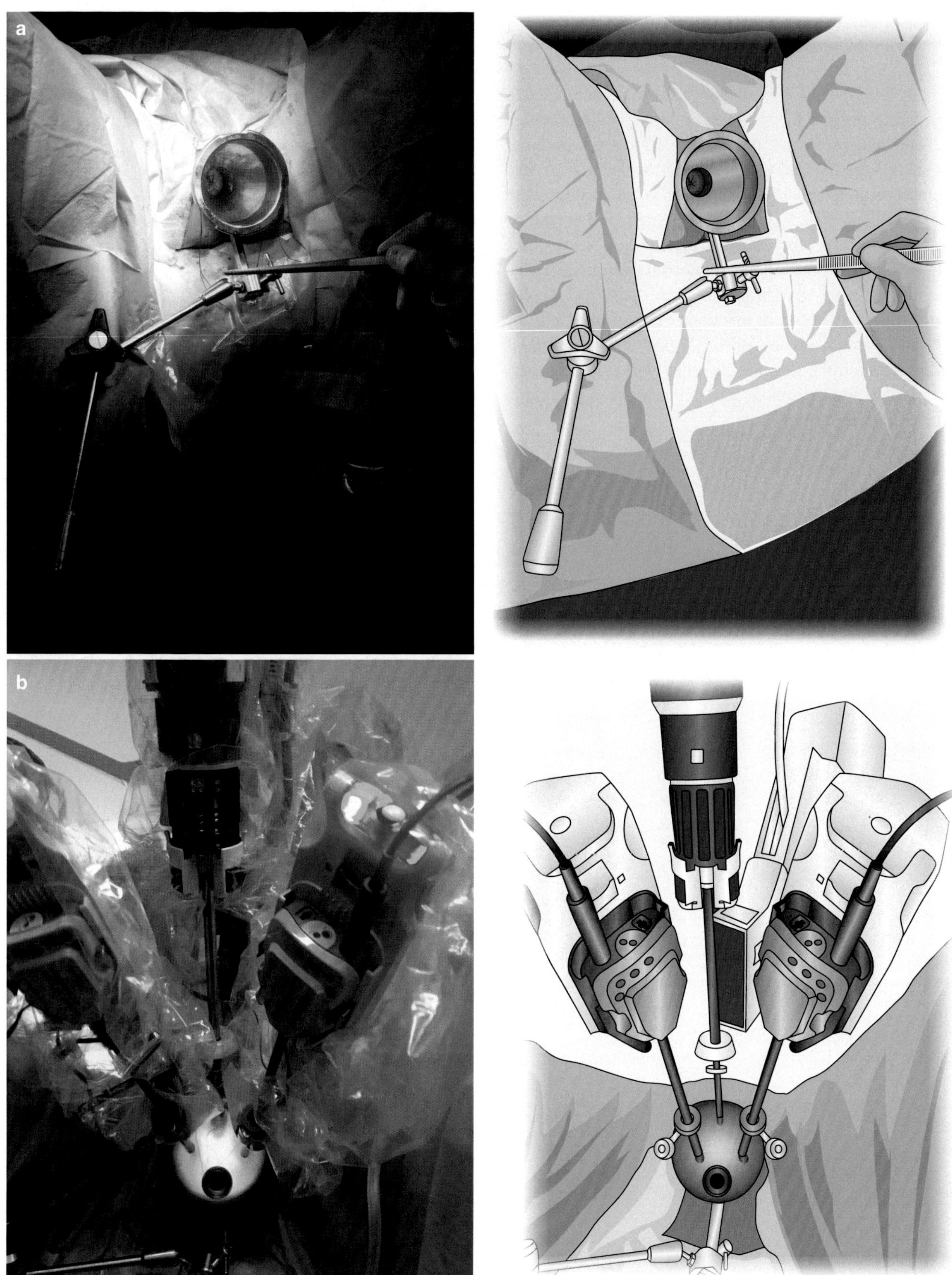

Fig. 25.7 (**a**) A customized rigid platform with a conical shape is shown. Designed for transanal surgery by Dr. Marcos Gómez Ruiz, the device is a hybrid cross between TAMIS and transanal endoscopic operation (TEO). (**b**) It utilizes a gelatinous cap designed for single-port laparoscopy, which measures 80 mm. This allows for improved triangulation and minimizes robotic arm collision because the diameter of the cap is twice the diameter of the standard TAMIS port (Photos courtesy of Marcos Gómez Ruiz)

Robotic Transanal Surgery for Local Excision of Neoplasia: Step-By-Step

For both TAMIS and RTS, patients are pharmacologically paralyzed to prevent rectal lumen collapse, and humidified CO_2 is typically used with the pressure set to a maximum of 15 mm Hg. With the GelPOINT path port seated in place and pneumorectum established, a laparoscope is introduced to perform cursory visualization of the target lesion and to assess the rectum for luminal expansion. Next, three GelPOINT path cannulas are introduced at an equilateral distance in such a way that triangulation is optimized. The da Vinci® robotic 8 or 5 mm trocars are then placed into the GelPOINT cannulas. The GelPOINT path gelatinous cap is next placed onto the sleeve, which has already been seated into position, and the robotic cart is then docked parallel to the operating table (Fig. 25.8).

Next, a robotic 5 mm hook with monopolar cautery and Maryland grasper are secured. Cautery is used to delineate the circumlinear resection margin, and a full-thickness local excision is then performed by the console surgeon (Fig. 25.9). For evacuation of smoke, a bedside assistant uses a 5 mm laparoscopic suction irrigation device, which may be passed directly through the GelPOINT path gelatinous cap, or, alternatively, an additional 5 mm trocar. We find that simple, short bursts of suction maintain image clarity without collapsing the rectal lumen, and the addition of a valveless trocar system helps maintain a stable pneumorectum. The specimen may be tented gently using a robotic Maryland grasper, while hook cautery allows for full-thickness excision. The best technique emphasizes minimal manipulation of the tumor itself, which can result in micro-fragmentation and potential tumor seeding. Importantly, the CO_2 insufflation provides a natural pneumo-dissection, thereby augmenting the ease and clarity of local excision using RTS.

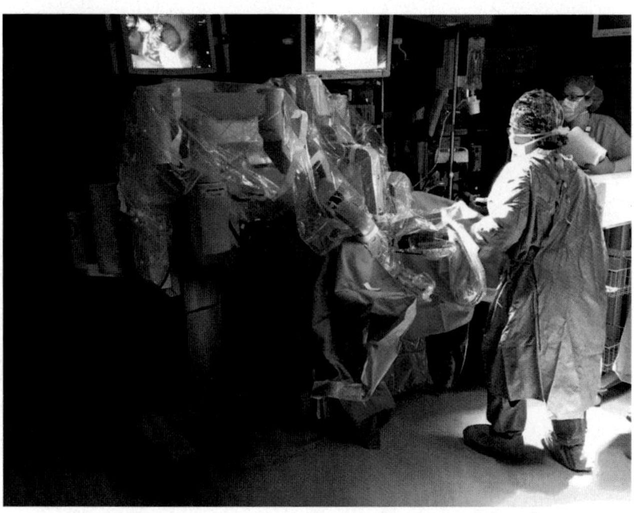

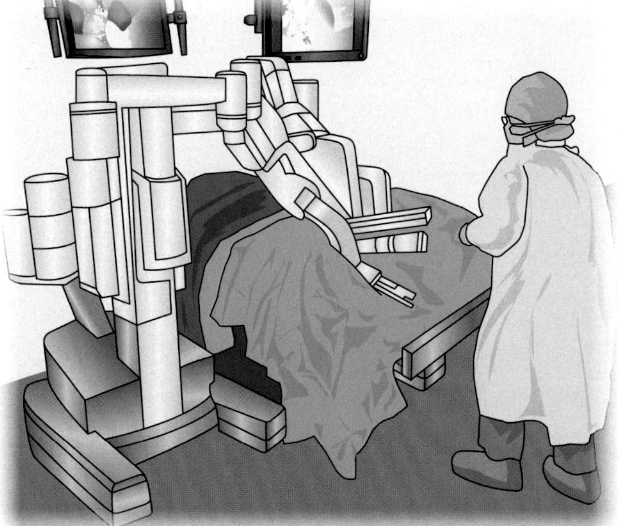

Fig. 25.8 This patient is in the modified Lloyd-Davies position with moderate Trendelenburg in Allen stirrups. The da Vinci® Si robotic cart is docked parallel and flush against the operating Table. A bedside assistant is able to operate a suction-irrigation device and assist as needed with smoke evacuation and specimen extraction

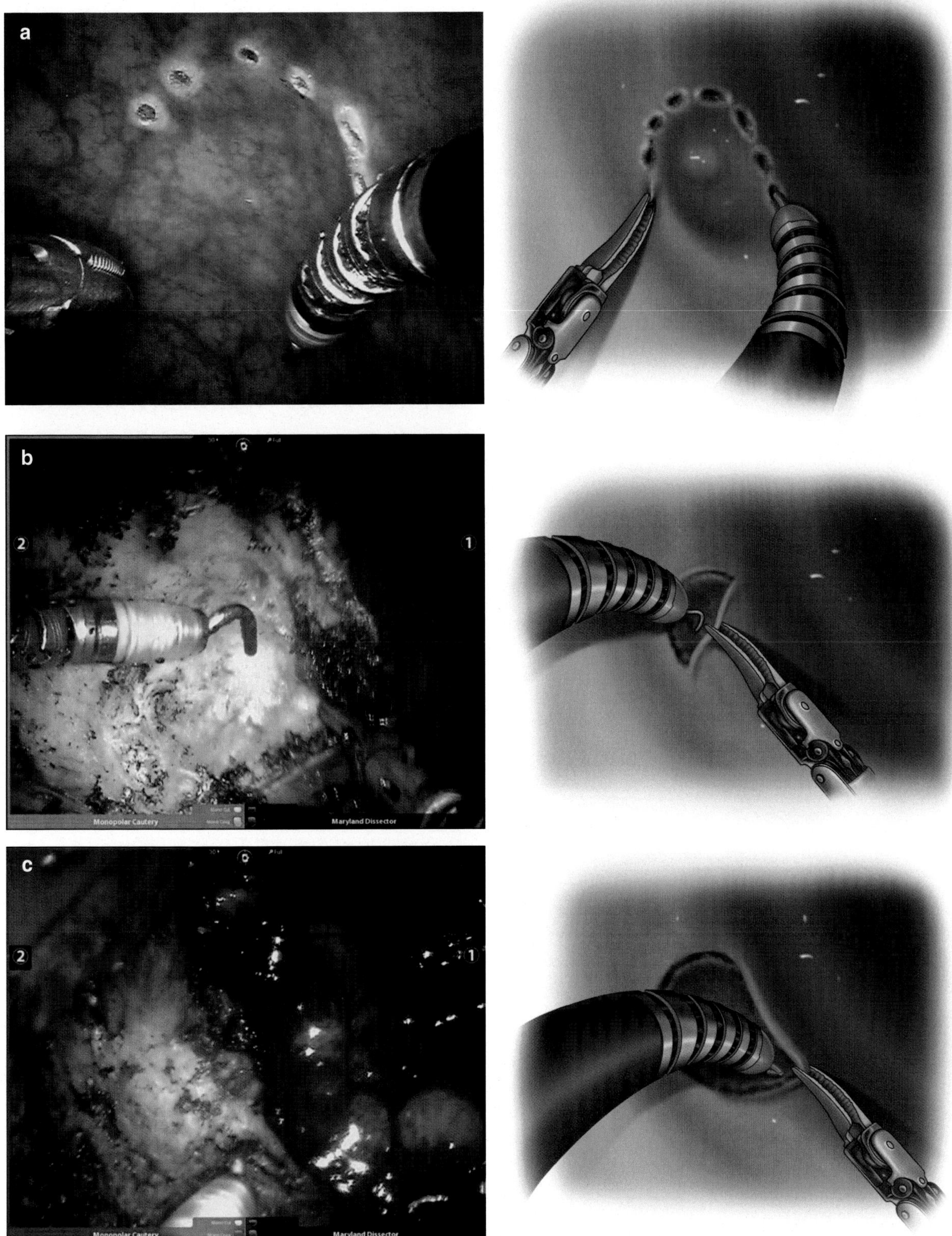

Fig. 25.9 (**a**) A pT1 lesion at the site of a polypectomy in the mid-rectum is circumscribed with electrocautery using a 5 mm robotic hook instrument. As with all advanced transanal approaches to local excision, this is always the first step, as it helps to ensure margin negativity. (**b** and **c**) A 3.7 cm distal tubulovillous adenoma is removed full-thickness using RTS

To retrieve the resected specimen, the robot must be dismounted from the GelPOINT path interface. The lesion can be retrieved with a 5 mm laparoscopic grasper operated by a bedside assistant (Fig. 25.10). Once this handoff has occurred and robot has been undocked, the lid to the port is simply removed to allow for specimen extraction.

The next step is closure of the full-thickness rectal wall defect, which is always recommended. The hook cautery is exchanged for a robotic needle driver, and the robotic cart is redocked in the same position as before. Robotic intraluminal suturing is then carried out using a V-Loc™ 180 absorbable wound closure device (Covidien; Mansfield, MA). This allows for suturing without the need for intraluminal knot tying, as the unidirectional barbs on the suture self-lock as they pass through the rectal wall. The defect can be closed with a single running, self-locking, absorbable suture, thereby completing the operation (Fig. 25.11). Alternatively, endoscopic visualization (*e*TAMIS) [19] can be used for closure of more proximal defects, with the aid of a dual-channel colonoscope and an automated suturing device such as Overstitch (Apollo Endosurgery; Austin, TX) (Fig. 25.12).

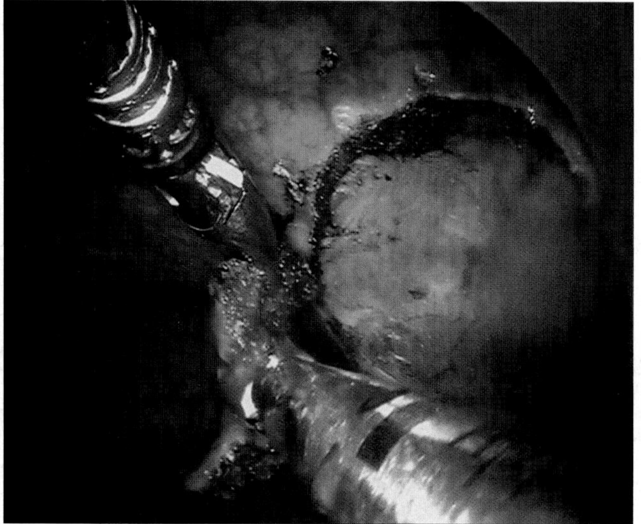

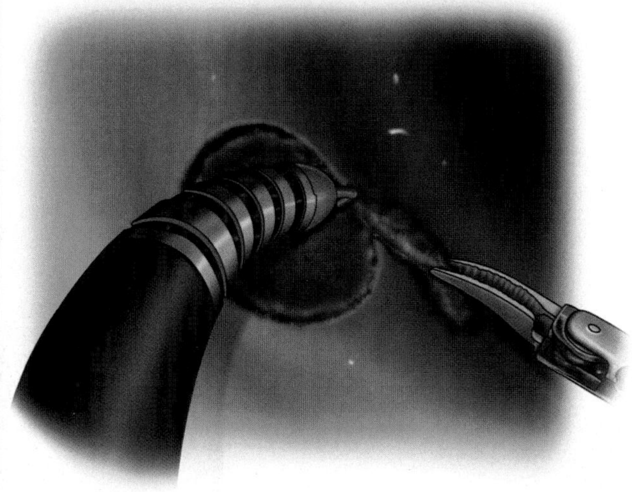

Fig. 25.10 The specimen has been completely resected using RTS. The robotic Maryland grasper is then used to pass off the surgical specimen to a 5 mm laparoscopic grasper, as shown. This grasper is operated by the bedside assistant

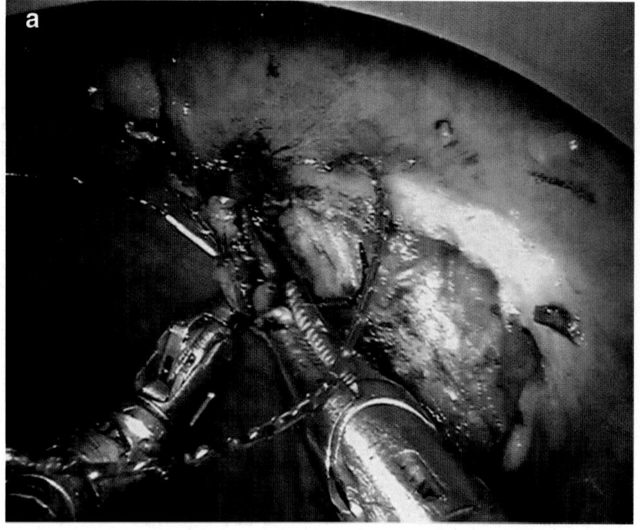

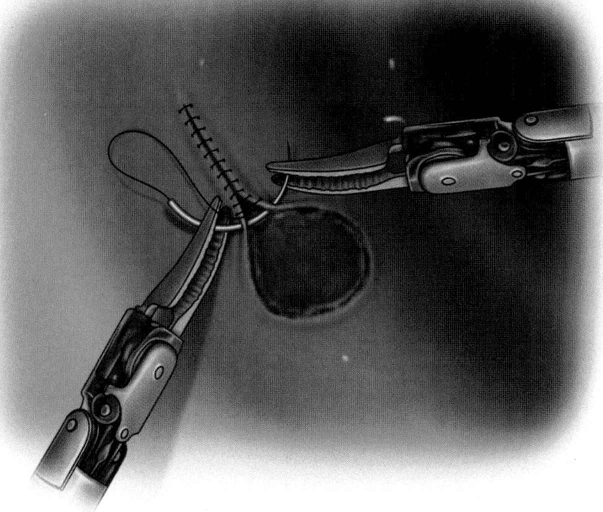

Fig. 25.11 (**a**) Robotic suturing of the surgical defect after resection using a 5 mm needle drive, Maryland grasper, and a 3 0 absorbable barbed suture. (**b**) Upon closure of the surgical defect, a bedside assistant uses laparoscopic scissors to divide the suture tail, and the procedure is completed. (**c**) The finished result

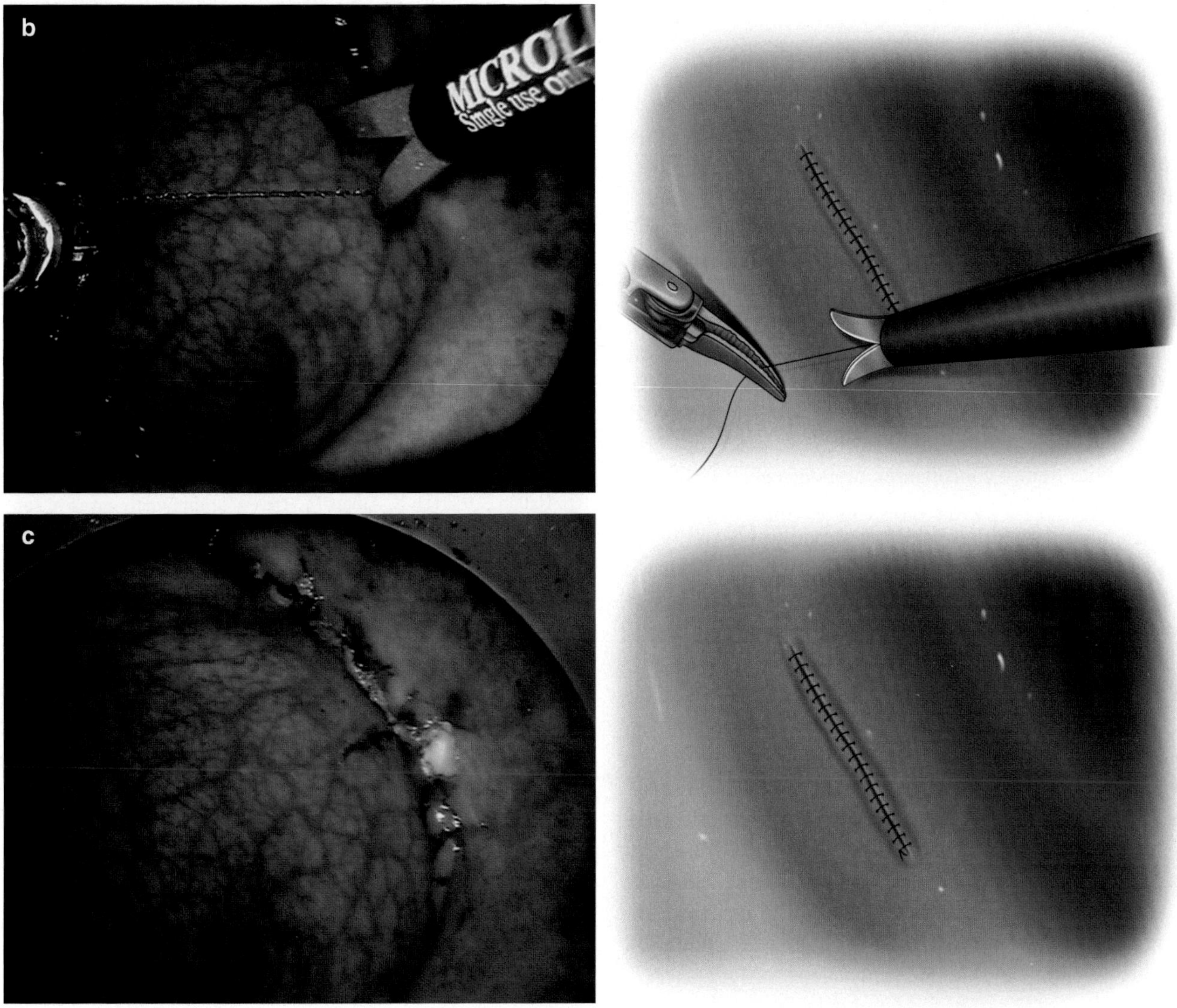

b

c

Fig. 25.11 (continued)

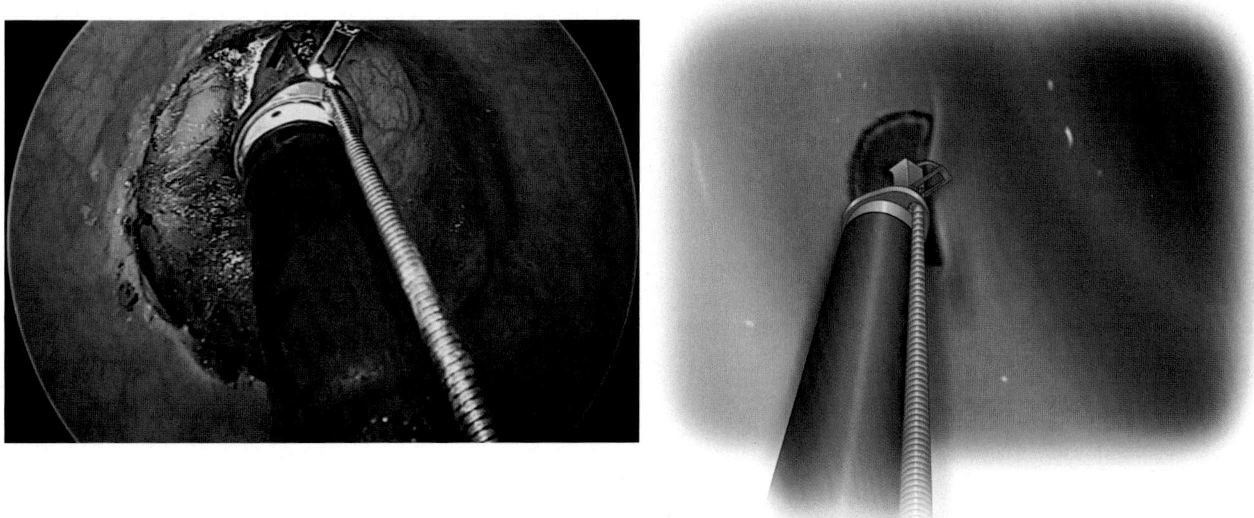

Fig. 25.12 An over-the-colonoscope suturing device is used to close a proximal defect after RTS. This hybrid approach borrows from the concept of endoscopic visualization to perform TAMIS (*e*TAMIS)

Discussion

Now that transanal access platforms used for TEM, TEO, and TAMIS are more widely accessible and available, the conventional Parks transanal excision for rectal neoplasms should be abandoned altogether [51]. RTS illustrates a novel approach to the resection of rectal neoplasia and is feasible for lesions located in the mid-rectum (5–10 cm from the anal verge). A theoretical advantage of robotic transanal excision over transanal endoscopic surgery (TEM, TEO, TAMIS) is that the surgeon at the robotic console is able to perform intricate surgery with articulating instruments within the narrow, cylindrical lumen. The EndoWrist (Da Vinci Robotic Surgical Platform; Intuitive Surgical, Sunnyvale, CA) movement allows for greater intraluminal dexterity and perceived precision. This, together with tremor cancellation, motion scaling, and magnified (10×–40×) 3D optics, enhances the surgeon's ability to perform transanal local excision with improved dexterity.

The RTS approach also improves the dexterity associated with more complex tasks during transanal endoscopic surgery, such as intraluminal suturing. RTS is a new approach to transanal endoluminal surgery, and its ability to facilitate intricate tasks with greater articulation and perceived precision makes this method attractive for complex cases in which local excision, defect suture closure, or other advanced transanal procedures (such as transanal repair of rectourethral or rectovaginal fistulae) may be more technically challenging with TEM, TEO, or TAMIS.

Although more ergonomic for the surgeon, RTS increases operative cost substantially, so this approach should be approached with reservation and preferably in a clinical trial institutional review board setting. RTS is a technique that remains in its infancy, and the applications for RTS in rectal surgery have not yet been fully evaluated or defined. RTS is currently undergoing further investigation, and more data are necessary to establish its practicality and benefit over transanal endoscopic surgery. In addition, as robotic platforms evolve and are further refined, the utility and practicality of RTS will likely increase, particularly with single-port robotic systems in the field of transanal total mesorectal excision [32, 52–57].

References

1. Buess G, Theiss R, Hutterer F, Pichlmaier H, Pelz P, Holfeld T, et al. Die transanale endoscopische Rektumoperation. Erprobung einer neuen Methode im Tierversuch. Leber Magen Darm. 1983;13:73–7.
2. Buess G. Review: transanal endoscopic microsurgery (TEM). J R Coll Surg Edinb. 1993;38:239–45.
3. Middleton PF, Sutherland LM, Maddern GJ. Transanal endoscopic microsurgery: a systematic review. Dis Colon Rectum. 2005;48:270–84.
4. Moore JS, Cataldo PA, Osler T, Hyman NH. Transanal endoscopic microsurgery is more effective than traditional transanal excision for resection of rectal masses. Dis Colon Rectum. 2008;51:1026–30.
5. Barendse RM, van den Broek FJ, Dekker E, Bemelman WA, de Graaf EJ, Fockens P, Reitsma JB. Systematic review of endoscopic mucosal resection versus transanal endoscopic microsurgery for large rectal adenomas. Endoscopy. 2011;43:941–9.
6. Tsai BM, Finne CO, Nordenstam JF, Christoforidis D, Madoff RD, Mellgren A. Transanal endoscopic microsurgery resection of rectal tumors: outcomes and recommendations. Dis Colon Rectum. 2010;53:16–23.
7. Salm R, Lampe H, Bustos A, Matern U. Experience with TEM in Germany. Endosc Surg Allied Technol. 1994;2:251–4.
8. Said S, Stippel D. Transanal endoscopic microsurgery in large, sessile adenomas of the rectum. A 10-year experience. Surg Endosc. 1995;9:1106–12.
9. Schäfer H, Baldus SE, Hölscher AH. Giant adenomas of the rectum: complete resection by transanal endoscopic microsurgery (TEM). Int J Color Dis. 2006;21:533–7.
10. Atallah S, Larach S, Albert M. Transanal minimally invasive surgery: a giant leap forward. Surg Endosc. 2010;24:2200–5.
11. Lorenz C, Nimmesgern T, Back M, Langwieler TE. Transanal single port microsurgery (TSPM) as a modified technique of transanal microsurgery (TEM). Surg Innov. 2010;17:160–3.
12. Lim SB, Seo SI, Lee JL, Kwak JY, Jang TY. Feasibility of transanal minimally invasive surgery for mid-rectal lesions. Surg Endosc. 2012;26:3127–32.
13. Slack T, Wong S, Muhlmann M. Transanal minimally invasive surgery: an initial experience. ANZ J Surg. 2014;84:177–80.
14. Rega D, Cardone E, Montesarchio L, Tammaro P, Pace U, Ruffolo F, et al. Transanal minimally invasive surgery with single-port laparoscopy for rectal tumors. Eur J Surg Oncol. 2012;38:982.
15. Albert M, Atallah S, Larach S, deBeche-Adams T. Minimally invasive anorectal surgery: from parks local excision to transanal endoscopic microsurgery to transanal minimally invasive surgery. Sem Colon Rectal Surg. 2013;24:42–9.
16. Albert M, Atallah S, deBeche-Adams T, Izfar S, Larach S. Transanal minimally invasive surgery (TAMIS) for local excision of benign neoplasms and early-stage rectal cancer: efficacy and outcomes in the first 50 patients. Dis Colon Rectum. 2013;56:301–7.
17. Barendse RM, Doornebosch PG, Bemelman WA, Fockens P, Dekker E, de Graaf EJ. Transanal employment of single access ports is feasible for rectal surgery. Ann Surg. 2012;256:1030–3.
18. Corman ML. Corman's colon and rectal surgery. 6th ed. Philadelphia: Lippincott Williams & Wilkins; 2013.
19. McLemore EC, Coker A, Jacobsen G, Talamini MA, Horgan S. *e*TAMIS: endoscopic visualization for transanal minimally invasive surgery. Surg Endosc. 2013;27(5):1842.
20. Martin-Perez B, Andrade-Ribeiro GD, Hunter L, Atallah S. A systematic review of transanal minimally invasive surgery (TAMIS) from 2010 to 2013. Tech Coloproctol. 2014;18:775–88.
21. McLemore EC, Weston LA, Coker AM, Jacobsen GR, Talamini MA, Horgan S, Ramamoorthy SL. Transanal minimally invasive surgery for benign and malignant rectal neoplasia. Am J Surg. 2014;208:372–81.
22. McLemore EC, Coker A, Leland H, Yu PT, Devaraj B, Jacobsen G, et al. New disposable transanal endoscopic surgery platform: longer channel, longer reach. Glob J Gastroenterol Hepatol. 2013;1:36–40.
23. Atallah S, Albert M, deBeche-Adams T, Larach S. Transanal minimally invasive surgery (TAMIS): applications beyond local excision. Tech Coloproctol. 2013;17:239–43.

24. Atallah SB, Albert MR, deBeche-Adams TH, Larach SW. Robotic transanal minimally invasive surgery in a cadaveric model. Tech Coloproctol. 2011;15(4):461.
25. Hompes R, Rauh SM, Hagen ME, Mortensen NJ. Preclinical cadaveric study of transanal endoscopic da Vinci® surgery. Br J Surg. 2012;99(8):1144.
26. Carrara A, Mangiola D, Motter M, Tirone A, Ghezzi G, Silvestri M, et al. Glove port technique for transanal endoscopic microsurgery. Int J Surg Oncol. 2012;2012:1. https://doi.org/10.1155/2012/383025.
27. Atallah S, Parra-Davilla E, deBeche-Adams T, Albert M, Larach S. Excision of a rectal neoplasm using robotic transanal surgery (RTS): a description of the technique. Tech Coloproctol. 2012;16:389–92.
28. Buchs NC, Pugin F, Volonte F, Hagen ME, Morel P, Ris F. Robotic transanal endoscopic microsurgery: technical details for the lateral approach. Dis Colon Rectum. 2013;56:1194–8.
29. Bardakcioglu O. Robotic transanal access surgery. Surg Endosc. 2013;27:1407–9.
30. Hompes R, Rauh SM, Ris F, Tuynman JB, Mortensen NJ. Robotic transanal minimally invasive surgery for local excision of rectal neoplasms. Br J Surg. 2014;101:578–81.
31. Atallah S. Robotic transanal minimally invasive surgery for local excision of rectal neoplasms (Br J Surg. 2014; 101: 578-581). Br J Surg. 2014;101:581. https://doi.org/10.1002/bjs.9467.
32. Atallah S, Martin-Perez B, Parra-Davila E, deBeche-Adams T, Nassif G, Albert M, Larach S. Robotic transanal surgery for local excision of rectal neoplasia, transanal total mesorectal excision, and repair of complex fistulae: clinical experience with the first 18 cases at a single institution. Tech Coloproctol. 2015;19:401–10.
33. Qi Y, Stoddard D, Monson JR. Indications and techniques of transanal endoscopic microsurgery (TEMS). J Gastrointest Surg. 2011;15(8):1306.
34. Nascimbeni R, Burgart LJ, Nivatvongs S, Larson DR. Risk of lymph node metastasis in T1 carcinoma of the colon and rectum. Dis Colon Rectum. 2002;45:200–6.
35. Garcia-Aguilar J, Shi Q, Thomas CR Jr, Chan E, Cataldo P, Marcet J, et al. A phase II trial of neoadjuvant chemoradiation and local excision for T2N0 rectal cancer: preliminary results of the ACOSOG Z6041 trial. Ann Surg Oncol. 2012;19:384–91.
36. Kundel Y, Brenner R, Purim O, Peled N, Idelevich E, Fenig E, et al. Is local excision after complete pathological response to neoadjuvant chemoradiation for rectal cancer an acceptable treatment option? Dis Colon Rectum. 2010;53:1624–31.
37. Kim CJ, Yeatman TJ, Coppola D, Trotti A, Williams B, Barthel JS, et al. Local excision of T2 and T3 rectal cancers after downstaging chemoradiation. Ann Surg. 2001;234:352–8. discussion 358–9
38. Bedrosian I, Rodriguez-Bigas MA, Feig B, Hunt KK, Ellis L, Curley SA, et al. Predicting the node-negative mesorectum after preoperative chemoradiation for locally advanced rectal carcinoma. J Gastrointest Surg. 2004;8:56–62.
39. Bujko K, Nowacki MP, Nasierowska-Guttmejer A, Kepka L, Winkler-Spytkowska B, Suwaski R, et al. Prediction of mesorectal nodal metastases after chemoradiation for rectal cancer: results of a randomised trial: implication for subsequent local excision. Radiother Oncol. 2005;76:234–40.
40. Yeo SG, Kim DY, Kim TH, Chang HJ, Oh JH, Park W, et al. Pathologic complete response of primary tumor following preoperative chemoradiotherapy for locally advanced rectal cancer: long-term outcomes and prognostic significance of pathologic nodal status (KROG 09-01). Ann Surg. 2010;252:998–1004.
41. Wang LM, Kevans D, Mulcahy H, O'Sulivan J, Fennelly D, Hyland J, et al. Tumor budding is a strong and reproducible prognostic marker in T3N0 colorectal cancer. Am J Surg Pathol. 2009;33:134–41.
42. Bond JH. Polyp guideline: diagnosis, treatment, and surveillance for patients with nonfamilial colorectal polyps. The Practice Parameters Committee of the American College of Gastroenterology. Ann Intern Med. 1993;119:836–43.
43. Farraye FA, Wallace M. Clinical significance of small polyps found during screening with flexible sigmoidoscopy. Gastrointest Endosc Clin N Am. 2002;12:41–51.
44. Schoen RE, Weissfeld JL, Pinsky PF, Riley T. Yield of advanced adenoma and cancer based on polyp size detected at screening flexible sigmoidoscopy. Gastroenterology. 2006;131:1683–9.
45. Haggitt RC, Glotzbach RE, Soffer EE, Wruble LD. Prognostic factors in colorectal carcinomas arising in adenomas: implications for lesions removed by endoscopic polypectomy. Gastroenterology. 1985;89:328–36.
46. Kikuchi R, Takano M, Takagi K, Fujimoto N, Nozaki R, Fujiyoshi T, Uchida Y. Management of early invasive colorectal cancer Risk of recurrence and clinical guidelines. Dis Colon Rectum. 1995;38:1286–95.
47. Winde G, Nottberg H, Keller R, Schmid KW, Bunte H. Surgical cure for early rectal carcinomas (T1). Dis Colon Rectum. 1996;39:969–76.
48. Monson JRT, Abbas MA, Chang GJ, Read TE, Rothenberger DA, Garcia-Aguilar J, Peters W. Optimizing rectal cancer management: analysis of current evidence. Dis Colon Rectum. 2014;57:252–9.
49. Heald RJ. The 'Holy Plane' of rectal surgery. J R Soc Med. 1988;81:503–8.
50. Bislenghi G, Wolthuis A, de Buck van Overstraeten A, D'Hoore A. AirSeal system insufflator to maintain a stable pneumorectum during TAMIS. Tech Coloproctol. 2015;19:43–5.
51. Atallah S, Keller D. Why the conventional parks transanal excision for early stage rectal cancer should be abandoned. Dis Colon Rectum. 2015;58:1211–4.
52. Sylla P, Rattner DW, Delgado S, Lacy AM. NOTES transanal rectal cancer resection using transanal endoscopic microsurgery and laparoscopic assistance. Surg Endosc. 2010;24:1205–10.
53. Atallah S, Nassif G, Polavarapu H, deBeche-Adams T, Ouyang J, Albert M, et al. Robotic-assisted transanal surgery for total mesorectal excision (RATS-TME): a description of a novel surgical approach with video demonstration. Tech Coloproctol. 2013;17:441–7.
54. Huscher CGS, Bretagnol F, Ponzano C. Robotic-assisted transanal total mesorectal excision. Ann Surg. 2015;261:e120–1.
55. Gómez Ruiz M, Parra IM, Palazuelos CM, Martín JA, Fernández CC, Diego JC, Fleitas MG. Robotic-assisted laparoscopic transanal total mesorectal excision for rectal cancer: a prospective pilot study. Dis Colon Rectum. 2015;58:145–53.
56. Verheijen PM, Consten ECJ, Broeders IAMJ. Robotic transanal total mesorectal excision for rectal cancer: experience with a first case. Int J Med Robot. 2014;10(4):423–6.
57. Hompes R. Robotics and transanal minimal invasive surgery (TAMIS): the "sweet spot" for robotics in colorectal surgery? Tech Coloproctol. 2015;19:377.

Robotic Distal Pancreatectomy

26

Anusak Yiengpruksawan

Robotic distal pancreatectomy using the da Vinci Si® platform (Intuitive Surgical, Sunnyvale, CA), although considered to be easier than pancreatoduodenectomy, is a challenging procedure from both strategic and technical standpoints. Careful planning for robotic setup is one of the first important steps that can lead to smooth surgery with less frustration. This step requires thorough knowledge of locoregional anatomy, tumor biology, and the planned extent of the procedure related to the particular patient. This chapter presents detailed technical steps together with tips and tricks that the author frequently employs. Although the techniques are based on the da Vinci Si® platform, the basic thought process and techniques should work as well with the da Vinci Xi® platform, except for the initial robotic setup.

Advantages and Disadvantages of Robotic Surgery

Robotic surgery with the da Vinci Si® has both advantages and disadvantages when compared with conventional open and laparoscopic surgery. Its disadvantages are lack of tactile feedback, the fixed platform, and the limited operative field. Its advantages are intuitive hand-eye coordination, which returns the "open surgery" experience to the surgeon, EndoWrist® instruments (intuitive surgical), high-definition 3D imaging, motion scaling, enhanced imaging capability using the TilePro™ display and Firefly™ fluorescence imaging (Intuitive Surgical, Sunnyvalle, CA), and infinite hardware-software upgradability. The combination of its upsides and downsides creates a unique decision-making process for a surgeon when planning for a surgery.

Unlike an open or laparoscopic approach, most of the robotic surgical process—especially the initial robotic setup—must be planned or choreographed carefully before the actual surgery begins. This requirement is due mostly to the fixed platform of the da Vinci Si® system, which does not allow for flexibility. Once the robot "surgeon" is fixed to the patient and its arms are docked to their respective ports, the operating table cannot be adjusted, or it can cause injury to the patient. The eye (camera) is arranged and integrated with the arms on each side, just as our eyes are with our arms; this arrangement provides a natural hand-eye coordination, but it also limits the flexibility of the system and the operative field because the camera and instrument ports are not interchangeable. Therefore, the robot setup is one of the most crucial steps and may determine the success or failure (conversion) of the surgery, especially when dealing with an organ that occupies a large space or more than a single quadrant. This problem may be less significant with the new Xi® system, which is a boom-mounted system allowing for four-quadrant access without having to reposition the surgical cart, but the Si® will continue to be the main system used worldwide for at least the next few years, so this discussion will remain relevant for some time.

Robotic Setup for Distal Pancreatectomy

Flexibility is the key when dealing with surgery of the left pancreas. Because the left pancreas lies almost horizontally across the left side of the retroperitoneal space, robot setup, positioning of the patient, and the technical approach can and should be varied. The setup of the Si® system and the patient's positioning depend not only on the location of the tumor in relation to the superior mesenteric vein (SMV) and splenic hilum but also by the patient's body habitus, the intent of the procedure, and the topographic anatomy of that individual.

Basic robotic setup and patient positioning for a simple distal pancreatectomy with or without splenectomy are shown in Fig. 26.1. In this example, the target lesion (*orange*) is in the left upper abdomen, and the robot (surgical/patient cart) is placed over the patient's left shoulder. For a lesion located close to the SMV or for those requiring radical lymphadenectomy, the port placements should be spread toward the right, focusing attention to the pancreatic neck region (Fig. 26.2).

A. Yiengpruksawan, MD
Department of Surgery, Faculty of Medicine, Siriraj Hospital, Mahidol University, Bangkok, Thailand

Y. Fong et al. (eds.), *The SAGES Atlas of Robotic Surgery*, https://doi.org/10.1007/978-3-319-91045-1_26

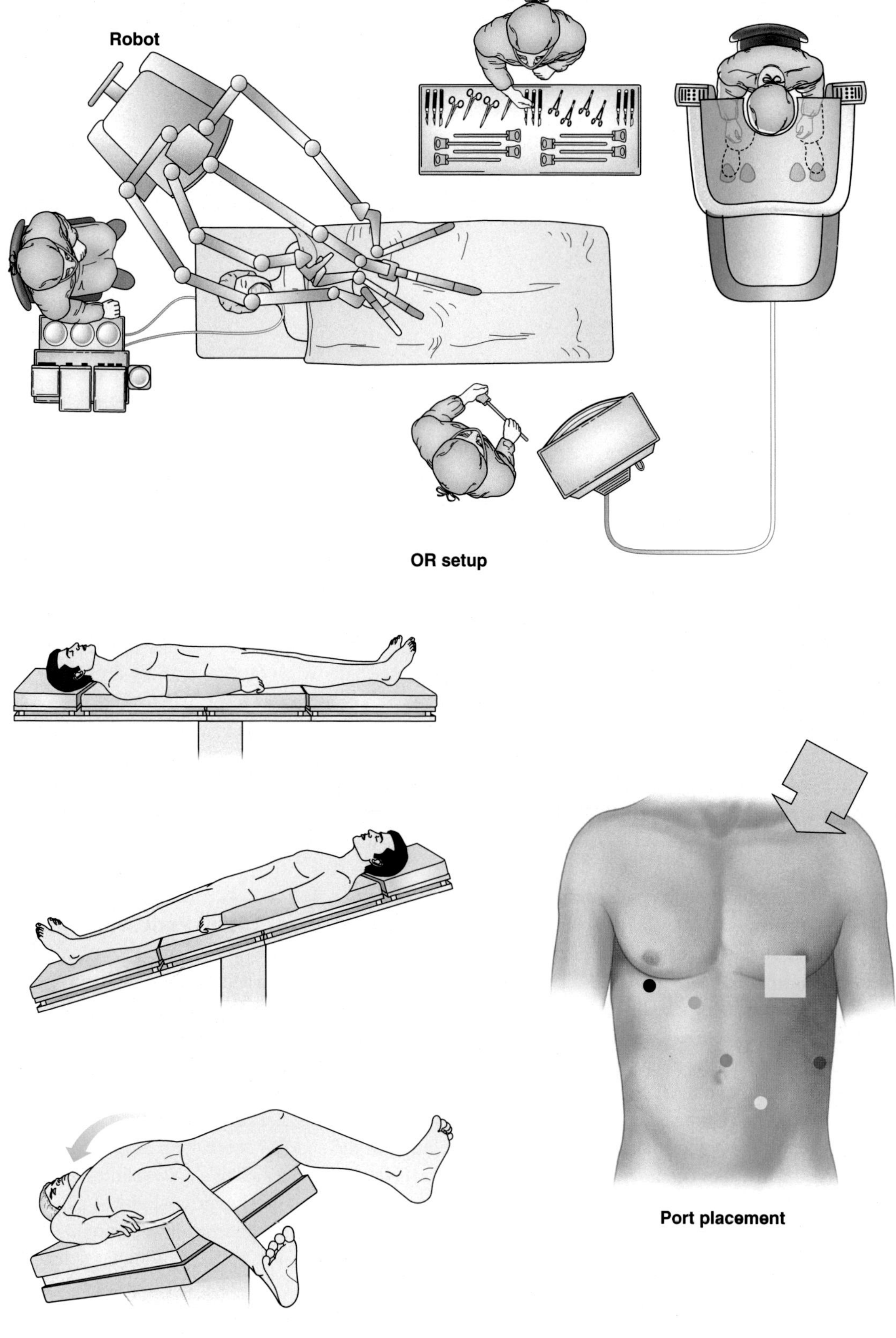

Fig. 26.1 Basic robotic setup for distal pancreatectomy. Port positions are depicted in the circle. *Blue*, camera port, above the umbilicus slightly toward the left pararectal line; *red*, instrument arm 1, left anterior axillary line below the costal margin; *green*, instrument arm 2, midline between the umbilicus and xiphoid; *black*, instrument arm 3, right midclavicular line below the costal margin; *yellow*, assistant port, between the camera port and the port for instrument arm 1

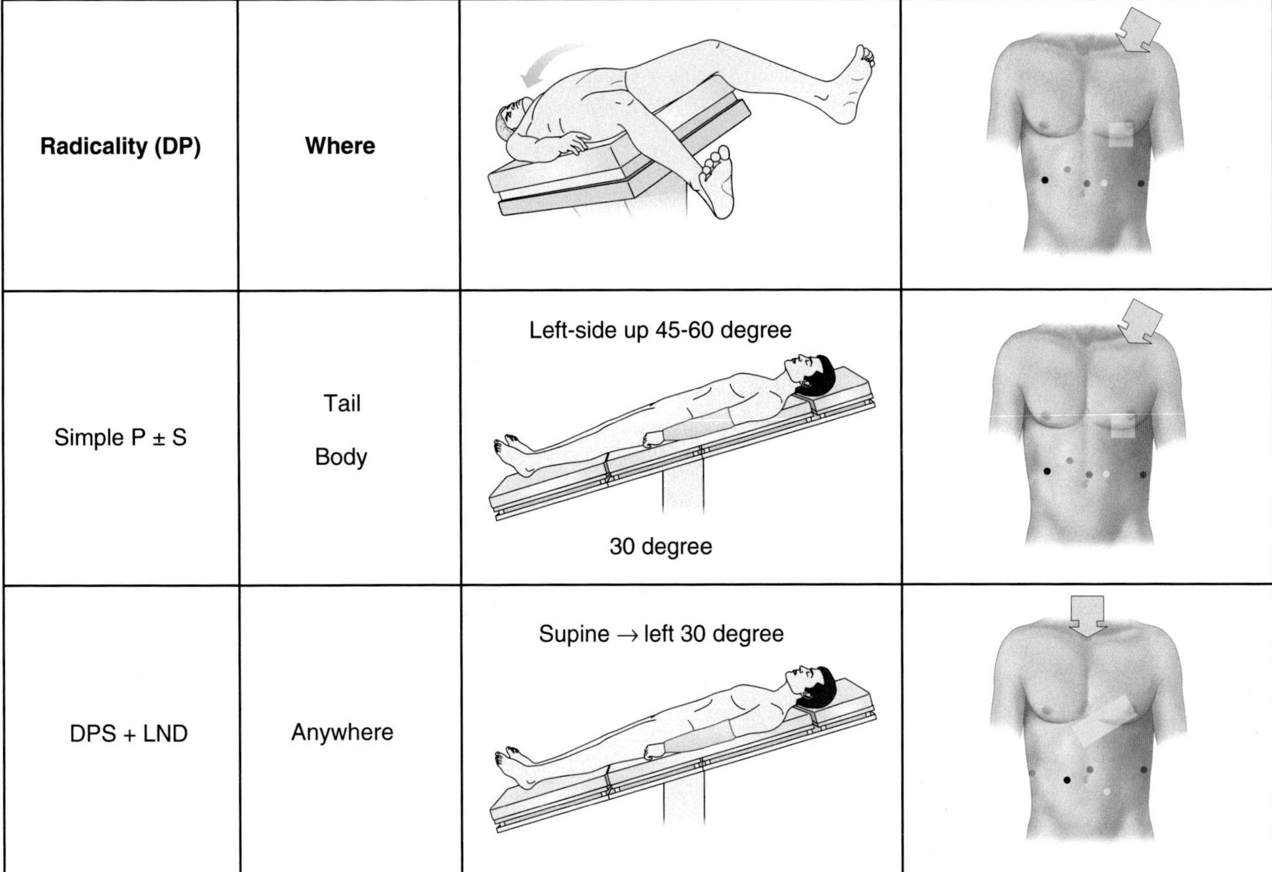

Fig. 26.2 Modification of robotic setup based on radicality of the procedure and tumor location. For simple pancreatectomy with or without splenectomy, the setup is as shown in Fig. 26.1, but for radical distal pancreatosplenectomy, the entire port setup is moved toward the right, following the camera port, which is relocated to the umbilicus. The patient is placed head up with the bed tilted at a 30-degree right lateral oblique position. The surgical cart is brought in directly over the head or toward the left side of the neck. *DPS* distal pancreatosplenectomy, *LND* lymphadenectomy, *P* pancreatectomy, *S* splenectomy

Choosing Robotic Instruments

Choices of instruments for arms 1 and 2 are based on the surgeon's preference and circumstances (Fig. 26.3). For dissection, an ideal combination consists of a bipolar energy instrument on one arm and a monopolar energy instrument on the other.

Commonly used instruments for arm 1 include a Harmonic® scalpel (Ethicon, Somerville, NJ), Maryland forceps, a cautery hook, scissors, or vessel sealers. Scissors provide sharp dissection and cause less collateral thermal injury than other devices when monopolar energy is used. A Harmonic® scalpel allows for simultaneous hemostasis and cutting, but it does not have EndoWrist® tips, so it is not ideal for dissection in a deep and angular area. A cautery hook is a good tool for dissection because of better wrist movement, but it is not a good cutting device because it can cause traction or laceration injury. Some surgeons use Maryland forceps in low cutting current to dissect, cauterize, and tear tissues around the vessels and lymph nodes with good effect. The vessel sealer is a recently introduced bipolar cutting and coagulating device that works well with the vessel and tissue bundles such as the mesentery and omentum.

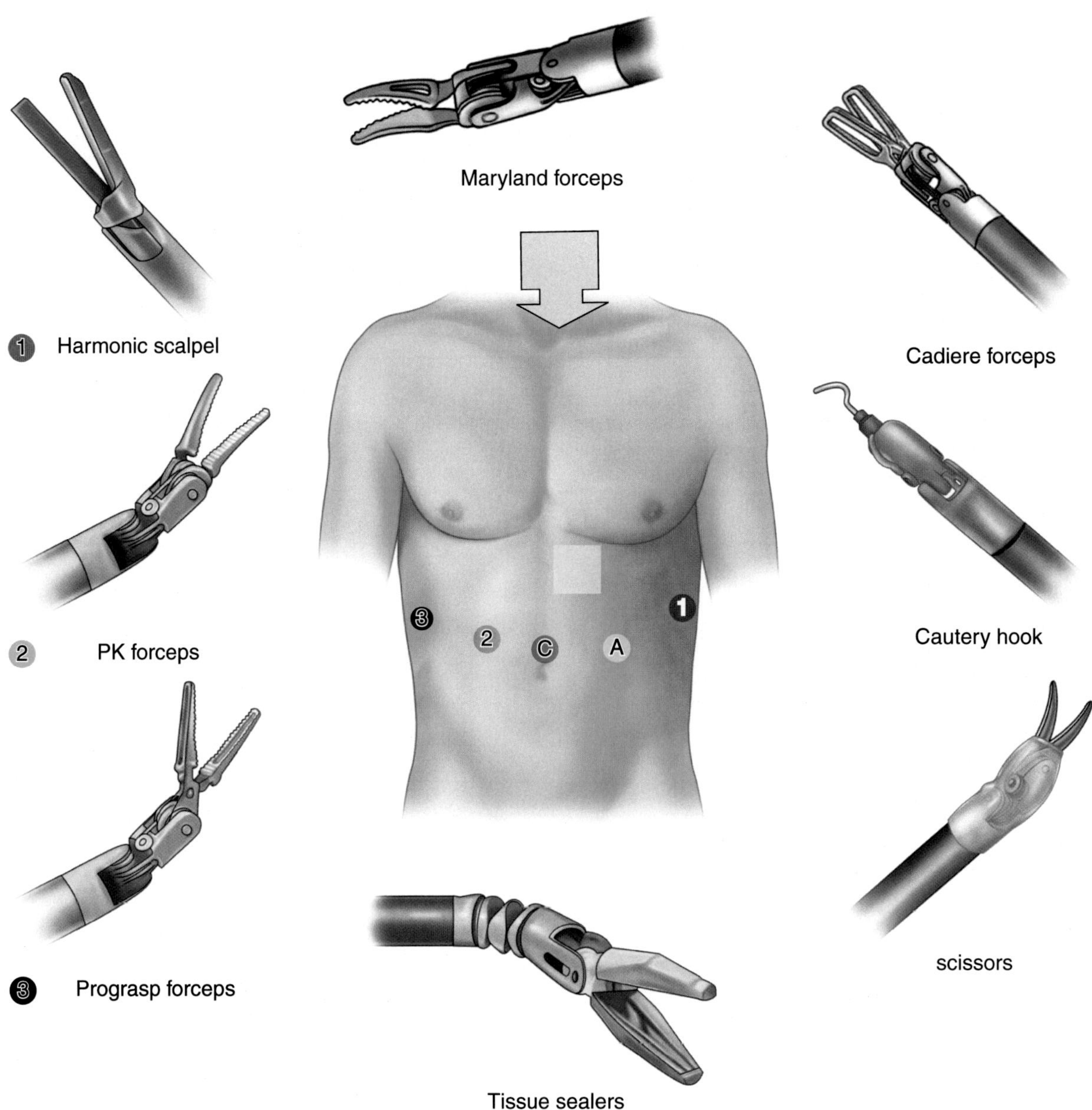

Fig. 26.3 Choosing robotic instruments for matched arms

For arm 2, bipolar forceps or PK forceps are frequently used. PK forceps have pointy, curved tips that can be used for blunt dissection; they are effective hemostatic instruments that are less traumatic as a grasper.

For the arm 3, which is used mostly for exposure and retraction purposes, a Cadiere or ProGrasp™ Forceps is frequently used.

The author's preferred combination is scissors on arm 1, PK forceps on arm 2, and Cadiere Forceps on arm 3. Many other available instruments can be used effectively in place of the instruments listed. Each surgeon should have his or her own routine combination of instruments but should be flexible and able to use other similar instruments if the preferred instrument is not available.

Surgical Steps for Robotic Distal Pancreatectomy

Distal pancreatic resection involves three basic steps:

1. Exposure of the pancreatic body and tail
2. Mobilization of the pancreas with or without the spleen
3. Pancreatic transection and specimen extraction

The extent of dissection in step 1 varies slightly depending on whether the intended procedure is distal pancreatectomy (DP) or distal pancreatosplenectomy (DPS). Step 2 is perhaps the most flexible step, in which various approaches and techniques can be applied based on tumor location and the extent of resection.

Step 1: Pancreatic Exposure

The point of this step is to enter the bursa cavity through the widest space. The stomach is grasped with the third arm (Cadiere or ProGrasp™ Forceps) close to the greater curvature, between the proximal third and half of the stomach, and is lifted upward and to the right. The assistant can help by pulling the distal omentum to create a tenting effect. The gastrocolic ligament (GCL) is then divided approximately 3–4 cm below the gastroepiploic arcade (Fig. 26.4). Only a few vertical crossing vessels must be divided.

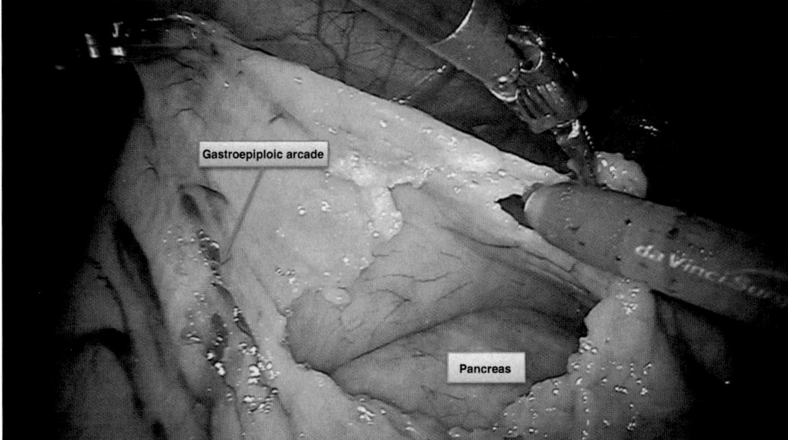

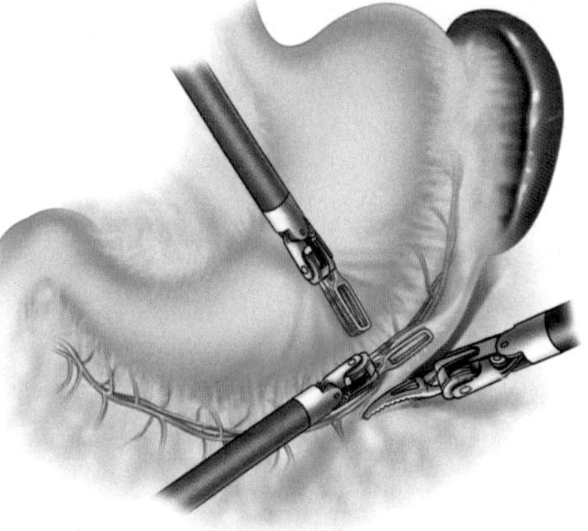

Fig. 26.4 The stomach was grasped at the midbody near the greater curvature with arm 3 and was lifted up to allow greater access to the bursa. The incision on the gastrocolic ligament was made 3–4 cm below the gastroepiploic arcade

The extent of dissection will vary depending on the case. If the spleen is to be preserved, GCL dissection should stop at gastrosplenic ligament, which contains short gastric vessels (Fig. 26.5). If possible, the splenocolic ligament (SCL) containing the artery to the lower pole should also be preserved. However, if pancreatic tail is close to the splenic hilum or embedded in it, both SCL and SRL (splenorenal ligament) must be divided in order to mobilize spleen and pancreatic tail prior to pancreatic dissection.

When a lesion is located close to the neck or at the neck, subtotal pancreatectomy or central pancreatectomy may be performed, depending on pathology. In this situation, the GCL should be divided widely toward the duodenum to expose the gastroduodenal artery (Fig. 26.6) and the right gastroepiploic artery and vein (Fig. 26.7); the latter can be traced back to the SMV.

The author prefers wide exposure of the operative field regardless of the tumor location, so that if accidental vascular injury occurs, it can be better managed. To free up the third arm for other use and to stabilize the operative field, the author always tags the stomach (after it is fully mobilized) to the diaphragm and falciform ligament with silk sutures (Fig. 26.8).

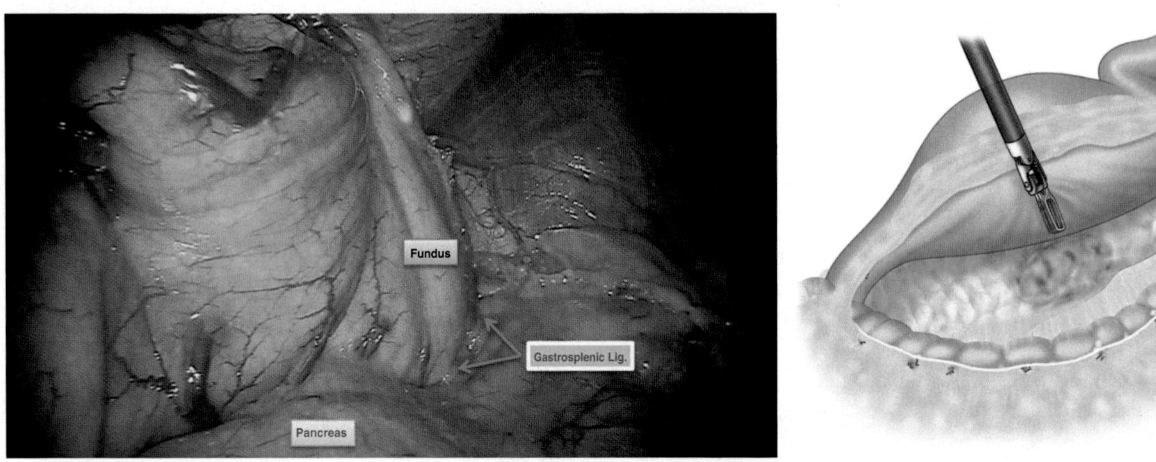

Fig. 26.5 This gastrocolic ligament was completely divided, leaving the gastrosplenic ligament intact, in preparation for a spleen-preserving distal pancreatectomy

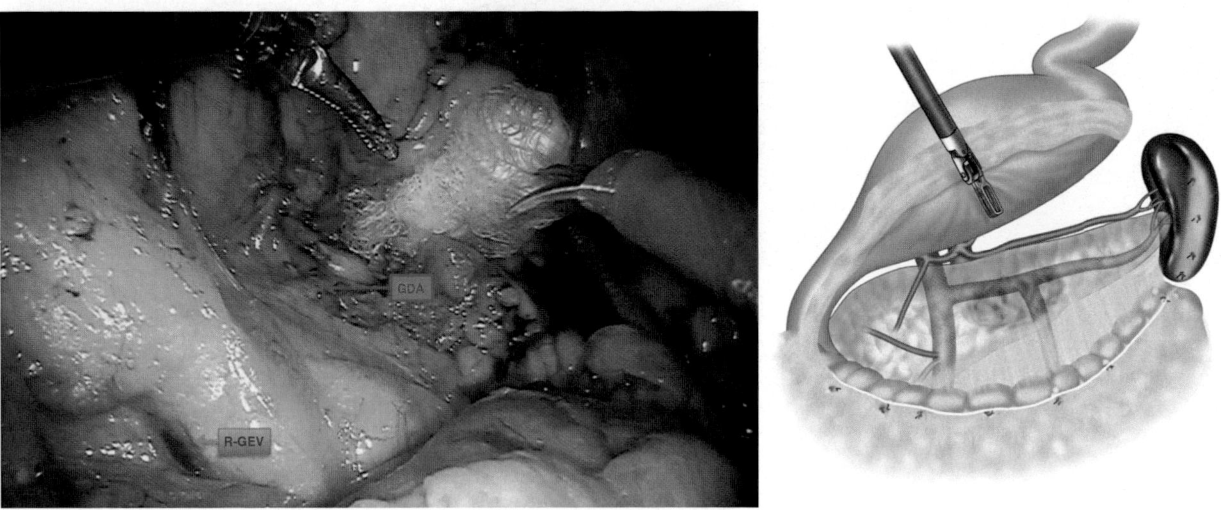

Fig. 26.6 For a central lesion, the right-sided dissection should extend to the duodenum in order to expose the gastroduodenal artery (GDA) and right gastroepiploic vein (RGEV)

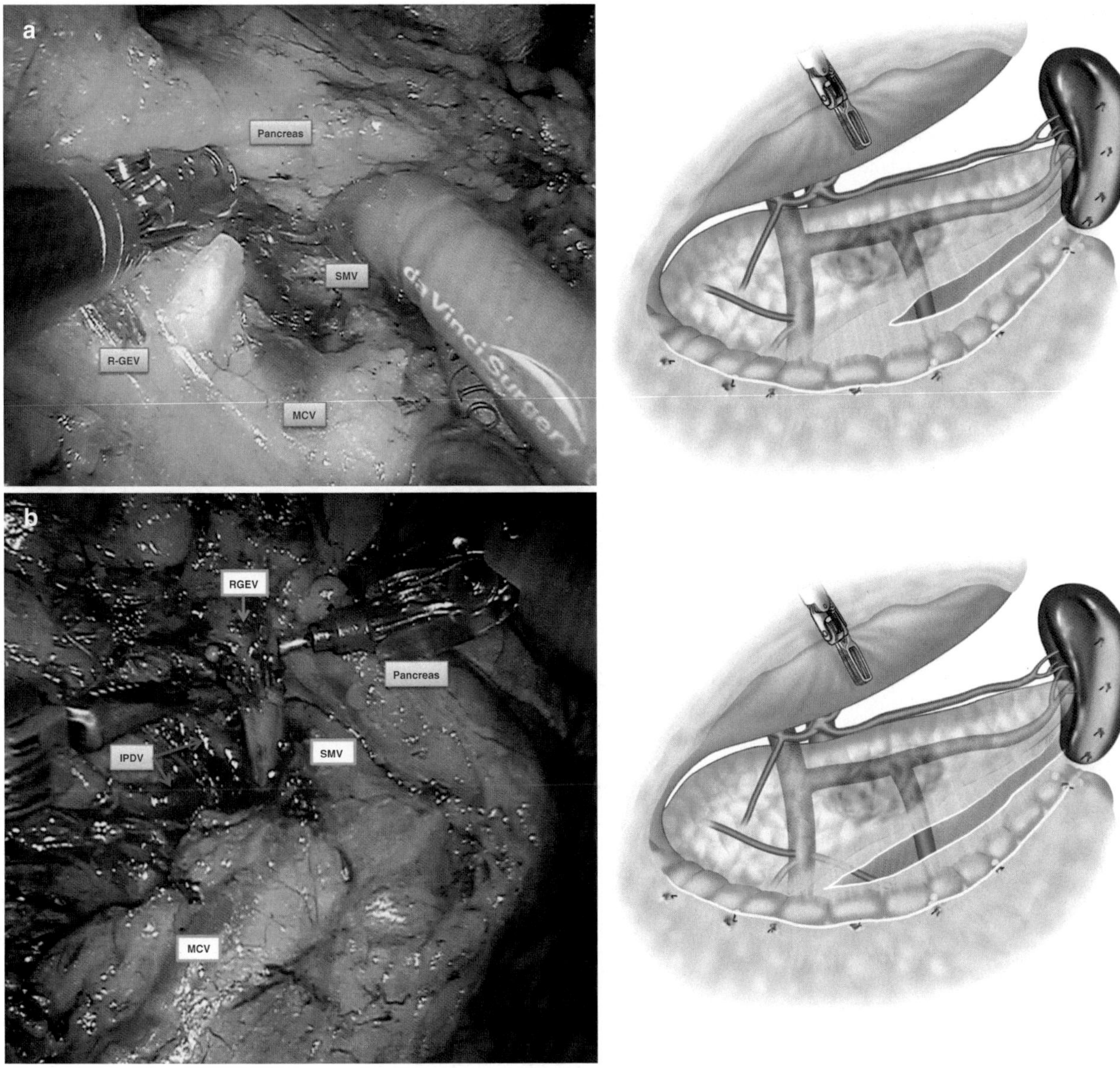

Fig. 26.7 (**a** and **b**) Identification of the right gastroepiploic vein (RGEV) or right colic vein (MCV) followed by dissection along the tissue plane could lead to the superior mesenteric vein (SMV) even in a patient with fatty omentum. *IPDV* inferior pancreaticoduodenal vein

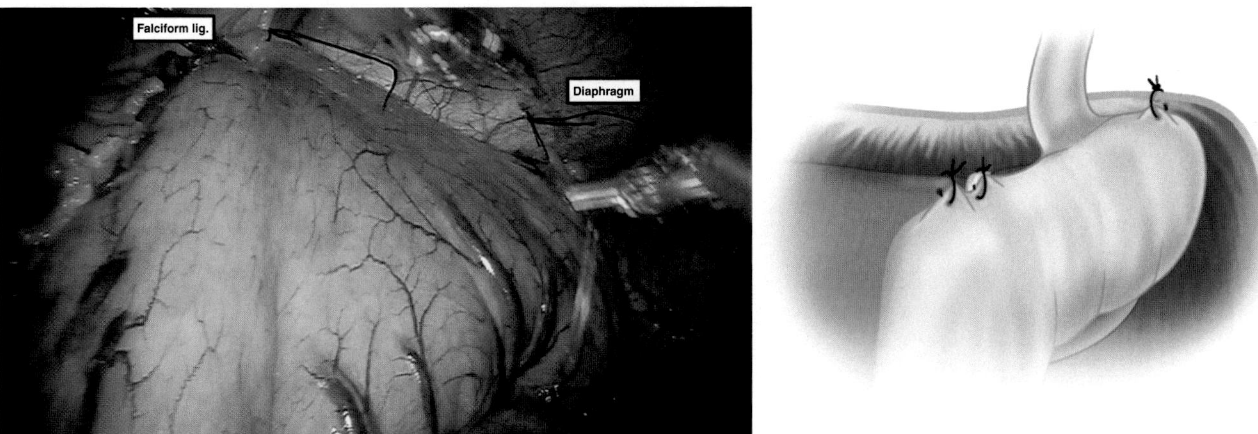

Fig. 26.8 The stomach was tagged to the diaphragm and falciform ligament with 2–0 silk sutures in order to provide stability of the operative field and to free the third instrument arm for other use

Step 2: Pancreatic Mobilization

With Splenectomy (DPS)

If the gastrosplenic ligament can be completely divided in step 1 (Fig. 26.9), the surgeon may continue to dissect toward the spleen to mobilize the upper pole off from the diaphragm by dividing the splenophrenic ligament at this step. If this dissection is not possible because of a deep fundus, it can be done later.

One may try to approach the proximal splenic artery first by dissecting the gastropancreatic fold, which contains the celiac trunk (Fig. 26.10). This step is important in a malignant tumor that requires lymphadenectomy. Tracing the common hepatic artery back to the celiac trunk may help to facilitate safe identification of splenic artery origin. The left gastric vein can be divided if necessary. Once the splenic artery is isolated, it can be encircled with a vessel loop (Fig. 26.11) and then divided using vascular staplers, suture ligatures, or clips.

Dissection of the pancreas begins medially along the inferior border at the neck or where the inferior mesenteric vein

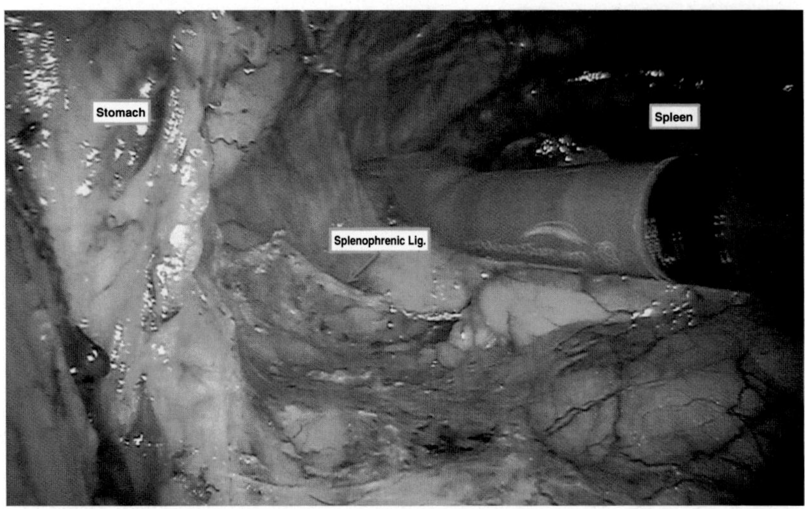

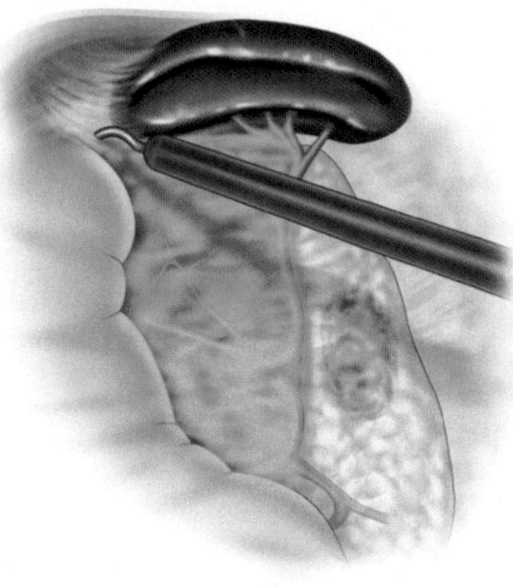

Fig. 26.9 In this case, the stomach was completely separated from the spleen. It is possible at this stage to continue dissection laterally to detach the spleen from the diaphragm and retroperitoneum

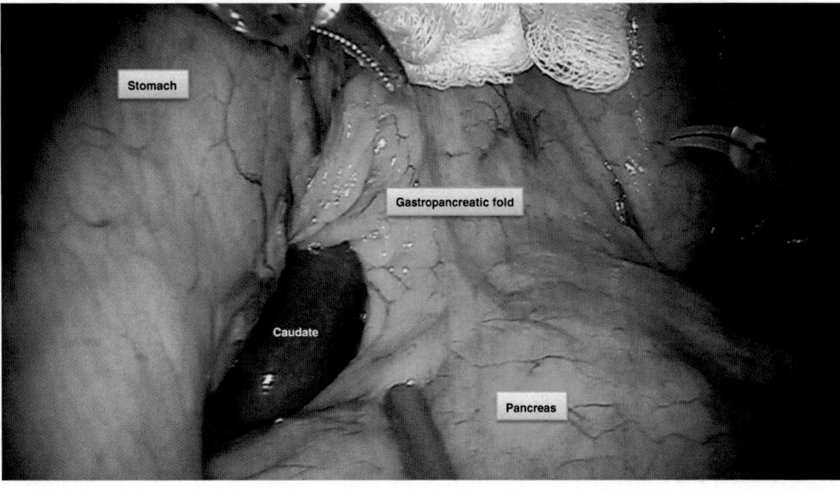

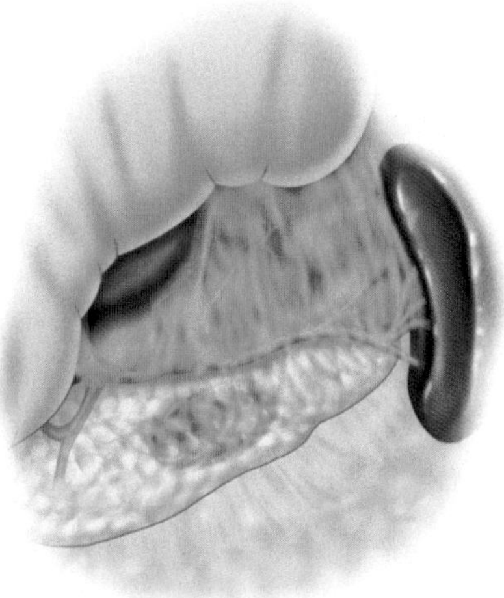

Fig. 26.10 The lesser curve of the stomach was pulled up to straighten the gastropancreatic fold. Before pancreatic dissection, control of the proximal splenic artery can be achieved by dissecting this fold, which envelops the celiac trunk and its branches

(IMV) is seen (Fig. 26.12). The peritoneum overlying the inferior pancreatic border is incised parallel to the pancreas and deepened down to reach the avascular plane on the preadrenal fascia, which continues onto the renal fascia (Fig. 26.13). Along this plane, the pancreas can be mobilized cephalad toward the tail with minimal bleeding.

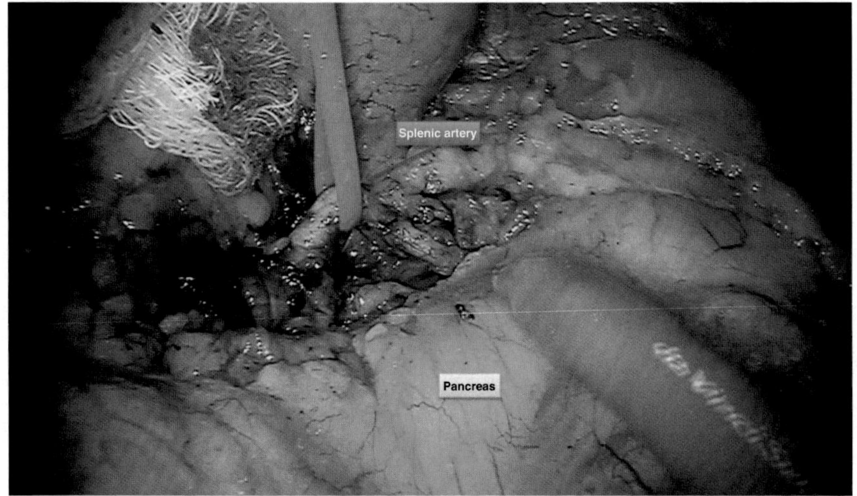

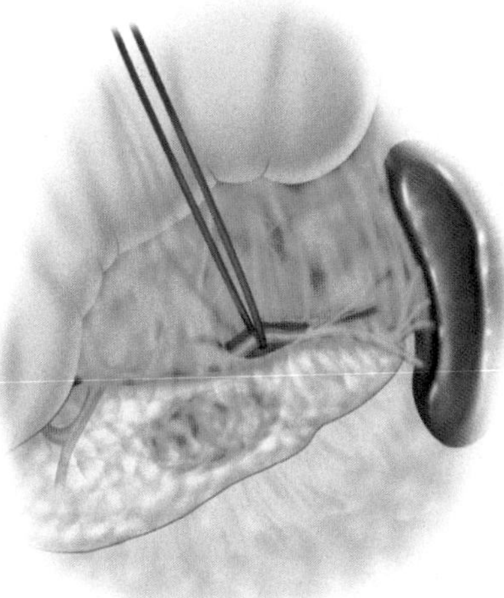

Fig. 26.11 The splenic artery was dissected circumferentially and encircled with vessel loop

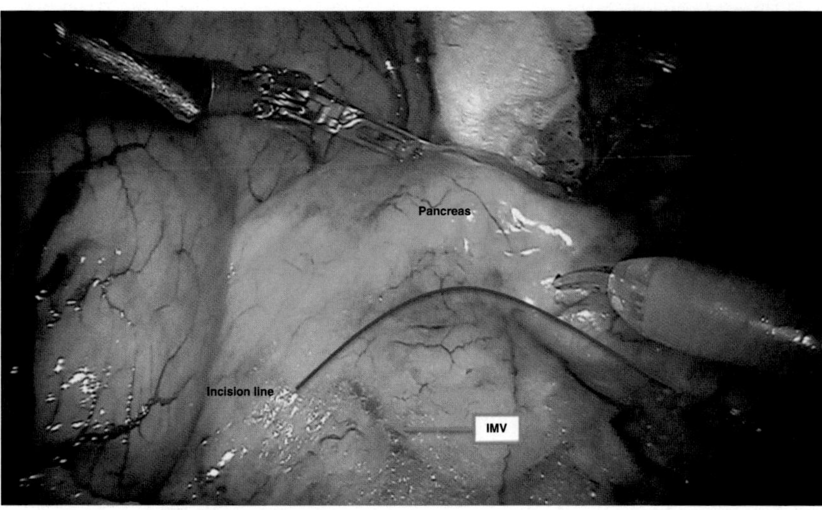

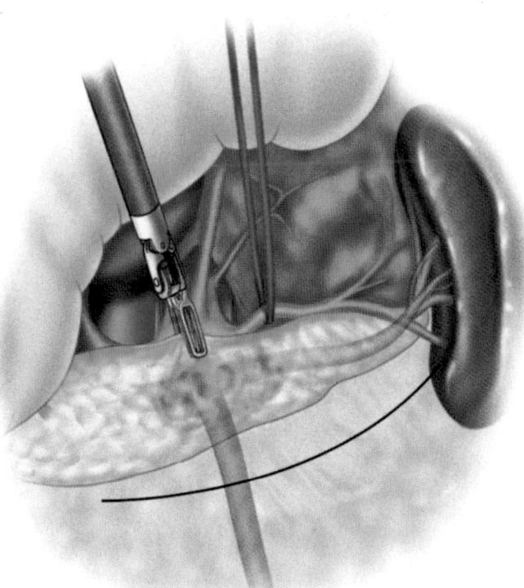

Fig. 26.12 The inferior border of the pancreatic body was exposed. *Blue line* indicates incision on the peritoneum to enter the avascular plane posterior to the pancreas. The inferior mesenteric vein (IMV) could be seen and was used as a starting point

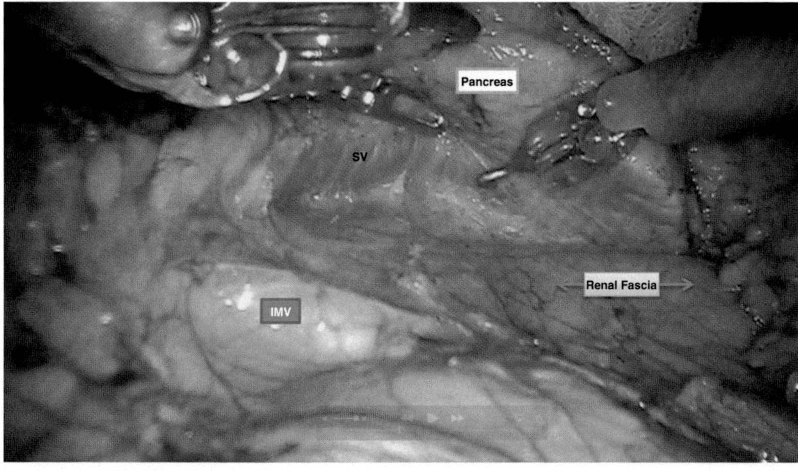

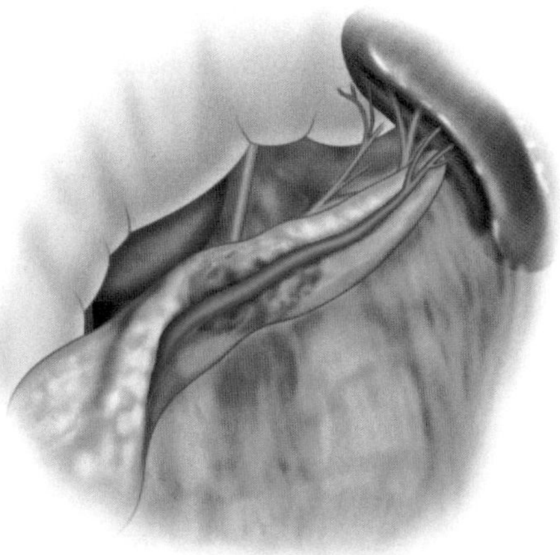

Fig. 26.13 Posterior view of the pancreas shows the splenic vein (SV) running closer to the superior border of the pancreas. The dissection plane was made in the loose avascular tissue above the preadrenal and renal fasciae for simple pancreatectomy

For a malignant lesion, the dissection plane should include these fasciae with the pancreas (Fig. 26.14). If the preadrenal fascia is involved, then en bloc adrenalectomy should be performed (Fig. 26.15).

The author prefers to mobilize both the spleen and pancreas completely (or as much as possible) at this stage, which can be done, once the pancreas body is mobilized, by changing the direction of dissection from

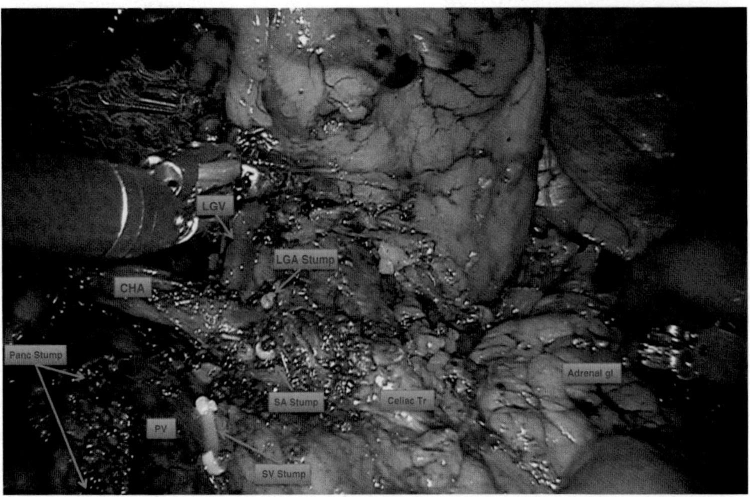

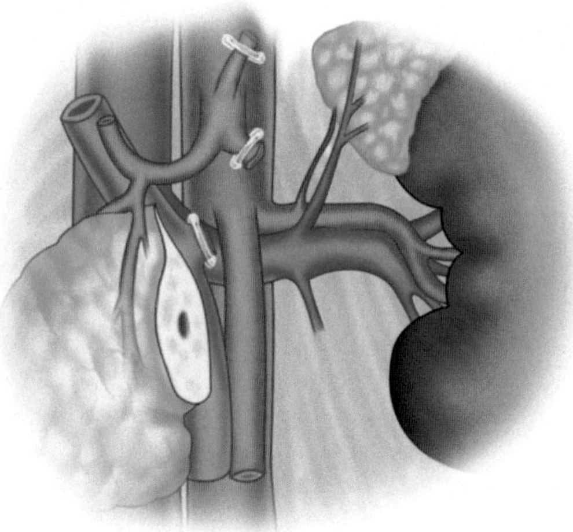

Fig. 26.14 Surgical bed following radical pancreatectomy that included fascia over the left adrenal gland. *CHA* common hepatic artery, *LGA* left gastric artery, *LGV* left gastric vein, *PV* portal vein, *SA* splenic artery, *SV* splenic vein

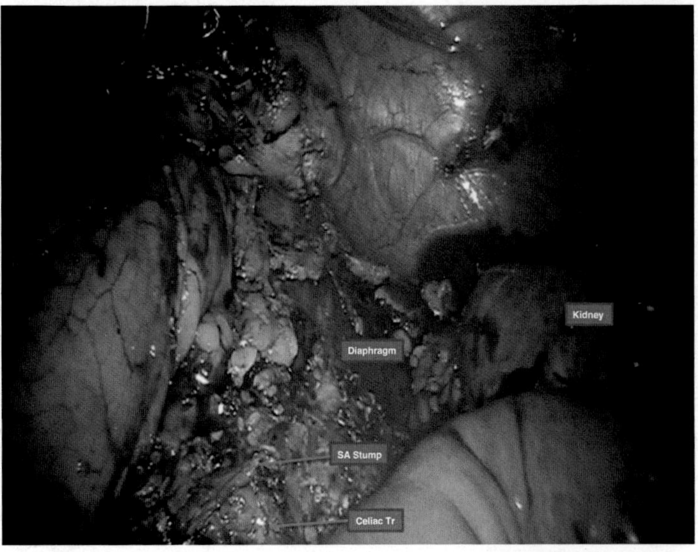

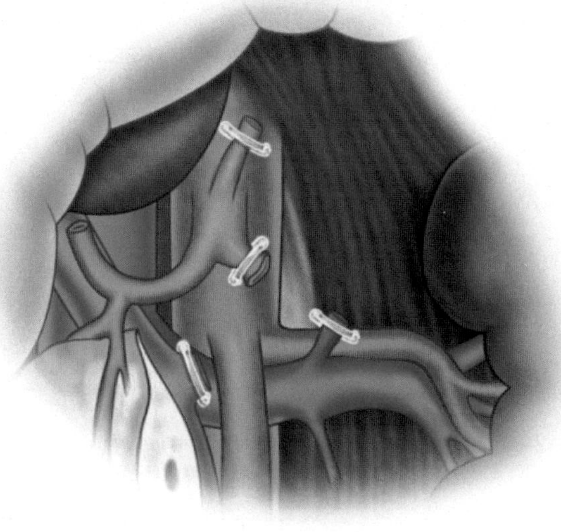

Fig. 26.15 Surgical bed following radical pancreatectomy that included the left adrenal gland and Gerota fat of the upper pole of the left kidney. The diaphragm (adrenal bed), upper renal pole, aorta, celiac trunk, and splenic artery (SA) stump were exposed

medial-lateral to lateral-medial. The splenocolic ligament is completely divided to expose the entire distal pancreas. The splenorenal ligament is next divided and used as a handle to mobilize the spleen medially along with the pancreatic tail until the previously dissected space is reached (Fig. 26.16).

The splenic vein can be found for dissection in two ways:

- By locating the SMV and tracing it upward behind the pancreas until it is seen joining the splenic vein (Fig. 26.17)
- By identifying the vein directly in the dorsal aspect of the pancreatic body during the posterior plane dissection, when it can be found nearer to the superior border of the pancreas

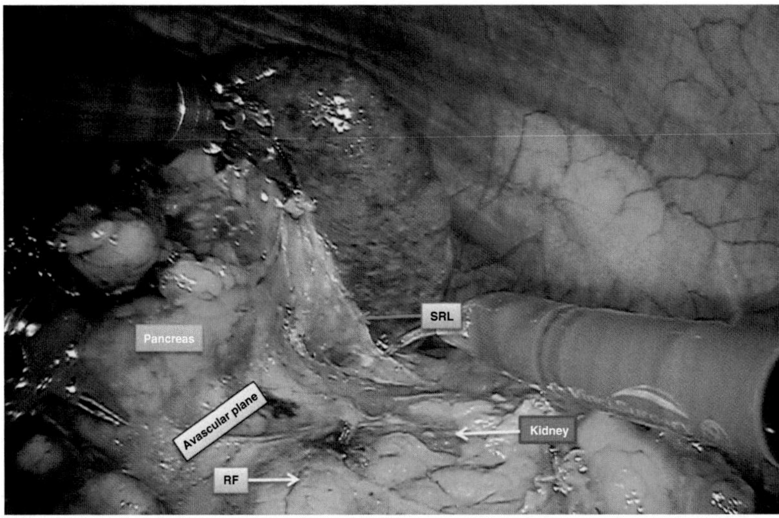

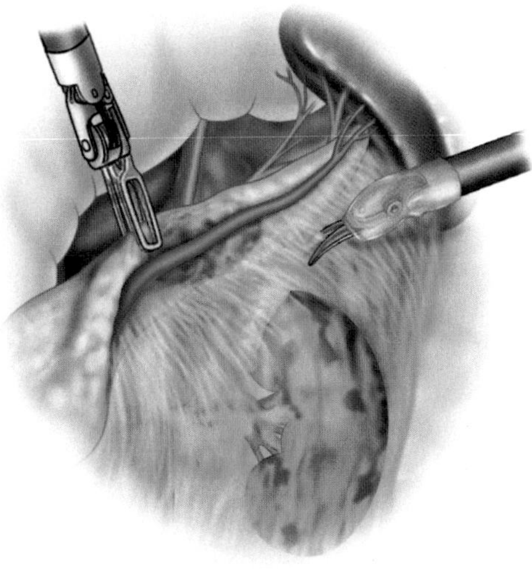

Fig. 26.16 Mobilization of the spleen and distal pancreas en bloc. Dissection was made above the renal fascia (RF). A portion of splenorenal ligament (SRL) was left on the spleen to be used for retraction

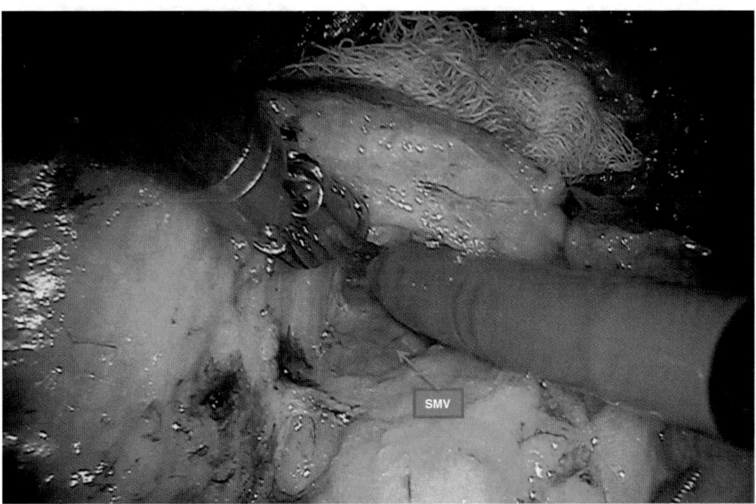

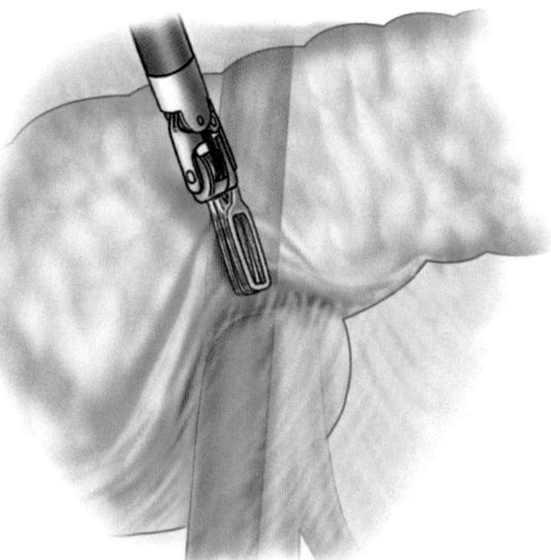

Fig. 26.17 A dissection tunnel was created at the pancreatic neck between the anterior wall of the SMV and the pancreas. In this case, the transection line was the pancreatic neck

The vein can be incorporated into the stapling transection line if the pancreas is thin. Otherwise it must be dissected free from the pancreas and can be divided after the pancreatic transection.

Without Splenectomy

For benign or low-grade malignant lesions, the spleen can be preserved, either together with the main splenic vessels or without them (Warshaw's technique). In the latter technique, the short gastric vessels should be preserved, along with a portion of splenocolic ligament that contains the lower pole artery (see step 1—spleen preservation). The viability of the spleen may be assessed with the naked eye or by using the Firefly™ fluorescence technique (Intuitive Surgical, Sunnyvalle, CA), which involves injecting 1 cc (2.5 mg) of indocyanine green (ICG) intravenously and, after 1–2 min, changing the scope mode from natural light to near-infrared light. The perfused splenic area will illuminate green (fluoresce). The need for splenectomy depends on the perfusion area. The author's first choice is always splenic vessel preservation, especially when the spleen is large, as it may not be adequately perfused via short gastric vessels.

Distal pancreatectomy (DP) with splenic vessel preservation requires meticulous dissection and careful handling of small and short vascular branches (Fig. 26.18). It is generally more time-consuming than straightforward DPS or Warshaw's DP and should be done only after the surgeon becomes comfortable with robotic surgery and especially with handling robotic instruments. Using preoperative imaging to understand the splenic vascular pattern of the patient helps to mentally prepare the surgeon, so injury to the vessels may be avoided. Management of the branches of splenic vessels requires delicate and meticulous dissection, especially at the splenic hilar region, as the vessels tend to cross over one another (Fig. 26.19). Wristed instruments with fine tips can be helpful with dissection in this area. When the

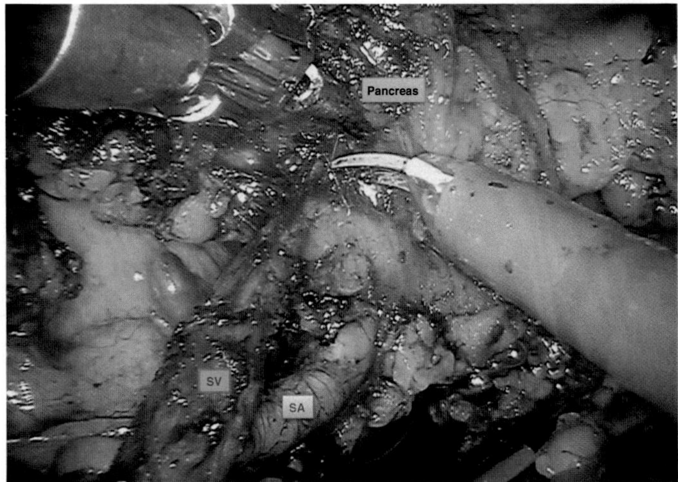

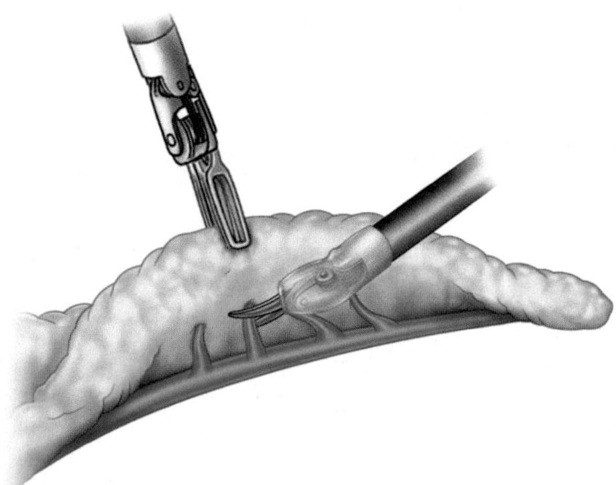

Fig. 26.18 The splenic vessels were carefully dissected from the pancreas. A combination of scissors and PK forceps facilitated safe dissection of fine venous branches. *SA* splenic artery, *SV* splenic vein

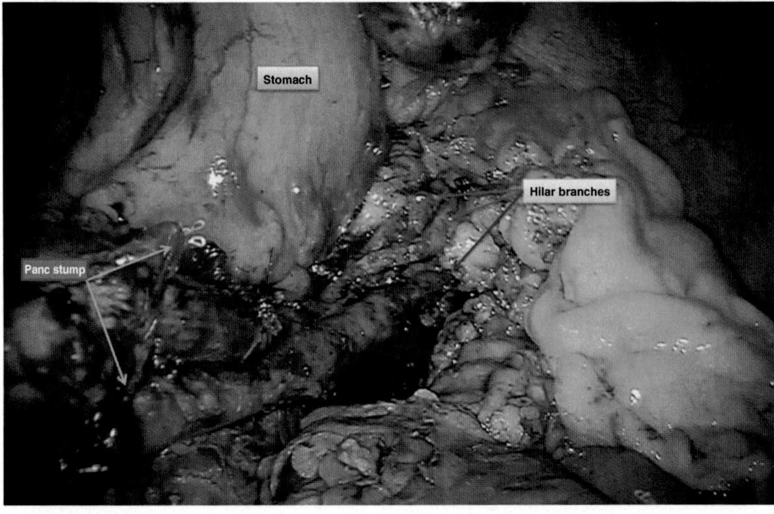

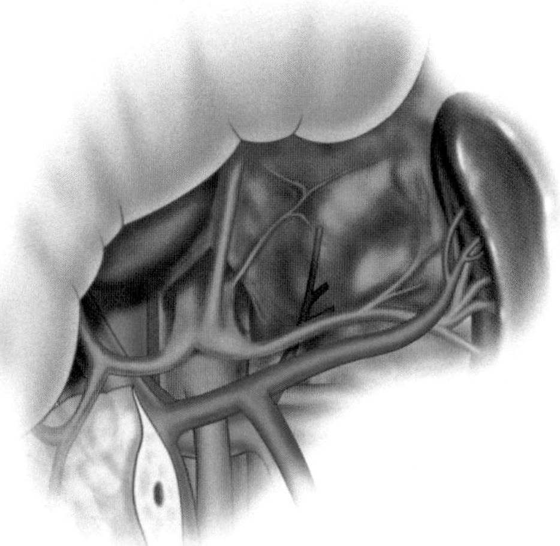

Fig. 26.19 Surgical bed following vessel preservation pancreatectomy shows multiple hilar vascular branches. The spleen was covered by omentum. *SA* splenic artery, *SV* splenic vein

Harmonic® scalpel is used, the cutting blade should not rest on the main vessel, as heat from the blade may cause injury to the wall, resulting in delayed perforation or pseudoaneurysm.

The author uses PK forceps to cauterize venous branches that are at least 1 cm long from the main vessel (or can be dissected to achieve that length) and then divides the cauterized vessel with robotic scissors toward the pancreas. Suture ligation is the option for shorter vessels. Clips are used only for larger arterial branches.

For a tail lesion, a lateral-to-medial approach is used, with the patient in an oblique right lateral position. The splenocolic ligament is divided, and the spleen, together with the pancreatic tail, is mobilized until the lesion is completely exposed (Fig. 26.20) and an adequate proximal margin is achieved. Pancreatic tail containing the lesion is then carefully dissected away from the spleen. All communicating vessels are carefully cauterized or ligated until the transection line is reached. Using stay suture on the tail for traction may help facilitate dissection.

Step 3: Pancreatic Transection and Specimen Extraction

There is no fixed rule as to when and how the pancreas should be divided. The surgeon's decision will depend on the circumstances encountered, which vary from patient to patient.

The author prefers to mobilize the pancreas (step 2) as much as possible before deciding on the transection line (proximal margin). At this stage, the splenic artery should be isolated and divided; otherwise, it can be left until after the pancreas and splenic vein are divided. If the artery must be divided after the vein, it should be done as soon as possible, as venous congestion could cause venous stump blowout.

Before pancreatic transection, a space should be carefully created between the pancreas and splenic vein. Through this space, an umbilical tape can be passed around the pancreas and lifted up (hanging maneuver) before applying the stapler to the pancreas (Fig. 26.21). If the pancreas is thin and small, the splenic vein may be divided together with the pancreas.

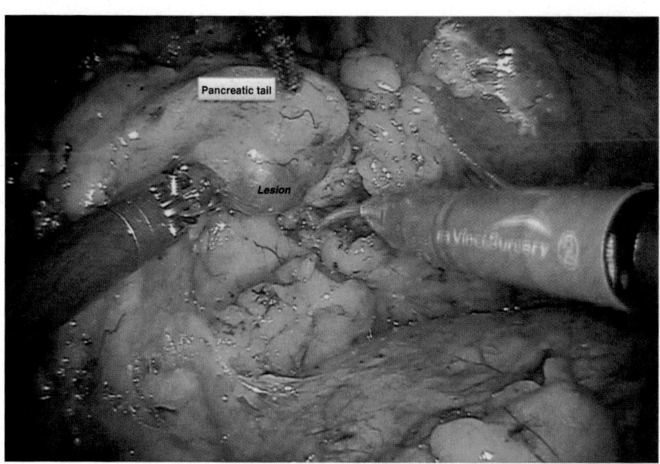

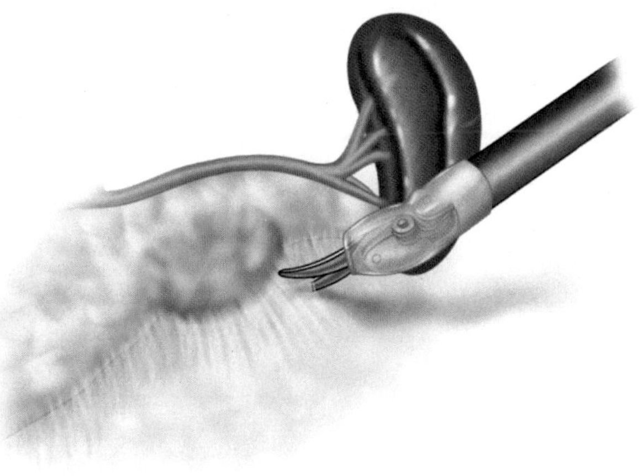

Fig. 26.20 Dissection and mobilization of the distal pancreas and spleen for a limited resection of a tail lesion

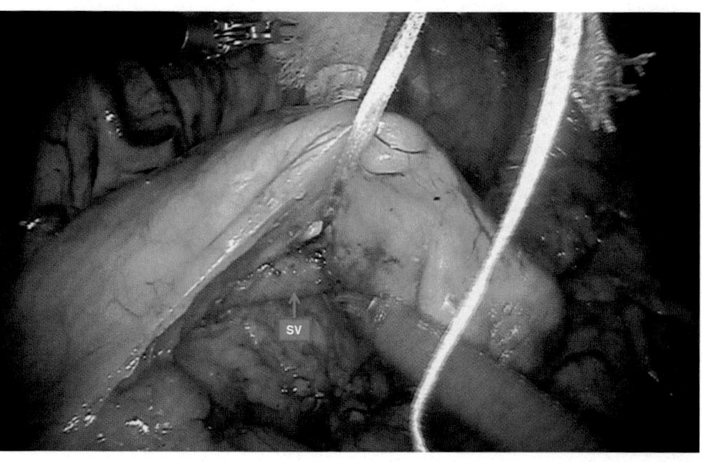

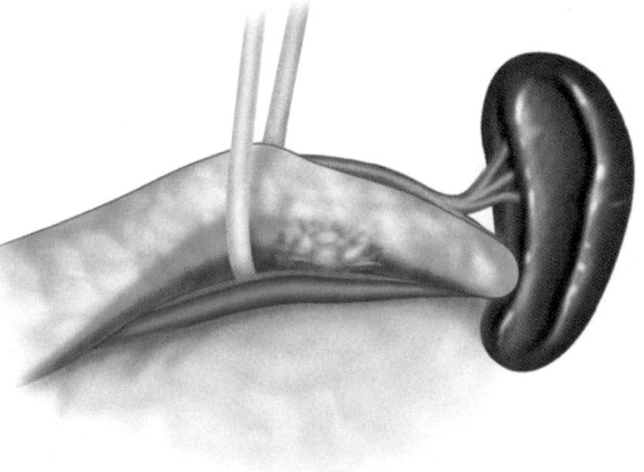

Fig. 26.21 The splenic vein (SV) was dissected away from the pancreas at the transection line, where an umbilical tape was passed through. The tape was used to lift the pancreas (hanging maneuver) to allow for safe application of endostaplers

Pancreatic Transection Methods

An endostapler with a vascular cartridge is used for thin and soft pancreas (Fig. 26.22). Staplers should be closed slowly to prevent tissue fracture and left closed for a few minutes to allow for tissue dehydration before cutting, which should also be slow.

Manual transection is recommended for thick or fibrotic pancreas or when splenic vessels are densely adherent to the pancreas. This can be done stepwise using the Harmonic® scalpel or a combination of scissors and bipolar forceps. The pancreatic stump can be sprayed with fibrin glue to reinforce the closure.

After pancreas and splenic vascular transection, the specimen is freed by dividing the remaining attachments along the superior border of the pancreas and spleen (Fig. 26.23). Care should be taken when dividing short gastric vessels, as applying heat directly on the gastric wall may result in delayed perforation. Bleeding from splenic injury at this point is not a cause for concern, as it is mostly from back bleeding. If the spleen is too big and cannot easily be mobilized together with the pancreas, it can be resected separately.

Specimen Extraction

A DP specimen with a benign lesion can be brought out directly via an enlarged port incision. A malignant lesion should be placed inside a bag before it is extracted. In the case of a larger DPS specimen, a Pfannenstiel incision is used to remove the bag that contains the specimen. If the spleen is too large to be brought out through the incision, it can be cut into small pieces inside the bag and then carefully removed.

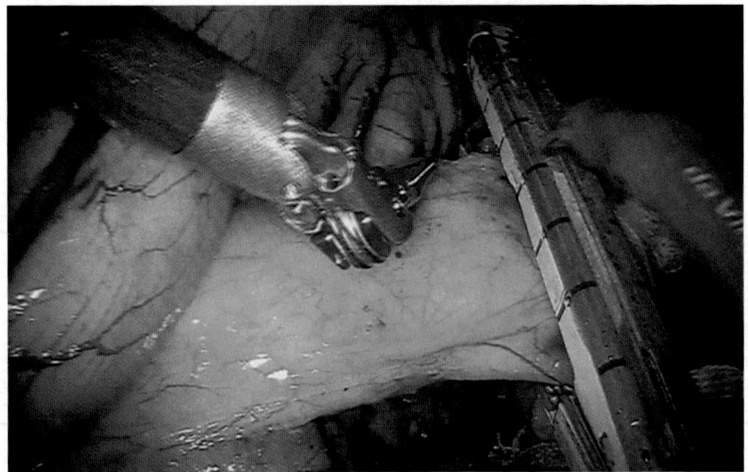

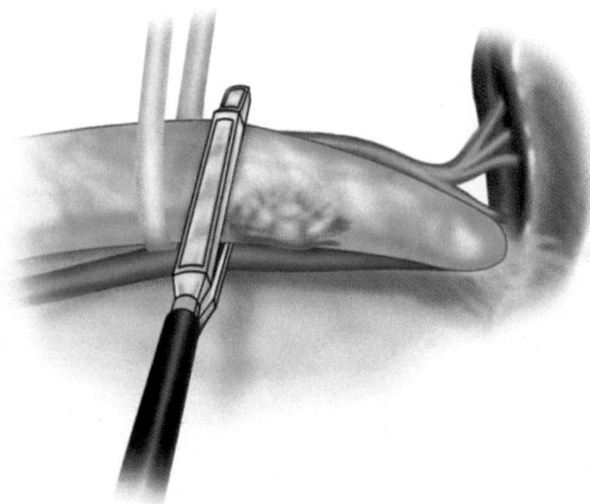

Fig. 26.22 Pancreatic transection using the endostapler with vascular cartridge

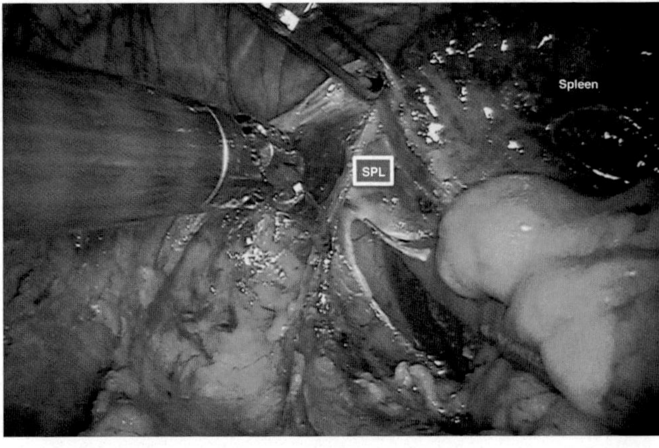

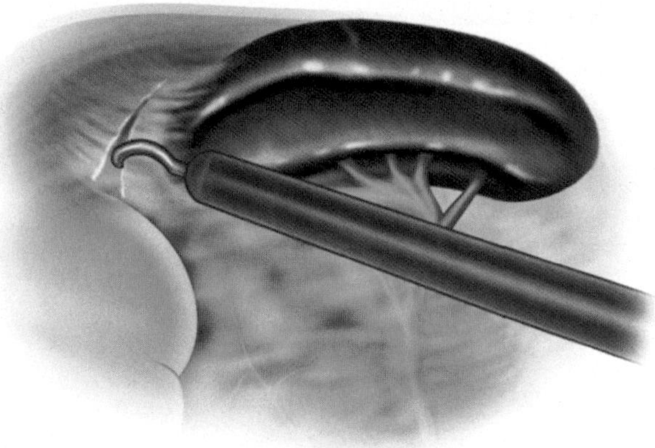

Fig. 26.23 The last attachment holding the spleen to the diaphragm is divided before the specimen is freed. *SPL* splenophrenic ligament

Further Reading

Giulianotti P, Sbrana F, Bianco F, Elli E, Shah G, Addeo P, et al. Robot-assisted laparoscopic pancreatic surgery: single-surgeon experience. Surg Endosc. 2010;24:1646–57.

Guerra F, Pesi B, Amore Bonapasta S, Di Marino M, Perna F, Annecchiarico M, Coratti A. Challenges in robotic distal pancreatectomy: systematic review of current practice. Minerva Chir. 2015;70:241–7.

Lai EC, Tang CN. Robotic distal pancreatectomy versus conventional laparoscopic distal pancreatectomy: a comparative study for short-term outcomes. Front Med. 2015;9:356–60.

Lee SY, Allen PJ, Sadot E, D'Angelica MI, DeMatteo RP, Fong Y, et al. Distal pancreatectomy: a single institution's experience in open, laparoscopic, and robotic approaches. J Am Coll Surg. 2015;220:18–27.

Liu Y, Ji WB, Wang HG, Luo Y, Wang XQ, Lv SC, Dong JH. Robotic spleen-preserving laparoscopic distal pancreatectomy: a single-centered Chinese experience. World J Surg Oncol. 2015;13:275.

Napoli N, Kauffman EF, Perrone VG, Miccoli M, Brozzetti S, Boggi U. The learning curve in robotic distal pancreatectomy. Updat Surg. 2015;67:257–64.

Shakir M, Boone BA, Polanco PM, Zenati MS, Hogg ME, Tsung A, et al. The learning curve for robotic distal pancreatectomy: an analysis of outcomes of the first 100 consecutive cases at a high-volume pancreatic Centre. HPB (Oxford). 2015;17:580–6.

Yiengpruksawan A. Technique for laparobotic distal pancreatectomy with preservation of spleen. J Robot Surg. 2011;5:11–5.

27 Robotic Pancreatoduodenectomy

Pier Cristoforo Giulianotti and Federico Gheza

Introduction

Pancreatoduodenectomy (PD) is the standard surgical treatment for tumors of the pancreatic head, ampulla, duodenum, and distal common bile duct. Nononcological resections (mainly for chronic pancreatitis) have fewer indications. In abdominal surgery, PD is considered the most complex surgical procedure. It was one of the last abdominal operations attempted, introduced by Whipple in 1935. Its high mortality rate has only recently decreased below 5% in major series, and it has one of the highest morbidity rates, ranging from 30 to 50%, with many clinically significant complications [2]. It also has the longest mean hospital stay for an elective procedure in general surgery. The pure laparoscopic approach was introduced in 1994 but has had a low penetrance [3], mostly due to technical difficulties; it is still limited to a few centers around the world [4]. It requires the surgeon to perform and manage a gastrointestinal anastomosis, pancreatic anastomosis, biliary reconstruction, and vascular isolation at the same time.

A minimally invasive approach could potentially offer better overall outcomes, but it must provide the same oncological results and a pancreatic fistula rate comparable with open surgery, which remains the gold standard. The robotic platform theoretically may provide some advantages compared with a total laparoscopic approach:

- During the dissection of the uncinate process, the third arm and the EndoWrist® technology provide stable retraction and expose the retroportal lamina.
- Enhanced suturing capabilities and stable magnified vision help during vascular ligation and node dissection.
- Increased range of motion allows a variety of technical solutions for the reconstruction, so the surgeon can choose the best anastomotic technique based on the patient's features and personal preference.

P. C. Giulianotti, MD (✉) · F. Gheza, MD
Division of General, Minimally Invasive and Robotic Surgery, Department of Surgery, University of Illinois at Chicago, Chicago, IL, USA
e-mail: piercg@uic.edu

Patient Selection

Our experience is a series of consecutive, unselected patients in a center (University of Illinois at Chicago) with an extremely high (>80%) penetrance of the robotic approach for elective cases in general surgery. The same surgeon had more than 5 years of previous experience, starting in 2001, as shown at the end of our chapter. In general, our suggestion to start a robotic program including PD is to begin with a wise patient selection, based on BMI, expected duct size, comorbidities, and tumor features (avoiding bulky lesions and those located in the uncinate process). The ideal path toward robotic PD should be progressive and focused; it requires a strong expertise in hepato-pancreatico-biliary surgery and a solid laparoscopic background. Our experience with proctoring led us to recommend attempting a robotic PD after other abdominal surgeries (with an increasing difficulty level), without relying too much on the open experience only.

Trocar Positioning and Docking

The patient is positioned supine in a 20-degree reverse Trendelenburg position with tucked arms and parted legs, using a bean bag and slightly tilted to the left side. The assistant surgeon is positioned between the patient's legs. Pneumoperitoneum is achieved with a Veress needle, preferably placed in the left subcostal area. A 5-mm trocar is positioned in the left upper quadrant for a diagnostic laparoscopy when the proper pressure is obtained (12–15 mm Hg), in order

Y. Fong et al. (eds.), *The SAGES Atlas of Robotic Surgery*, https://doi.org/10.1007/978-3-319-91045-1_27

to exclude any contraindications to surgery (e.g., peritoneal metastases, carcinosis) and place the ports under direct vision. Standardization of the trocar positioning is essential, with minor modifications according to the patient anatomy. For the Si system, the robotic cart is coming from the patient's head.

A 12-mm camera port is placed on the right pararectal line, at the intersection with the transverse umbilical line, which marks the center of the operative field. This location allows a better vision angle and exposure of the uncinate process, superior mesenteric vein (SMV), superior mesenteric artery (SMA), and portal vein. Another 12-mm trocar is placed on the left side of the navel for the assistant. The first robotic arm (R1) is placed in the left side, 3–4 in. lateral to the assistant port. The second robotic arm (R2) follows at the same distance, but on the right side. A 5-mm assistant port is placed between the camera port and R2. Depending on the body habitus of the patient, the third arm (R3) will be placed laterally on either the right or the left side. To avoid collisions, R3 is typically placed far laterally to the right flank in patients with a large body habitus (Fig. 27.1); in thin patients, R3 is placed as lateral as possible on the left side.

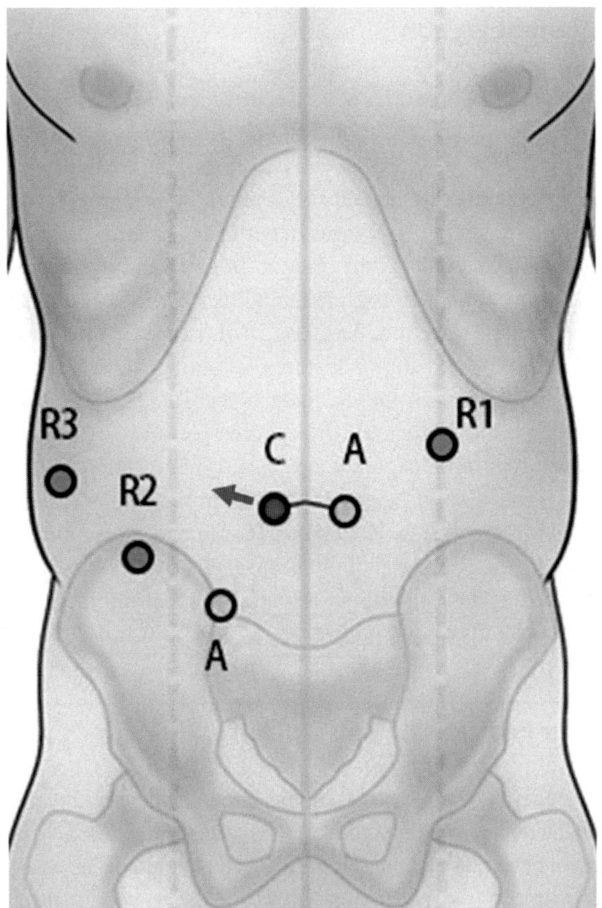

Fig. 27.1 Port setting. Shown are locations for the robotic arms (R1, R2, R3) and the assistant ports (*A*), as explained in the text. In this example, R3 is represented on the right side. The camera port (*C*) could be placed even more on the right side. Its placement is decided during the first laparoscopic exploration with pneumoperitoneum

With the Xi system, our port placement differs in few details: four 8-mm robotic trocars are placed along a straight line, similar to what is described for Si. The shorter distance between robotic trocars helps avoid collisions. The Xi cart does not have to come from the patient's head.

Surgical Technique

Mobilization of the Right Colic Flexure

The first step of the procedure is the mobilization of the right colonic flexure. It is performed with a combination of hook cautery (R1) and bipolar forceps (R2). The slight left rotation and the reverse Trendelenburg position facilitate the retraction of the colon. Our suggestion is to perform a wide mobilization of the right colonic flexure, reaching the origin of the right colonic vessels medially and sometimes the cecum inferiorly, to expose the duodenum, the SMV, and the head of the pancreas. This preliminary dissection is sometimes considered an easy step, but it has underestimated pitfalls: The venous anatomy of the right colon, including the presence of a Henle's trunk, could be difficult to evaluate (mostly in obese patients); limited mobilization could be the main reason for a difficult duodenal mobilization and a poor exposure of the ventral pancreas.

Kocher Maneuver

The Kocher maneuver is formally considered the second step, but a progressive dissection needs to be performed during the entire procedure and must be completed before dividing the pancreas. This maneuver should be more extensive than in open surgery, allowing complete detachment from the retroperitoneum and mobilization toward the left side and making the dissection of the uncinate process easier and safer. Our anatomical landmark as the dissection limit is the visualization of the left side of the aorta. The goal is the direct visualization of the posterior aspect of the pancreatic head.

As in open surgery, this maneuver is part of surgical exploration to assess resectability, as involvement of the SMA or SMV is considered in most cases to be a sign of unresectable lesions.

Opening of the Gastrocolic Ligament

Exposure is achieved using a grasper in the third arm to retract the stomach upward, tensioning the gastrocolic ligament and allowing its opening with the Harmonic® scalpel based on Ethicon Endo-Surgery Harmonic ACE technology (Ethicon, Somerville, NJ, USA) or the vessel sealer (Intuitive Surgical; Sunnyvale, CA, USA).

The anterior aspect of the pancreatic body and neck, as well as the posterior stomach, can be examined at this stage to look for carcinosis or signs of local cancer spread.

If a pylorus-preserving PD (PPPD) is planned, the right gastroepiploic arcade must be identified and carefully preserved. The dissection should be extended laterally, reaching and preserving the short gastric vessels.

Hepatic Hilum Exploration and Arterial Control

During the exploration of the liver hilum (still assessing resectability), a very careful evaluation of vascular anatomy is required, looking particularly for the presence of a right accessory hepatic artery coming from the SMA. If this variant is found, the procedure is still feasible, as we have shown [5], but the dissection will be more complex.

At this point, usually scan is performed using an ultrasound laparoscopic probe. Before irreversible steps are carried out, we need to rule out the presence of undetected metastases in the liver and to evaluate local extension and vascular involvement.

During this phase, the node dissection is performed according to tumor position and type. Some nodes can be divided and sent separately or left en bloc with the specimen.

The common hepatic artery is identified and dissected to reach the origin of the gastroduodenal artery (GDA). The right gastroepiploic artery dissection is a crucial point: The goal is to balance an accurate node dissection with the preservation of good vascularization for the first duodenal part. Lifting up the antrum vertically using the third arm could be useful to better visualize the vascular anatomy through some traction. The gastroepiploic artery transection is typically performed 1 cm from the origin, leaving a short stump attached to the pancreas.

The right gastric artery is sutured and divided at its origin. This artery can originate from the proper hepatic, common hepatic, or left gastric artery. Understanding this variation of the anatomy is important in order to achieve a better lymphadenectomy.

Cholecystectomy and Common Bile Duct Transection

If the gallbladder is in place, an anterograde cholecystectomy is performed, starting from the fundus. This allows a complete en bloc resection, leaving the cystic duct attached to the common bile duct. The cystic artery is preferably divided with scissors in between sutures, without applying Hem-o-lok®, which can interfere with further dissections. The common bile duct (CBD) is transected with cold scissors above the cystic duct origin; we consider this level the best compromise between a good vascularization and an easy reconstruction. A gentle robotic bulldog is applied on the CBD stump to avoid biliary spillage during dissection, and its proximal margin is sent to pathology for frozen-section evaluation. The distal bile duct is sutured and kept attached to the specimen. A long stay suture may help in retracting the CBD and exposing the portal vein underneath.

Division of the Duodenum

To perform the PPPD, we need to preserve innervation and vascular supply of the pylorus. The right gastroepiploic and right gastric arteries have been already transected. Minor vascular and lymphatic connections are cleared in order to have enough space to place the laparoscopic stapler and divide the first duodenal portion 1 cm distal to the pylorus. After transection, better exposure of the cephalic peripancreatic lymph node stations and better control of the hepatoduodenal ligament are achieved.

Transection of the Gastroduodenal Artery

This is a difficult step, and the stump of the GDA may be a major source of bleeding complications in the postoperative period [6]. The vascular stapler is our preferred technique. To place the jaws of the stapler correctly, some fine dissection may be necessary, entering and dividing a few collaterals. If there is not enough room for the stapler, suture/ligation is the second option. Clips should be avoided for the GDA.

First Jejunal Loop Transection

Before attempting any division of the pancreatic neck, the duodenojejunal flexure should be divided, derotating the duodenum on the right side.

To transect the first jejunal loop at the Treitz ligament, we move to the inframesocolic space. The third arm lifts and pushes cephalad the mesocolon to get some tension on the suspension ligament. The monopolar hook (and sometimes the Harmonic® device) is used to reach from below the previous dissection on the supramesocolic and retroperitoneal space to totally free the fourth duodenal part. After a stapler transection, a derotating maneuver allows us to push the duodenojejunal flexure through this natural passage posteriorly to the mesenteric vessels, with the pancreatic head in the supramesocolic space.

Pancreatic Neck Transection

Before dividing the pancreas, octreotide infusion at 50 μg/h is started. In the common PD, the pancreatic neck is transected in front of the portal vein. To perform this in the safest way, good exposure of the inferior and superior pancreatic neck and body must be achieved. Two stay sutures (one on each side of the transection line) of polypropylene are passed on the inferior edge for lifting and retraction. Using the Harmonic® scalpel, the neck is transected, proceeding slowly to ensure hemostasis and the visualization of the pancreatic duct. The stay sutures are moved laterally to open the surgical plane while advancing with neck transection. A complete tunnel in front of the portal vein is needed only if it is easy. If there are inflammatory adhesions, we prefer to split the neck anterogradely, reaching the periadventitial plane and gradually opening up the space.

Once the pancreatic duct is identified, we typically place a stent and secure it with a 5–0 polydioxanone (PDS) suture. If the pancreatic duct is accidentally closed with the Harmonic®, it should be immediately reopened and stented.

A section of the pancreatic duct is sent for frozen-section analysis to confirm negative margins prior to reconstruction, as we do for the CBD.

Dissection of the Uncinate Process

This represents the last dissection step and is considered the most controversial aspect of the minimally invasive approach. Detractors of this technique assert that open surgery could allow a more extensive and complete resection. We consider this step one of the clearest advantages of robotic versus laparoscopic surgery, because of third arm retraction and EndoWrist® use behind the portal axis. Another major advance is the possibility of selectively closing with stitches venous branches coming from the SMV (Fig. 27.2). The Harmonic® scalpel is the preferred tool for this task but used in a very discerning way for dissection and closure of small branches; stitches are used for bigger vessels.

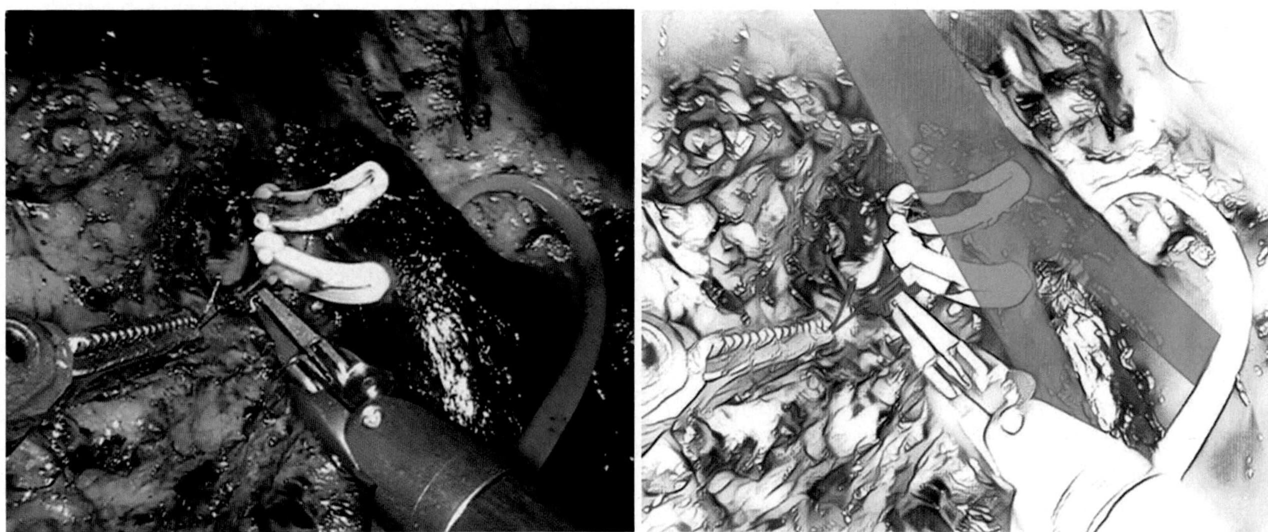

Fig. 27.2 Dissection of the superior mesenteric vein (SMV). Two different ways to dissect small branches for the uncinate process are shown: fine cutting with round-tip scissors between sutures or Hem-o-lok®

A vessel loop surrounding the SMV is placed for vascular control and retraction ("hanging maneuver"). The dissection begins distally, following the SMV upward. Branches from the SMV to the pancreas should be divided, either between sutures or using the Harmonic® scalpel. The anterior and right border of the SMA is reached; this represents our landmark for a complete dissection (Fig. 27.3). The hanging maneuver allows safe access to the critical space between the SMV and SMA.

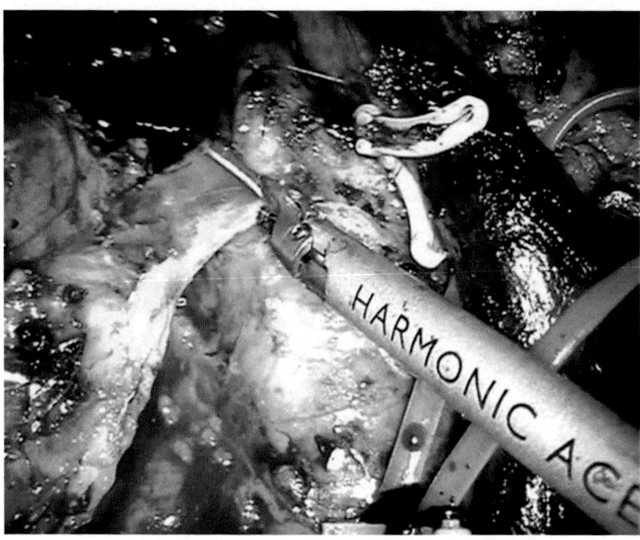

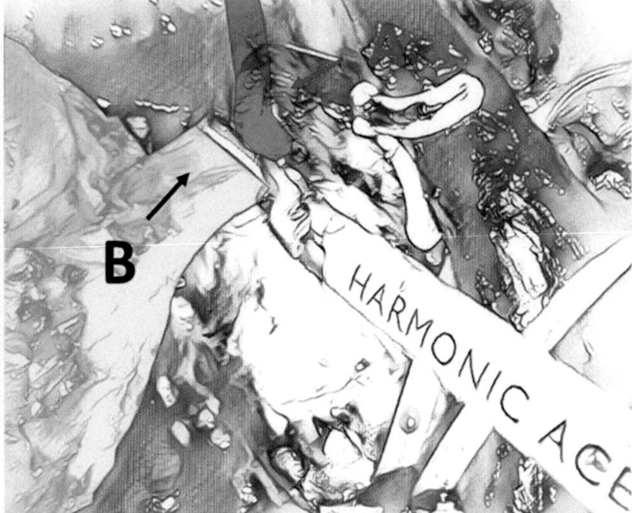

Fig. 27.3 Uncinate process dissection. With our port setting, the Harmonic® device is coming in the optimal position to separate the uncinate from the retroperitoneal space. The scheme at the right shows the transection of the last attachment (*B*) from an accessory right hepatic artery coming from the SMA (*A*)

Anastomosis

As with the open technique, the reconstruction varies depending on whether the pylorus is being preserved and on the quality of the pancreas and the pancreatic duct size. If a gastric resection is performed (as for the classic Whipple technique, in patients with tumors too close to the first duodenal portion), the pancreatic reconstruction is better done with a jejunostomy on the same biliopancreatic loop. Our usual technique includes the passage of the jejunal loop exactly where the fourth duodenal portion was crossing the mesocolic root. The type of pancreatic anastomosis is based mainly on the consistency of the parenchyma and the duct dimension. In cases with a fragile, soft pancreas and/or small duct (less than 3 mm in diameter), transgastric pancreaticogastrostomy is preferred. In cases with a hard, fibrotic pancreas and a bigger duct, a pancreaticojejunostomy could also provide good results (see below). The glue injection that was adopted at the beginning of our experience has been completely abandoned.

Pancreaticojejunostomy

There are several techniques for a pancreaticojejunostomy. The main point is that the robot allows surgeons to replicate the same technique they are comfortable with in open surgery, adding scaling effect and magnification. The result is a setting very close to the use of a surgical microscope.

When the pancreatic duct is greater in size, we opt for an end-to-side, duct-to-mucosa reconstruction: the posterior capsule of the pancreatic stump is sutured to the jejunal serosa with polypropylene. A small opening is made in the mucosa of the jejunum, and the pancreatic duct is sutured on its edge, using interrupted stitches of PDS 4–0 (or two half running stitches in case of big ducts). A small stent is placed in the duct and secured with a 5–0 PDS stitch. Another row of running suture of 4–0 polypropylene is used to fix the anterior capsule of the pancreas to the jejunum, and sometimes more interrupted stitches are added to reinforce the suture (Fig. 27.4).

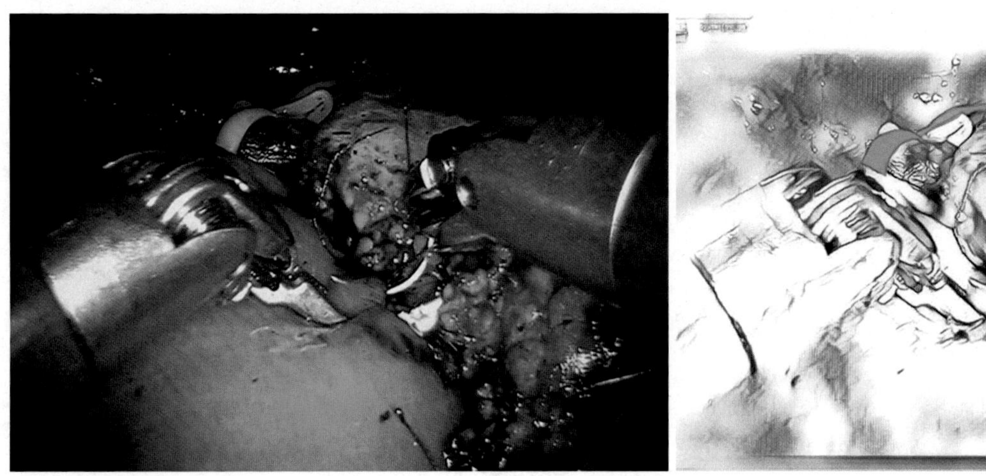

Fig. 27.4 Pancreatojejunostomy. The pancreatic duct is joined to the mucosal layer, using a small stent (*red*) as a guide

Pancreaticogastrostomy with Anterior Gastrotomy

This is our preferred technique in patients with a high-risk pancreatic stump. This anastomosis presents two main technical issues: the need for extensive pancreatic stump mobilization (about 2 in.) to allow the dunking technique and accurate hemostasis of the pancreatic transection line to reduce postoperative anastomotic bleeding.

The pancreatic stump is prepared and mobilized, dividing between sutures all the collateral branches of the splenic artery and vein. A longitudinal incision is performed on the anterior aspect of the stomach. The pancreas is brought inside the gastric cavity through a second small opening on the posterior wall, by pulling from the anterior gastrotomy the two stay sutures placed on the gland. Multiple interrupted stitches of 4/0 PDS are placed around the pancreas to secure it to the gastric wall. Once the anastomosis is completed, the anterior gastrotomy is closed with a running 3/0 PDS suture (Fig. 27.5).

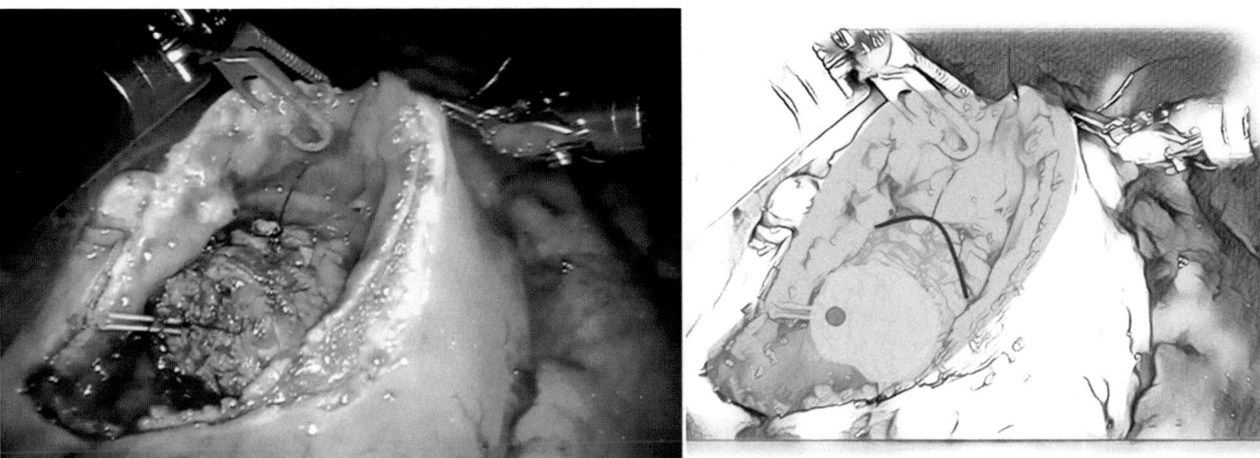

Fig. 27.5 Pancreaticogastrostomy, anterior approach. The pancreatic stump is dunked inside the stomach and sutured with interrupted stitches from the inside (*blue line*)

Biliary Reconstruction

An end-to-side hepaticojejunostomy is performed with a short running PDS suture on the posterior wall (with or without a *parachute technique*) and interrupted stitches on the anterior wall. The anterior layer is reconstructed, starting from each side of the duct, with stitches at a 1-mm distance from each other. After every stitch is passed, a Hem-o-lok® clip is placed to momentarily secure the tails and keep them separated. Once all the stitches are in place, they are tied one by one starting from the corner. For a very dilated and thick bile duct, another running suture is also used for the anterior wall.

Duodenojejunal Reconstruction

In the PPPD, this anastomosis is performed on the same loop, 50–60 cm distal to the hepaticojejunostomy. An end-to-side anastomosis is performed, commonly by two half running stitches of 3/0 PDS. Interrupted polypropylene stitches are commonly placed to reinforce the anterior wall and the corners. Indocyanine green (ICG) fluorescence could be used to assess adequate perfusion of the distal enteric stump.

Specimen Extraction and Closure

The specimen is placed in an Endobag (Medtronic; Minneapolis, MN) and extracted using a small Pfannenstiel incision. Other options could be adopted in cases with previous laparotomies. The timing of the extraction could be either before starting the reconstruction or at the very end of the procedure (depending on the pathology requirements for the fresh tissue).

Two drains are left in place at the end of the procedure: one close to the pancreatic anastomosis and the second close to the biliary anastomosis.

Our Experience

Our overall experience includes more than 150 robotic PD operations, 92 of which were done at the University of Illinois at Chicago. These are consecutive, single-surgeon, unselected robot-assisted PD, 64% of which were pylorus-preserving procedures and 36% Whipples. The mean operative time was 472.1 min, with a mean estimated blood loss of 331.5 mL.

The mean hospital stay was 13.9 days. The overall morbidity rate was 29%, with a 2.2% mortality rate.

The conversion rate was 8.6%, but conversion never occurred for acute bleeding or other emergencies. The main reason for conversion was the presence of bulky lesions, often encasing main vessels. In our experience, we have cases of associated vascular resection and reconstruction [7], but we still consider vascular involvement to be a formal indication for conversion. A vascular resection and reconstruction could be done in these cases through a small laparotomy.

References

1. Giulianotti PC, Coratti A, Angelini M, Sbrana F, Cecconi S, Balestracci T, Caravaglios G. Robotics in general surgery: personal experience in a large community hospital. Arch Surg. 2003;138:777–84.
2. Kutlu OC, Lee JE, Katz MH, Tzeng CD, Wolff RA, Varadhachary GR, et al. Open pancreaticoduodenectomy case volume predicts outcome of laparoscopic approach: a population-based analysis. Ann Surg. 2018;267(3):552–60.
3. Gagner M, Pomp A. Laparoscopic pylorus-preserving pancreatoduodenectomy. Surg Endosc. 1994;8:408–10.
4. Fong ZV, Chang DC, Ferrone CR, Lillemoe KD, Fernandez Del Castillo C. Early national experience with laparoscopic pancreaticoduodenectomy for ductal adenocarcinoma: is this really a short learning curve? J Am Coll Surg. 2016;222:209.
5. Kim JH, Gonzalez-Heredia R, Daskalaki D, Rashdan M, Masrur M, Giulianotti PC. Totally replaced right hepatic artery in pancreaticoduodenectomy: is this anatomical condition a contraindication to minimally invasive surgery? HPB (Oxford). 2016;18:580–5.
6. Miura F, Asano T, Amano H, Yoshida M, Toyota N, Wada K, et al. Management of postoperative arterial hemorrhage after pancreatobiliary surgery according to the site of bleeding: re-laparotomy or interventional radiology. J Hepato-Biliary-Pancreat Surg. 2009;16:56–63.
7. Giulianotti PC, Addeo P, Buchs NC, Ayloo SM, Bianco FM. Robotic extended pancreatectomy with vascular resection for locally advanced pancreatic tumors. Pancreas. 2011;40:1264–70.

Robotic Pylorus-Preserving Pancreaticoduodenectomy

28

Sharona B. Ross, Darrell J. Downs, Iswanto Sucandy, and Alexander S. Rosemurgy

Introduction

The application and adoption of minimally invasive techniques in hepatopancreaticobiliary (HPB) surgery have been much slower when compared to other surgical disciplines such as urology, gynecology, colorectal, and bariatric surgery. Notably, HPB operations are uncommon, and they involve unusual complexity, with relatively high risk and "many moving parts." The complexity of surgical steps undertaken during pancreaticoduodenectomy includes the precise dissection along major mesenteric vessels and reconstruction of biliary, pancreatic, and enteric anastomoses. To date, there have been just more than a handful of centers in the world that have accumulated a notable experience with laparoscopic pancreaticoduodenectomy [1–9].

The advent and development of robotic platforms, such as the da Vinci Xi® system (Intuitive Surgical, Sunnyvale, CA, USA), provide an avenue to obtain MIS proficiency due to the robotic features that overcome many of laparoscopy's shortcomings of visualization of the surgical field and manipulation of tissue. The da Vinci Xi® system, through EndoWrist™ motion technology, offers instruments that mimic the natural dexterity of the human hand, with seven degrees of freedom, more than that of the human wrist. The vision system offers the first immersive vision system, which is aided by the 3D laparoscope. The surgeon console synchronizes two images produced by optics at the tip of the laparoscope to produce a higher resolution and a more natural view of the operating field. Furthermore, the robotic system provides surgeons with improved ergonomics and improved manipulation by reducing physiologic tremor and scaling movements into smaller, more precise maneuverings. For these reasons, enthusiasm for minimally invasive pancreaticoduodenectomy has entered a new phase, especially among pancreatic surgeons at high-volume centers worldwide.

Zureikat et al. reported similar perioperative outcomes achieved by robotic pancreaticoduodenectomy when compared to open pancreaticoduodenectomy in a recent multi-institutional study consisting of 1028 patients [10]. On multivariate analysis, the robotic approach was associated with longer operative times but reduced operative blood loss and reduced rate of major complications. Ninety-day mortality, clinically relevant postoperative pancreatic fistula, infection rate, postoperative length of stay, and 90-day readmission rate were comparable to the open approach. In a subset analysis of 522 patients who underwent pancreaticoduodenectomy for pancreatic ductal adenocarcinoma, operative approach was not an independent predictor of margin status or suboptimal lymphadenectomy (<12 lymph nodes harvested).

There have been several variations of surgical techniques among centers that offer robotic pancreaticoduodenectomy. Fully robotic, hand-assisted, and hybrid laparoscopic-robotic techniques (laparoscopic resection and robotic reconstruction) have been developed and described [1, 11–16]. Reconstruction techniques, including "classical" versus pylorus-preserving pancreaticoduodenectomy, are also varied among centers and surgeons [1, 10]. Our group has a tremendous experience with both pancreaticoduodenectomy, laparoscopic operations, advanced laparoendoscopic single-site (LESS) foregut operations, and robotic surgery [17–22]. Our technique for pancreaticoduodenectomy is an outgrowth of our experience; herein, we describe our current technique for undertaking robotic pylorus-preserving pancreaticoduodenectomy. It must be realized that robotic pancreaticoduodenectomy is still in its relative infancy, and the technique and its application will continue to evolve in the years to come.

S. B. Ross, MD (✉) · D. J. Downs, BS · I. Sucandy, MD
A. S. Rosemurgy, MD
Department of Surgery, Florida Hospital Tampa, Tampa, FL, USA
e-mail: ddowns2@mail.usf.edu

Y. Fong et al. (eds.), *The SAGES Atlas of Robotic Surgery*, https://doi.org/10.1007/978-3-319-91045-1_28

Indications and Contraindications

Indications

- Malignant pancreatic lesions of the head, uncinate process, and/or neck of the pancreas, including pancreatic ductal adenocarcinoma, pancreatic islet cell carcinoma, malignant intraductal papillary mucinous neoplasm (IPMN), peri-ampullary adenocarcinoma, cholangiocarcinoma, and duodenal carcinoma

Contraindications

- Patients with locally advanced disease
- Patients with metastatic disease
- Patients with presumed significant intraperitoneal adhesions from multiple prior open abdominal operations
- Patients who underwent neoadjuvant chemotherapy and/or radiation therapy for locally advanced disease now with resectable disease that requires major vascular resection and reconstruction

Preparation and Operative Strategy

- Computed tomography (CT) of the chest, abdomen, and pelvis, 1-mm thin-cut high-quality triphasic with oral and IV contrast (pancreatic protocol)—for the diagnosis and staging of malignant lesions
  - We also utilize Surgical Planner™ (Surgical Theater LLC, Mayfield Village, OH) to reconstruct patient-specific 3D models, which is helpful to evaluate for resectability, surgical planning, as well as patient and family education.
- MRCP—to delineate the pancreatic and biliary ducts (not always necessary)
- Comprehensive laboratory examination (i.e., CA 19–9 tumor marker levels, etc.)
- Endoscopic ultrasound (EUS) and fine-needle aspiration (FNA)—preoperative tissue biopsy for histologic diagnosis and staging
- Endoscopic retrograde cholangiopancreatography (ERCP)—with the placement of an intraductal stent when necessary (i.e., obstruction of the distal common bile duct with hyperbilirubinemia)
- Risk analysis —cardiac, pulmonary, liver, and kidney function
- Enhanced recovery after surgery (ERAS) pathway
  - Patient education and nutritional status

Our indications for conversion to "open" pancreaticoduodenectomy include, but are not limited to:

1. Failure to progress for greater than 20 min for whatever reason
2. Significant intraoperative bleeding or uncontrolled bleeding
3. Intolerance to carbon dioxide pneumoperitoneum
4. Major vascular invasion
5. Any factors that promote an R1 resection
6. Excess difficulties to complete safe biliary, pancreatic, or enteral reconstruction

We follow an enhanced recovery after surgery (ERAS) protocol for robotic pancreaticoduodenectomy. Patients are given preoperative education of the protocol by a team member in clinic after a plan to operate is made. The multidisciplinary team of surgeons, physician extenders, perioperative nursing staffs, residents, fellows, and anesthesiologists (and their certified registered nurse anesthetists) must all be familiar with the ERAS protocol. Briefly, preoperatively, the patient agrees to smoking/alcohol cessation, a new preoperative weight loss and diet regiment, exercise, diabetes education classes, preoperative use of incentive spirometry, and the intake of Impact Advanced Recovery® (Nestle HealthCare Nutrition, Florham Park, NJ) (a nutritional drink taken three times a day for 5 days and ending the night before the operation to boost their immune system).

Additionally, patients meet with members of the anesthesiology team to discuss their perioperative analgesia management plan (i.e., intrathecal injection of 10 cc of Duramorph® prior to induction, oral Celebrex/gabapentin, and IV Tylenol postoperatively). Alvimopan is administered preoperatively, and it is continued twice daily for 7 days, as needed, for perioperative postoperative nausea and vomiting control. It is our opinion that diligent preoperative education (by all members of the multidisciplinary team) of the patient on what to expect has led to early recovery and increased patient satisfaction. With this ERAS plan, we have been able to reduce our length of stay after robotic pancreaticoduodenectomy to 3–5 days.

Operating Room Setup

The patient is placed in the supine position on the operating table. Compression stockings and sequential compression devices (SCD) are used in all patients to prevent deep vein thrombosis (DVT). After general endotracheal anesthesia is established, a nasogastric tube and a Foley catheter are placed. Both arms are extended and all pressure points are padded. The patient's abdomen is widely prepped with alcohol, and a Betadine-impregnated plastic drape is applied. The surgical table is then positioned in reverse Trendelenburg position with a slight left lateral tilt. The da Vinci Xi® robotic system is docked with the boom coming over the patient's right shoulder. The bedside surgeon stands on the patient's right, and the scrub tech stands to the patient's left. This arrangement enables easy access to the robotic arms for instrument exchange. Two surgeon consoles are placed in such a way that the surgeon at the console has a direct visualization of the patient. We utilize dual consoles for the education and training of fellows and residents. Intraoperatively, the 3D image system is utilized for surgical navigation. The Surgical Navigation Advanced Platform™ (SNAP, Surgical Theater LLC, Mayfield Village, OH) images are displayed on a portable monitor and placed next to the surgeon console for easy reference by all the team members during the operation.

Operative Steps

Step 1. Operating Room Setup (Fig. 28.1) and Port Placement

Prior to making the incision, approximately 5–8 cc of 0.25% Marcaine™ (AstraZeneca, Wilmington, DE) with epinephrine (1:1000) is injected into the umbilicus and all robotic port sites for local anesthesia. We believe this helps to decrease postoperative pain. The abdomen is entered via 8-mm incision in the umbilicus, and pneumoperitoneum is established (up to 15 mmHg). After diagnostic laparoscopy, without notable findings, three 8-mm robotic trocars, an Advanced Access Gelport® (Applied Medical, Rancho Santa

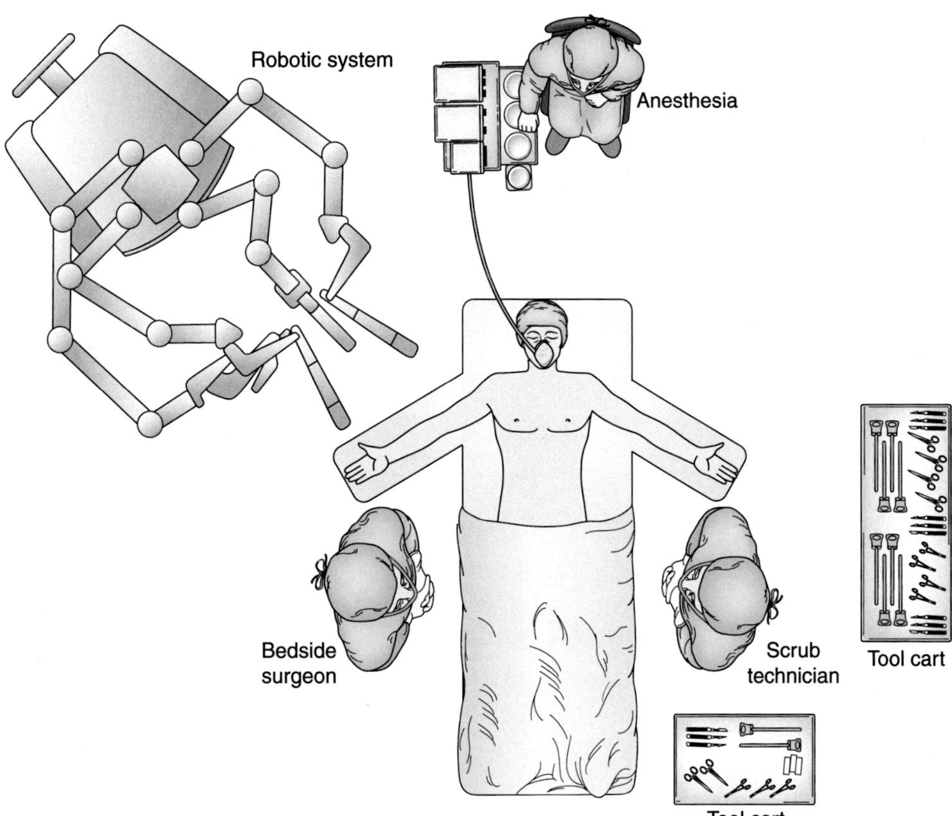

Fig. 28.1 Operating room setup

Margarita, CA), and one 5-mm AirSeal® Access Port (ConMed Inc., Utica, NY) are then placed under laparoscopic visualization. The placement site for each trocar is very important. The liver retractor is placed via the right upper quadrant AirSeal® port and secured to the surgical drape using Kocher clamps. The da Vinci Xi® robotic system is brought from the patient's right shoulder, and it is docked with the bed in the reverse Trendelenburg position with a slight left lateral tilt.

- Trocar placement (Fig. 28.2):
  - At the right midclavicular line, same level as the umbilicus, for 8-mm robotic trocar (robotic arm # 1)
  - At the umbilicus: 8-mm trocar for the robotic camera (robotic arm # 2)
  - At the left midclavicular line, slightly above the level of the umbilicus, for 8-mm robotic trocar (robotic arm # 3)
  - At the left anterior axillary line, midway between the umbilicus and the costal margin, for 8-mm robotic trocar (robotic arm # 4)
  - At the right anterior axillary line about 4 cm caudal to the costal margin for the AirSeal® Access Port
  - Between the midclavicular line and the umbilicus caudal to the umbilicus for Advanced Access Gelport® (not interfering with robotic arm # 1)

Step 2. Porta Hepatis Dissection

Robotic arm # 1—Fenestrated bipolar device.
Robotic arm # 2—Camera.
Robotic arm # 3—Hook cautery.
Robotic arm # 4—Atraumatic bowel grasper.
The Advanced Access Gelport® is used for a suctioning device and atraumatic graspers utilized by bedside surgeon.
The AirSeal® Access Port for liver retractor.

The robotic camera remains in robotic arm # 2 until we begin closing trocar incisions. The gastrohepatic ligament is opened (Fig. 28.3) in a stellate fashion utilizing robotic hook cautery. The common hepatic artery is identified, despite the characteristic overlying lymph node, and followed distally toward the porta hepatis. The common hepatic artery lymph node (Fig. 28.4a, Station VIIIa node) is removed and sent to pathology for frozen section examination if it is substantial or suspicious. The gastroduodenal artery (GDA) is identified and circumferentially dissected prior to placement of two (or three) Hem-o-lok clips both proximally and distally. A thorough review of a triphasic CT scan and/or 3D imaging preoperatively is mandatory to rule out the presence of an accessory or replaced right hepatic artery, which is anticipated in this location. In our experience, the use of 3D virtual imaging has helped immensely in this regard.

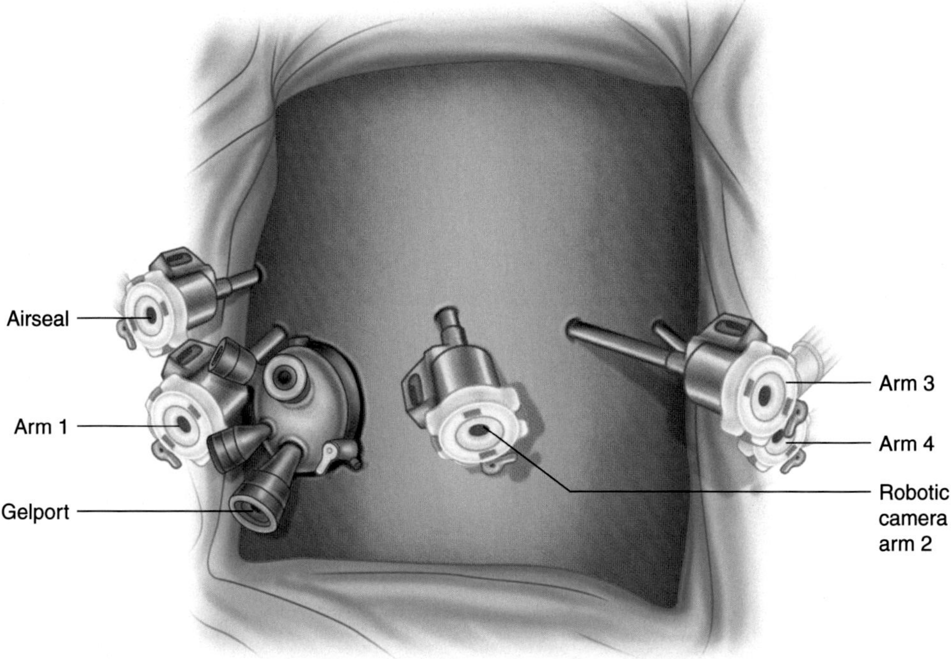

Fig. 28.2 Trocar/port placement

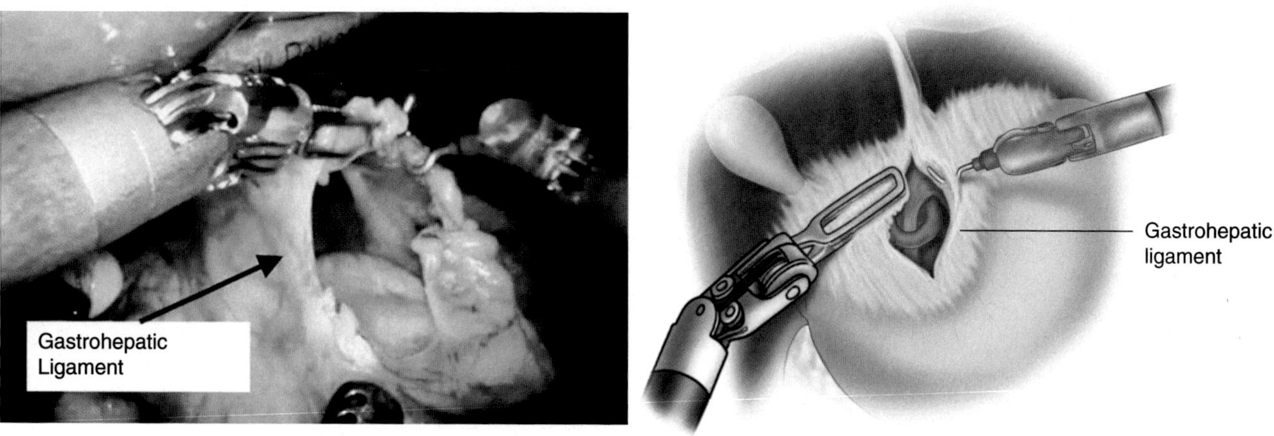

Fig. 28.3 Porta hepatis dissection, opening of the gastrohepatic ligament

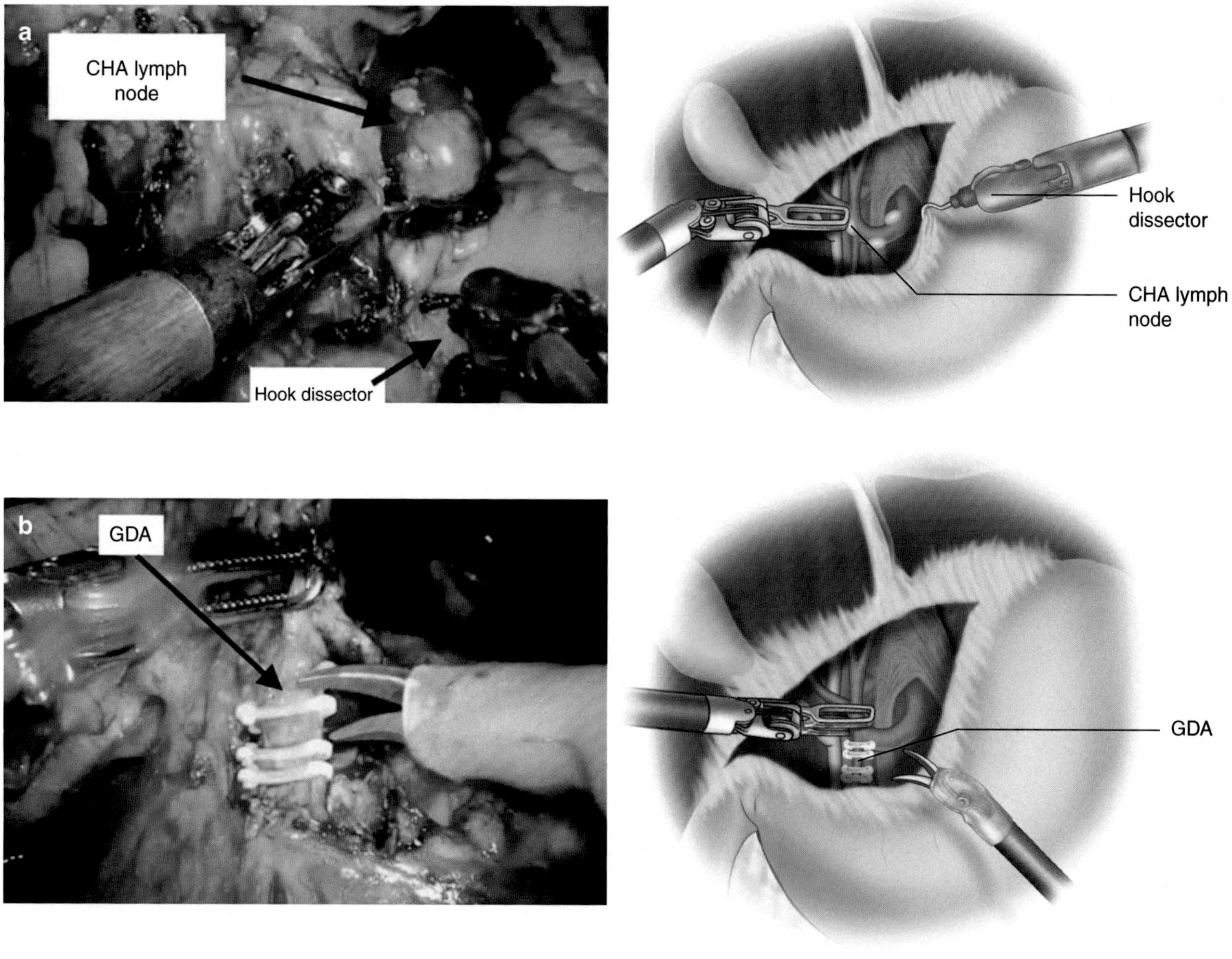

Fig. 28.4 (**a**) Dissection and removal of the common hepatic artery (CHA) lymph node. (**b**) Ligation and transection of the gastroduodenal artery (GDA)

Prior to division, the GDA is routinely test-clamped, and the pulse in the hepatic artery is visually assessed to confirm the artery being divided is not a replaced hepatic artery and to exclude a significant celiac artery stenosis. Once the GDA has been divided using robotic scissors (Fig. 28.4b), the portal vein, which is located posteriorly, comes into view with a bit of dissection dorsal to and medial to the GDA. The common hepatic duct is circumferentially dissected proximal to the cystic duct (before or after undertaking cholecystectomy). The distal common bile duct is identified and separated away from the portal vein by developing an avascular plane between them. The common bile duct lymph nodes, which are located along the right posterolateral aspect of the duct, are carefully taken with the specimen with hook cautery. The dissection is carried down the distal common bile duct (Fig. 28.5).

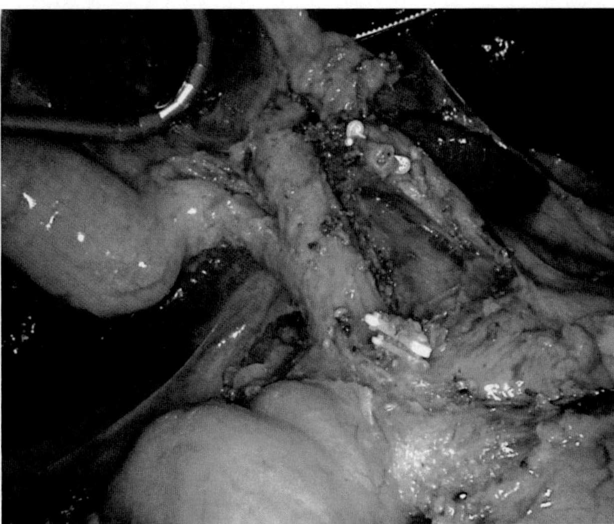

Fig. 28.5 Dissection carried down the distal common bile duct

Step 3. Kocher Maneuver

Robotic arm # 1—Fenestrated bipolar device.
Robotic arm # 2—Camera.
Robotic arm # 3—Hook cautery.
Robotic arm # 4—Atraumatic bowel grasper.

Because the nature of any written report does not allow for simultaneous activities, it is important for us to note that a Kocher maneuver may be undertaken first in the operation. With adequate anterosuperior retraction of the liver, the hepatic flexure of the colon is mobilized caudally as needed. The c-loop of the duodenum is exposed and widely mobilized, working proximal to distal along the lateral edge of the duodenum. The duodenum is grasped with an atraumatic bowel grasper in the robotic arm # 4 and retracted ventrally and, especially, to the left, with great care to avoid injury to the duodenum. The dissection continues until the left renal vein is easily identified and the ligament of Treitz is divided (Fig. 28.6). Next, the proximal jejunum is exposed. The jejunum is then delivered to the right of the superior mesenteric vein and divided with a robotic stapling device. The jejunum should be placed so that it can easily be retrieved later.

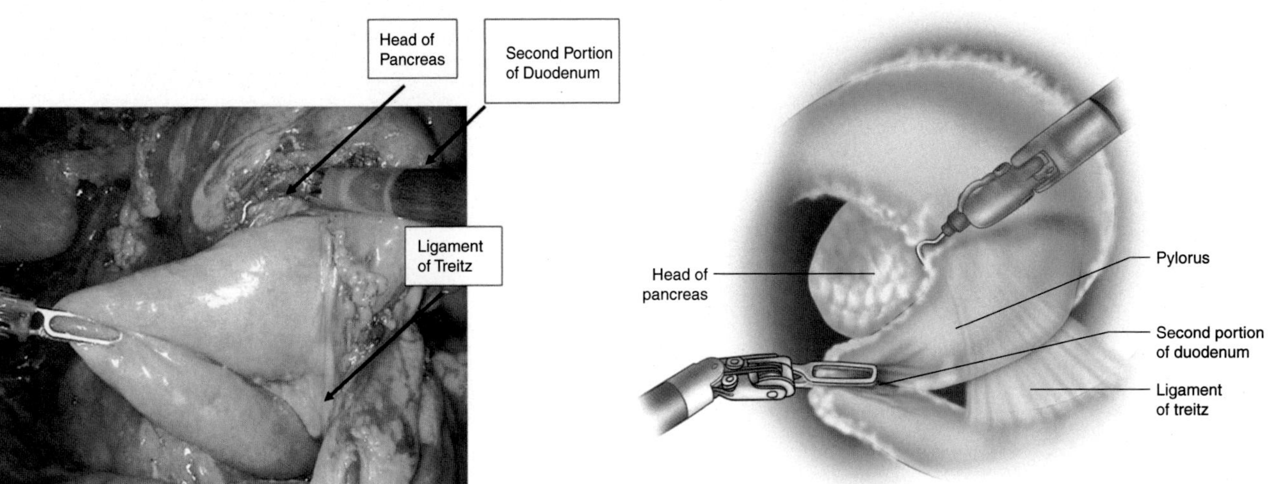

Fig. 28.6 Kocherization of duodenum

Step 4. Pancreatic Exposure

Robotic arm # 1—Fenestrated bipolar device.
Robotic arm # 2—Camera.
Robotic arm # 3—Vessel sealer (alternating with hook cautery).
Robotic arm # 4—Atraumatic bowel grasper.

We begin to divide the gastrocolic omentum, while the stomach is reflected in the cephalad direction. The gastrocolic omentum is opened somewhere near the midpoint along the greater curve of the stomach, probably closer to the pylorus. This exposure places the right gastroepiploic vein at a near-right angle to the superior mesenteric vein, to facilitate later clipping and division. As the omentum is opened, the pancreas comes into view. The inferior border of the pancreas is identified and dissected along utilizing hook cautery going carefully toward the superior mesenteric vein; in general, we like to dissect away from critical vessels to avoid injury. The right gastroepiploic vein may be double-clipped and divided at this time. In unusual circumstances of morbidly obese patients or when a significant amount of adipose tissue is encountered in this location, a robotic ultrasound device can be used to help identify the exact location of the superior mesenteric vein.

Once the superior mesenteric vein is identified, the dissection is carried along its ventral surface going cephalad (Fig. 28.7). A tunnel behind the neck of the pancreas is carefully developed using robotic hook cautery while gently elevating the pancreas anteriorly using a fenestrated bipolar grasper and an atraumatic bowel grasper. A suction device placed through the gel port pushes gently down on the portal vein to keep it from harm's way. Once the tunnel is developed, we determine that the tumor mass is resectable with "clean" margins, and, if resection is the plan, we proceed with pancreatic transection.

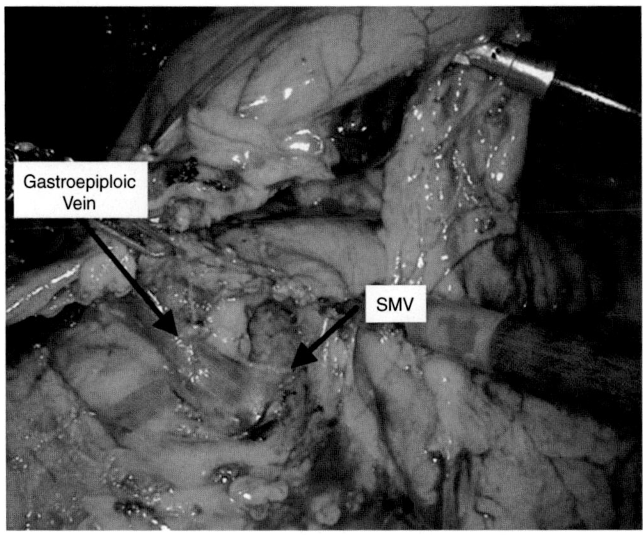

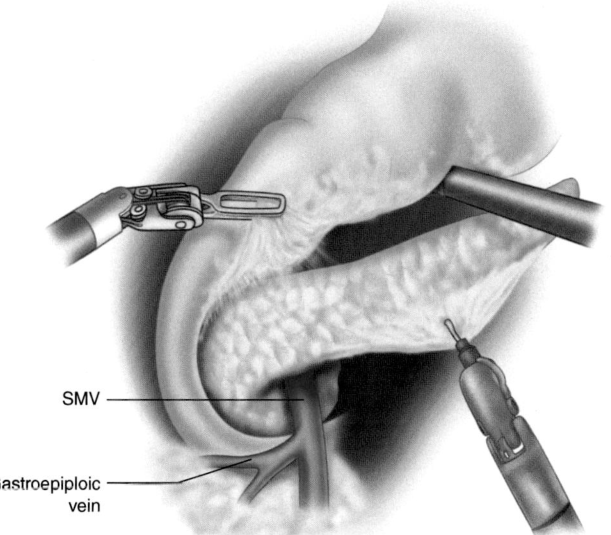

Fig. 28.7 Pancreatic exposure and transection of the neck of the pancreas

Step 5. Transection of the First Portion of Duodenum

Robotic arm # 1—Fenestrated bipolar device.
Robotic arm # 2—Camera.
Robotic arm # 3—Vessel sealer.
Robotic arm # 4—Atraumatic bowel grasper.

The gastrocolic omentum is further divided while avoiding the transverse mesocolon. Transection of the right gastroepiploic vessels occurs during this dissection. The distal stomach, pylorus, and first portion of duodenum are mobilized. The identification of the pylorus is aided by the recognition of the vein of Mayo. A point of transection for a stapling device is chosen approximately 2 cm distal to the pylorus (Fig. 28.8), but we work to get as much length along the duodenum as possible; dusky duodenum can always be trimmed back later. After transection, the stomach and duodenum are then deflected to the left upper quadrant, and the neck of the pancreas is now clearly visualized.

Step 6. Pancreatic Transection

Robotic arm # 1—Fenestrated bipolar device.
Robotic arm # 2—Camera.
Robotic arm # 3—Vessel sealer (alternating with hook cautery).
Robotic arm # 4—Atraumatic bowel grasper.

The pancreatic parenchyma is divided using robotic hook cautery (Fig. 28.9) or bipolar scissors. A laparoscopic suctioning device is introduced into the Advanced Access Gelport®. The suctioning device is utilized for suctioning and retracting tissue. Hemostasis must be obtained as the pancreatic transection advances, because excessive bleeding in this area can obscure the view of the operative field very quickly. Most of the pancreatic transection is undertaken with the hook cautery; the main pancreatic duct is identified. The pancreatic duct is then sharply divided with robotic scissors (which helps identify the pancreatic duct for later construction of the pancreaticojejunal anastomosis). The use of ther-

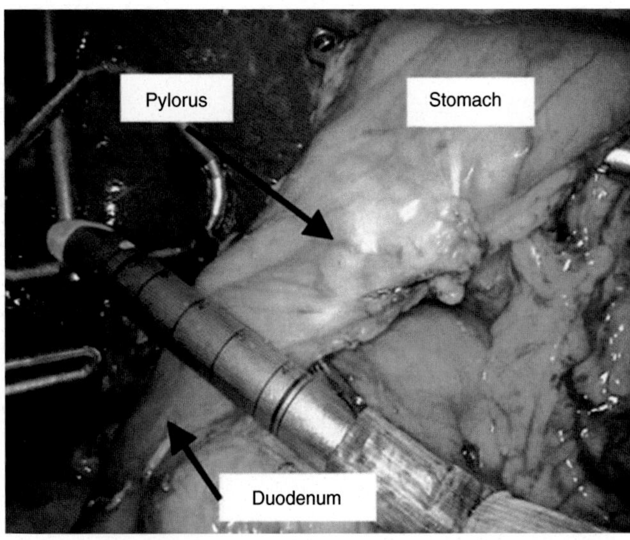

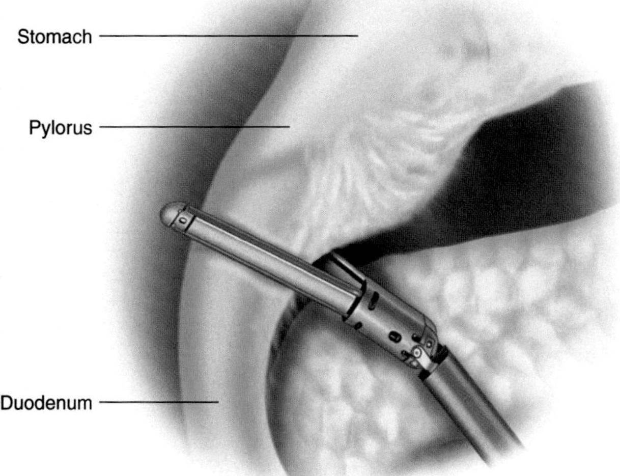

Fig. 28.8 Transection of duodenum

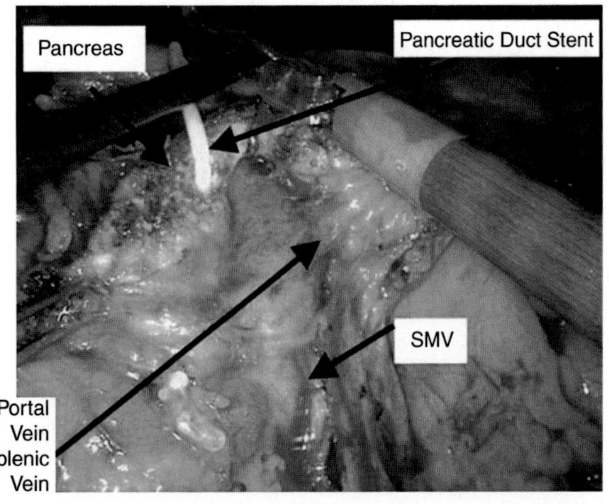

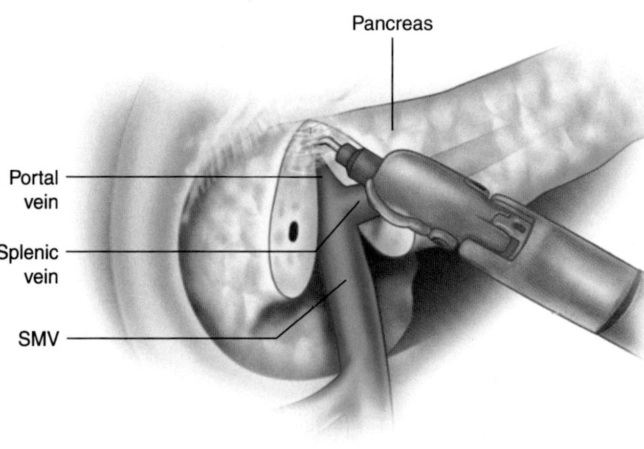

Fig. 28.9 Pancreatic transection and identification of the pancreatic duct

mal energy in dividing the pancreatic duct can seal the duct closed. The right lateral portion of the superior mesenteric vein/portal vein is bluntly teased away from the pancreatic head. The position of the superior mesenteric artery is identified by knowing its position to the left of the superior mesenteric vein. After the Kocher maneuver (described in the next section), the uncinate process and duodenal mesentery are separated from the portal vein/superior mesenteric vein. The vessel sealer instrument of the robot is helpful in this portion of the operation and is our preferred choice. It is uncommon to have to use clips for vascular control. Division of the uncinate process/duodenal mesentery begins caudal and proceeds cephalad until the pancreas and duodenum are freed (i.e., until the common hepatic artery is reached). The dissection continues along the lateral and posterior aspect of the portal vein to the common hepatic duct, which is finally transected.

Step 7. Pancreaticoduodenectomy Specimen Removal

Robotic arm # 1—Fenestrated bipolar device (alternating with a vessel sealer).

Robotic arm # 2—Camera.

Robotic arm # 3—Vessel sealer (alternating with hook cautery).

Robotic arm # 4—Atraumatic bowel grasper.

Once the head of the pancreas is separated from the body and tail, the mesentery of the third and fourth portions of the duodenum is divided, and the uncinate process is freed using the robotic vessel sealer along the superior mesenteric vein. The bedside surgeon may provide a dynamic gentle lateral retraction of the specimen to the patient's right using a laparoscopic atraumatic bowel grasper, though this is generally unnecessary. The laparoscopic suctioning device, through the Advanced Access Gelport®, may facilitate this dissection as well by providing some tissue retraction as needed. The lymphatic basin is included with the specimen.

The superior mesenteric artery must be carefully identified and protected from any injury as the dissection is carried along it. The specimen is also freed from the portal vein and superior mesenteric vein (Fig. 28.10). Once the specimen dissection of the superior mesenteric vein, superior mesenteric artery, and the portal vein attachments is complete, the distal common bile duct is encountered as it enters the head of the pancreas. The hepatic duct is divided with

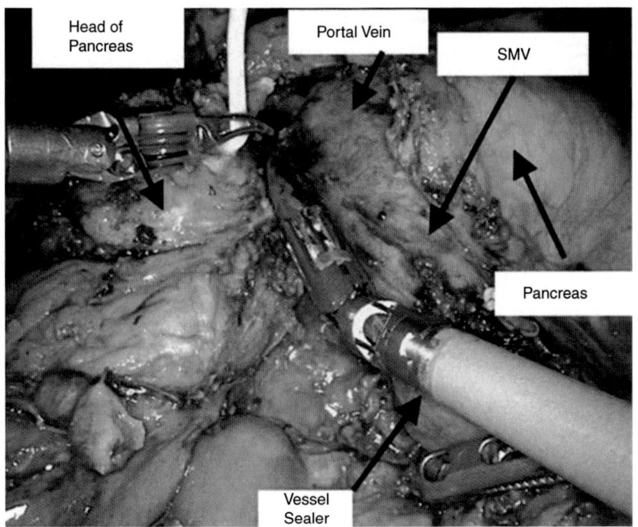

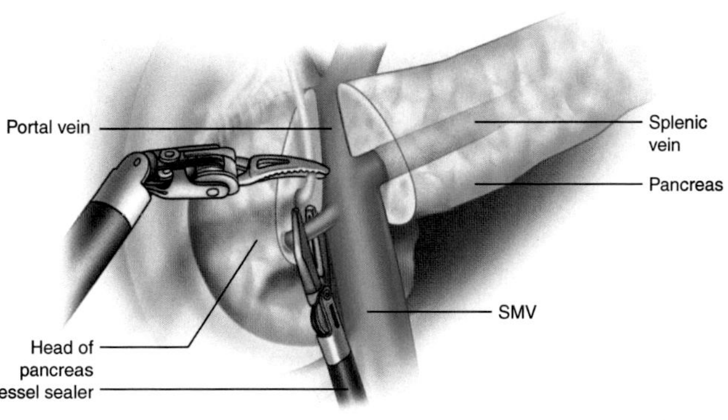

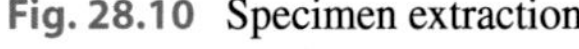
Fig. 28.10 Specimen extraction

either robotic hook cautery or scissors (Fig. 28.11). The bile duct lumen is identified and the bile effluent is suctioned off. If present, a bile duct stent is removed with the specimen. A cholecystectomy is undertaken next; this is often an opportunity for a younger, more inexperienced surgeon to participate and gain robotic experience. The gallbladder and the pancreaticoduodenectomy specimen are then placed into a laparoscopic EndoCatch Bag (Applied Medical, Rancho Santa Margarita, CA) and removed via the Advanced Access Gelport®. Water-soluble gel applied in the gel port and on the extraction bag helps "slip" the specimen out through the gel port. With lubrication, it is possible to deliver a specimen the size of a "lemon" through an incision the size of a "lemon drop."

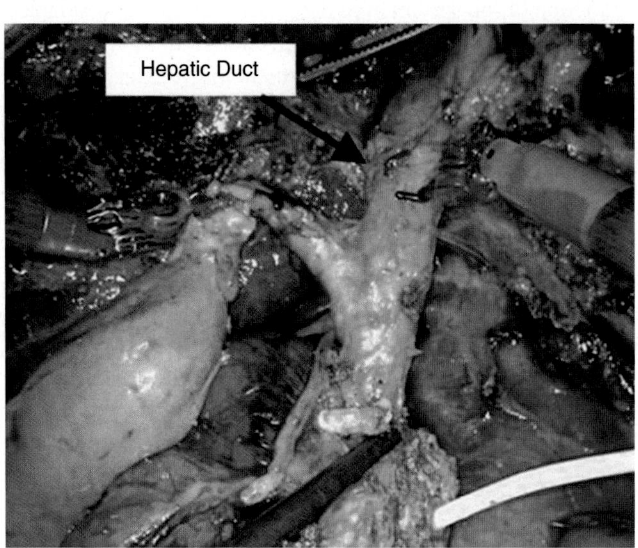

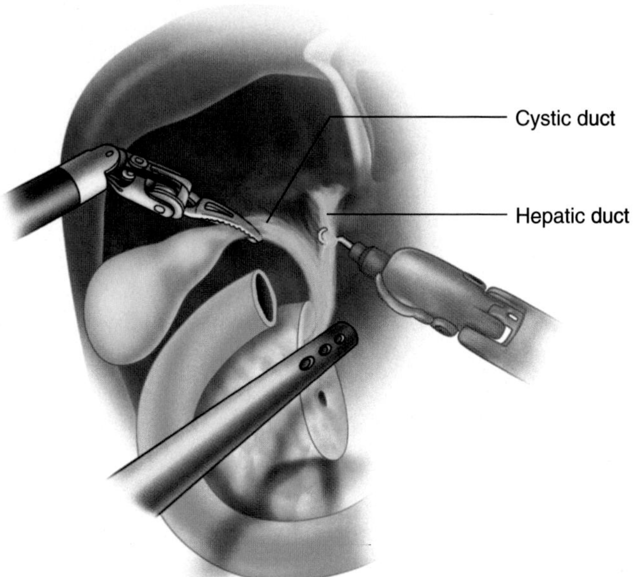

Fig. 28.11 Hepatic duct transection

Reconstruction

All sutures utilized in the reconstruction (i.e., hepaticojejunostomy, pancreaticojejunostomy, and duodenojejunostomy) are introduced into the peritoneal cavity through the Advanced Access Gelport®.

Step 8. Construction of the Hepaticojejunostomy

Robotic arm # 1—Needle driver.
Robotic arm # 2—Camera.
Robotic arm # 3—Needle driver.
Robotic arm # 4—Atraumatic bowel grasper.

A suitable length of proximal jejunum is brought under the root of the mesentery and advanced cephalad toward the porta hepatis and the cut edge of the pancreas. The laparoscopic liver retractor should be positioned in such a way to easily visualize the hepatic duct lumen. The proximal jejunal limb is held in position using an atraumatic bowel grasper in the robotic arm # 4; it holds the bowel in position by grasping it proximal to the anastomosis. Doing the hepaticojejunostomy before the pancreaticojejunostomy is our strong preference.

The cut end of the bile duct is further opened along the ventral surface of the bile duct if the duct is small (less than 1 cm) to increase the cross-sectional area of the bile duct anastomosis to help prevent a clinically apparent stricture. Construction of a single-layer anastomosis is started at the 9-o'clock position using a 3–0 V-Loc™ (Medtronic, Minneapolis, MN) suture in a running fashion (Fig. 28.12). The stitch is run dorsally toward the 3-o'clock position and kept tight after each needle passes. Another V-Loc™ suture (starting at the 9-o'clock position) is used to construct the ventral aspect of the anastomosis. Both stitches are tied, on the outside of the duct lumen, at the 3-o'clock position, after ensuring that the suture is snug. The anastomosis is inspected and additional sutures are placed as needed.

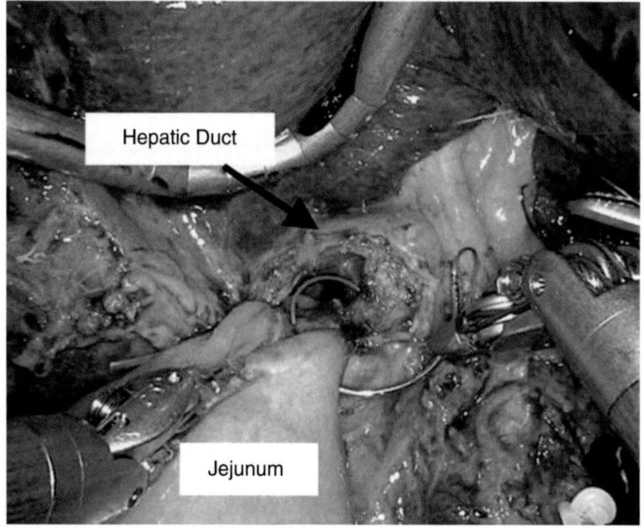

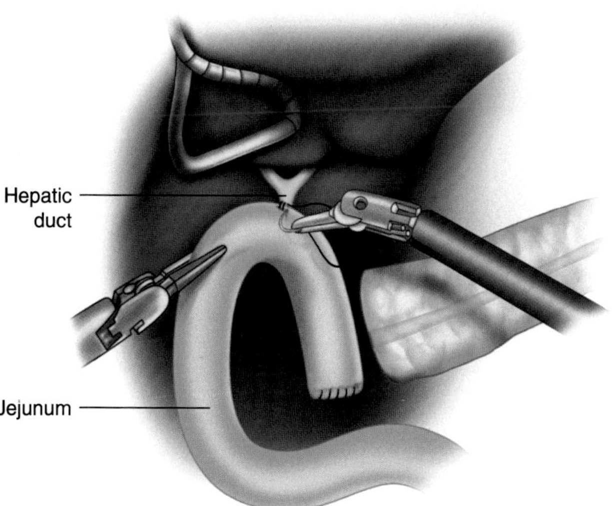

Fig. 28.12 Hepaticojejunostomy

Step 9. Construction of the Pancreaticojejunostomy

Robotic arm # 1—Needle driver.
Robotic arm # 2—Camera.
Robotic arm # 3—Needle driver.
Robotic arm # 4—Atraumatic bowel grasper.

The pancreaticojejunostomy is constructed using a two-layer anastomosis with 3–0 V-Loc™ sutures (Fig. 28.13). The posterior layer is undertaken by bringing the pancreatic parenchyma to the seromuscular layer of the jejunum in a running fashion. The pancreatic duct is then identified. The duct is generally quite posterior, so don't include it in the posterior layer of the anastomosis. The duct-to-jejunum anastomosis is undertaken after making a *small* enterotomy by placing interrupted sutures (at the 6-,9-, 3-, and 12-o'clock positions) using 4–0 or 5–0 polypropylene sutures. All the knots are tied on the outside of the pancreatic duct anastomosis (i.e., outside the lumen). The anterior layer of the pancreaticojejunostomy anastomosis is constructed by bringing the anterior capsule of the pancreas to the seromuscular layer of the jejunum in a running fashion. The posterior and anterior layer stitches are then tied together, which completes the pancreaticojejunal anastomosis.

Step 10. Reconstruction of the Ligament of Treitz

Robotic arm # 1—Needle driver (alternating with an atraumatic bowel grasper).
Robotic arm # 2—Camera.
Robotic arm # 3—Needle driver.
Robotic arm # 4—Atraumatic bowel grasper.

The transverse colon is elevated ventral and cephalad with atraumatic bowel graspers which exposes the prior location of the ligament of Treitz, i.e., the defect under the mesenteric vessels. The jejunal limb coming from the bile duct is identified and secured to the root of the transverse colon mesentery with a 3–0 V-Loc™ suture. The goal of reconstructing the ligament of Treitz is to avoid potential small bowel herniation under the root of mesentery alongside the jejunal limb. Careful attention must be paid not to include any mesenteric vessel branches during placement of the stitches. It is also important to avoid excessive distal traction on the jejunal limb, which in turn can promote mechanical tension on the hepaticojejunostomy and pancreaticojejunostomy.

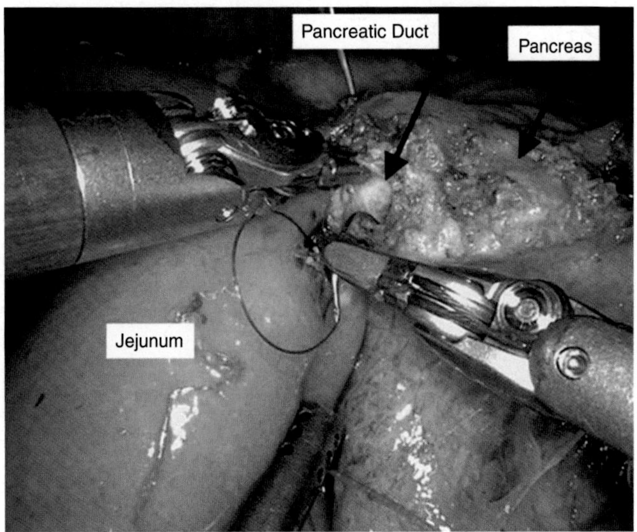

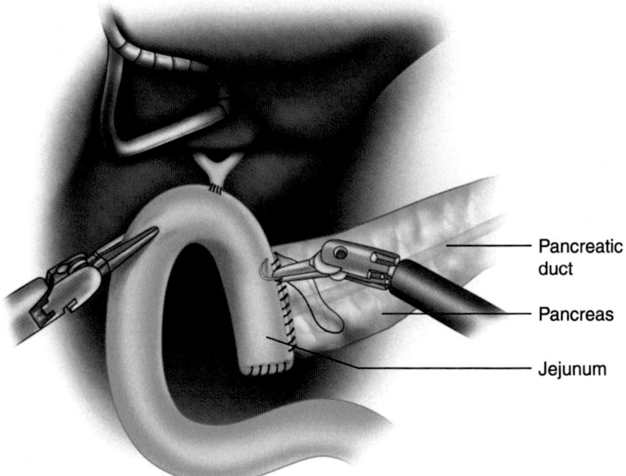

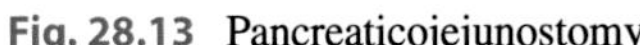
Fig. 28.13 Pancreaticojejunostomy

Step 11. Construction of the Duodenojejunostomy

Robotic arm # 1—Needle driver.
Robotic arm # 2—Camera.
Robotic arm # 3—Needle driver.
Robotic arm # 4—Atraumatic bowel grasper.

The surgical bed is leveled (from reverse Trendelenburg position). The duodenojejunostomy is constructed using a single-layer running anastomosis with 2 3–0 V-Loc™ sutures in a similar fashion to the hepaticojejunostomy (Fig. 28.14). Construction is started at the 9-o'clock position (looking at the cut end of the duodenum) using a 3–0 V-Loc™ suture in a running fashion. The stitch is ran dorsally to the 3-o'clock position and kept tight after each needle pass. Utilizing a Gambee technique may aid in making a nice, clean anastomosis. Another V-Loc™ suture, which also begins at the 9-o'clock position, is used to construct the ventral aspect of the anastomosis. Both stitches are tied at the 3-o'clock position after ensuring that the sutures are tight. The afferent and efferent limbs are anchored to the distal stomach to avoid tension or twisting of the duodenojejunostomy.

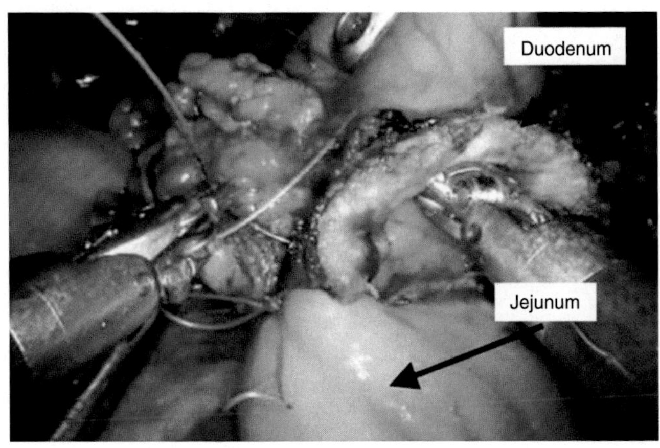

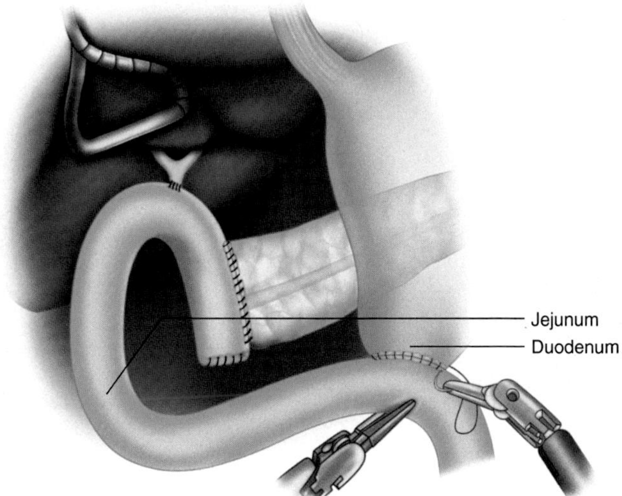

Fig. 28.14 Duodenojejunostomy

Step 12. Placement of Drain and Closure

A closed suction 10F Jackson-Pratt drain is routinely placed about the hepaticojejunostomy and pancreaticojejunostomy. The Jackson-Pratt drain is brought out through the right upper quadrant 5 mm AirSeal® Access Port incision (Fig. 28.15). The drain is sutured to the skin with a nylon suture.

To help decrease postoperative pain, the diaphragm is irrigated bilaterally and liberally with a solution of 7.5 mL of 0.25% Marcaine™ in 250 mL of normal saline. All incisions are closed along anatomic layers. Absorbable monofilament sutures are used for fascial closure, and the skin is approximated with interrupted 3–0 absorbable sutures and Steri-Strips. To further aid in postoperative pain control, we routinely inject all incisions with a solution of 20 mL of Exparel® (Pacira Pharmaceuticals, Parsippany, NJ) in 30 mL of normal saline. A sterile 1.5 × 6 silver dressing (Therabond® 3D, Alliqua Biomedical, Langhorne, PA) is applied to all incisions followed by sterile 2 × 2 gauze; it is covered with a Tegaderm™ (Tegaderm transparent dressing, 3M™, St Paul, MN) dressing. This watertight dressing allows patients to shower at home. The dressing is removed at 5–7 days postoperatively.

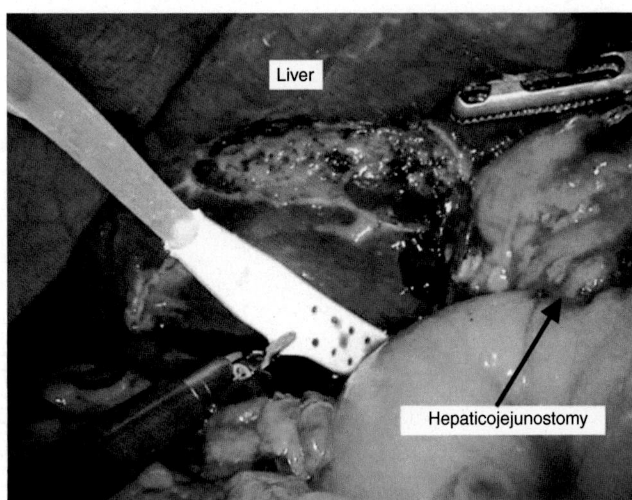

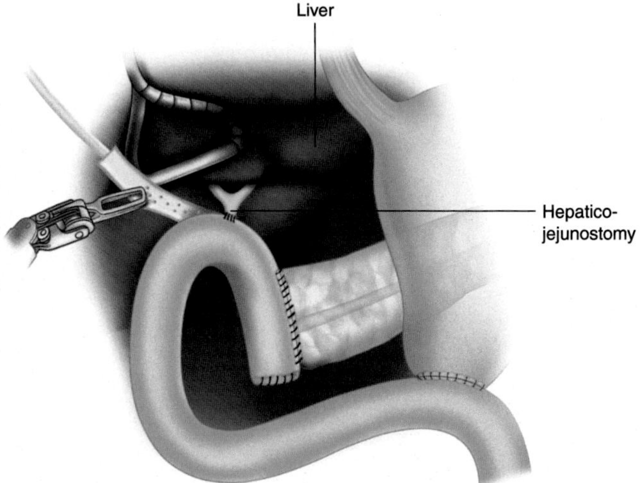

Fig. 28.15 Placement of drain

Intraoperative Care

Judicious intraoperative fluid administration is emphasized. We follow perioperative goal-directed fluid therapy (PGDFT) principles, guided by the ClearSight™ EV1000 System (Edwards Lifesciences, Irvine, CA). Utilizing this system, hemodynamic metrics (i.e., cardiac output, stroke volume, stroke volume variation, etc.) are continuously monitored within a strict protocol to allow for precise volume administration. Percentage of stroke volume variations is followed to estimate fluid status and used to determine whether intravenous albumin/fluid bolus is needed. All the steps and points are strictly adhered to by the anesthesia team in our enhanced recovery after surgery (ERAS) protocol.

Postoperative Care

- POD 1: CBC and CMP daily.
- POD 2: Foley out, NGT out, start clear liquid diet.
- POD 3: Intraperitoneal drain amylase levels, if it's within normal value, drain is removed.
- Physical therapy: twice a day.
- Pain control: intravenous Tylenol (1000 mg every 6 h for 3 days) in addition to intravenous ketorolac (15 mg every 6 h for 3 days), oral gabapentin, and oral celecoxib. Breakthrough pain is managed with intravenous 0.5–1 mg hydromorphone (when patients are still unable to tolerate a diet).
- Patients are encouraged to chew gum during recovery to help stimulate gut function/motility.

Postoperative Complications

- Atelectasis
- Pneumonia
- Urinary tract infection
- Wound infection
- Pancreatic anastomosis leak
- Intra-abdominal abscess
- Hepaticojejunostomy stricture

Tricks of the Master

- With the intuitive da Vinci Xi® system, the operating room bed is paired with the robotic system, which enables easy positional changes throughout the operation without constant undocking and redocking of the robotic system (effective way to use gravity to provide adequate exposure).
- The role of an experienced bedside surgeon cannot be over emphasized. The bedside surgeon is crucial in providing appropriate traction and organ manipulation to maintain optimal exposure and keeping the operative field bloodless.
- Early/swift conversion to open pancreaticoduodenectomy if failure to progress (for more than 20 min due to difficult dissections), significant intraoperative bleeding, and intolerance to carbon dioxide pneumoperitoneum.
- The current da Vinci Xi® system utilizes an 8-mm laparoscope (instead of a 15 mm) as the robotic camera, which allows the utilization of the camera in any trocar.
- We prefer to use V-Loc™ barbed sutures for the robotic anastomoses since they provide and maintain tension across the tissue interface after each needle passes. We found this to be very useful since loosening of the running anastomotic stitches is unlikely. In both open and robotic operations, corners are points where anastomotic leaks are commonly seen. Therefore, we routinely reinforce both corners with additional full-thickness stitches. Careful attention must be given after completion of any anastomosis to ensure the absence of any mechanical twisting or tension.
- We routinely place a closed suction drain about the hepaticojejunostomy and pancreaticojejunostomy. Drain amylase level is checked on postoperative day 3, 24 h after the patient was started on a clear liquid diet. The drain is removed at the bedside when drain amylase levels are within normal levels.
- On postoperative day 2, nasogastric tubes are removed. We begin our patients on Ensure Clear and then advance to clear liquid diet.
- On postoperative day 3, patients are advanced to full liquid diet. Patients are discharged home.
- Postoperative clinic visit in our office occurs in 7–10 days following discharge.

One of the major concerns about robotic surgery is the cost of purchasing and maintaining a robotic surgical system. Data about costs are lacking and have been explored for single procedures such as distal pancreatectomy [23]. Short hospital stays deriving from minimally invasive procedures do translate into cost cuts for health-care institutions; whether the robotic platform is overall cost-effective is difficult to evaluate. However, we have reported that costs can become affordable and cost-effective if used to the maximum potential (i.e., in high-volume centers) [9]. The robotic platform will eventually become more affordable over time, and institutions with the latest technologies may hold a competitive edge over other institutions with regard to patients seeking treatment. Pancreatic surgery remains one of the most successful fields of application of the robotic platform, and its use is growing at a remarkable pace.

References

1. Fernandes E, Giulianotti PC. Robotic-assisted pancreatic surgery. J Hepatobiliary Pancreat Sci. 2013;20(6):583–9.
2. Kendrick ML, Cusati D. Total laparoscopic pancreaticoduodenectomy: feasibility and outcome in an early experience. Arch Surg. 2010;145(1):19–23.
3. Kim SC, Song KB, Jung YS, Kim YH, do Park H, Lee SS, et al. Short-term clinical outcomes for 100 consecutive cases of laparoscopic pylorus-preserving pancreatoduodenectomy: improvement with surgical experience. Surg Endosc. 2013;27(1):95–103.
4. Palanivelu C, Rajan PS, Rangarajan M, Vaithiswaran V, Senthilnathan P, Parthasarathi R, et al. Evolution in techniques of laparoscopic pancreaticoduodenectomy: a decade long experience from a tertiary center. J Hepato-Biliary-Pancreat Surg. 2009;16(6):731–40.
5. Dulucq JL, Wintringer P, Mahajna A. Laparoscopic pancreaticoduodenectomy for benign and malignant diseases. Surg Endosc. 2006;20(7):1045–50.
6. Gumbs AA, Gayet B. The laparoscopic duodenopancreatectomy: the posterior approach. Surg Endosc. 2008;22(2):539–40.
7. Pugliese R, Scandroglio I, Sansonna F, Maggioni D, Costanzi A, Citterio D, et al. Laparoscopic pancreaticoduodenectomy: a review of 19 cases. Surg Laparosc Endosc Percutan Tech. 2008;18(1):13–8.
8. Gagner M, Palermo M. Laparoscopic Whipple procedure: review of the literature. J Hepato-Biliary-Pancreat Surg. 2009;16(6):726–30.
9. Ross SB, Downs D, Saeed SM, Dolce JK, Rosemurgy AS. Robotics in surgery: is a robot necessary? For what? Minerva Chir. 2017;72(1):61–70.
10. Traverso LW, Longmire WP Jr. Preservation of the pylorus in pancreaticoduodenectomy. Surg Gynecol Obstet. 1978;146(6):959–62.
11. Walsh RM, Chalikonda S. How I do it: hybrid laparoscopic and robotic pancreaticoduodenectomy. J Gastrointest Surg. 2016;20(9):1650–7.
12. Zureikat AH, Moser AJ, Boone BA, Bartlett DL, Zenati M, Zeh HJ 3rd. 250 robotic pancreatic resections: safety and feasibility. Ann Surg. 2013;258(4):554–9. discussion 559–62
13. Nguyen TK, Zenati MS, Boone BA, Steve J, Hogg ME, Bartlett DL, et al. Robotic pancreaticoduodenectomy in the presence of aberrant or anomalous hepatic arterial anatomy: safety and oncologic outcomes. HPB (Oxford). 2015;17(7):594–9.
14. Koops A, Wojciechowski B, Broering DC, Adam G, Krupski-Berdien G. Anatomic variations of the hepatic arteries in 604 selective celiac and superior mesenteric angiographies. Surg Radiol Anat. 2004;26(3):239–44.
15. Boone BA, Zenati M, Hogg ME, Steve J, Moser AJ, Bartlett DL, et al. Assessment of quality outcomes for robotic pancreaticoduodenectomy: identification of the learning curve. JAMA Surg. 2015;150(5):416–22.
16. Fisher WE, Hodges SE, Wu MF, Hilsenbeck SG, Brunicardi FC. Assessment of the learning curve for pancreaticoduodenectomy. Am J Surg. 2012;203(6):684–90.
17. Rosemurgy AS, Downs D, Swaid F, Ross SB. Laparoendoscopic Single-Site (LESS) Nissen fundoplication: how we do it. J Gastrointest Surg. 2016;20(12):2093–9.
18. Sukharamwala P, Teta A, Ross S, Co F, Alvarez-Calderon G, Luberice K, et al. Over 250 Laparoendoscopic Single Site (LESS) Fundoplications: lessons learned. Am Surg. 2015;81(9):870–5.
19. Mathur A, Luberice K, Ross S, Choung E, Rosemurgy A. Pancreaticoduodenectomy at high-volume centers: surgeon volume goes beyond the leapfrog criteria. Ann Surg. 2015;262(2):e37–9.
20. Ryan CE, Ross SB, Sukharamwala PB, Sadowitz BD, Wood TW, Rosemurgy AS. Distal pancreatectomy and splenectomy: a robotic or LESS approach. JSLS. 2015;19(1):e2014.00246.
21. Ryan CE, Wood TW, Ross SB, Smart AE, Sukharamwala PB, Rosemurgy AS. Pancreaticoduodenectomy in Florida: do 20-year trends document the salutary benefits of centralization of care? HPB (Oxford). 2015;17(9):832–8.
22. Rosemurgy A, Cowgill S, Coe B, Thomas A, Al-Saadi S, Goldin S, Zervos E. Frequency with which surgeons undertake pancreaticoduodenectomy continues to determine length of stay, hospital charges, and in-hospital mortality. J Gastrointest Surg. 2008;12:442–9.
23. Waters JA, Canal DF, Wiebke EA, Dumas RP, Beane JD, Aguilar-Saavedra JR, et al. Robotic distal pancreatectomy: cost effective? Surgery. 2010;148(4):814–23.

29 Liver Resection: Right Lobectomy

Pier Cristoforo Giulianotti and Pablo Quadri

Introduction

Safe liver surgery has been performed for the past three decades. Before the 1980s, the mortality rate associated with liver resections was above 20%, mostly related to massive hemorrhage. Improved anesthesia and postoperative care, in addition to a better understanding of the liver's anatomy, reduced mortality rates to less than 5% in specialized centers. Laparoscopic liver surgery started in the mid-1990s [1]. The recent advances in laparoscopic devices and the development of liver parenchymal transection equipment led to an increased performance of laparoscopic liver resections in recent years. Although laparoscopy has been shown to be a safe and feasible approach [2–9], major hepatectomies are being performed in few centers [1]. In expert hands, oncologic and clinical outcomes have proven to be equivalent to those of the open technique [10–13], with the benefits of minimally invasive surgery (early recovery, shorter hospitalization, and better cosmetic outcomes) [14]. Limitations of laparoscopic surgery such as the restricted movement of the instruments and two-dimensional view, the complexity of these procedures, and the potential risk of major bleeding during the parenchymal transection are some of the obstacles preventing a wider application of laparoscopy in liver resections [1].

Robotic surgery has been introduced to enhance the surgeon's dexterity through a magnified, three-dimensional view, instruments with seven degrees of freedom, and intuitive hand-control movements [1], overcoming limitations of laparoscopy [14]. Since the initial commercialization of the da Vinci Surgical System® (Intuitive Surgical, Sunnyvale, CA), the robotic approach has revolutionized the field of minimally invasive surgery and is being used in the most complex minimally invasive surgeries [14, 15].

Indications

There are several indications for robotic hepatectomy:

- Liver metastasis
- Hepatocellular carcinoma
- Cholangiocarcinoma/Klatskin tumor

Contraindications

A few conditions are considered relative contraindications:

- Bulky lesions
- Diaphragm involvement
- Previous liver resections

Vascular invasion is an absolute contraindication for robotic hepatectomy.

P. C. Giulianotti (✉) · P. Quadri
Division of General, Minimally Invasive and Robotic Surgery, Department of Surgery, University of Illinois at Chicago, Chicago, IL, USA
e-mail: piercg@uic.edu; pquadri@uic.edu

Y. Fong et al. (eds.), *The SAGES Atlas of Robotic Surgery*, https://doi.org/10.1007/978-3-319-91045-1_29

Robotic Right Hepatectomy: Technique

Patient Positioning

The patient is placed in the supine position on a bean bag, with parted legs wearing intermittent compression devices. The patient's operative bed is set in reverse Trendelenburg position (20°–30°) with mild tilting to the left side (15°). Figure 29.1 shows the operative room disposition for a right robotic hepatectomy. The first assistant is positioned between the patient's legs, and the scrub nurse is on the patient's left side.

Induction of the Pneumoperitoneum and Preliminary Exploration

Veress technique is the preferred approach for induction of the pneumoperitoneum. A Veress needle is placed in the left subcostal margin, and once adequate pressure inside the abdominal cavity is obtained, the first trocar, a 5-mm Optiview®, is inserted into the left upper quadrant. Using a 5-mm, 30° scope, a preliminary exploration of the abdomen is performed. The role of this simple diagnostic laparoscopy is dual:

- To rule out contraindications or reasons to change the procedure, such as adhesions or cancer spread
- To plan fine adjustments of the final trocar setting according to the patient's anatomy

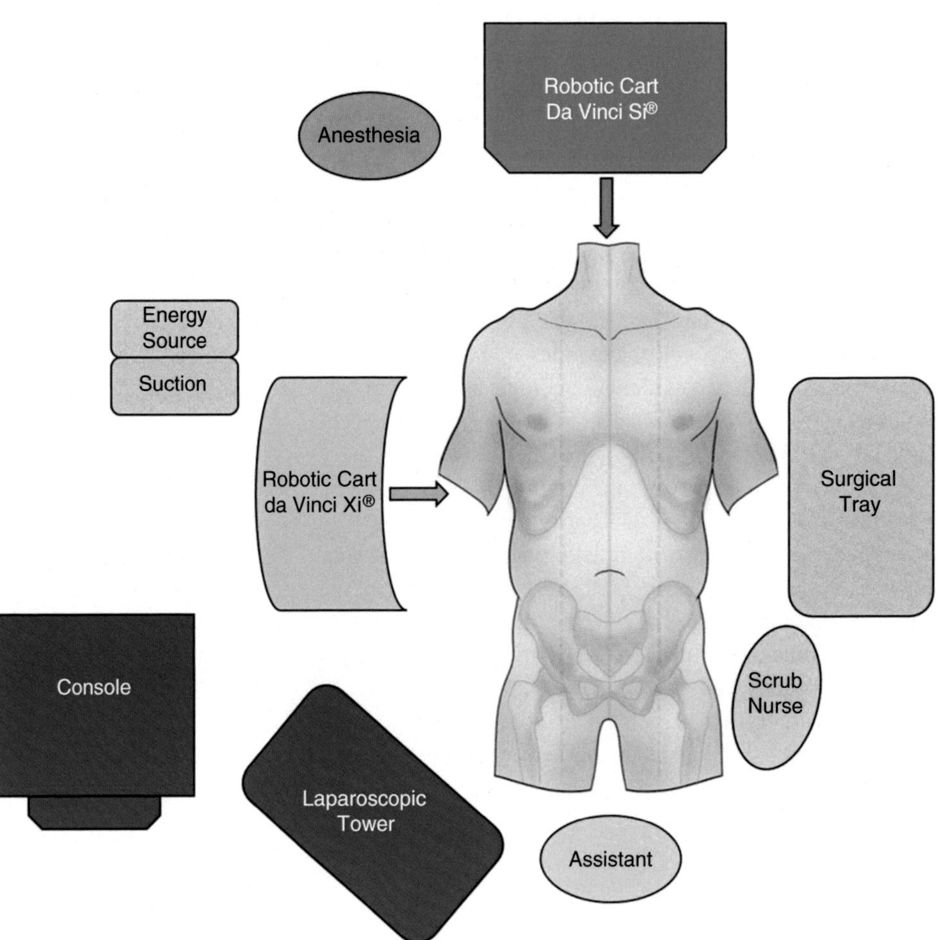

Fig. 29.1 Operative room disposition for a right robotic hepatectomy

Port Setting

Figure 29.2 shows the port setting for a right robotic hepatectomy. All ports are placed under direct laparoscopic vision. If using the da Vinci Si® system, a set of four 4- or 8-mm ports are positioned along a straight line 2 in. above the transverse umbilical line. The scope (C) is located at the insertion of the right pararectal line. The third robotic arm (R3) is placed laterally, below the left costal line. Two 10- or 12-mm assistant ports (A) are positioned at each side of the scope.

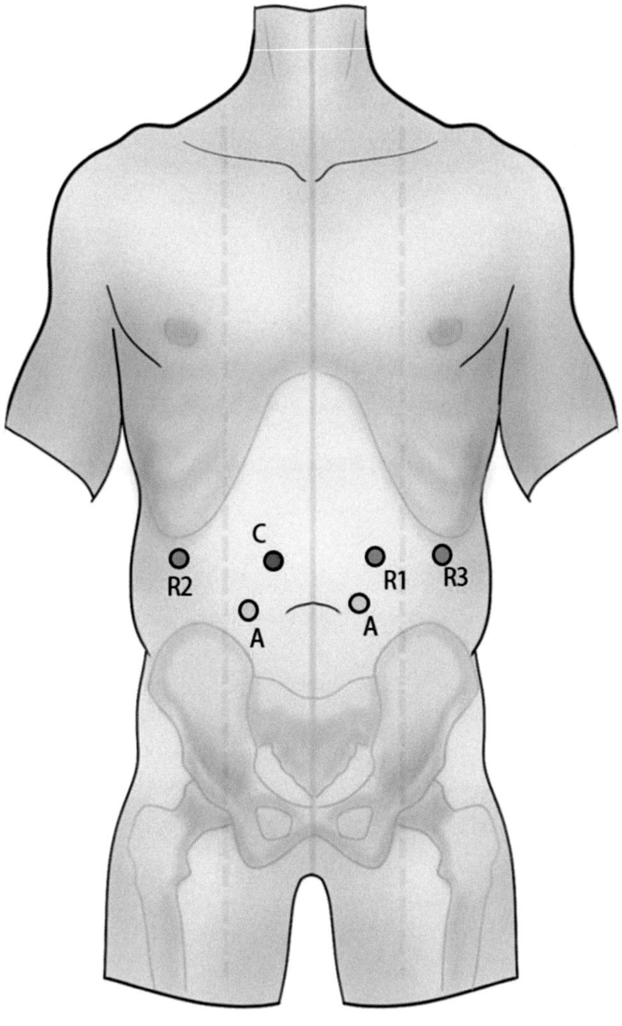

Fig. 29.2 Port setting for a right robotic hepatectomy: camera port (C), assistant ports (A), and ports for robotic arms 1, 2, and 3 (R1, R2, R3)

Surgical Technique

The operation can be divided into three technical steps:

1. Hilum dissection
2. Vena cava preparation
3. Parenchymal transection

The first two steps are significantly improved with the use of the robotic system.

Hilum Dissection

Before starting this step, the falciform ligament is taken down and an ultrasound (US) scan is performed using a laparoscopic probe. The US can confirm the liver anatomy and the number and location of the lesions and can define the tumor margins.

A grasper with a sponge in the third robotic arm is positioned to retract the liver segment IV B and open up the hilar space, achieving optimal visualization of the different hilar structures. A retrograde cholecystectomy is performed to obtain better exposure. The right hepatic artery is identified, dissected, and divided in between 3–0 and 4–0 polypropylene sutures.

The right biliary duct is divided next. Figure 29.3 shows the dissected right hepatic duct. Indocyanine green fluorescence is used to assess the biliary anatomy. The distal stump is tied with Vicryl® 4–0 or sutured with polydioxanone (PDS®) 4–0. The right hepatic duct can be divided at this stage, but only if the anatomy of the bifurcation is low and easy. If there are unfavorable conditions, the right hepatic duct can be divided intraparenchymally during the final steps.

The dissection of the portal vein comes next. In Fig. 29.4, the vein is prepared on a vessel loop. The vein can either be transected with a vascular stapler, or of there is not enough room for a stapler, it can be tied and suture ligated with polypropylene 3–0. Tiny venous branches to segment 1 sometimes need to be sutured with 5–0 polypropylene and taken down.

At the end of this step, a good ischemic demarcation of the right lobe is achieved, outlining the section line (the cholecysto-cava line).

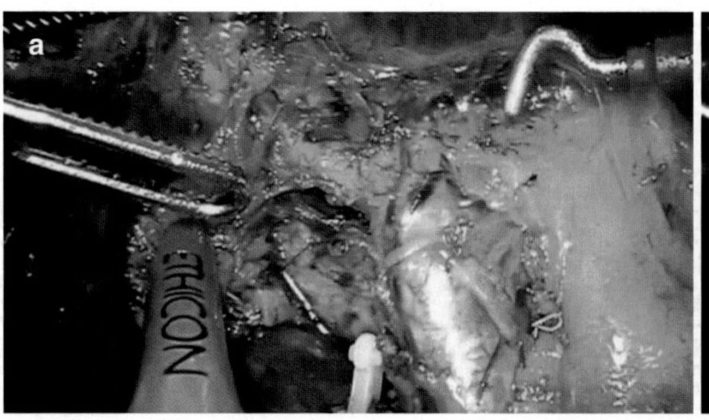

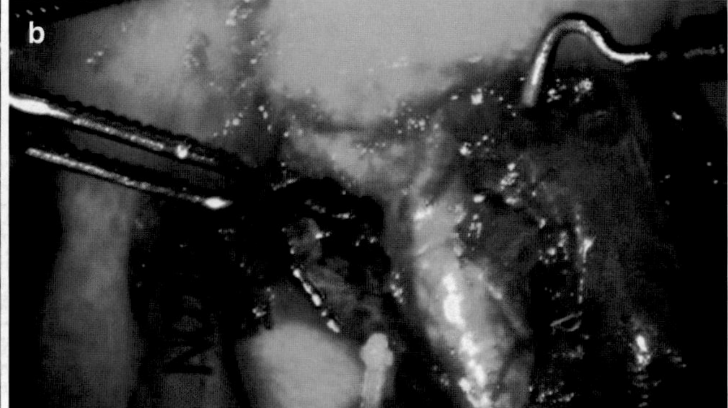

Fig. 29.3 Dissection of the right hepatic duct (**a**) and indocyanine green fluorescence assessment (**b**)

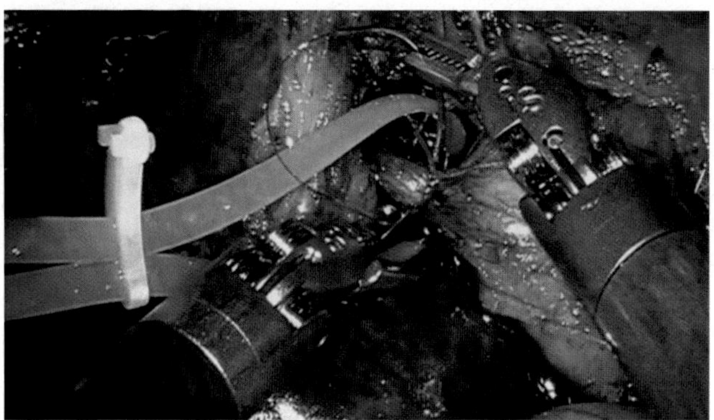

Fig. 29.4 Preparation and suture ligation of the right portal vein

Vena Cava Preparation

At this point the third arm is repositioned, retracting the inferior face of the right lobe. The ligaments that are anchoring the right lobe to the diaphragm are divided, exposing the right side of the vena cava. Then, retracting the hepatoduodenal ligament and the caudate lobe, the anterior aspect of the retrohepatic vena cava is exposed. The accessory short hepatic veins are prepared (using the hook as a right angle), suture ligated, and divided.

The preparation of the vena cava continues until the main right hepatic vein is reached. At this point, it is usually not taken down. It will be divided intracapsularly as the last step of the parenchymal transection. A hanging maneuver can be performed using an umbilical tape, placing the loop between the right and median veins, or simply immediately to the right side of the vena cava.

Parenchymal Transection

This part of the procedure remains the most challenging for many reasons:

- Lack of specialized tools for the transection
- Difficulty in assessing tumor margin
- Bleeding control

In our experience, there are two distinct phases of the parenchymal transection:

1. Subcortical layers, which are well controlled with the Harmonic® shears
2. Core dissection, where major hepatic veins are encountered and the staplers can be very effective, fast, and safe

After defining the section line (monopolar coagulation tattoo), strong 2–0 polypropylene stay sutures are placed on both sides of the section line, and the third robotic arm is used to retract the left side.

The Harmonic® shears are moved to the assistant port (telescopic technique), closer to the midline, in order to have a more favorable angle to approach the liver, as vessels are best met with a 90° angle (Fig. 29.5).

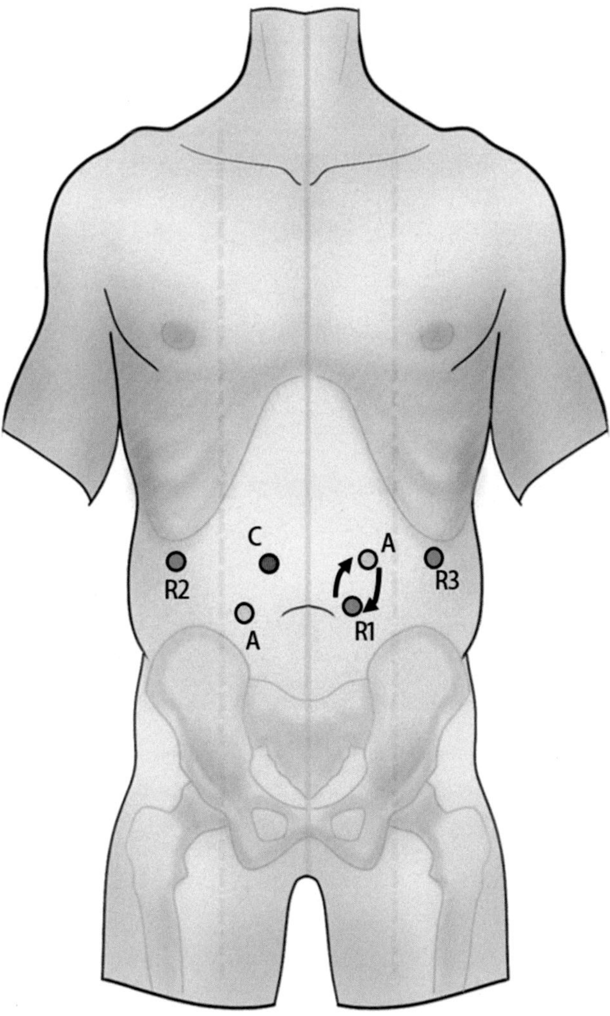

Fig. 29.5 Port setting modification for the parenchymal transection

The dissection proceeds layer by layer, avoiding the need to go too deep into a narrow field. While proceeding with the dissection, more stay sutures are placed in the section line, and the third robotic arm is used to retract them laterally (Fig. 29.6).

One of the most important tricks is to "superficialize" the working area, always keeping the dissected tissue at the surface so that it is easy to suture bleeding spots. Once the core of the liver is reached, a few vascular stapler loads are needed to complete the transection and divide and seal the main right hepatic vein and some branches that communicate with the median vein.

It is important to remember that during the parenchymal transection, the anesthesiologist must keep a very low central venous pressure (less than 6-mm Hg). High pressures may considerably increase the overall blood loss. Another important tip is related to the use of the stapler during the final steps of the parenchymal transection: the direction of the stapling should always go away from the vena cava (right side). The role of the umbilical tape in the hanging maneuver is to allow a clear landmark for the transection (Fig. 29.7).

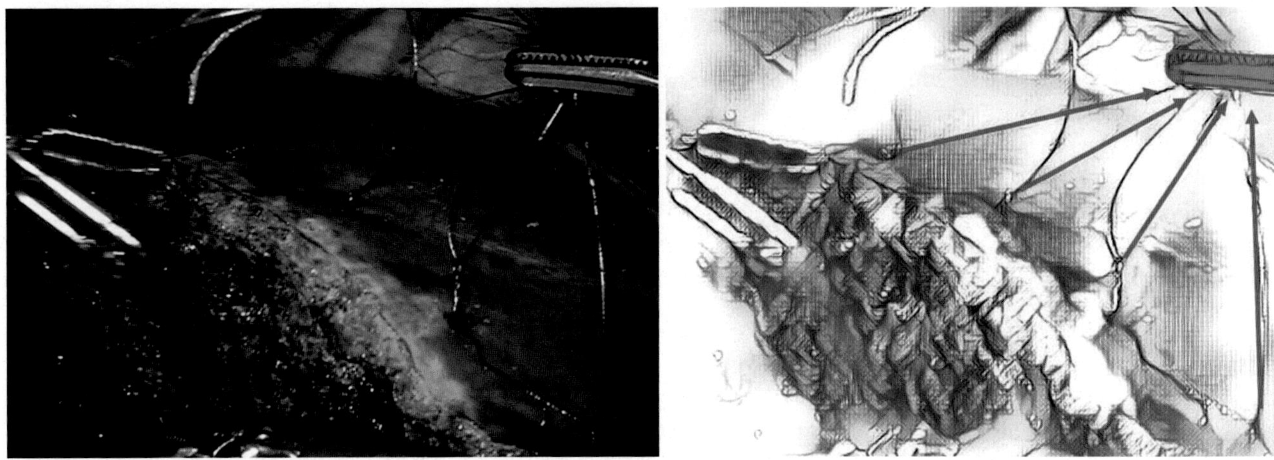

Fig. 29.6 Retraction of the left hepatic lobe with the stay sutures and the third robotic arm

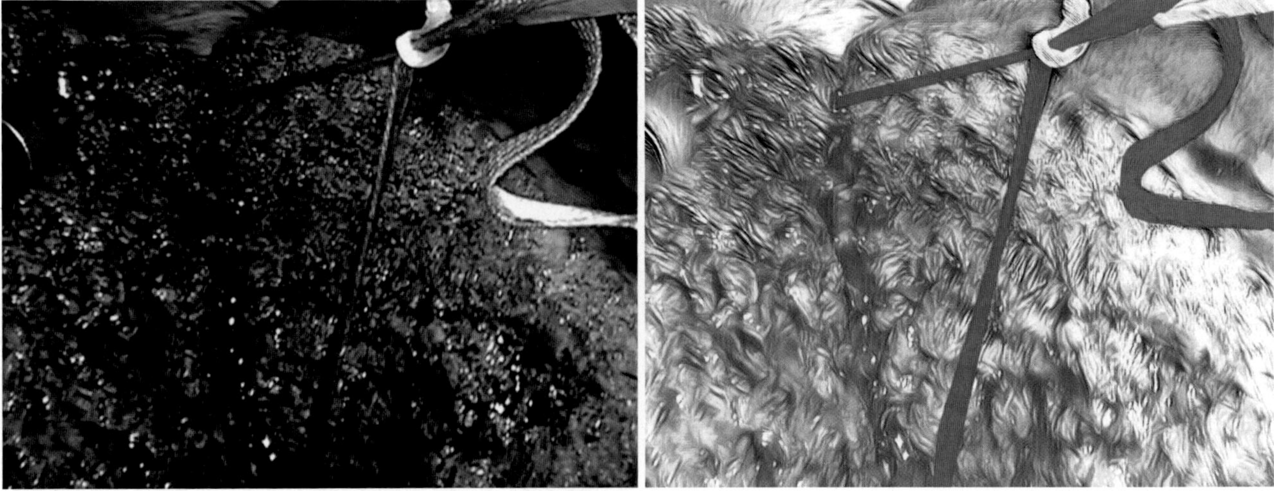

Fig. 29.7 Deep parenchymal transection and hanging maneuver to allow stapling and the completion of the transection

Extraction/Retrieval of the Specimen

Usually, the specimen is placed in a big Endobag™. Before undocking the robot for the extraction of the specimen, the hemostasis is carefully reviewed, sometimes adding more stitches of polypropylene 3–0. The anesthesiologist is requested to increase the central venous pressure above 12–14-mm Hg and to perform some Valsalva maneuvers.

A hemostatic agent (fibrin glue or a fibrin sealant patch) may help to improve the coagulation of the cut surface. The falciform ligament is used to anchor the left lobe to the diaphragm using interrupted stitches of polypropylene 2–0. Stabilizing the liver remnant prevents the kinking or twisting of the main left hepatic vein and the development of an acute outlet obstruction syndrome.

Once good and stable hemostasis is achieved, the robot is undocked from the surgical field. A Pfannenstiel incision is the preferred extraction site.

Our Experience: Outcomes

A total of 165 robotic liver resections were performed by the senior author of this chapter between April 2001 and February 2017. These include 53 (32.1%) right lobectomies, 10 (6.1%) left lobectomies, 38 (23.0%) bisegmentectomies, 42 (25.45%) segmentectomies, 12 (7.25%) wedge resections, and 10 (6.1%) enucleations. The series comprised 91 (55.2%) women and 74 (44.8%) men. The mean age at the date of surgery was 54.8 years (SD = 15.5), and the mean body mass index (BMI) was 29.2 kg/m^2 (SD = 6.2). The mean operative time was 316.3 minutes (SD = 134.4). The estimated blood loss was 422.6 mL (SD = 601.3). The conversion rate to open surgery was 9.8%. The reasons for conversion for most of the patients corresponded to the relative contraindications for robotic hepatectomies: bulky lesions, diaphragm infiltration, difficulty in assessing tumor margins, friable liver with a high risk of bleeding, and inaccessible lesions that were posteriorly located. The reoperation rate was 0%. The mean length of hospitalization was 6.5 days (SD = 4.2). The 30-day morbidity rate was 24.9%, and the 30-day mortality rate was 0% in the overall series.

References

1. Choi GH, Choi SH, Kim SH, Hwang HK, Kang CM, Choi JS, Lee WJ. Robotic liver resection: technique and results of 30 consecutive procedures. Surg Endosc. 2012;26:2247–58.
2. Nguyen KT, Gamblin TC, Geller DA. World review of laparoscopic liver resection--2,804 patients. Ann Surg. 2009;250:831–41.
3. Nguyen KT, Marsh JW, Tsung A, Steel JJ, Gamblin TC, Geller DA. Comparative benefits of laparoscopic vs open hepatic resection: a critical appraisal. Arch Surg. 2011;146:348–56.
4. Milone L, Daskalaki D, Fernandes E, Damoli I, Giulianotti PC. State of the art in robotic hepatobiliary surgery. World J Surg. 2013;37:2747–55.
5. Giulianotti PC, Sbrana F, Coratti A, Bianco FM, Addeo P, Buchs NC, et al. Totally robotic right hepatectomy: surgical technique and outcomes. Arch Surg. 2011;146:844–50.
6. Soubrane O, Goumard C, Laurent A, Tranchart H, Truant S, Gayet B, et al. Laparoscopic resection of hepatocellular carcinoma: a French survey in 351 patients. HPB (Oxford). 2014;16:357–65.
7. Packiam V, Bartlett DL, Tohme S, Reddy S, Marsh JW, Geller DA, Tsung A. Minimally invasive liver resection: robotic versus laparoscopic left lateral sectionectomy. J Gastrointest Surg. 2012;16:2233–8.
8. Tsung A, Geller DA, Sukato DC, Sabbaghian S, Tohme S, Steel J, et al. Robotic versus laparoscopic hepatectomy: a matched comparison. Ann Surg. 2014;259:549–55.
9. Bhojani FD, Fox A, Pitzul K, Gallinger S, Wei A, Moulton CA, et al. Clinical and economic comparison of laparoscopic to open liver resections using a 2-to-1 matched pair analysis: an institutional experience. J Am Coll Surg. 2012;214:184–95.
10. Jackson NR, Hauch A, Hu T, Buell JF, Slakey DP, Kandil E. The safety and efficacy of approaches to liver resection: a meta-analysis. JSLS. 2015;19:e2014.00186.
11. Vanounou T, Steel JL, Nguyen KT, Tsung A, Marsh JW, Geller DA, Gamblin TC. Comparing the clinical and economic impact of laparoscopic versus open liver resection. Ann Surg Oncol. 2010;17:998–1009.
12. Memeo R, de'Angelis N, Compagnon P, Salloum C, Cherqui D, Laurent A, Azoulay D. Laparoscopic vs. open liver resection for hepatocellular carcinoma of cirrhotic liver: a case-control study. World J Surg. 2014;38:2919–26.
13. Dagher I, Belli G, Fantini C, Laurent A, Tayar C, Lainas P, et al. Laparoscopic hepatectomy for hepatocellular carcinoma: a European experience. J Am Coll Surg. 2010;211:16–23.
14. Lai EC, Tang CN, Li MK. Robot-assisted laparoscopic hemihepatectomy: technique and surgical outcomes. Int J Surg. 2012;10:11–5.
15. Levi Sandri GB, de Werra E, Mascianà G, Colasanti M, Santoro R, D'Andrea V, Ettorre GM. Laparoscopic and robotic approach for hepatocellular carcinoma--state of the art. Hepatobiliary Surg Nutr. 2016;5:478–84.

30 Robotic Partial Hepatectomy

Susanne G. Warner and Yuman Fong

Minimally invasive liver resection is accepted as standard for peripheral hepatic lesions [1]. Many surgeons are comfortable with laparoscopic wedge resections as well as left lateral sectionectomies, but minimally invasive lobectomies are generally only performed at specialty centers [2–4]. Still fewer centers are attempting these resections robotically. Many minimally invasive surgeons who prefer laparoscopic to robotic techniques for minimally invasive liver surgery point to the cumbersome nature of robotic instrumentation and the necessity of a skilled bedside assistant. However, recent development of improved robotic instrumentation, such as articulated instruments, sealers, and staplers, allows liver surgeons to exploit the benefits of robotic surgery—like binocular vision, ease of suturing, and decreased surgeon fatigue and tremor—without some of the previous drawbacks. Moreover, even prior to the introduction of newer robotic systems, evidence suggested that lobectomies were much more likely to be completed without conversion to open when they are performed robotically instead of laparoscopically [5, 6].

The development of instrumentation by da Vinci® Xi (*Intuitive Surgical, Sunnyvale, CA*) has eliminated many of the cumbersome limitations that were off-putting to surgeons considering adoption of robotic techniques, namely, lower profile robotic arms, enhanced ease of robotic alignment and docking, and, finally, positioning of the robot at the patient's side rather than at the head of the bed, where anesthesia might have trouble accessing the airway. The benefits of robotic resection using either da Vinci® system are perhaps most obvious in right posterior sectionectomy. This chapter will review the preoperative considerations for partial hepatic resection as well as positioning and steps of right posterior sectionectomy in detail. Differences when using the Xi system will be highlighted and helpful tips will be provided.

S. G. Warner, MD · Y. Fong, MD (✉)
Department of Surgery, City of Hope National Medical Center, Duarte, CA, USA
e-mail: suwarner@coh.org

Indications

As with any liver resection, indications include primary hepatic malignancies, metastatic lesions, benign tumors at risk for rupture or causing compressive symptoms, symptomatic cysts, and abscesses. Examples of these indications can be found in Table 30.1. In recent years, many liver surgeons have pushed the envelope in terms of what were traditionally considered acceptable indications for malignancy resection. Many patients with metastatic disease who would previously have been ruled out for surgical management are now offered surgery, provided their oligometastatic disease demonstrates stability and thus favorable biology [7–9].

Aside from medical comorbidities, relative contraindications to robotic resection include, but are not limited to, history of prior extensive abdominal surgery, prior hepatic resection, history of upper abdominal radiation, and surgeon discomfort with robotic techniques. The importance of having multiple attending surgeons scrub the first several robotic partial resection techniques cannot be overemphasized. It is

Table 30.1 Indications for robotic partial hepatic resection

Primary hepatic malignancy Hepatocellular carcinoma Intrahepatic cholangiocarcinoma
Metastatic lesions Colorectal Neuroendocrine Breast Melanoma Adrenal Renal Lung
Benign tumors at risk for rupture Hepatic adenoma Enlarging hemangioma
Tumors or cysts causing compressive symptoms Enlarging focal nodular hyperplasia Cystadenoma Simple cysts
Liver abscess not amenable to percutaneous treatment

Y. Fong et al. (eds.), *The SAGES Atlas of Robotic Surgery*, https://doi.org/10.1007/978-3-319-91045-1_30

critical that patient safety be prioritized over a surgeon's desire to push the envelope. This includes setting time limits and having a low threshold for converting to open if the case is failing to progress.

Preoperative Preparation and Staging

As with any major surgery, patients should be medically optimized for the procedure. When possible, institutional enhanced recovery protocols should be employed at every perioperative stage [10]. Thorough preoperative work-up should include consideration of liver function, cardiopulmonary comorbidities, and overall frailty. Additionally, multidisciplinary discussions regarding the oncologic efficacy of resection should be undertaken. This extends to the preoperative area, where anesthesia colleagues should be reminded that central venous pressure (CVP) of less than 5 mmHg is desired until the parenchymal transection is completed.

Table 30.2 details preoperative investigations that are requisite for most resections. Radiologic staging investigations vary by malignancy, but should always include a CT scan to check for resectability and vascular anatomy, particularly if hepatic arterial infusion pump placement is planned. Additional preoperative studies may include MRI with appropriate contrast agents and timing for the disease process in question. MRI is especially important in patients with hepatic steatosis.

Contraindications for surgery include but are not limited to severe coronary artery disease, congestive heart failure, severe pulmonary disease, and limited mobility that would hinder postoperative recovery. Additionally, elderly patients whose comorbidities yield a life span shorter than that presented by the relevant malignancy should be advised against surgery in most instances.

Table 30.2 Preoperative studies

Test	Justification
CT scan	Assess resectability Plan hepatic arterial infusion pump Be aware of vascular anatomy
MRI	Assess resectability in patients with steatosis Identify lesions not seen on CT
Pulmonary evaluation	CXR to assess for metastases where appropriate (CT chest may be best modality depending on disease) Pulmonary function testing depending on comorbidities
Cardiac evaluation	Preoperative cardiac risk assessment per ASA guidelines
Liver function evaluation	CBC, CMP, INR Calculate MELD or Child's score

ASA American Society of Anesthesiologists, *CT* computed tomography, *MRI* magnetic resonance imaging, *CBC* complete blood count, *CMP* complete metabolic panel (includes liver panel with transaminases, alkaline phosphatase, and bilirubin), *INR* international normalized ratio, *MELD* model for end-stage liver disease

Room Setup and Patient Positioning

Unless a right posterior resection is planned, supine patient positioning is preferred. Prior to docking, the operating table is airplaned opposite the target lesion (if target lesion is on the left, airplane to patient's right). Doing this suspends the portion of the liver to be removed from the ipsilateral triangular ligament. Moreover, reverse Trendelenburg position is often beneficial, again to make use of gravity both in terms of intestinal retraction and to provide countertraction as the liver hangs from suspensory ligaments. In cases of right posterior resections, left lateral decubitus positioning is utilized to allow for best exposure (Fig. 30.1).

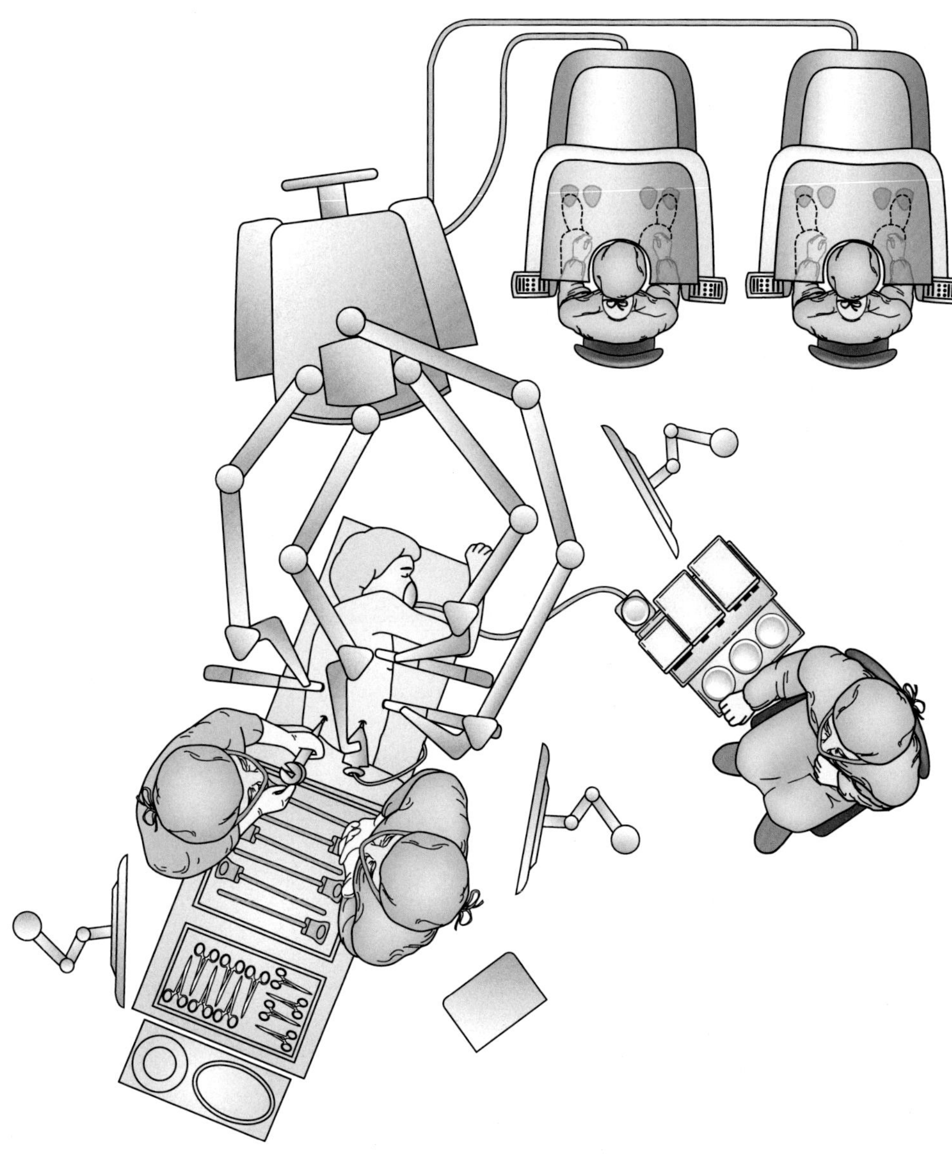

Fig. 30.1 Positioning and room setup for right posterior liver resection (Segment 6, 7 surgeries) (using da Vinci Si® system, Intuitive Surgical, Sunnyvalle, CA))

When utilizing the da Vinci Si® system, the robot will be docked so that the patient-side cart camera arm is aligned with the anticipated line of liver transection. This means that the cart is brought over the patient's left shoulder for left-sided resections, and over the right shoulder for right-sided resections. If resections are planned for both lobes of the liver and do not include the need for patient repositioning (as with a posterior lesion where a posterior approach is preferred), then the cart can be brought directly over the patient's head (Fig. 30.2). Anesthesia intubates and places lines as is standard, and then the bed is turned 90 degrees to facilitated docking, leaving the anesthesiologist positioned at the patient's side.

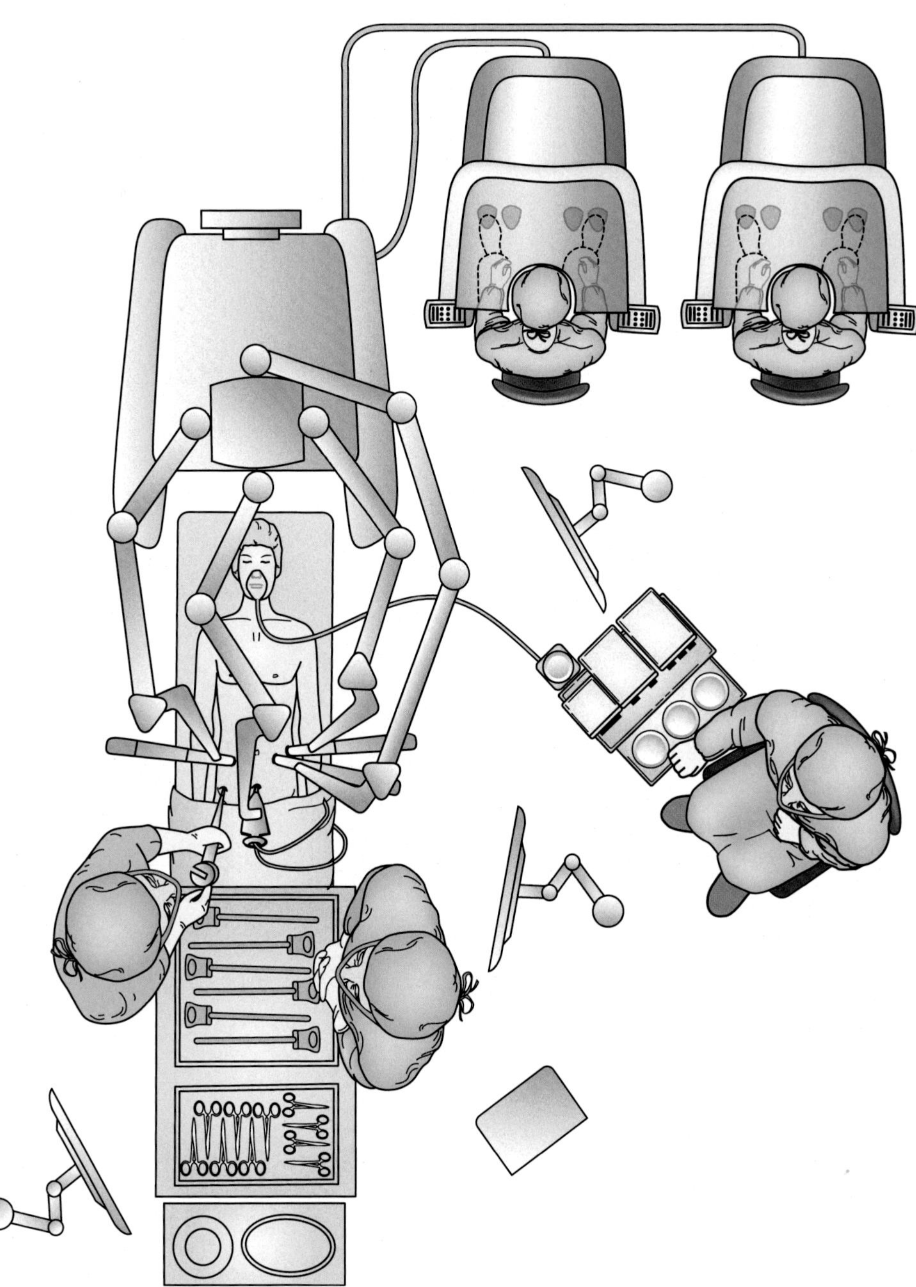

Fig. 30.2 Positioning and room setup if bilateral resections are planned (using da Vinci Si system)

Procedure Steps

Si port placement for standard right or left hepatectomy is shown (Fig. 30.3). Typically, the camera port is placed at the umbilicus. A balloon port works well as the camera port and in accessory ports and keeps air from leaking around the port. For minor resections, the authors typically use four ports. For major resections, one or two additional assistant ports can be utilized.

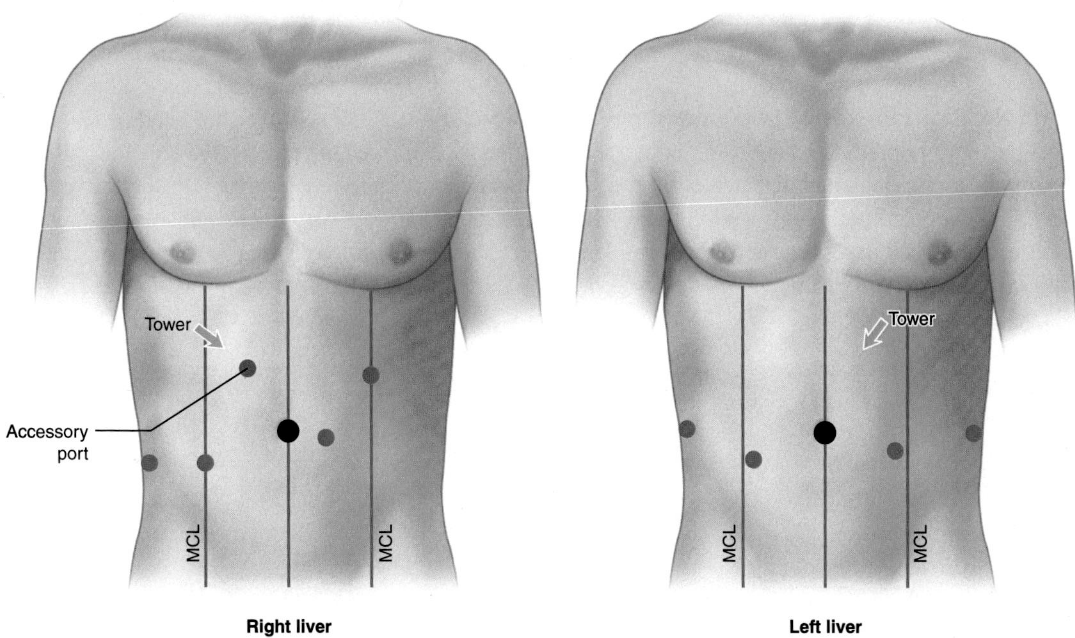

Fig. 30.3 Standard port placement for left and right hepatectomy

Staging

Detailed examination of the peritoneum is performed. Visual inspection of the liver surface is also performed. Ultrasound inspection of the liver is then performed, preferably with a "drop-in" type probe (Fig. 30.4a). Landmarks and transection planes are then marked on the liver surface (Fig. 30.4b).

Detailed Example: Right Posterior Sectionectomy

In cases of malignancy, prior to docking, the abdomen is inspected for signs of ascites and unanticipated peritoneal or nodal metastases. Location of pathology is confirmed with laparoscopic ultrasound when necessary, and resection planning, including any necessary adjustments of standard port placement, is performed. Again, the camera is aligned as closely as possible with the line of liver transection. For right posterior resections, patients are positioned in left lateral decubitus with a break in the table corresponding with the area between the ribs and the iliac crest. Typical port placement is similar to that of standard right hepatectomy, but the lateral-most port positioning is crucial (Fig. 30.5). Of note, as above, both the umbilical and midclavicular assistant ports should be 12 mm in order to allow the use of the camera and vascular staplers via either port. Once all ports are in place and the robot is docked over the head of the patient, ultrasound is performed to verify lesion location and confirm relationship of the lesion to major vasculature. Of note, the ultrasound can be laparoscopic, but a drop-in robotic probe is very easily manipulated with robotic graspers and is preferred by the authors. With ultrasound assistance, an instrument of

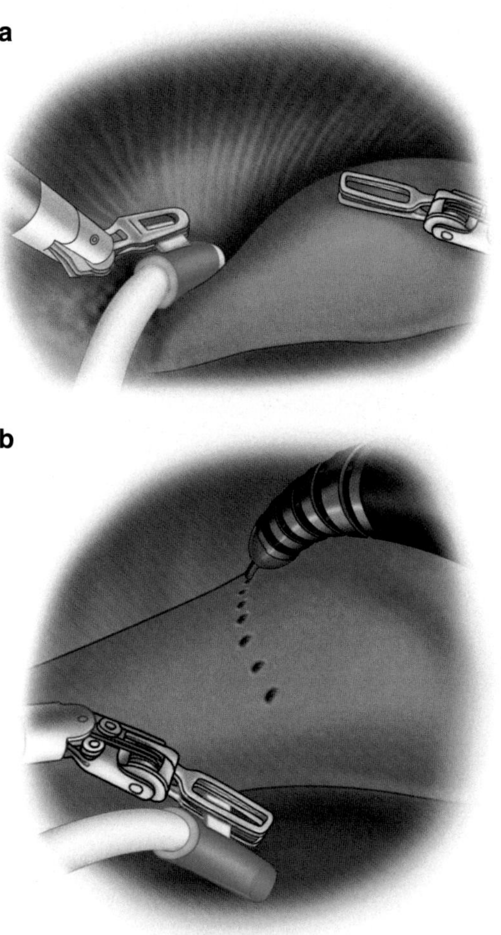

Fig. 30.4 Ultrasound staging and assessment of the liver. A "drop-in" probe is preferred for ultrasound assessment (Panel **a**). The liver surface is then marked to show internal landmarks and to show the line of transection (Panel **b**)

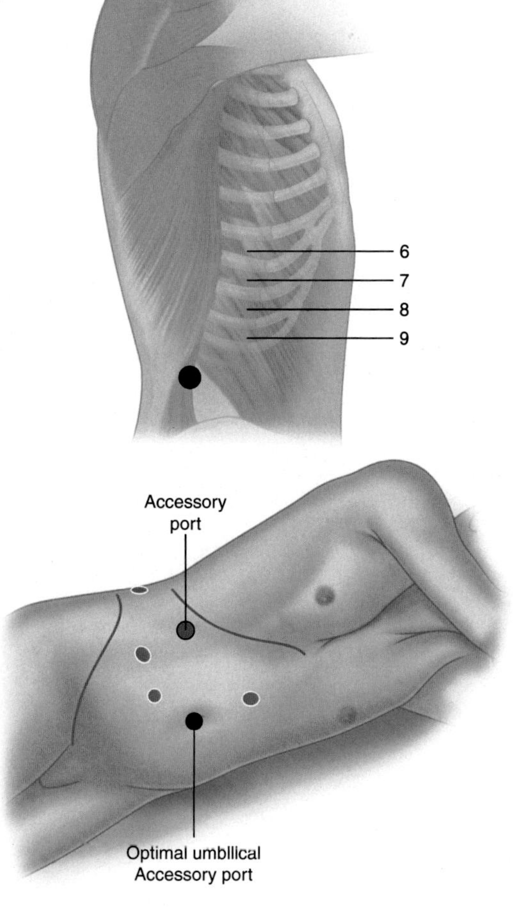

Fig. 30.5 Lateral-most port placement near the midaxillary line for right posterior resection

monopolar cautery is used to mark off the plane of transection (Fig. 30.6). Many surgeons advocate a Pringle maneuver during parenchymal transection. The authors generally do not employ this for robotic partial resections, but the potential need for the maneuver is evaluated on a case-by-case basis. Parenchymal transection can proceed safely by any number of techniques. The authors prefer to use a vessel sealer with a built-in blade (Laparoscopic LigaSure by *Covidien, Mansfield, MA*, or the robotic vessel sealer). Vessel sealers can be used as a blunt crushing instrument to assist with crush-clamp tech-

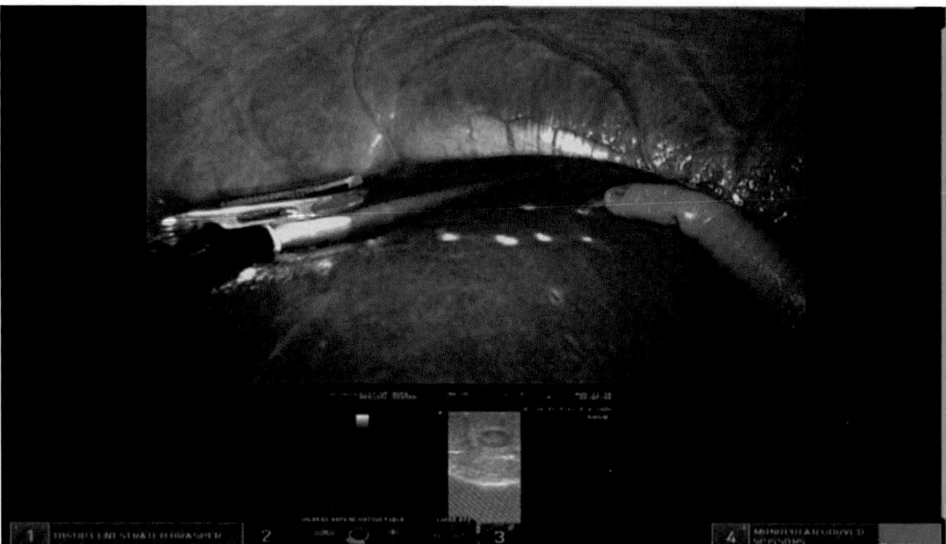

Fig. 30.6 Ultrasound confirms lesion location in relation to relevant vasculature; monopolar cautery marks off plane of transection

nique. The crush-clamp is then followed by sealing with vessel sealer and then transecting with the blade in the case of vessels smaller than 5 mm (Fig. 30.7). Larger vessels can be stapled, clipped, or tied with silk. The use of a stapler is shown (Fig. 30.8). The safest way to staple a large portal pedicle is to apply countertraction on the pedicle by an umbilical tape, which protects the junction of the pedicle to be stapled and the immediate portion to be saved (Fig. 30.8b).

a **Photo** **Drawing**

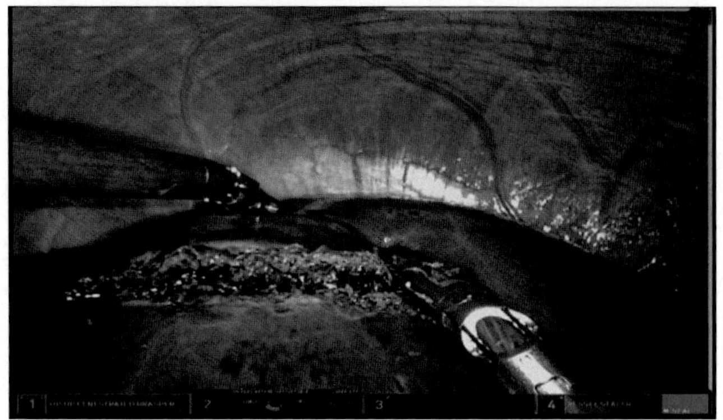

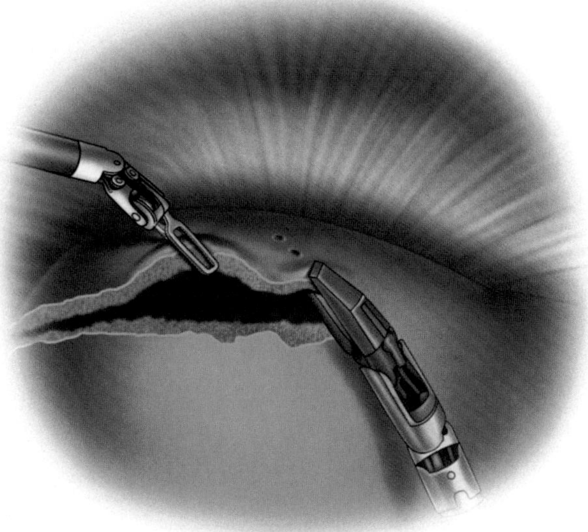

b

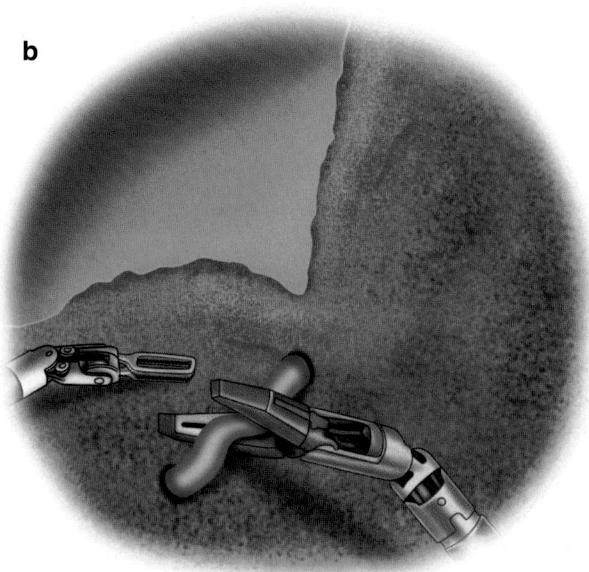

Fig. 30.7 Robotic vessel sealer is used for liver transection. It can be used to transect the capsule (Panel **a**: *left*, photo; *right*, drawing) or as a crush-clamp to identify smaller blood vessels which can then be sealed and divided (Panel **b**)

a **Photo** **Drawing**

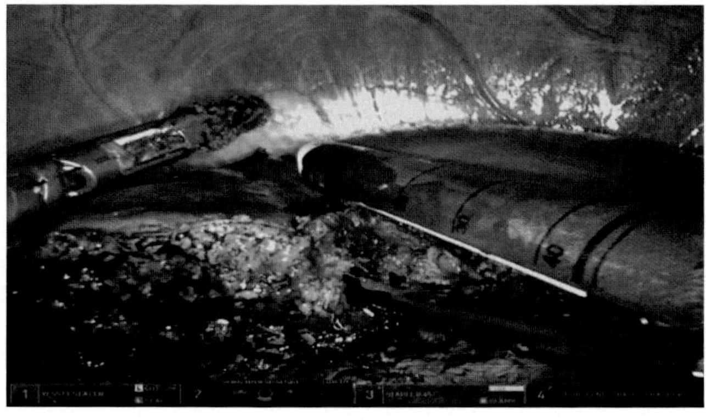

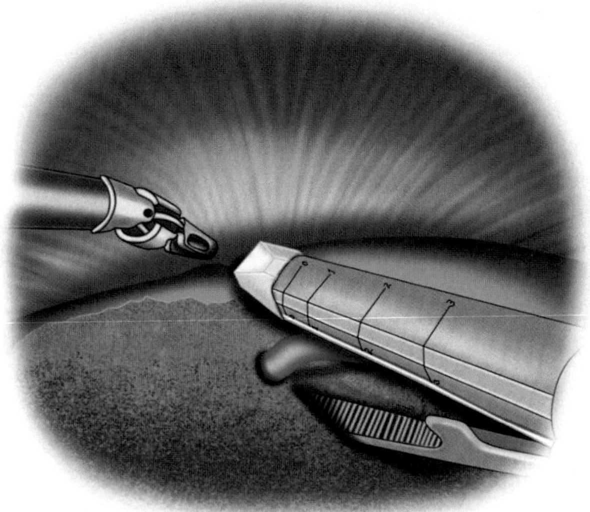

b

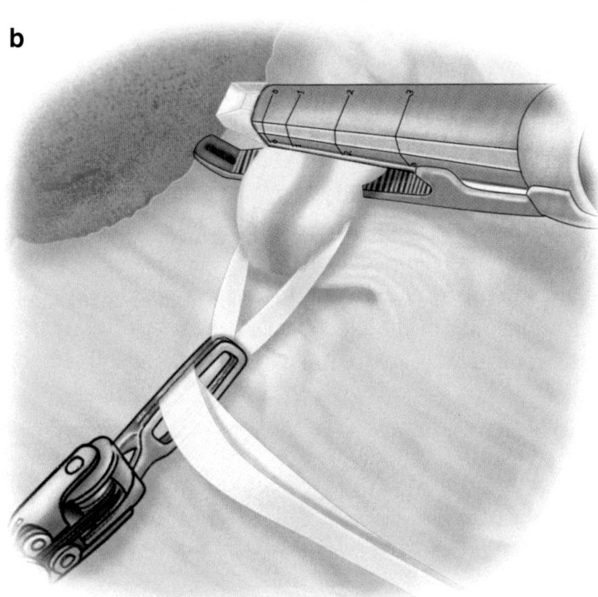

Fig. 30.8 Either robotic or handheld staplers can be used to ligate larger vessels (Panel **a**: *left*, photo; *right*, drawing). For large pedicles, umbilical tape is used as countertraction for stapler (Panel **b**)

If clips are used, the authors prefer robotic Weck clips which, unlike metal clips, do not create a failed seal when in contact with a vessel sealer. Similarly, silk ties and sutures are preferred to polypropylene because silk does not melt when in contact with cautery or vessel sealers. Parenchymal transection proceeds until the right hepatic vein is identified and stapled or suture ligated.

With parenchymal transection complete, attention is turned to division of the triangular and falciform ligaments. The authors generally prefer to leave these intact until the resection is mostly complete, as they provide added retraction, especially in reverse Trendelenburg position. With the ligaments divided, the specimen is placed in a laparoscopic retrieval bag and brought to the level of the umbilicus at the assistant port for later removal. With parenchymal transection complete, hemostasis and biliary stasis are achieved using either high-energy monopolar cautery or argon beam coagulation. The authors also prefer to place a sheet of Surgicel® (*Ethicon Inc., Cincinnati, OH*) along the parenchymal resection bed. The authors do not leave a drain.

In cases of formal anatomic lobectomy, the authors prefer to secure and ligate inflow vasculature. While individual components of portal pedicles can be identified and ligated separately, the simplest method of inflow ligation is to leave the Glissonian sheath of the portal pedicle unviolated and staple it en masse. In general, the pedicle is identified and encircled with an umbilical tape. The tape can conveniently be used for counter-tension during stapler positioning. The lack of pliability of the tape makes it a superior retraction tool as compared to a vessel loop, which thereby yields the least chance of damage to nearby structures that are not intended for division. A summary of case steps is found in Table 30.3.

Xi Differences

For Xi, port placement should generally be in more of a straight line rather than curvilinear. However, curvilinear configurations can be quite helpful in more slender patients (Fig. 30.9). That being said, more freedom is allowed in terms of port placement. Whereas Si robotic ports needed to be at least 8–10 cm apart, the Xi ports can often be 5–8 cm apart without creating too many problems. Moreover, the Xi camera can fit through standard 8 mm robotic ports, which is very helpful when there are multiple planes of transection. However, for those who are used to the flexibility of alternating between the 12 mm camera port and 12 mm assistant port for staple firing, being limited to one 12 mm assistant port for staple firing can be an adjustment. For this reason, the authors enjoy employing the robotic stapler. Staple articulation yields flexibility and can eliminate the need for more than one stapler port. This requires a 12 mm camera, and stapler position must be anticipated at port placement.

Table 30.3 General procedure steps

Patient positioning
Laparoscopic abdominal exploration ± ultrasound
Robotic port placement and docking
Robotically-assisted ultrasound and mark out line of transection
In cases of lobectomy, isolate ± secure and divide vascular inflow
Parenchymal transection
Examination of hepatic remnant and establishment of hemostasis
Specimen extraction and fascial closure

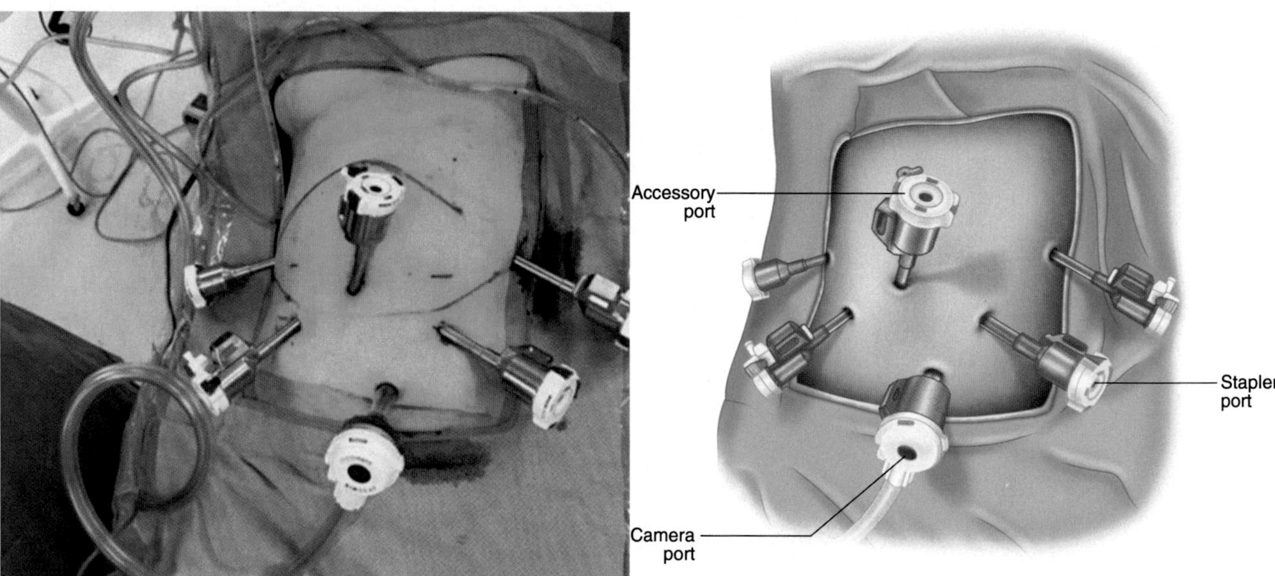

Fig. 30.9 Port placement in slender patient using Xi. For major lobectomies, the two ports nearest midline can be 1–12 mm ports placed to act as interchangeable camera/stapler ports

Table 30.4 Summary of tricks of the master

Set time limits for procedure components and convert to open if they are exceeded
Convert to open early in case of bleeding or loss of orientation
Plan and prepare for emergent conversion to open
Use Gelport for large extraction site/can place robot and assistant ports here
Transcutaneous sutures can be used to suspend the liver for exposure
Small vessel bleeding can be controlled with sutures or vessel sealer

Tricks of the Master

- A 7 mm bariatric robotic port can be placed within a standard 12 mm laparoscopic assistant port for robot docking. When using the Si system, this allows for moving the camera from midline to midclavicular line as needed, and the 12 mm port is helpful for stapling, suction, and added retraction, as well as for smoke evacuation as needed.
- Pringle maneuver is largely unnecessary for partial resections. Thus, the authors do not typically place Rumel tourniquets prior to parenchymal transection. However, if during dissection Pringle maneuver is needed, a laparoscopic bulldog can be used, as can umbilical tape or vessel loop. The surgeon should have his/her preferred instrument at the ready prior to the start of the case.
- If a large specimen extraction site is anticipated, a Gelport can be used. During dissection, up to two Xi ports and one assistant port can be placed in the Gelport. If using the Si, one robotic port and one assistant port can be placed. The surgeon should ensure an adequately sized fascial defect in order to facilitate necessary port use without conflicting ranges of motion.
- Set time limits during the initial learning curve for each phase of the procedure. Convert to open if/when time limits expire, and use your times to track your progress.
- Always discuss the emergency undocking plan in case of bleeding or code, and ensure that necessary sutures and staple loads are open and ready prior to beginning a portion of the case that might result in heavy bleeding.

The above tips are summarized in Table 30.4.

Postoperative Care

Anticipating potential postoperative complications is critical to identifying them in a timely manner. Complications to watch for include bleeding, biloma, liver failure, injury from positioning, pulmonary insufficiency secondary to effusion or pneumothorax, pneumonia, venous thromboembolic complications, and arrhythmia. The authors agree with recently published AHPBA guidelines for venous thromboembolic prophylaxis and routinely employ subcutaneous heparin preoperatively and postoperatively [11]. The intensity of postoperative monitoring is determined by the extent of resection and patient comorbidities. In more extensive resections, where aggressive fluid resuscitation is required and electrolyte balances are anticipated, telemetry monitoring is used.

In the immediate postoperative setting, the authors obtain a complete blood count (CBC), coagulation studies (INR), phosphorous and magnesium levels, as well as a complete metabolic panel (CMP). For more extensive resections, where arterial lines are utilized, an arterial blood gas is also obtained (ABG) in order to monitor acidosis and base deficit to guide aggressive fluid resuscitation. The authors use blood urea nitrogen (BUN) and central venous pressure (CVP) as guides to adequate resuscitation. After 24 h of isotonic fluid resuscitation, fluids are switched to include phosphorous supplementation. Unless hemodynamic or laboratory changes suggest concern, labs are checked twice daily in the initial postoperative period. In general, following aggressive fluid resuscitation, aggressive dieresis is initiated on postoperative day 2. Some patients are ready to go home on postoperative day 2, and many are ready for discharge by postoperative day 3 and enjoy a quicker return to functionality secondary to minimally invasive surgical techniques.

Conclusion

Robotic liver surgery offers the benefits of minimally invasive resection with the added benefit of wristed movement and binocular vision. With appropriate preparation and caution, the learning curve is easily surmounted, and even extensive robotic resections can be performed safely.

References

1. Buell JF, Cherqui D, Geller DA, O'Rourke N, Iannitti D, Dagher I, et al. The international position on laparoscopic liver surgery: the Louisville statement, 2008. Ann Surg. 2009;250(5):825–30.
2. Buell JF, Thomas MT, Rudich S, Marvin M, Nagubandi R, Ravindra KV, et al. Experience with more than 500 minimally invasive hepatic procedures. Ann Surg. 2008;248(3):475–86.
3. Nguyen KT, Laurent A, Dagher I, Geller DA, Steel J, Thomas MT, et al. Minimally invasive liver resection for metastatic colorectal cancer: a multi-institutional, international report of safety, feasibility, and early outcomes. Ann Surg. 2009;250(5):842–8.
4. Dagher I, O'Rourke N, Geller DA, Cherqui D, Belli G, Gamblin TC, et al. Laparoscopic major hepatectomy: an evolution in standard of care. Ann Surg. 2009;250(5):856–60.
5. Ocuin LM, Tsung A. Robotic liver resection for malignancy: current status, oncologic outcomes, comparison to laparoscopy, and future applications. J Surg Oncol. 2015;112(3):295–301.
6. Leung U, Fong Y. Robotic liver surgery. Hepatobiliary Surg Nutr. 2014;3(5):288–94.
7. Fitzgerald TL, Brinkley J, Banks S, Vohra N, Englert ZP, Zervos EE. The benefits of liver resection for non-colorectal, non-neuroendocrine liver metastases: a systematic review. Langenbeck's Arch Surg. 2014;399(8):989–1000.

8. D'Angelica M, Brennan MF, Fortner JG, Cohen AM, Blumgart LH, Fong Y. Ninety-six five-year survivors after liver resection for metastatic colorectal cancer. J Am Coll Surg. 1997;185(6):554–9.
9. Fong Y, Cohen AM, Fortner JG, Enker WE, Turnbull AD, Coit DG, et al. Liver resection for colorectal metastases. J Clin Oncol. 1997;15(3):938–46.
10. Hughes MJ, McNally S, Wigmore SJ. Enhanced recovery following liver surgery: a systematic review and meta-analysis. HPB (Oxford). 2014;16(8):699–706.
11. Aloia TA, Geerts WH, Clary BM, Day RW, Hemming AW, D'Albuquerque LC, et al. Venous thromboembolism prophylaxis in liver surgery. J Gastrointest Surg. 2016;20(1):221–9.

Robot-Assisted Roux-en-Y Gastric Bypass

31

Vivek Bindal and Enrique E. Elli

This chapter reviews the technique and outcomes of robot-assisted Roux-en-Y gastric bypass (RYGB). With the rise in obesity and bariatric procedures, surgeons are encountering patients with high body mass index (BMI) and revisional bariatric procedures. The use of digital platforms holds great promise for these complex procedures. Many specialists consider RYGB, which involves two anastomoses (gastrojejunostomy and jejunojejunostomy), to be the gold-standard surgical procedure for morbid obesity. Robotic surgery is currently considered to be an attractive technology that could help tperform RYGB, given its well-described advantages. It is also the most-studied robotic bariatric procedure. This chapter describes the instrumentation, patient positioning, operating room setup, surgical technique, and outcomes of robot-assisted RYGB.

Introduction

With the rise in the prevalence of obesity, the field of bariatric surgery is witnessing an ever-increasing demand. Laparoscopic Roux-en-Y gastric bypass (LRYGB) was described in the 1990s [1], and it is estimated that more than 100,000 procedures are being performed annually in United States alone [2]. According to an estimate published in July 2015 by the American Society for Metabolic and Bariatric Surgery (ASMBS), Roux-en-Y gastric bypass (RYGB) constitutes 26.8% of total bariatric surgery volume [3]. Performing bariatric surgery can be technically demanding in many situations, as large patients, large livers, thick abdominal walls, and substantial visceral fat make exposure, dissection, and reconstruction difficult [4]. Super-obese (SO) patients with a BMI of 50 kg/m^2 or higher are difficult to manage because of limited working space, excessive torque on instruments due to thick abdominal walls, super-obese patients' comorbidities, and high risk for anesthesia [5]. The maneuvering of instruments while performing LRYGB becomes challenging, especially while doing intracorporeal suturing. The learning curve of LRYGB has been estimated to be about 75–100 cases [6, 7]. Moreover, surgeons encounter very difficult ergonomic positions that can potentially shorten their careers, so surgeons have been looking for methods that will improve patient outcomes and surgical technique, decrease complications, and also reduce the learning curve.

The use of robotics in bariatric surgery has been evolving since Cadiere et al. reported the first such case in 1999 [8]. Robotic surgery has provided surgeons with the advantage of three-dimensional vision and has increased dexterity and precision by downscaling the surgeon's movements, enabling fine tissue dissection, and filtering out physiological tremor [9, 10]. It overcomes the restraint of torque on ports from the thick abdominal wall and minimizes port site trauma by remote center technology [11]. According to the consensus document on robotic surgery prepared by the SAGES-MIRA Robotic Surgery Consensus Group, robotic surgery holds particular value for gastric bypass among general surgical procedures.

The main limitation of robotic surgery is the perceived higher cost and setup time, compared with laparoscopy [12]. With increased experience, however, it is seen that setup times are reduced, and as other players enter the market, the cost of robotic surgery is likely to come down.

Advantages of Roux-en-Y Gastric Bypass

Many specialists consider RYGB to be the gold-standard surgical procedure for morbid obesity [13, 14]. The overall results are good in terms of both weight loss and comorbidity

V. Bindal, MS, FNB
Institute of Minimal Access, Metabolic and Bariatric Surgery, Sir Ganga Ram Hospital, New Delhi, India

E. E. Elli, MD, FACS (✉)
Department of Surgery, Mayo Clinic Florida, Jacksonville, FL, USA
e-mail: elli.enrique@mayo.edu

Y. Fong et al. (eds.), *The SAGES Atlas of Robotic Surgery*, https://doi.org/10.1007/978-3-319-91045-1_31

resolution [15]. RYGB leads to 65.7% excess weight loss and remission rates of 66.7% for type 2 diabetes mellitus and 60.4% for dyslipidemia [16]. As RYGB involves two anastomoses (gastrojejunostomy and jejunojejunostomy), robotic surgery is currently considered as an attractive technology that could help perform RYGB, given its well-described advantages [17]. It is also the most-studied robotic bariatric procedure [18, 19].

Surgical Technique

The many ways by which robotic RYGB can be performed include a number of major variations:

- Single docking versus double docking
- Hybrid versus totally robotic
- Antecolic versus retrocolic
- Handsewn, linear, or circular stapler anastomosis for gastrojejunostomy
- Staple line reinforcements or oversewing

The technique of choice at the University of Illinois Health System is to perform a single docking, totally robotic RYGB with a handsewn gastrojejunostomy. This technique is described in the following paragraphs.

Instrumentation

The following 8-mm robotic instruments are used for a robotic RYGB in a da Vinci® Si system (Intuitive Surgical, Sunnyvale, CA):

- Cadiere forceps
- Large needle driver
- da Vinci Harmonic® scalpel
- Permanent cautery hook
- Fenestrated bipolar forceps
- Laparoscopic/robotic staplers

All three arms of the robotic system are used, with the third arm coming from the left side of the patient.

Patient Positioning and Operating Room Setup

The patient, under general anesthesia, is positioned in supine position with 15–20° reverse Trendelenburg tilt. This small tilt helps complete the procedure in a single docking fashion, as one is able to perform both infracolic and supracolic portions of the procedure without changing the patient position. The abdomen is cleaned and draped, and an orogastric tube and urinary catheter (optional) are placed. The assistant surgeon stands by the side of the patient with scrub nurse (Fig. 31.1). The master console is placed so that the surgeon can freely visualize the operative field while sitting on the console. Two video monitors are placed on either side of the patient to enable the assistants to easily watch and help at every step of procedure, with ergonomic comfort. The anesthesia machine is kept on one side of the head end, as the patient cart comes in from the head end.

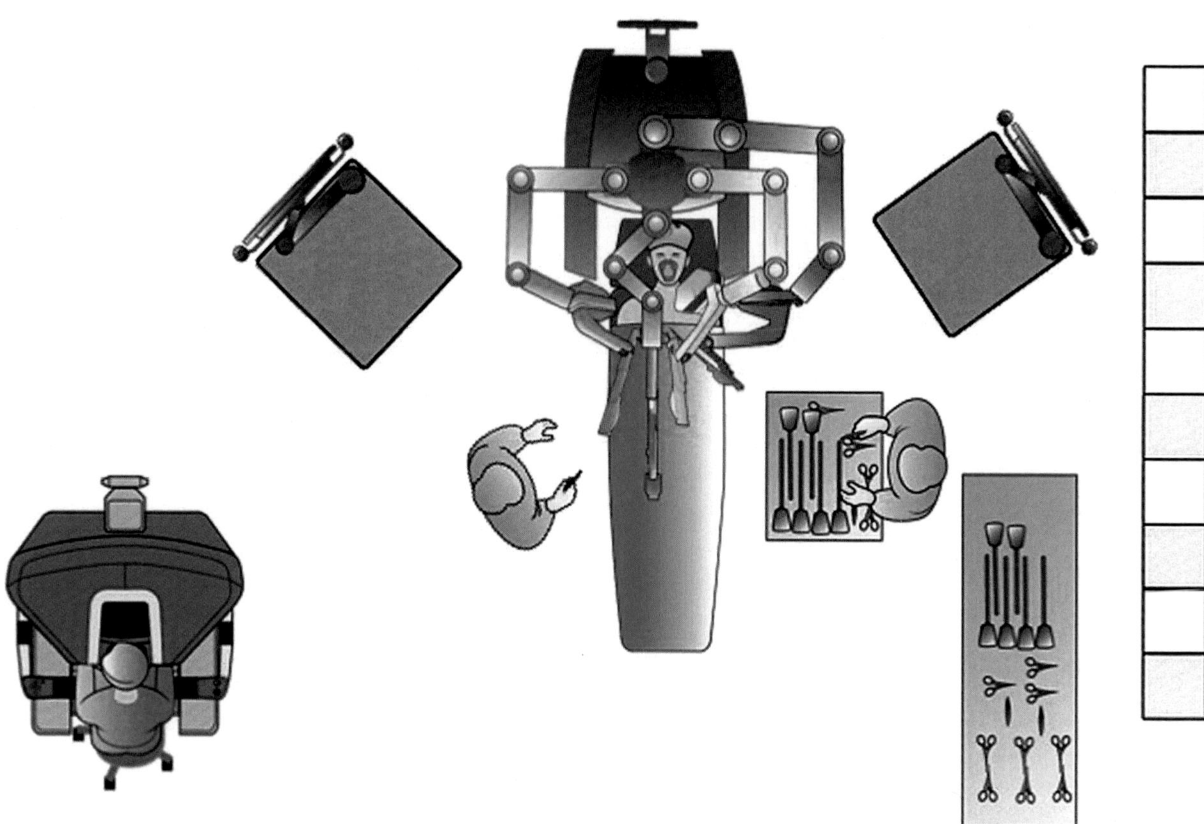

Fig. 31.1 Operating room setup and patient cart positioning for robot-assisted Roux-en-Y gastric bypass (RYGB)

Port Position and Docking

Pneumoperitoneum is achieved to 15 mm Hg using a Veress needle at Palmer's point. (We prefer closed technique.) All the distances are measured after insufflation of the abdomen, as they significantly change after pneumoperitoneum is created, especially in morbidly obese patients, because of the pendulous abdominal wall. The minimum intertrocar distance recommended in robotic surgery is 8–10 cm, but the actual distance intraperitoneally in morbidly obese individuals is significantly shorter than the distance measured on the skin. This factor must be taken into account, and the trocars should be placed at the maximum possible distance to avoid external clashing of the robot arms.

The camera port (12-mm-diameter, 150-mm-long trocar) is placed 20 cm below the xiphisternum, slightly to the left of midline under vision, using a zero-degree, 10-mm scope to avoid any inadvertent visceral injury (Fig. 31.2). Next, three da Vinci® trocars and one assistant trocar are placed:

- R1 (8-mm da Vinci® cannula) is placed in the left midclavicular line about 20 cm from the xiphisternum.
- R2 (8-mm da Vinci® cannula) is placed in the right hypochondrium in the midclavicular line, taking care that the entry of the port is below the margin of the liver.
- R3 (8-mm da Vinci® cannula) is placed in the left flank at the level of the camera port.
- Assistant port (12 mm diameter) is placed between the camera port and R2, at a distance of at least 10 cm from both of them.

A 5-mm epigastric port is used to place a Nathanson liver retractor to retract the left lobe of the liver.

The port placement must be adjusted based on the body habitus of the patient, so as to prevent external arm collision and provide optimal exposure. A diagnostic laparoscopy is done to look for any adhesions, hernias, or inadvertent injury during abdominal wall access.

The da Vinci® patient cart is brought from the head end of the patient, and the arms are docked to the ports placed. The third arm of the robot comes from the left side of the patient. To start the procedure, a permanent cautery hook is taken in R1, fenestrated bipolar forceps in R2, and a Cadiere forceps in R3. As illustrated in Fig. 31.1, the assistant surgeon stands by the side for complementary maneuvers such as suction, stapling, or retraction.

Creation of Gastric Pouch

Initial dissection is started from the left crus by taking down the phrenoesophageal membrane, using a hook, after retracting the fundus of the stomach caudally (Fig. 31.3). A

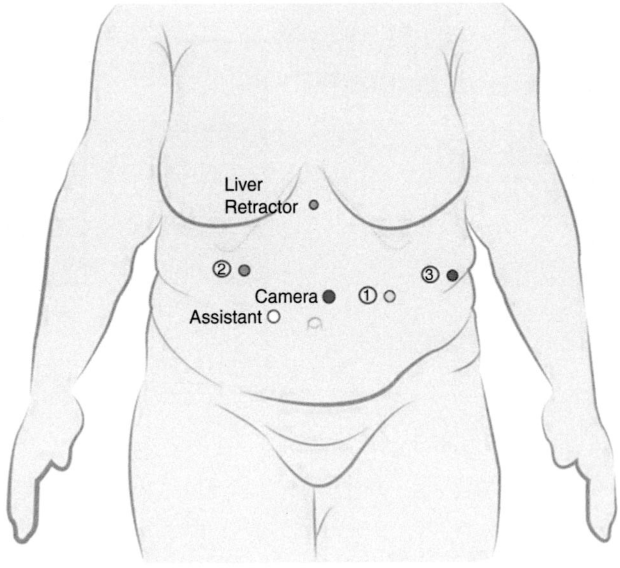

Fig. 31.2 Port positions for robot-assisted RYGB

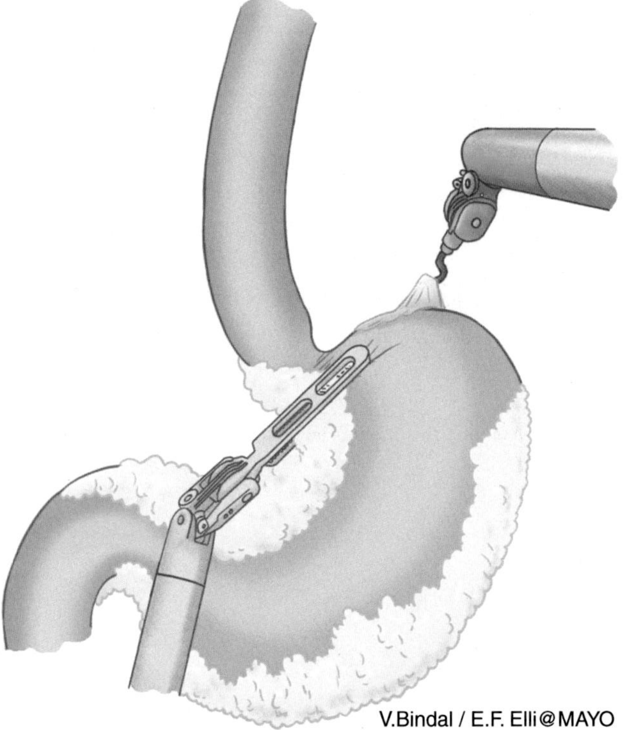

Fig. 31.3 Initial dissection around the left crus. The bowel grasper in the left hand retracts the fundus caudally, while the monopolar hook divides the phrenoesophageal membrane, simplifying the final step of gastric pouch creation

small gastric pouch is created using perigastric dissection starting at the second vessel from the gastroesophageal junction. The third arm is used to retract the stomach laterally, while the Harmonic scalpel is used to open up the gastrohepatic ligament. Perigastric dissection is commenced using the hook, avoiding injury to the vagus nerve, and the lesser sac is reached (Fig. 31.4). A horizontal fire of the stapler is done by the assistant using a 60-mm blue cartridge. Further dissection is continued superiorly to free the posterior adhesion of the stomach. One may place a bougie at this time to size the pouch. The vertical firing is done (usually a single 60-mm fire, but two may be needed), and pouch creation is completed (Fig. 31.5). The seven degrees of freedom help dissect in this area, especially around the left crus. We prefer staple line reinforcements in the vertical firings.

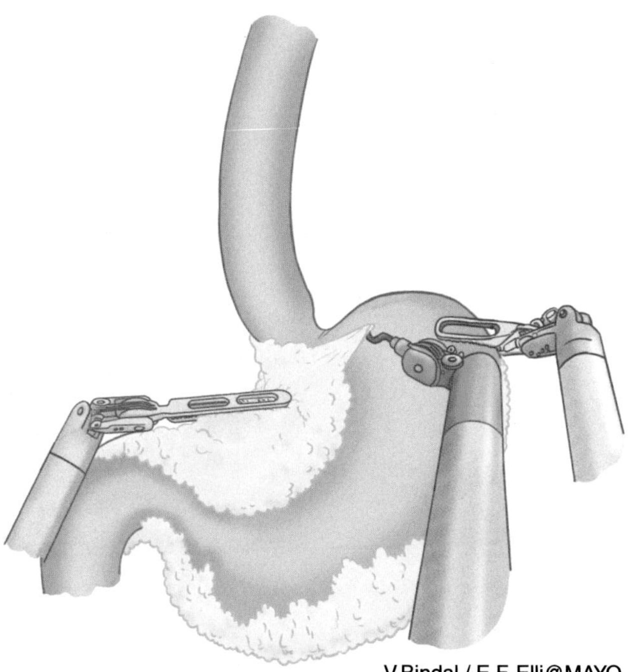

Fig. 31.4 Perigastric dissection is commenced at the level of second vessel from GE junction using the monopolar hook, avoiding injury to the vagus nerve. The third arm is used to retract the stomach anterolaterally, while fat is retracted medially by second arm

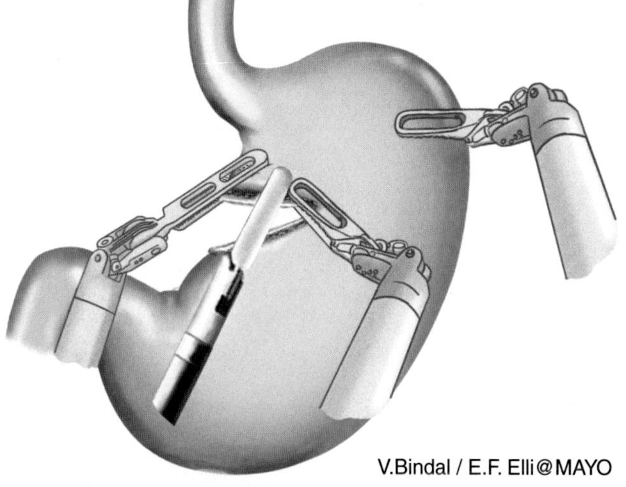

Fig. 31.5 A small gastric pouch is created by first horizontal fire followed by vertical firings using an endoscopic stapler with 60-mm cartridge

Creation of Jejunojejunostomy

Now the camera is focused on the infracolic part of the procedure. The transverse colon is lifted up, the ligament of Treitz is identified, and 60 cm of jejunum is measured from the ligament of Treitz and divided using the stapler. The third arm holds the biliopancreatic limb static, while 120 cm of Roux limb is measured and the site for the jejunojejunostomy (JJ) is identified. The third arm holds the two bowel loops together while an enterotomy is created with the cautery hook (Fig. 31.6). By using the third arm to hold the limbs together, the time for a stay suture is saved and the operation runs more efficiently.

A JJ is created using a 60-mm stapler. The enterotomy is closed using PDS 3–0 running suture with large needle driver. Then the omentum is divided using the Harmonic scalpel, and the Roux limb is taken up to the gastric pouch for the gastrojejunostomy (GJ) (Fig. 31.7). The JJ mesenteric defect is closed using polypropylene suture after GJ creation to avoid tension on the mesentery while the Roux limb is taken up to the gastric pouch.

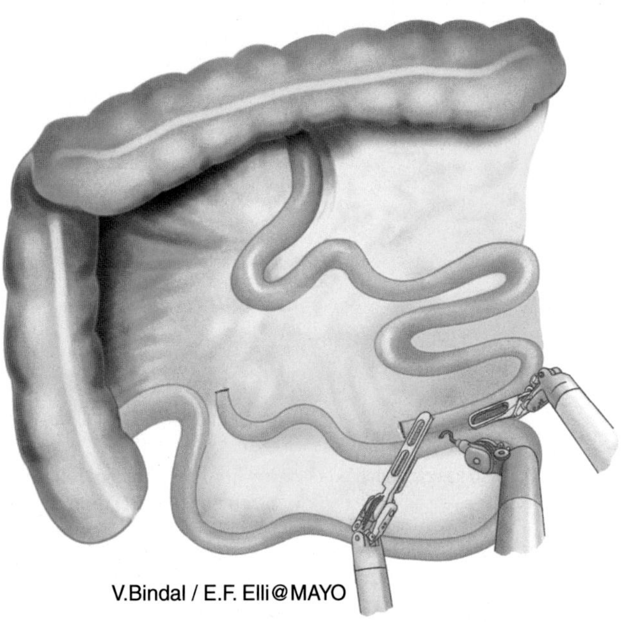

Fig. 31.6 Creation of the jejunojejunostomy. The second and third arms are holding both the loops of jejunum together. A monopolar hook is being used to create an enterotomy

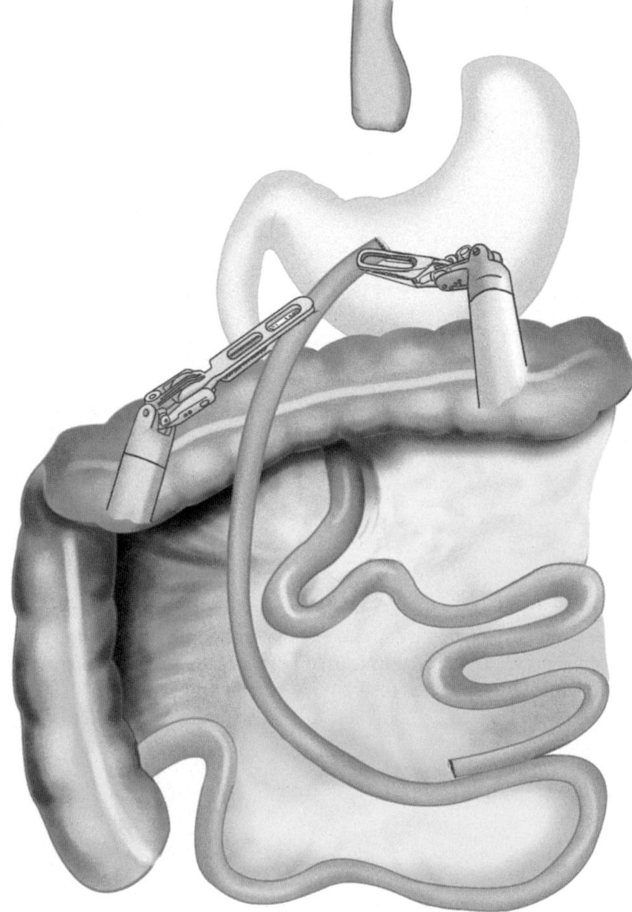

Fig. 31.7 The Roux limb is taken up to gastric pouch for gastrojejunostomy, using second and third arm

Creation of Gastrojejunostomy

A totally handsewn GJ is done using PDS 3–0 suture. We do not use nonabsorbable sutures, as they increase the risk of marginal ulceration and stricture formation. Two needle drivers are taken in R1 and R2. While constructing the GJ, the third arm will hold the gastric pouch and small bowel together to release tension. A through-and-through running suture is taken across the staple line and the Roux limb of jejunum, in a left-to-right fashion, making the posterior-most layer of the anastomosis and distributing the tension evenly across the staple line. Now a 1.5-cm gastrotomy and enterotomy is created using the cautery hook (roughly equal to three lengths of the horizontal portion of the hook). The anastomosis is started by securing the left corner and continuing with a running, full-thickness suture forming the posterior wall of the GJ, ending on the right corner of the anastomosis (Fig. 31.8). A similar full-thickness anterior layer of GJ is completed from left to right, and the ends of the sutures are knotted securely. Then the anterior sero-serosal layer is completed from left to right. The robotic platform allows the surgeon to be ambidextrous and drive the needle effectively in all directions required during creation of the GJ. We use four pieces of 6-in. PDS 3–0 to complete the four-layered GJ.

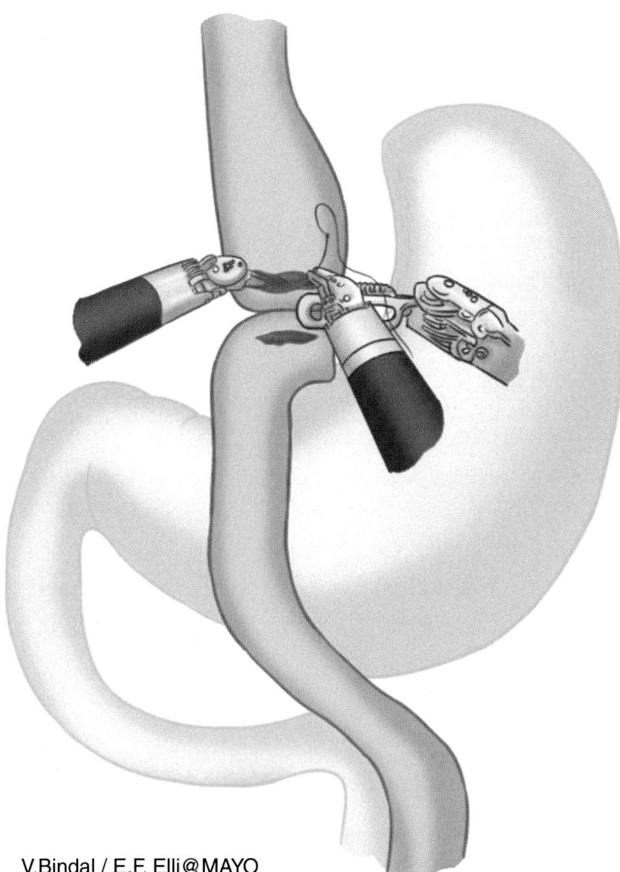

Fig. 31.8 Creation of the gastrojejunostomy (GJ). A handsewn GJ is being created using PDS 3–0 suture. The third arm is holding the gastric pouch and Roux limb together

The Petersen's defect is closed starting from the base of the defect by lifting up the transverse mesocolon and working toward the top, using polypropylene suture and taking care that no mesenteric vessel is injured. An intraoperative check esophagogastroscopy is done with an air leak test at the end of the procedure in all cases.

Perioperative Care

Patients are given prophylaxis for deep venous thrombosis by mechanical (sequential compression devices, ambulation) and pharmacological (low molecular weight heparin) methods. They are given a single shot of cephalosporin before induction for antimicrobial prophylaxis. Patients are encouraged to walk in the evening of surgery and are started on a liquid diet. No upper GI gastrografin study is done, except in patients with intolerance to liquids or prolonged nausea. Patients are kept on a liquid diet for 1 week, followed by a week of a soft diet. Thereafter, they are progressed to a normal diet.

Results

We have been performing robot-assisted RYGB (RRYGB) with excellent results at Mayo Clinic Florida. A total of 429 patients (377 females, 52 males) with a mean age of 42.5 ± 10.2 years have undergone RRYGB. The mean BMI was 46.6 ± 7.2 kg/m^2. Mean operative time was 173 ± 0.9 min, and length of stay was 2.3 ± 0.9 days. The percentage excess weight loss was 53.4 ± 17.4 (n = 152) at 6 months, 68.3 ± 22 (n = 97) at 1 year, and 71 ± 24.9 (n = 49) at 2 years. There were no anastomotic leaks or GJ strictures in the entire series. Three patients required reoperation for bowel obstruction because of internal hernia.

Robot-Assisted RYGB: Its Current and Future Role

Many significant published series have compared outcomes of robotic RYGB versus laparoscopic RYGB (LRYGB) [20–29]. Most of the published studies suggest a lower rate of anastomotic complications like leak and stricture formation with the use of the robotic technique as compared with laparoscopic technique. Bindal et al. [30] reviewed the published literature with a total of 3337 patients (1381 RRYGB and

1956 LRYGB). They found that mean OR time was 211.9 min in the robotic arm versus 185.1 min in the laparoscopic arm. This difference may be compounded by the fact that in all the studies, a sutured GJ was done in the robotic arm whereas a stapled GJ was done in the laparoscopic arm in six of nine studies. The average length of stay was 5 days for the robotic group versus 7.1 days for the laparoscopic group. The overall complication rate was 12.2% in the robotic group versus 13.3% in the laparoscopic group. Buchs et al. [28] found a significantly lower incidence of complications in the robotic group (11.6 vs. 16.1%). The average leak rate across studies was 0.9% in RRYGB versus 1.6% in LRYGB, and the GJ stricture rate was 3.1% in the robotic arm and 3.2% in the laparoscopic arm. Snyder et al. [21] and Buchs et al. [28] found significantly lower leak rates in RRYGB. The overall mortality in both groups was 0.05%. In our own series, there has been no leak or stricture formation after RRYGB in 429 patients, a result that compares favorably with the published literature on LRYGB, and we believe that a handsewn GJ done in a precise way decreases the anastomotic complication rate.

A surgeon skill bias is at play in most of these studies, as it is very difficult to find a surgeon equally skilled in both robotic and laparoscopic techniques. Most surgeons and their teams become proficient in either of the two techniques. But large comparative studies and systematic reviews do offer some tendencies for robotic bariatric surgery [31–33].

The learning curve has been studied for both LRYGB and RRYGB. The learning curve for LRYGB has been reported to be 75–100 cases in order to normalize complications [5, 33]. Buchs et al. [17] analyzed the learning curve for RRYGB and found it to be 14 cases in order to achieve mastery for a surgeon well versed in laparoscopic surgery but not in bariatric procedures. Yu et al. [34] studied complications in the first 100 cases of RRYGB and found no leaks and one reoperation. The published literature seems to suggest that the learning curve for RRYGB is shorter than for the laparoscopic technique.

Robotic surgery is a team effort, and this is even more true for bariatric surgery. The entire team learns with the surgeon and develops experience in patient safety precautions, OR setup, and the type of instruments needed, thus leading to better OR times and better patient outcomes. As the main surgeon is separated from the patient while performing robotic surgery, the assistant surgeon at the bedside is responsible for stapling (if robotic staplers are not used) and must be trained enough to help with difficult tasks and to take care of any emergency situation arising during the procedure. The scrub nurse and OR technician are also very important in streamlining the conduct of the procedure and preventing any waste of time and resources.

Another advantage which comes with use of the robotic system is improved ergonomics and reduced operator fatigue. Ergonomics in laparoscopic surgery can be very challenging, as big patients and uncomfortable postures lead to surgeon fatigue and work-related musculoskeletal symptoms [35]. Robotics also provides the advantage of more degrees of freedom, a help in performing difficult dissection and sutured anastomosis.

There has been a concern about cost every time the use of a robotic system is considered, as the direct costs are generally higher for the robotic approach in bariatric procedures like RYGB [36]. However, Hagen et al. [25] took into consideration the total costs, including complications and readmissions, and found that the cost of RRYGB was lower than the cost of LRYGB when all the factors were accounted for. A decrease in the number of laparoscopic staplers used in robotic procedures by doing a handsewn anastomosis also results in a saving.

Ultimately, the big question to be answered is whether the use of robotics is going to stay or whether it will perish with time like many other fancy technologies. Looking at the basic concept of computer-assisted navigational surgery, robotics provide an enabling platform between the surgeon and the patient. It provides augmented and higher-quality inputs from the patient to the surgeon, and the surgeon's output is refined to a superior quality before reaching back to the target. We believe that the final analysis should not be limited to the features of the systems currently available for use, but rather should consider the potential in the concept of using a digital interface to enhance the performance of the surgeon in interacting with patients. With the advent of newer technologies in robotics, such as fluorescence, integration of images, virtual and augmented reality, telesurgery, single-site platforms, natural orifice surgery, and haptic feedback, we believe that digital platforms will provide an empowering tool to surgeons that potentially may change the way surgery is practiced today.

References

1. Wittgrove AC, Clark GW, Tremblay LJ. Laparoscopic gastric bypass, Roux-en-Y: preliminary report of five cases. Obes Surg. 1994;4:353–7.
2. Nguyen NT, Masoomi H, Magno CP, Nguyen XM, Laugenour K, Lane J. Trends in use of bariatric surgery, 2003–2008. J Am Coll Surg. 2011;213:261–6.
3. Ponce J, Nguyen NT, Hutter M, Sudan R, Morton JM. American Society for Metabolic and Bariatric Surgery estimation of bariat-

ric surgery procedures in the United States, 2011-2014. Surg Obes Relat Dis. 2015;11(6):1199–200.

4. Wilson EB, Sudan R. The evolution of robotic bariatric surgery. World J Surg. 2013;37:2756–60.
5. Parikh MS, Shen R, Weiner M, Siegel N, Ren CJ. Laparoscopic bariatric surgery in super-obese patients (BMI>50) is safe and effective: a review of 332 patients. Obes Surg. 2005;15:858–63.
6. Schauer P, Ikramuddin S, Hamad G, Gourash W. The learning curve for laparoscopic Roux-en-Y gastric bypass is 100 cases. Surg Endosc. 2003;17:212–5.
7. Shikora SA, Kim JJ, Tarnoff ME, Raskin E, Shore R. Laparoscopic Roux-en-Y gastric bypass: results and learning curve of a high-volume academic program. Arch Surg. 2005;140:362–7.
8. Cadiere GB, Himpens J, Vertruyen M, Favretti F. The world's first obesity surgery performed by a surgeon at a distance. Obes Surg. 1999;9:206–9.
9. Talamini MA, Chapman S, Horgan S, Melvin WS. The academic robotic group. A prospective analysis of 211 robotic-assisted procedures. Surg Endosc. 2003;17:1521–4.
10. Bindal V, Bhatia P, Kalhan S, Khetan M, John S, Ali A, et al. Robot-assisted excision of a large retroperitoneal schwannoma. JSLS. 2014;18:150–4.
11. Cadiere GB, Himpens J, Vertruyen M, Bruyns J, Germay O, Leman G, et al. Evaluation of telesurgical (robotic) Nissen fundoplication. Surg Endosc. 2001;15:918–23.
12. Nakadi IE, Melot C, Closset J, DeMoor V, Betroune K, Feron P, et al. Evaluation of da Vinci Nissen fundoplication clinical results and cost minimization. World J Surg. 2006;30:1050–4.
13. Schauer PR, Ikramuddin S. Laparoscopic surgery for morbid obesity. Surg Clin North Am. 2001;81:1145–79.
14. Buchwald H, Williams SE. Bariatric surgery worldwide 2003. Obes Surg. 2004;14:1157–64.
15. Sjostrom L, Lindroos AK, Peltonen M, Torgerson J, Bouchard C, Carlsson B, et al. Lifestyle, diabetes, and cardiovascular risk factors 10 years after bariatric surgery. N Engl J Med. 2004;351:2683–93.
16. Puzziferri N, Roshek TB, Mayo HG, Gallagher R, Belle SH, Livingston EH. Long-term follow-up after bariatric surgery: a systematic review. JAMA. 2014;312:934–42.
17. Buchs NC, Pugin F, Bucher P, Hagen ME, Chassot G, Koutny-Fong P, et al. Learning curve for robot-assisted Roux-en-Y gastric bypass. Surg Endosc. 2012;26:1116–21.
18. Bindal V, Gonzalez-Heredia R, Masrur M, Elli EF. Technique evolution, learning curve, and outcomes of 200 robot-assisted gastric bypass procedures: a 5-year experience. Obes Surg. 2015;25:997–1002.
19. Bindal V, Gonzalez-Heredia R, Elli EF. Outcomes of robot-assisted Roux-en-Y gastric bypass as a reoperative bariatric procedure. Obes Surg. 2015;25:1810–5.
20. Sanchez BR, Mohr CJ, Morton JM, Safadi BY, Alami RS, Curet MJ. Comparison of totally robotic laparoscopic Roux-en-Y gastric bypass and traditional laparoscopic Roux-en-Y gastric bypass. Surg Obes Relat Dis. 2005;1:549–54.
21. Snyder BE, Wilson T, Leong BY, Klein C, Wilson EB. Robotic-assisted Roux-en-Y gastric bypass: minimizing morbidity and mortality. Obes Surg. 2010;20:265–70.
22. Ayloo SM, Addeo P, Buchs NC, Shah G, Giulianotti PC. Robot-assisted versus laparoscopic Roux-en-Y gastric bypass: is there a difference in outcomes? World J Surg. 2011;35:637–42.
23. Park CW, Lam ECF, Walsh TM, Karimoto M, Ma AT, Koo M, et al. Robotic-assisted Roux-en-Y gastric bypass performed in a community hospital setting: the future of bariatric surgery? Surg Endosc. 2011;25:3312–21.
24. Scozzari G, Rebecchi F, Millo P, Rocchietto S, Allieta R, Morino M. Robot-assisted gastrojejunal anastomosis does not improve the results of the laparoscopic Roux-en-Y gastric bypass. Surg Endosc. 2011;25:597–603.
25. Hagen ME, Pugin F, Chassot G, Huber O, Buchs N, Iranmanesh P, et al. Reducing cost of surgery by avoiding complications: the model of robotic Roux-en-Y gastric bypass. Obes Surg. 2012;22:52–61.
26. Benizri EI, Renaud M, Reibel N, Germain A, Ziegler O, Zarnegar R, et al. Perioperative outcomes after totally robotic gastric bypass: a prospective nonrandomized controlled study. Am J Surg. 2013;206:145–51.
27. Myers SR, McGuirl J, Wang J. Robot-assisted versus laparoscopic gastric bypass: comparison of short-term outcomes. Obes Surg. 2013;23:467–73.
28. Buchs NC, Morel P, Azagury DE, Jung M, Chassot G, Huber O, et al. Laparoscopic versus robotic Roux-en-Y gastric bypass: lessons and long-term follow-up learned from a large prospective monocentric study. Obes Surg. 2014;24:2031–9.
29. Markar S, Karthikesalingam A, Venkat-Ramen V, Kinross J, Ziprin P. Robotic vs. laparoscopic Roux-en-Y gastric bypass in morbidly obese patients: systematic review and pooled analysis. Int J Med Robot. 2011;7:393–400.
30. Bindal V, Bhatia P, Dudeja U, Kalhan S, Khetan M, John S, Wadhera S. Review of contemporary role of robotics in bariatric surgery. J Minim Access Surg. 2015;11:16–21.
31. Fourman MM, Saber AA. Robotic bariatric surgery: a systematic review. Surg Obes Relat Dis. 2012;8:483–8.
32. Kim K, Hagen ME, Buffington C. Robotics in advanced gastrointestinal surgery: the bariatric experience. Cancer J. 2013;19:177–82.
33. Toro JP, Lin E, Patel AD. Review of robotics in foregut and bariatric surgery. Surg Endosc. 2015;29:1–8.
34. Yu CJ, Clapp BI, Lee MJ, Albrecht WC, Scarborough TK, Wilson EB. Robotic assistance provides excellent outcomes during the learning curve for laparoscopic Roux-en-Y gastric bypass: results from 100 robotic-assisted gastric bypasses. Am J Surg. 2006;192:746–9.
35. Esposito C, El Ghoneimi A, Yamataka A, Rothenberg S, Bailez M, Ferro M, et al. Work-related upper limb musculoskeletal disorders in paediatric laparoscopic surgery. A multicenter survey. J Pediatr Surg. 2013;48:1750–6.
36. Curet MJ, Curet M, Soloman H, Lui G, Morton JM. Comparison of hospital charges between robotic, laparoscopic stapled, and laparoscopic handsewn Roux-en-Y gastric bypass. J Robot Surg. 2009;3:75–8.

Robotic Roux-en-Y Gastric Bypass

32

Michele L. Young and Keith Chae Kim

Introduction

Indications for the Roux-en-Y gastric bypass (RYGB) remain the same as they have been since the 1991 publication of the NIH Consensus Guidelines: BMI ≥ 40 or BMI 35–39 with one or more obesity-related comorbidities [1]. There are data, however, that support the benefits and safety of the RYGB in patients with a lower BMI with metabolic burden, particularly diabetes, suggesting that these indications should be reconsidered [2]. In reviews of comparative studies looking at robotic versus laparoscopic approaches to the RYGB, two trends seem to consistently stand out: (1) major complications, particularly leaks, tend to be lower in the robotic groups; and (2) the operative times tend to be longer in the robotic groups [3]. The longer operative times should be a consideration in terms of minimizing added risks to the patient and minimizing impact on productivity; the operative times can be considerably longer. In transitioning to a robotic approach to the RYGB, the intention should be to progress to performing all RYGBs robotically, so the indications for a robotic RYGB should be the same as for RYGB in general.

Indications

The RYGB is an ideal procedure for robotic surgery. RYGB is a moderately complex procedure that requires a high degree of minimally invasive dexterity, including suturing, the ability to maneuver in small working areas, and the need to overcome the challenges of an obese anatomy, including thick abdominal walls. Additionally, most surgeons have a very consistent approach to the procedure, which lends itself to a very standardized robotic technique. Nevertheless, adoption of the robotic approach has been slow in bariatric surgery because of the high penetration of the laparoscopic approach and the remarkably low associated morbidity and mortality, which speak to the generally high skill level of bariatric surgeons.

Preoperative Preparation

The preoperative preparation for robotic RYGB consists of three elements: the patient, the surgeon, and the surgical team. The patient preparation is critical not only for mitigating the challenges of operating on a morbidly obese patient but also for best preparing the patient for lifelong commitment to combating obesity. The elements that we stress in our program are preoperative diet, nutritional repletion, and patient responsibility. On the first encounter with our program, patients are placed on a diet that emphasizes small portions, the elimination of sugars and starches, and a focus on good sources of protein and fresh fruits and vegetables. Generally, 2 weeks prior to their surgery, they are placed on a liquid protein-based, low-calorie diet, which generally results in diminished liver volume and decreased intra-abdominal fat. Patients are also placed on a complete adult multivitamin twice daily and instructed to walk twice daily. Complete nutrition labs are drawn, and supplementation is started to correct any deficiencies.

As with laparoscopic RYGB, the surgeon is responsible for ensuring that the patient is appropriately evaluated and prepared for surgery. With robotic RYGB, the surgeon has the added responsibility of understanding the robotic system and trying to ensure that the OR team is also appropriately trained. The surgeon should try to become familiar with the particular robotic system so that he or she is able to handle most of the basic troubleshooting if problems occur with the system. These may involve issues associated with docking the arms, instrument registration, recognition and proper functioning of energy sources, and console-related calibrations, including ergonomic adjustments to the console, scaling of motion, and sound and visual inputs. Additionally, the surgeon should be able to

M. L. Young, PA-C (✉) · K. C. Kim, MD
Center for Metabolic and Obesity Surgery, Florida Hospital Celebration Health, Celebration, FL, USA
e-mail: michele.young.pac@flhosp.org; Keith.Kim.md@flhosp.org

Y. Fong et al. (eds.), *The SAGES Atlas of Robotic Surgery*, https://doi.org/10.1007/978-3-319-91045-1_32

make appropriate internal or external arm adjustments in the event that external arm collisions limit internal instrument mobility. If a more complex problem occurs, the surgeon should be familiar with the online clinical support team, which has access to the robotic performance data and can troubleshoot remotely in real time. Task-oriented simulation modules are available, and increasing data support the idea that a "preoperative warm-up" enhances motor skills and performance [4].

The OR team is critical to safety and efficiency. Unlike laparoscopic RYGB, in which the surgeon typically performs all of the critical elements of the surgery—particularly the stapling aspects—the robotic approach requires a skilled assistant at the bedside to perform the stapling portions of the procedure. With robotic RYGB, the bedside assistant has the added burden of negotiating not only the internal robotic arms but also the external portions of the robotic arms, which can limit the range of motion available to navigate the stapler into position. The surgeon must provide adequate exposure and instructions from the console and trust that the assistant is not pushing the stapler through resistance and risking trauma to critical structures. This close coordination and anticipation of one another's actions comes with working together consistently. For this reason, it is ideal to have the same person assisting on all cases.

Time should be invested in training a dedicated robotic perioperative staff. At least one member should serve as the coordinator, who should be responsible for making sure that the system and the instruments are in appropriate working order. Each instrument has a limited number of uses, and the instruments should be checked at the end of each case to make sure the instrument does not have to be replaced. The circulator should be specifically trained in steering the patient console cart into position. Finally, the scrub tech ideally should be trained in docking and undocking the robotic arms and performing instrument exchanges. Time and energy invested in training the robotic team can make a significant difference in OR efficiency. With a dedicated robotic team, the entire robotic docking process can be consistently completed in less than 5 min.

Room Setup

The da Vinci® Si robotic system (Intuitive Surgical; Sunnyvale, CA) is used as the model for this discussion. With the robotic RYGB, there are five items to consider when setting up the room: the patient, the anesthesiologist, the robotic patient cart, the surgeon and surgeon console, and the bedside assistant. If the room is not a square, the patient should be positioned so that the head-to-feet axis corresponds to the long axis of the room, in order to allow room to maneuver the patient cart into place. The patient cart is docked straight over the patient's head. The anesthesiologist is positioned to the left of the patient's upper half. Because the entire robotic system encompasses a relatively large footprint, if the operating room is relatively small, the surgeon console is positioned anywhere that the room will accommodate it. Ideally the surgeon console should be positioned in a manner that allows the surgeon to look up from the console and view the patient and the patient cart. The assistant is positioned on the patient's right side, because all of the stapling for the procedure is typically done from that side. The video monitor is positioned opposite the assistant, on the patient's left. The scrub tech is positioned toward the foot of the bed beside the assistant (Fig. 32.1).

The anesthesiologist may resist giving up the position at the head of the patient. If this issue cannot be resolved, there is a parallel docking technique in which the patient cart is docked off to the left of the patient's head, giving the anesthesiologist access to the patient's head. This docking technique may be preferable for those surgeons who perform routine endoscopy at the end of the case to evaluate the gastric pouch and gastrojejunal anastomosis.

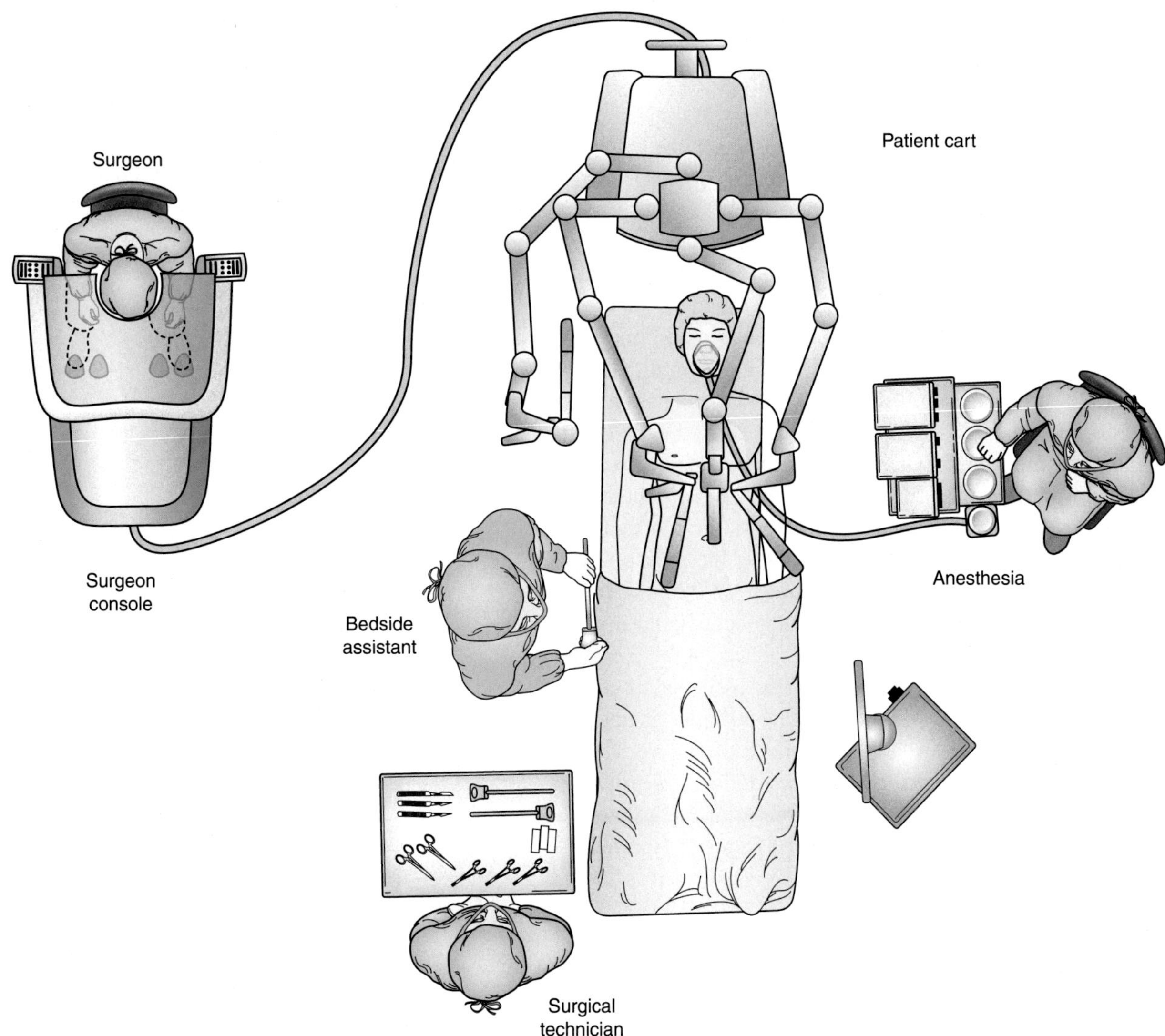

Fig. 32.1 Positioning of the patient, surgical team, and equipment

Procedure by Steps

Trocar Placement, Patient Positioning

Trocars are placed with the goal of trying to achieve maximal horizontal separation among the trocars, in order to create spacing among the external portions of the arms of the robotic system so that external clashing of the arms can be minimized. The patient cart of the robot is docked from directly over the head of the patient. Two robotic arms are assigned to the patient's left of the camera arm and one is assigned to the patient's right. This configuration dictates that the elbow of the camera arm be bent out to the patient's right side. The camera trocar is positioned 28 cm below the midpoint of the sternal notch and xiphoid process, just to the left of midline. The two robotic arms on the patient's left are positioned at the same level from a craniocaudal standpoint and are separated maximally in the horizontal plane. This places the most lateral trocar at the anterior axillary line and the medial trocar at the midclavicular line. The robotic arm on the patient's right is placed at the costal margin at the anterior axillary line. The assistant trocar, which is a 12-mm trocar to accommodate a stapler, is positioned at the midpoint in both the horizontal and vertical axis between the camera trocar and the robotic arm trocar on the patient's right (Fig. 32.2). All four arms are utilized in the procedure. Two working arms are assigned to the surgeon's right hand, and one working arm is assigned to the surgeon's left hand.

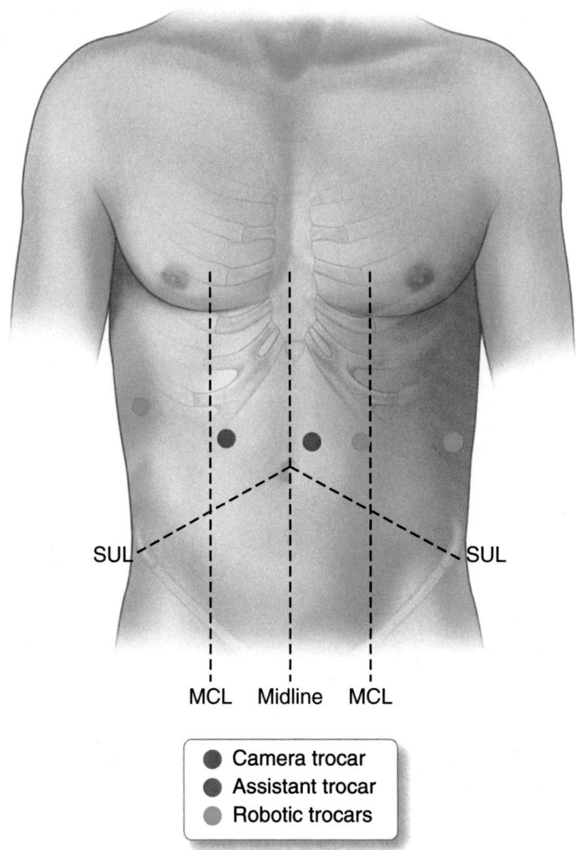

Fig. 32.2 Trocar placement

The patient is positioned with both arms out, and a retractor holder is positioned at the patient's left axilla to hold the liver retractor. A Nathanson liver retractor is used to retract the liver. The patient is positioned in mild reverse Trendelenburg position (10–15 degrees) for the procedure. Once the patient is docked to the robot, the patient's position cannot be adjusted. Access to the head of the patient can be limited once the robot is docked.

Gastric Pouch

The hiatus is carefully inspected for a hiatal hernia. If one is present, the hiatus is dissected free and a posterior hiatal hernia repair is performed. The fat pad at the angle of His is dissected free, and the anterior portion of the left crus is exposed. Using the articulation of the grasper, the left crus is exposed posteriorly as much as possible. The gastric pouch is created using a perigastric technique. A Maryland dissector is used in the surgeon's right hand to expose branches of vessels going into the lesser curvature. A harmonic scalpel is used in the surgeon's left hand to divide the vessel and perigastric fat to access the lesser sac. Once the window is created into the lesser sac, the harmonic scalpel on the left hand is changed to a tissue grasper. It is important to ensure clear exposure of the lesser sac, and the lesser sac should be evaluated to ensure that there are no retrogastric adhesions. The assistant staples from the patient's right side, and the first transverse fire is straight, without any articulation of the stapler (Fig. 32.3). The subsequent vertical staple fire is performed with the stapler fully articulated, with the surgeon at the console holding the two ends of the transverse staple line and angling the staple line so that the vertical staple line is perpendicular to

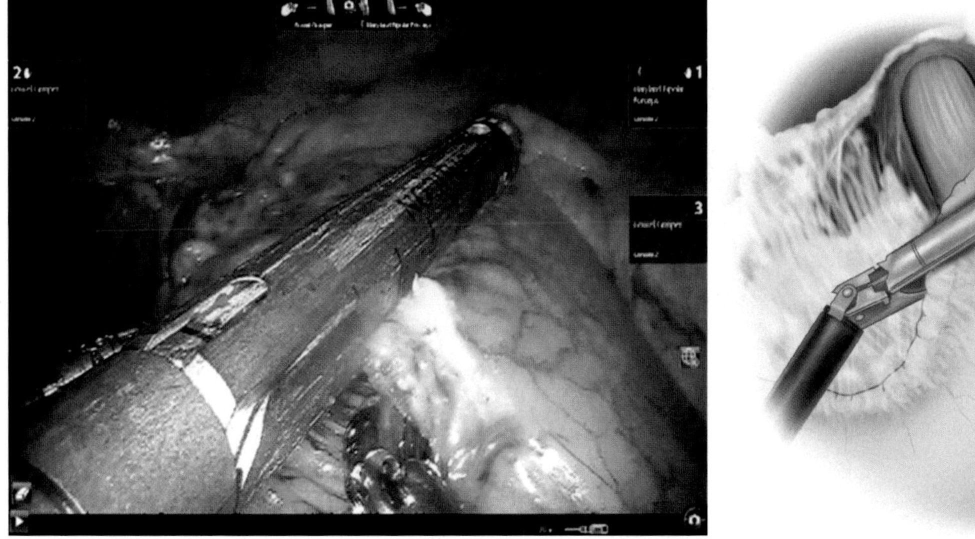

Fig. 32.3 The assistant staples from the patient's right side; the first transverse fire is straight, without any articulation of the stapler

the transverse staple line and is aimed toward the angle of His (Fig. 32.4). A bougie is positioned once the stapler has been closed, before it is fired. After the first vertical staple fire, the pouch and remnant stomach are retracted anteriorly to expose the dimple posteriorly in the gastric attachment at the level of the left crus, and the base of the left crus is carefully exposed. The grasper in the right hand is then used to push straight up along the left crus; this action should create a retrocolic window at the angle of His. Lateral retraction then exposes the window at the angle of His and facilitates the completion of the division of the vertical staple line (Fig. 32.5).

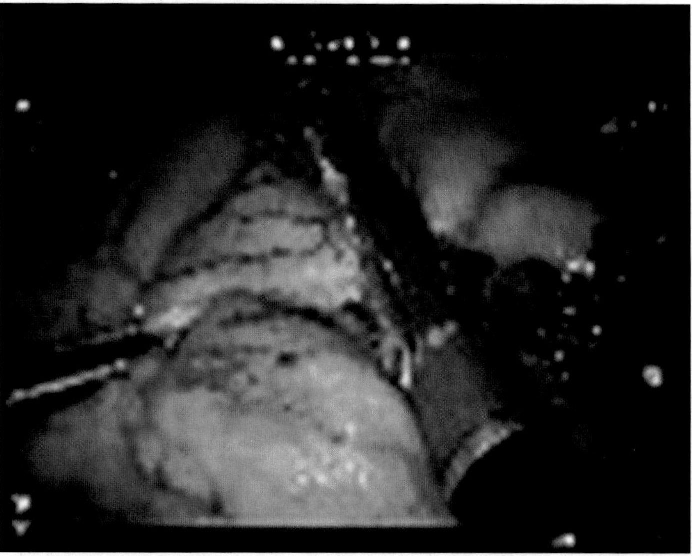

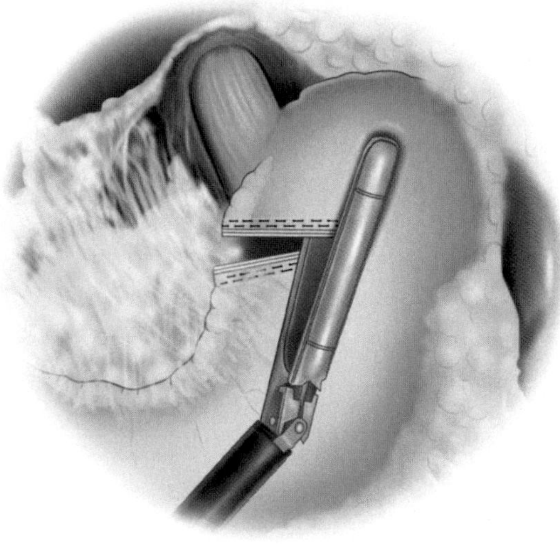

Fig. 32.4 The subsequent vertical staple fire is performed with the stapler fully articulated, with the surgeon at the console holding the two ends of the transverse staple line and angling the staple line so that the vertical staple line is perpendicular to the transverse staple line and aimed toward the angle of His

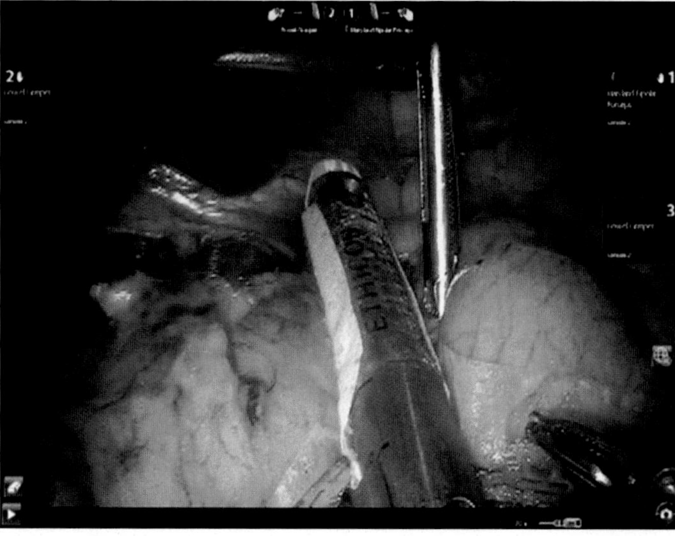

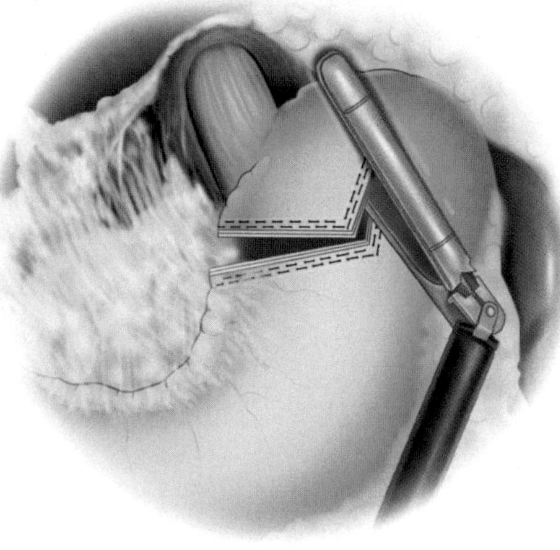

Fig. 32.5 The grasper in the right hand is used to push straight up along the left crus to create a retrocolic window at the angle of His. This is then used to retract laterally to expose the window at the angle of His and facilitate the completion of the division of the vertical staple line

Gastrojejunal Anastomosis

The omentum is retracted cephalad and is divided in the midline, starting from the transverse colon to avoid inadvertent injury to the colon (Fig. 32.6). The ligament of Treitz is then identified, and the jejunum is measured for a distance of 50 cm from the ligament of Treitz, measuring the loop out in a clockwise fashion to orient the proximal limb, or what will become the biliopancreatic limb, to the left. This loop is brought in an antecolic, antegastric fashion. The lateral arm on the right hand is used to hold the loop of bowel in position. The ambidexterity facilitated by the robot allows two needle drivers to be used to suture the anastomosis. A posterior outer row is completed from the end of the gastric pouch to the side of the jejunal loop, incorporating the end transverse staple line of the gastric pouch and the antimesenteric side of the jejunal limb (Fig. 32.7). Next, the harmonic scalpel is used to create a gastrotomy in the gastric pouch and an

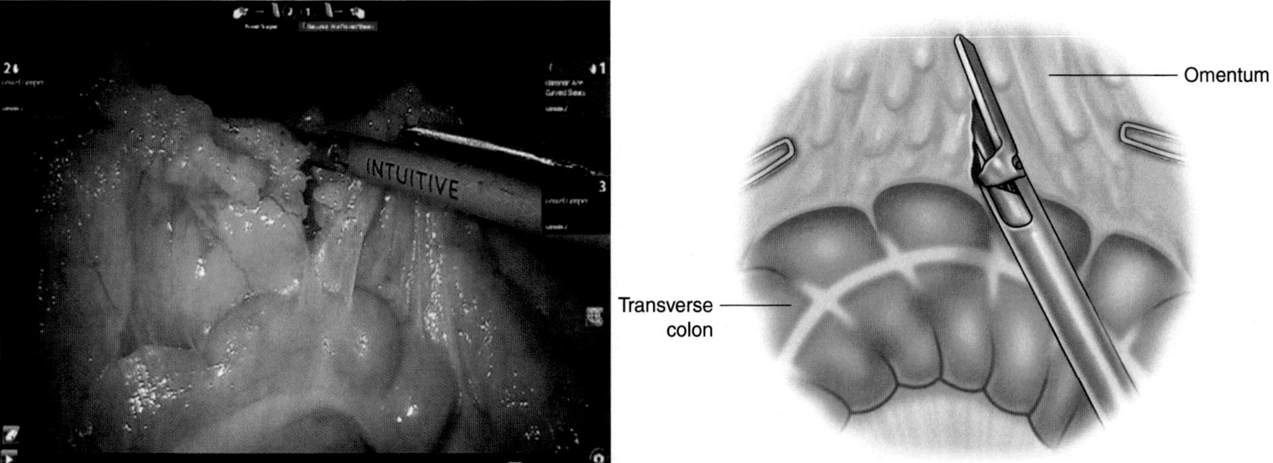

Fig. 32.6 The omentum is retracted cephalad and is divided in the midline, starting from the transverse colon to avoid inadvertent injury to the colon

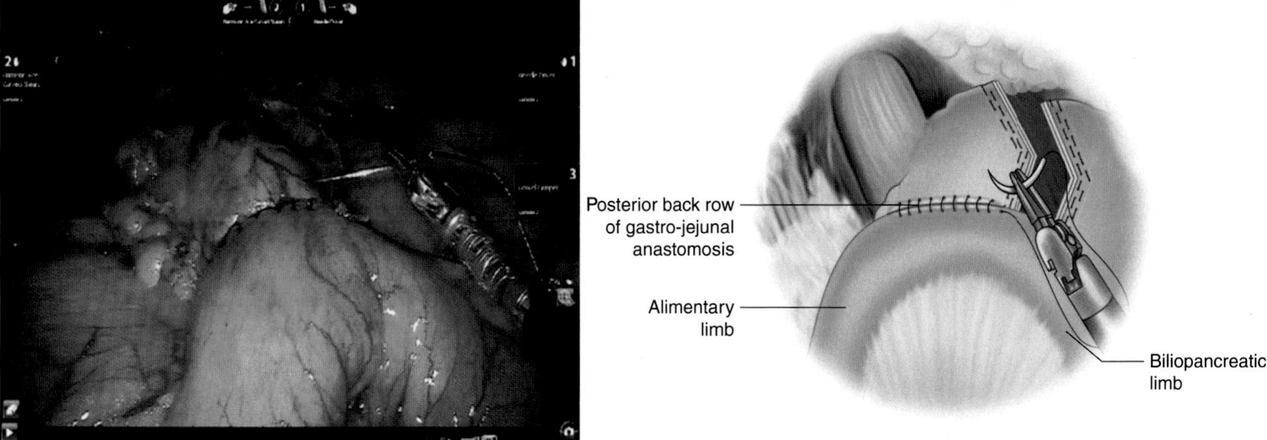

Fig. 32.7 A posterior outer row is completed in an end-gastric-pouch to side-jejunal-loop fashion, incorporating the end transverse staple line of the gastric pouch and the antimesenteric side of the jejunal limb

enterotomy in the jejunal loop (Fig. 32.8). The inner layer is then completed using a 34-Fr bougie to calibrate the stoma. The bougie is brought across the anastomosis once the posterior inner layer and a portion of the anterior inner layer have been completed (Fig. 32.9). The outer anterior layer is completed to finish the gastrojejunal anastomosis as a sutured two-layer anastomosis, leaving a loop gastrojejunostomy (Fig. 32.10).

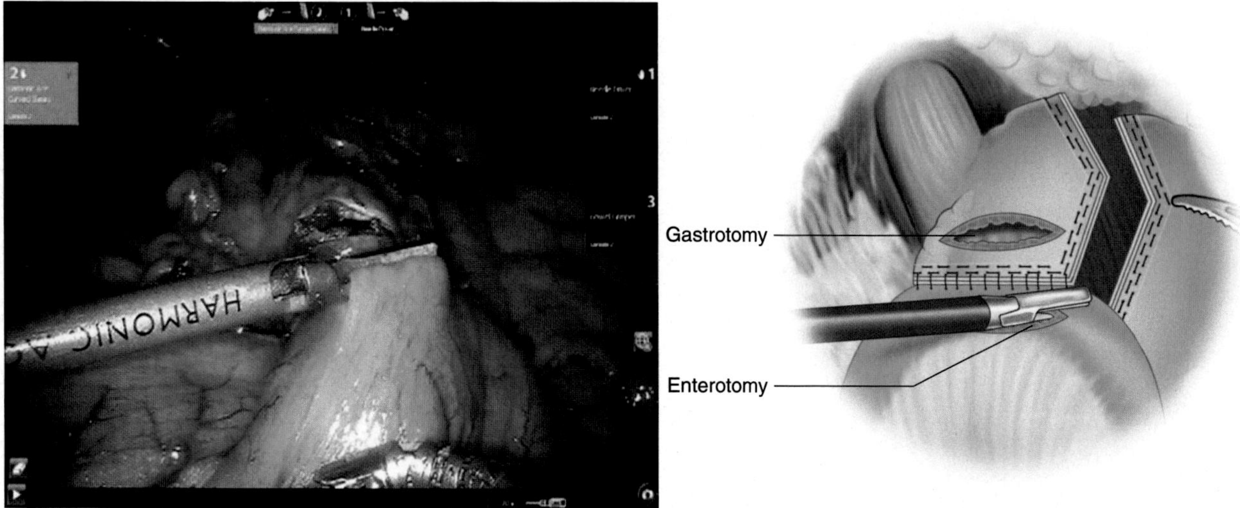

Fig. 32.8 The harmonic scalpel is used to create a gastrotomy in the gastric pouch and an enterotomy in the jejunal loop

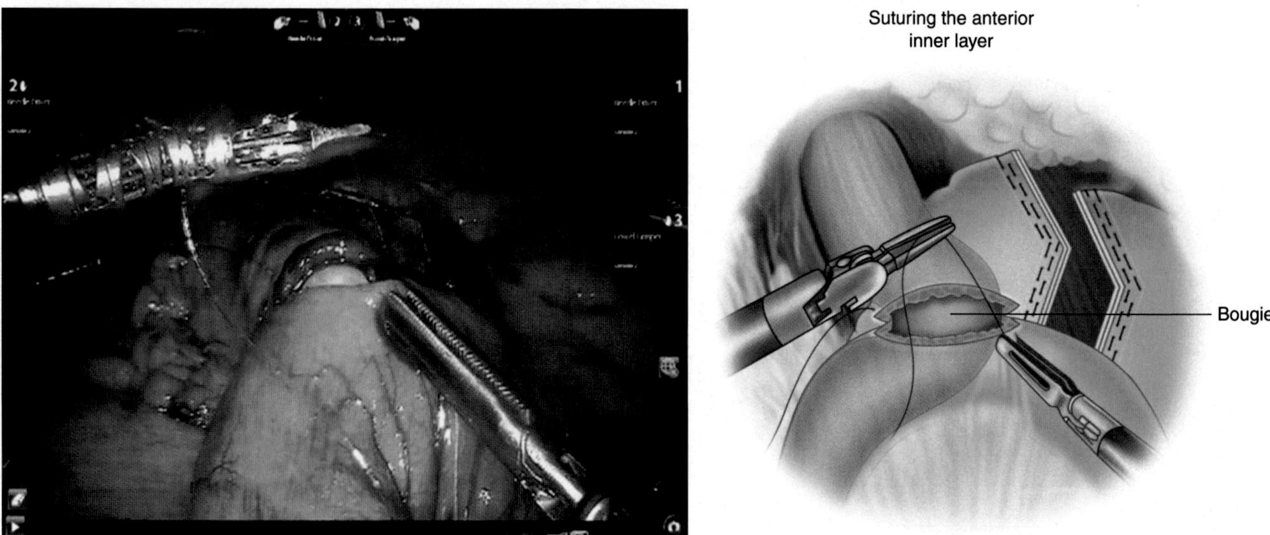

Fig. 32.9 The bougie is brought across the anastomosis once the posterior inner layer and a portion of the anterior inner layer have been completed

Jejuno-Jejunal Anastomosis

The jejunal loop is divided on the biliopancreatic side of the gastrojejunal anastomosis. The loop is oriented so that the biliopancreatic side should be to the patient's left of the gastrojejunal anastomosis. Division of the loop is accomplished by creating a small window in the mesentery just adjacent to the bowel, so that a minimal amount of the mesentery is divided (Fig. 32.11). The biliopancreatic limb is thus suspended in a relatively cephalad position, facilitating the cre-

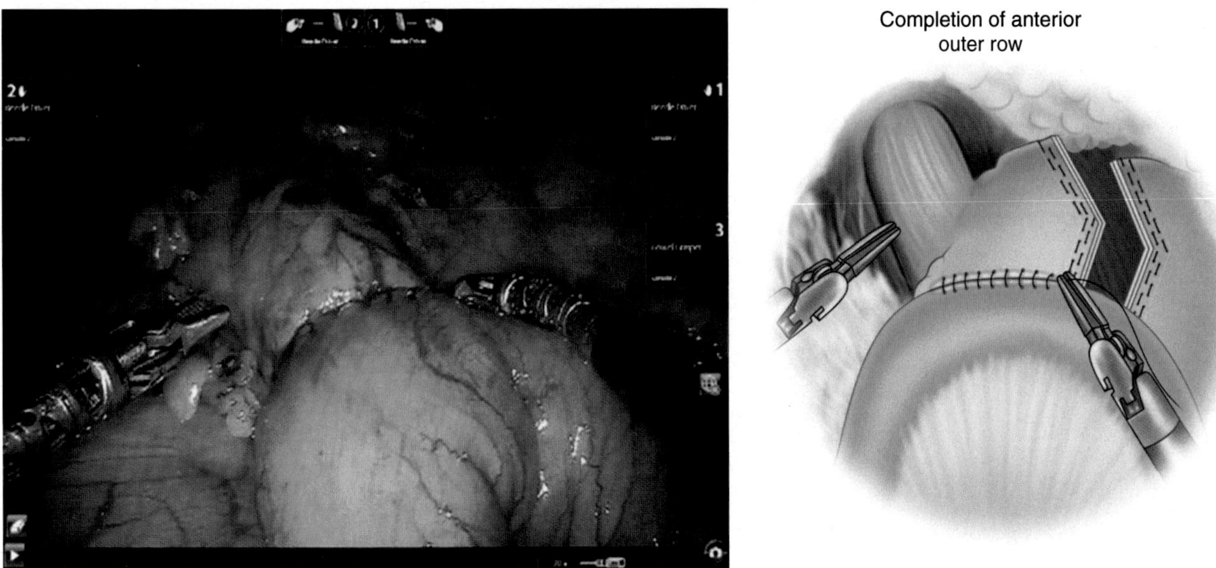

Fig. 32.10 The outer anterior layer is completed to finish the gastrojejunal anastomosis as a sutured two-layer anastomosis, leaving a loop gastrojejunostomy

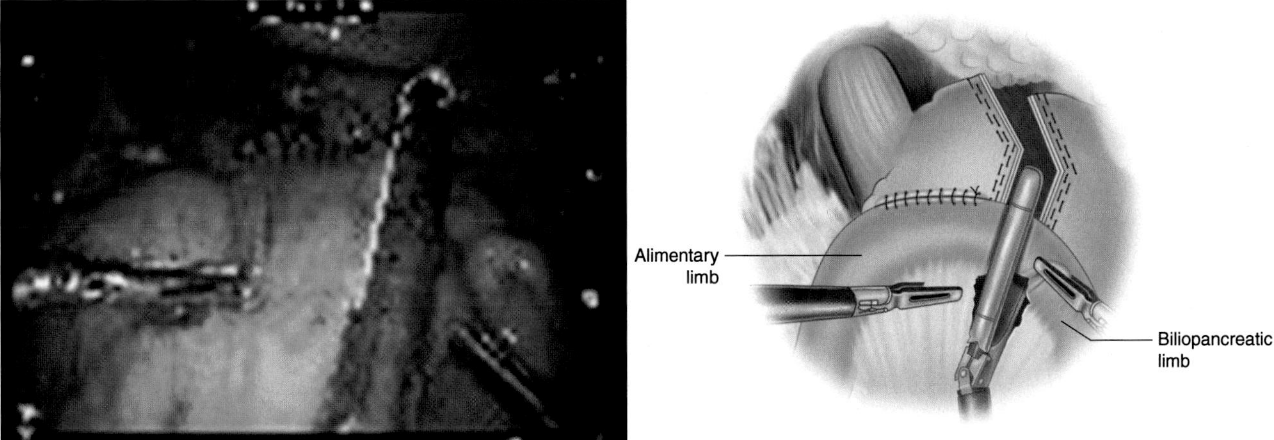

Fig. 32.11 The jejunal loop is divided on the biliopancreatic side of the gastrojejunal anastomosis, oriented so the biliopancreatic side is to the left of the gastrojejunal anastomosis. Division of the loop is accomplished by creating a small window in the mesentery just adjacent to the bowel, so that a minimal amount of the mesentery is divided

ation of the jejuno-jejunal anastomosis. The divided stump attached to the gastric pouch is the alimentary limb, and the free jejunal stump is the biliopancreatic limb. The alimentary limb is measured for another 100–150 cm distal to the gastrojejunal anastomosis, and the biliopancreatic limb is anastomosed to the 100- or 150-cm mark in a side-to-side fashion with a linear stapler (Fig. 32.12). The resulting enterotomy is closed with 2–0 Vicryl in a single-layered, running fashion starting from the mesenteric side of the enterotomy. Starting from the antimesenteric side of the enterotomy can make exposure of the end of the closure difficult.

Closure of Mesenteric Defects and Leak Test

The mesenteric defect is exposed by grasping the medial aspect of the alimentary limb at the proximal end of the jejuno-jejunal anastomosis, rotating it slightly outward, and retracting it slightly toward the left shoulder (Fig. 32.13). The closure can be started either from the top or the bottom, but it is important to seal the entire defect in a running fashion with suture, particularly at the crotch of the defect. Next, taking the alimentary limb and rotating it to the patient's left will reveal Petersen's space defect, which is best exposed by

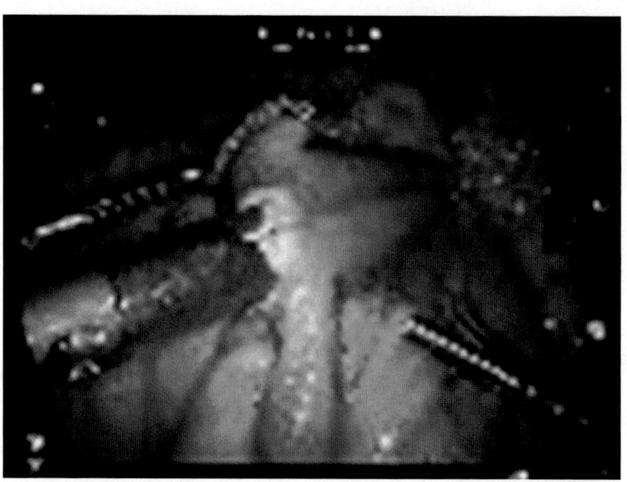

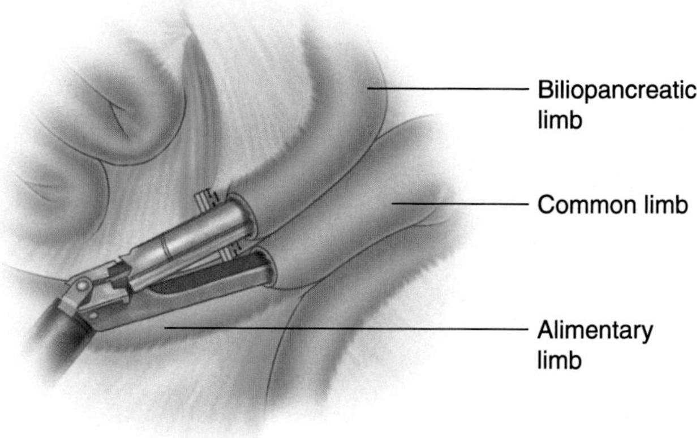

Fig. 32.12 The alimentary limb is measured for another 100–150 cm distal to the gastrojejunal anastomosis, and the biliopancreatic limb is anastomosed to the 100- or 150-cm mark in a side-to-side fashion with a linear stapler

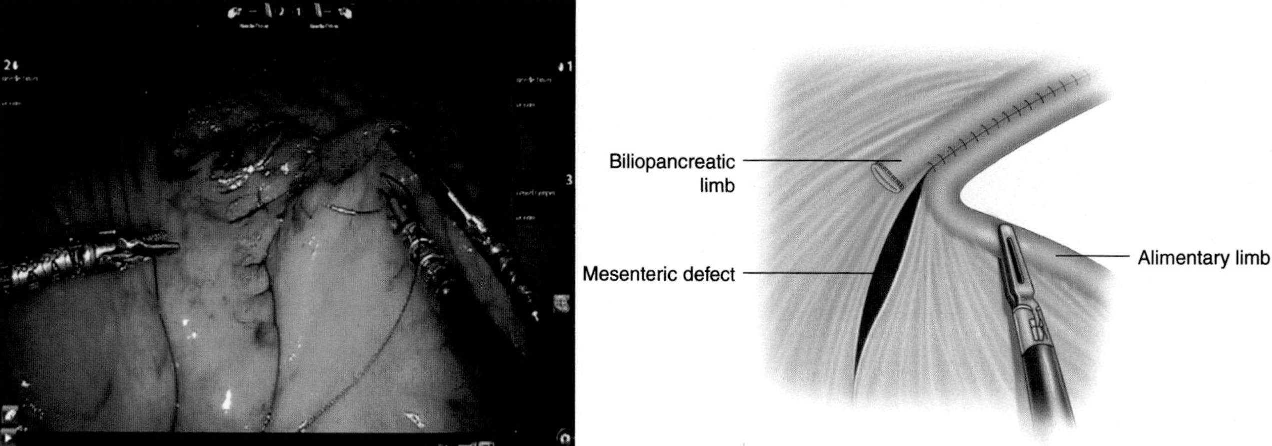

Fig. 32.13 The mesenteric defect is exposed by grasping the medial aspect of the alimentary limb at the proximal end of the jejuno-jejunal anastomosis, rotating it slightly outward, and retracting it slightly toward the left shoulder

grasping the transverse mesocolon just below the mid transverse colon and retracting it up to the gastrojejunal anastomosis (Fig. 32.14). The closure of Petersen's space is easier if started at the bottom. Taking several bites to close the crotch in a purse-string fashion is a nice way to start the running closure of this defect.

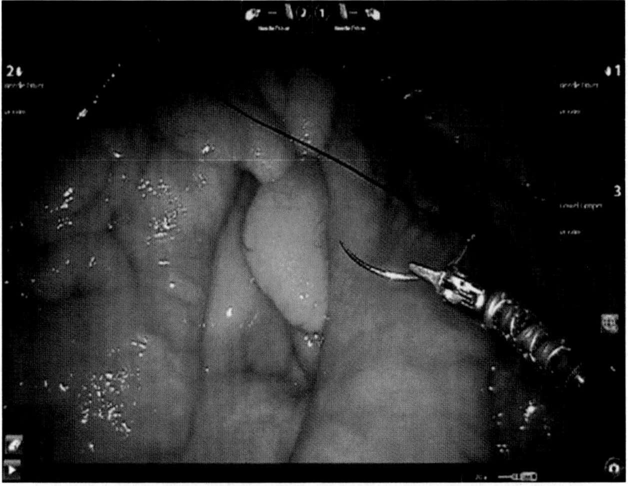

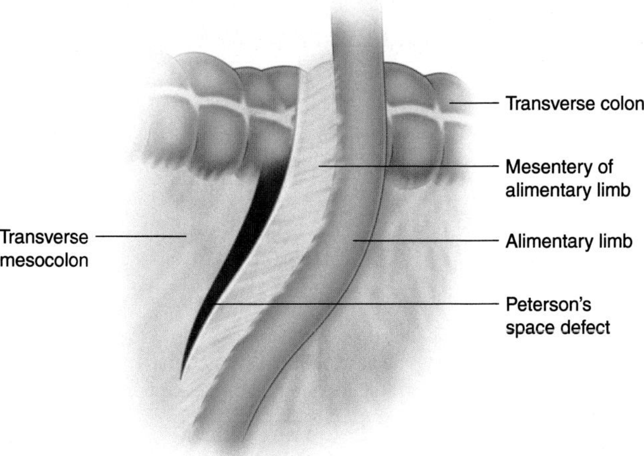

Fig. 32.14 Taking the alimentary limb and rotating it to the patient's left will reveal Petersen's space defect, which is best exposed by grasping the transverse mesocolon just below the mid transverse colon and retracting it up to the gastrojejunal anastomosis

Finally, a leak test is performed by passing an oral gastric tube across the gastrojejunal anastomosis, occluding the alimentary limb with a bowel clamp, and insufflating the gastric pouch and proximal alimentary limb with air. One of the left-side robotic arms is undocked to allow a suction irrigator to instill saline to check for air bubbles.

Postoperative Care

The postoperative care for robotic RYGB patients should be the same as that for laparoscopic RYGB patients. There are variations in what surgeons use to prevent deep vein thrombosis, as well as to mitigate nausea and pain with RYGB. Some studies have demonstrated that the robotic RYGB results in shorter length of stay, which is likely related to decreased complications with the robotic approach [3, 5, 6]. There have been suggestions as well that the robotic approach leads to decreased pain, although objective evidence demonstrating this result is lacking.

There is a mechanical difference in how the laparoscopic and robotic instruments transmit force to the abdominal wall. The robotic arms are designed with a remote center, which creates a fixed pivot point for the instrument. The remote center, or the fixed pivot point, is indicated on the trocar and, if positioned appropriately at the level of the fascia, minimizes trauma to the fascia. Conversely, if the remote center is not in the appropriate position, it can potentially cause more damage to the fascia because the robotic arms can transmit more force through the instrument shaft than is generally generated by the surgeon during laparoscopy.

There is a clear trend for a greater tendency in robotic RYGB to perform the gastrojejunal anastomosis in a sutured fashion rather than as a stapled anastomosis in the laparoscopic approach [3]. When a circular stapler is used for the anastomosis, the fascial defect created by the introduction of the circular stapler is usually closed to prevent a hernia. This closure is often the source of the greatest pain and can be eliminated by performing this anastomosis as a sutured anastomosis.

Tips and Tricks

RYGB is considered to be a moderately difficult procedure, and there are patient factors that can make this procedure very difficult. Having performed nearly 2000 robotic RYGB to date, I have learned a few tricks that help to make this procedure simpler:

- When exposing the angle of His and resecting the fat pad, take the additional step of exposing down on the left crus as far posterior as you can. This will facilitate the creation of the window at the angle of His from below for the last staple fire in creating the gastric pouch.
- If you encounter difficulties because of patient anatomy in creating the window at the angle of His, use a gauze to pack down at the angle of His. This gauze serves the purpose of pushing the spleen away to help avoid inadvertent injury and also serves as a marker to look for when dissecting from below.
- When creating the gastrotomy and enterotomy for the gastrojejunal anastomosis, use a needle to tent up the gastric pouch or jejunum (Fig. 32.15).
- Two Vicryl or PDS sutures can be tied together to create a double-armed suture for the inner row of the gastrojejunal anastomosis. Two sutures cut to 7 in. and tied together with at least two knots is an ideal suture length for the anastomosis. If the first stitch is taken in an inside-out fashion, the knot ends up inside the lumen and serves to stop the suture at the midpoint.
- Creation of an initial loop gastrojejunostomy will shift the operation more cephalad, particularly the creation of the jejuno-jejunal anastomosis. Additionally, the flow of the operation seems more efficient to create the loop anastomosis, divide the loop, create the jejuno-jejunal anastomosis, and then close the two defects. All of these steps are contained in a relatively small space in the abdomen, so it is not necessary to reposition anything.
- Sometimes exposing Petersen's space can be difficult. Grasping the transverse mesocolon just below the colon at approximately the midpoint of the transverse colon and retracting it toward the gastric pouch as far up as it will go with the lateral arm on the right hand is a simple way to consistently provide nice exposure of this defect for closure.

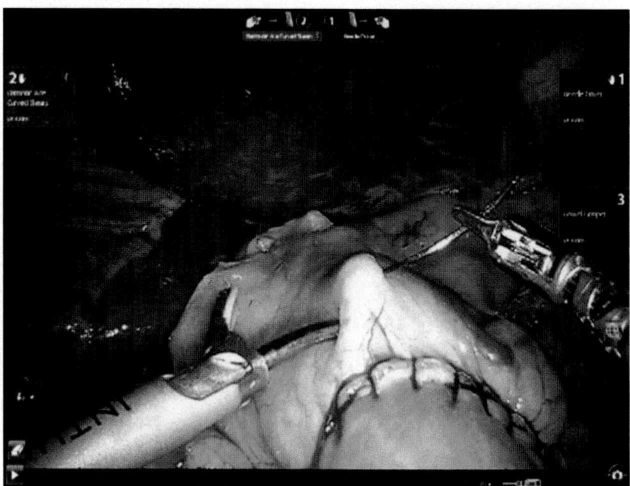

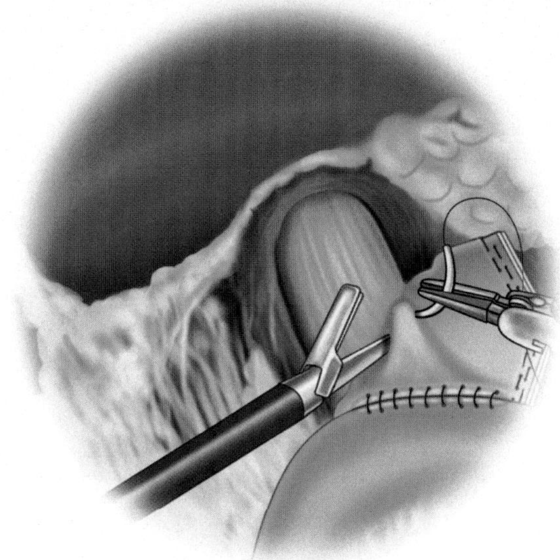

Fig. 32.15 When creating the gastrotomy and enterotomy for the gastrojejunal anastomosis, use a needle to tent up the gastric pouch or jejunum

Procedural Differences Using the da Vinci® Xi System

The Xi system represents the fourth generation of the da Vinci® robotic system. It also represents the most significant change in its platform, with boom-mounted arms instead of the pedestal-mounted arms that were featured in the three previous generations. Other notable changes to the system make it easier to position and dock the patient cart (particularly for novice users), allow for closer positioning of trocars, reduce external collision, allow for greater flexibility in positioning the patient cart relative to the patient anatomy, and facilitate multiquadrant surgery. Additionally, the Xi system can be coupled with a specially designed bed that moves in coordination with the robotic arms, so that the patient position can be changed without having to undock the arms. Here is a list of specific features of the Xi system:

- Robotic arms mounted on an overhead boom that allows the arms to rotate as a group.
- Smaller, lighter arms with an extended range of motion.
- Longer instruments for extended reach inside the abdomen.
- Docking facilitated by a laser targeting system; the endoscope can be pointed at the target anatomy, and when the targeting button is pushed, the system will configure itself to the optimal position for the procedure.
- A smaller, lighter 8-mm endoscope that is self-calibrating, can be sterilized, and can be docked to any of the arms, so this endoscope can be switched to any of the four arms during the procedure.
- Availability of a specialty bed that communicates and moves with the robotic arms so that the patient can be repositioned without undocking the arms.
- Availability of a white load on the robotic stapler in addition to the green and blue loads available on the Si system.
- An additional motor built into the robotic arms, which drives the stapler on the Xi, allowing the stapler to be lighter, smaller, and potentially more economical. In contrast, the stapler on the Si has the motor contained within the stapler itself.

Although these changes can have a dramatic impact on a procedure such as biliopancreatic diversion with duodenal switch, which requires multiquadrant access, their impact on the RYGB, which is performed with a single docking, is less significant. The overhead boom-mounted arms do allow the patient cart to be positioned at the side of the patient opposite the assistant, giving anesthesia access to the head of the patient and facilitating intraoperative endoscopy. Additionally, the smaller arms and the different joint orientation allow for more flexibility in trocar positioning and closer positioning of the trocars, which can be very helpful in patients with lower BMI. Lastly, the addition of the white load to the robotic stapler makes it more attractive to use the robotic stapler for the RYGB, making this a truly totally robotic procedure. This change is very appealing for surgeons who are uncomfortable with having a bedside assistant perform the stapling portions of the case.

References

1. NIH Conference. Gastrointestinal surgery for severe obesity. Consensus development conference panel. Ann Intern Med. 1991;115:956–61.
2. Cohen RV, Pinheiro JC, Schiavon CA, Salles JE, Wajchenberg BL, Cummings DE. Effects of gastric bypass surgery in patients with type 2 diabetes and only mild obesity. Diabetes Care. 2012;35:1420–8.
3. Bailey JG, Hayden JA, Davis PJ, Liu RY, Haardt D, Ellsmere J. Robotic versus laparoscopic Roux-en-Y gastric bypass (RYGB) in obese adults ages 18 to 65 years: a systematic review and economic analysis. Surg Endosc. 2014;28:414–26.
4. Rosser JC Jr, Gentile DA, Hanigan K, Danner OK. The effect of video game "warm-up" on performance of laparoscopic surgery tasks. JSLS. 2012;16:3–9.
5. Fourman MM, Saber AA. Robotic bariatric surgery: a systematic review. Surg Obes Relat Dis. 2012;8:483–8.
6. Markar SR, Karthikesalingam AP, Venkat-Ramen V, Kinross J, Ziprin P. Robotic vs. laparoscopic Roux-en-Y gastric bypass in morbidly obese patients: systematic review and pooled analysis. Int J Med Robot. 2011;7:393–400.

Robotic Operations for Gastroesophageal Reflux Disease

33

Daniel H. Dunn, Eric M. Johnson, Tor C. Aasheim, and Nilanjana Banerji

Introduction

Gastroesophageal reflux disease (GERD) is a common affliction treated in most instances with over-the-counter antireflux medications, generic proton pump inhibitors (PPIs), and various combinations of these treatments. In the past, surgical interventions for uncomplicated GERD have been reserved for patients who have severe symptoms without relief over prolonged periods of treatment [7]. More recently, the cost of medical treatment and the detrimental effect of uncontrolled heartburn on quality of life, in certain instances, validate surgical management as a superior and more reliable alternative for patients. In addition, there are concerns regarding upper gastrointestinal tract cancer risks with prolonged use of PPIs [8, 9]. Minimally invasive operations for GERD are safe and relatively easily tolerated, with short hospital stays and minimal discomfort [3, 4]. Patients usually are able to return to work in most instances within 1–2 weeks for desk work and 4 weeks for more physically demanding work.

In certain instances, significant side effects have been noted with surgical interventions for GERD management. Nissen fundoplication (full, 360-degree wrap) and Toupet (partial, 270-degree wrap) surgical procedures have reliable, reproducible short-term and long-term results [10–12]. These procedures can be (and typically are) performed with minimally invasive techniques. Laparoscopic techniques result in promising outcomes in most cases, but recurrent symptoms of heartburn, dysphagia, stricture, and recurrent hiatus hernia requiring reoperation have been noted within 5 years in 25–35% of individuals in published literature [7, 13]. Vexing side effects of dysphagia (e.g., gas-bloat syndrome, an inability to belch or vomit) prevent many patients from pursuing surgical management.

The LINX® magnetic esophageal sphincter augmentation system (Torax Medical, St. Paul, MN) received approval from the US Food and Drug Administration (FDA) in 2013 [14–16]. LINX® is a considerably simpler, easier, and a more predictable surgical intervention for GERD management than Nissen or Toupet procedures. It is an outpatient procedure, with 95% of patients being discharged on the same day. Return to work is faster and postoperative restrictions are fewer. At 5 years, 95% of patients are off PPIs [14, 15]. There is minimal gas bloat, and patients are able to vomit. However, the novelty of the procedure and challenges with insurance coverage have hampered the adoption of LINX® placement as a standard procedure in most surgical centers (personal communication, 2015).

Robot-assisted operations for GERD yield results that are comparable to those of laparoscopic procedures—and, in some instances, better. Consequently, use of robotic technology by gastrointestinal surgeons has become more prevalent, especially in general surgery [17]. General surgeons have adopted the robotic technology to the point that general surgery is the fastest growing specialty using robotic technology [18–20]. Utilizing robotic surgical procedures is advantageous for a surgeon, as 3D visualization has strong advantages, especially for large paraesophageal hernias or more complicated anatomy. The instrumentation continues to improve, with staplers that are substantially easier to manipulate. The latest da Vinci® model XI (Intuitive Surgical, Sunnyvalle, CA) allows visualization of all abdominal quadrants with equal ease and definition [21, 22]. Such advancements in knowledge have changed the indications for robotic technology from operating on one focused area of the abdomen to equal visualization of all quadrants, which is required for many gastrointestinal procedures.

D. H. Dunn, MD (✉) · E. M. Johnson, MD · T. C. Aasheim, MD
Department of Surgery, Abbott Northwestern Hospital, Minneapolis, MN, USA
e-mail: docdunn3@comcast.net; embjohnson@comcast.net

N. Banerji, MS, PhD
Neuroscience and Rehabilitation Research, Abbott Northwestern Hospital, Minneapolis, MN, USA

Y. Fong et al. (eds.), *The SAGES Atlas of Robotic Surgery*, https://doi.org/10.1007/978-3-319-91045-1_33

Preoperative Evaluations

Patients who have symptoms consistent with GERD should be carefully evaluated before considering operation. Heartburn-like symptoms do not necessarily come from acid reflux. Cardiac chest pain can be indistinguishable from heartburn. Heartburn that does not improve with medical management may not be reflux and may not improve if an antireflux procedure is performed. The patient may have a large hiatus hernia and partial outlet obstruction, which can present with similar GERD symptoms, such as chest pain. Gastritis, peptic ulcer disease, esophageal dysmotility, or even achalasia may present with similar symptoms. Thus, a clinical workup to prove GERD or determine the anatomy of the upper gastrointestinal tract is essential.

A barium upper gastrointestinal study provides important information about the anatomy and motility of the esophagus and stomach and will document GERD [23]. If gastroesophageal reflux is not seen on an adequate upper gastrointestinal tract study, GERD cannot essentially be eliminated, however, and additional testing must be performed to ascertain GERD.

The gold standard for documentation of GERD is the use of a pH probe or pH monitoring. This test gives a qualitative and a quantitative response as to the degree of reflux present, whether the reflux is postprandial, and the rate of acid clearance from the esophagus. Multichannel intraluminal impedance-pH monitoring is an alternative test that yields similar results but can also distinguish nonacid reflux [6].

Esophageal manometry is used in the workup of patients with presumed GERD. Manometry is especially important if patients have dysphagia and a symptom of heartburn or atypical symptoms with no evidence of reflux in the upper gastrointestinal tract. Patients with achalasia are often misdiagnosed with GERD before they undergo a complete workup. Such patients are often treated for reflux for extended periods before they undergo manometry.

Robotic Surgeries for GERD

Nissen Fundoplication

For a Nissen fundoplication, the patient is anesthetized in a normal supine position. After necessary lines are placed, the operating room table is shifted such that the patient's head is away from the anesthesiologist and the tubing is tracked along the side of the operating table. Throughout the operation, the anesthesiologist remains at the foot of the OR table. Frequently, especially with patients who have comorbid conditions, arterial and venous monitoring lines are placed. The first trocar is placed 12 cm below the xiphoid and 4 cm to the left in women, and 15 cm below the xiphoid and 4 cm to the left in men. The reason for placement off the midline to the left is to be in line with the hiatus. The remaining trocars are placed in relation to the first trocar, which is the camera port. Two trocars are placed 4 cm cephalad and 8 cm to the left and right, on either side of the camera port. A separate trocar is placed below the right costal margin for liver retraction, and the last port is placed as an assistant port, to the left at a place suitable, usually laterally below the costal margin. These trocars are placed under direct laparoscopic control after the camera port has been placed. In addition, the liver retractor is placed laparoscopically.

The robot is then brought into the operative field and positioned using the camera port to center the robot. The patient is then placed in a reverse Trendelenburg position and the robotic arms are attached to the trocars, followed by introduction of the robotic camera. The operator subsequently proceeds to the robot and begins the operation. The surgical procedure starts with a dissection of the lesser curvature, exposing the right crus of the diaphragm (Fig. 33.1). Of note, mobilization of the esophagus and stomach off the diaphragm may be challenging in obese patients with excess upper abdominal fat. Afterward, the dissection continues

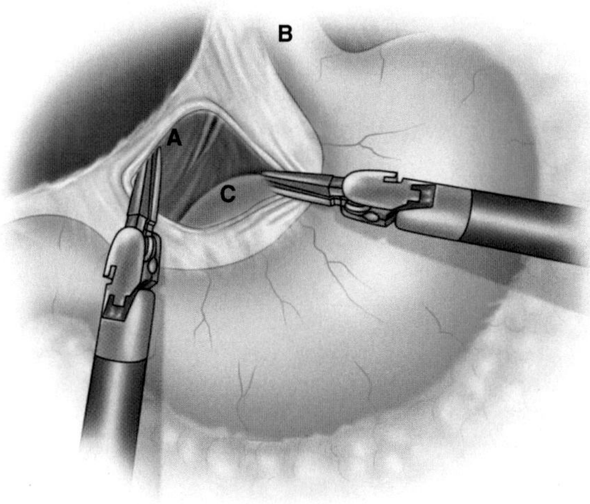

Fig. 33.1 Dissection of the lesser curvature. *A*, Right crus. *B*, Esophagus. *C*, Hernia sac over left crus

along the anterior hiatus and left crus. Once the anterior diaphragm is cleared of all attachments to the esophagus, the dissection is carried posteriorly to free up the esophagus and stomach circumferentially (Fig. 33.2). At this stage, identification and preservation of the posterior vagus nerve is imperative (Fig. 33.3). Subsequently, the anterior vagus nerve is dissected off the esophagus with the associated gastroesophageal fat pad. It remains attached to the stomach at the gas-

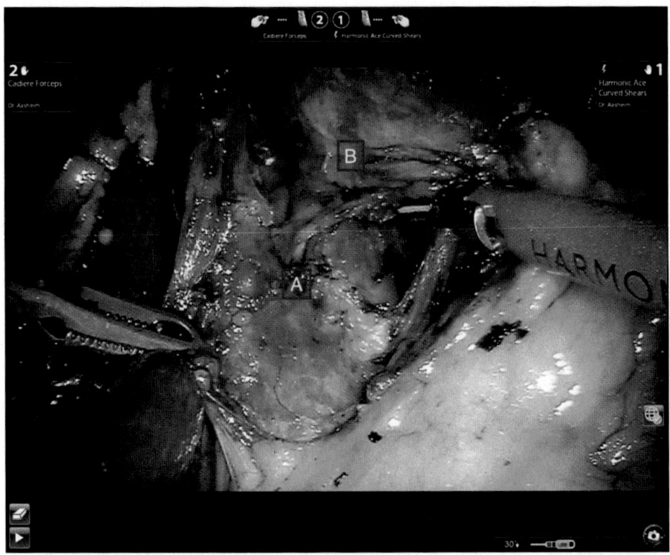

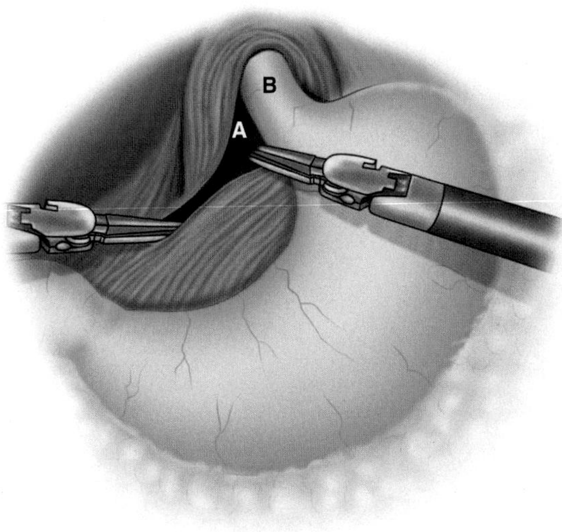

Fig. 33.2 Dissection carried posteriorly to free up the esophagus and stomach. *A*, Posterior junction of the left and right crura. *B*, Esophagus

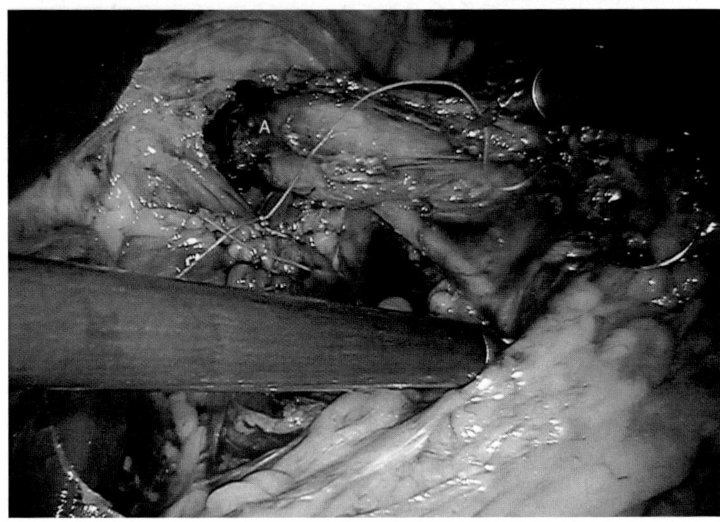

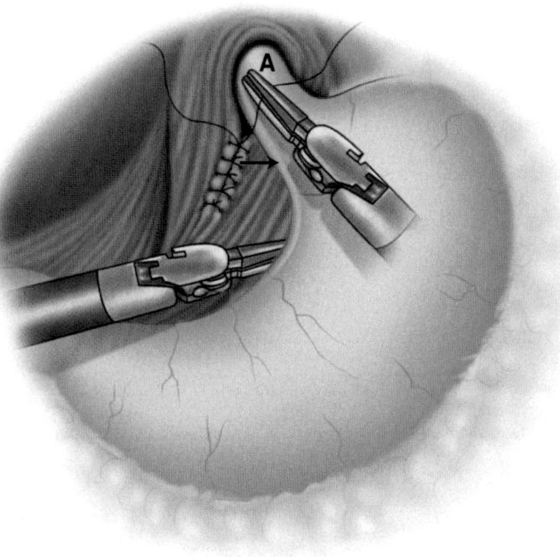

Fig. 33.3 Closure of diaphragm with preservation of the posterior vagus nerve (*arrow*). *A*, Esophagus without dilator.

troesophageal (GE) junction and provides a sling that assists in holding the wrap in position as the fundoplication is brought under the dissected anterior vagus (Fig. 33.4). It is important to dissect the gastroesophageal fat pad, as this dissection defines the GE junction and clears it of any fat, which may cause the wrap to loosen or even slip over time (Fig. 33.5).

If the esophagus is foreshortened, it must be mobilized in the mediastinum. This dissection is performed more easily with the robot than with a laparoscopic approach. The 3D visualization of structures provided by robotic technology results in a more meticulous dissection. The goal of the mediastinal dissection is to provide at least a 3-cm length of esophagus in the abdomen inferior to the hiatus, without

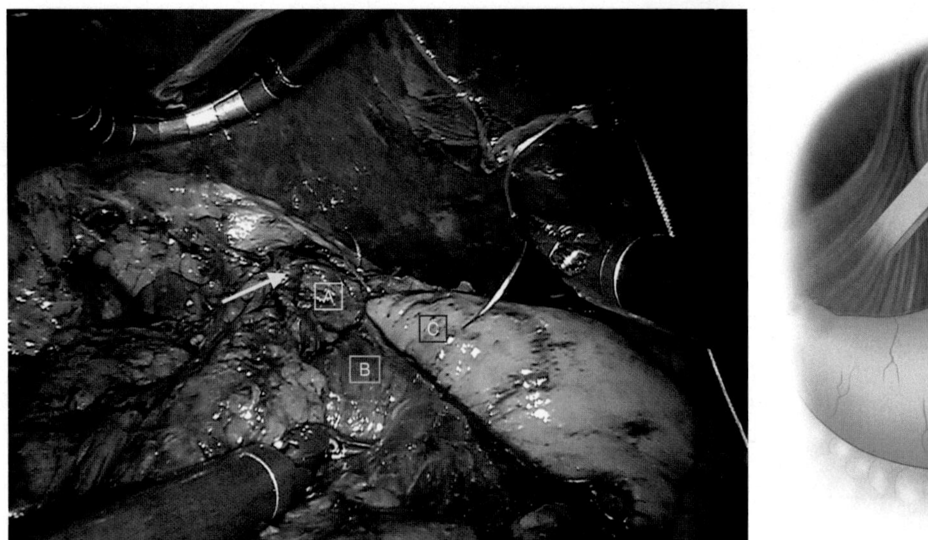

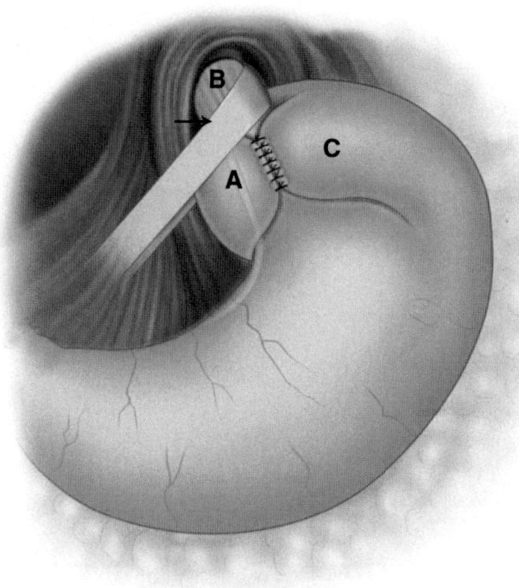

Fig. 33.4 'Sling' of anterior vagus to prevent slipping of the wrap (*arrow*). *A*, Right-sided fundus beneath the sling. *B*, Esophagus. *C*, Left-sided fundus

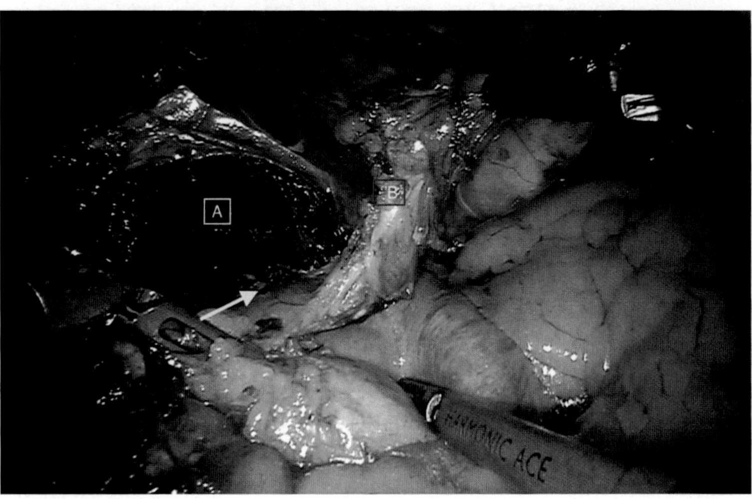

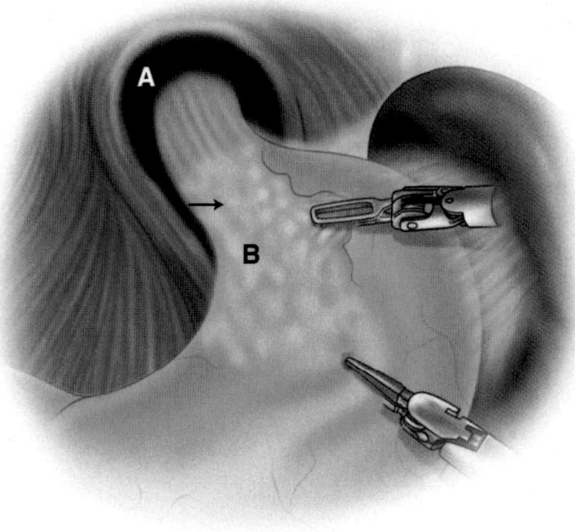

Fig. 33.5 Gastroesophageal (GE) junction with gastroesophageal fat pad and hernia sac (*arrow*). *A*, Hiatal hernia cavity. *B*, Residual gastroesophageal fat pad and hernia sac

requiring tension to hold it there. Once this dissection is completed, the short gastric vessels must be divided to mobilize the fundus enough to wrap around the esophagus without tension. The number of short gastric vessels that need to be divided may vary depending on the individual's anatomy, the size of the hernia, and the volume of stomach contained in the hernia sac (Fig. 33.6).

After clearing of the hiatus and adequate mobilization of the esophagus and the fundus of the stomach, the hiatus must be repaired. Dissection of the hiatus itself creates a larger defect, and dissection of the phrenoesophageal ligaments results in fewer attachments to retain the esophagus in place. The fundoplication itself assists with holding the esophagus below the diaphragm and with closing the hiatus.

Repair of the diaphragm is performed over a dilator. The size of the dilator generally ranges from 50 to 60 Fr and should be chosen with the patient's size and body habitus in mind. Surgeons' preferences generally determine the size of the dilator; there is no "one size fits all" paradigm. It is imperative to have an experienced anesthesiologist pass the dilator. It is also important that the surgeon and anesthesiologist work in tandem during the passing of the dilator to ensure that the surgeon is aware of the dilator's visibility as it moves through the hiatus. Perforating the esophagus with the dilator is a catastrophic complication that is always avoidable if care is taken.

Once the dilator is in place, the hiatus can be closed (Fig. 33.7). This suturing is significantly easier with the robot

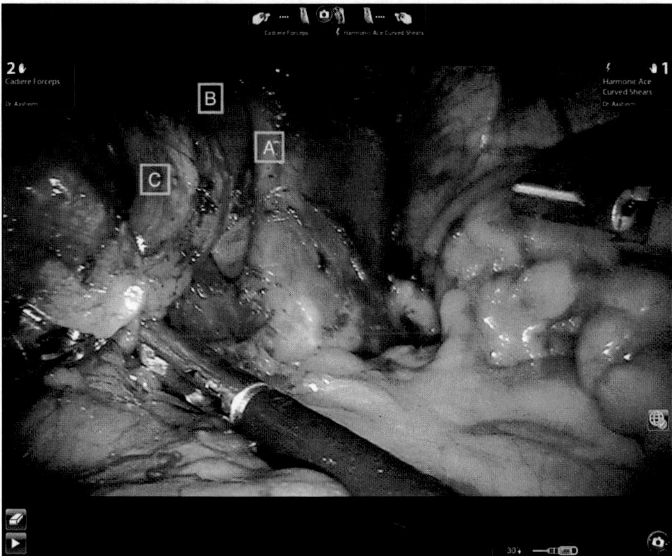

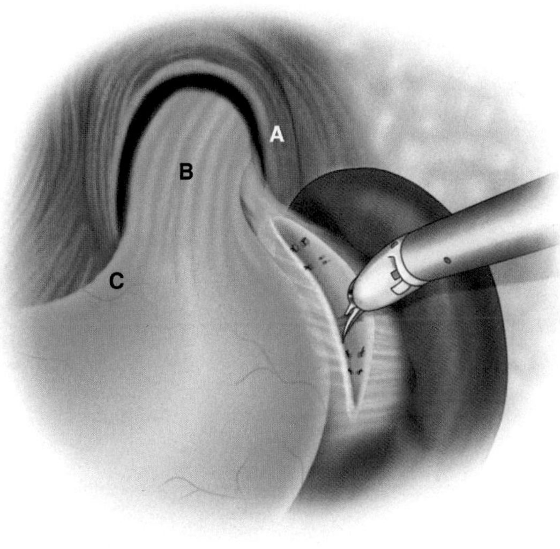

Fig. 33.6 Division of short gastric vessels. *A*, Left crus. *B*, Esophagus. *C*, Fundus of stomach after removal of short gastric vessels

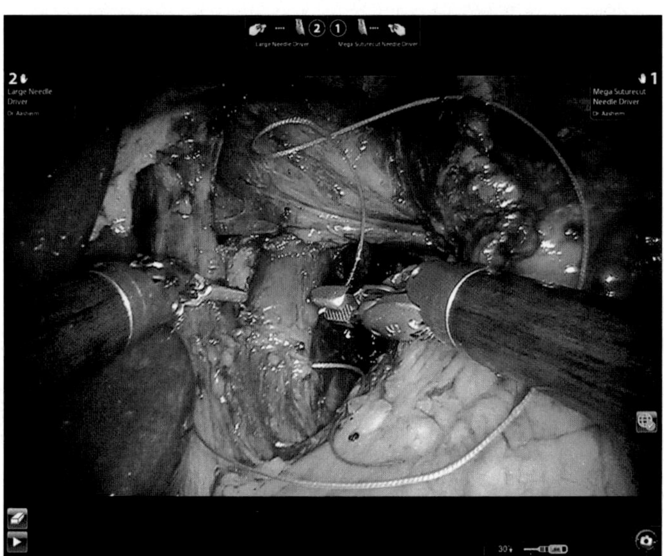

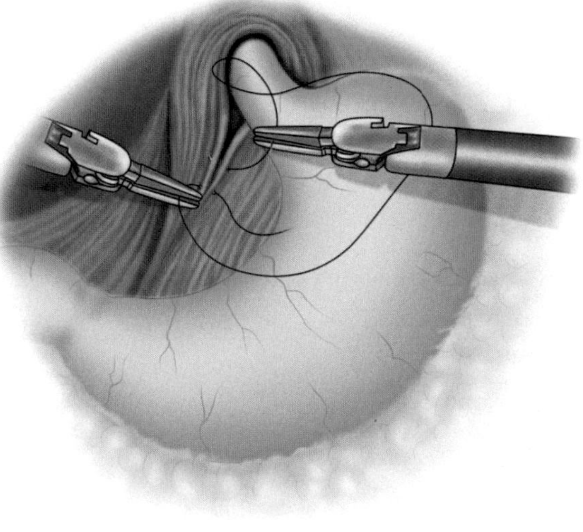

Fig. 33.7 Closure of the hiatus

than suturing with laparoscopic technology. Stitches can be placed similarly to those during an open technique. A figure-of-eight suture is more secure than single stitches (Fig. 33.8). In addition, this process ensures minimal muscle manipulation, thereby making certain that the muscle is not shredded. If possible, the peritoneum attached to the diaphragm should be left attached to the crura to prevent shredding of the crural muscle. If the hiatus defect is large or the crura are thin, then pledgets are helpful to provide additional strength to the closure. If pledgets are to be used, the suturing method should be slightly different. Instead of a figure-of-eight closure, a "U"-type stitch should be used, which will provide a more secure closure (Fig. 33.9). Additionally, reinforcement with an onlay biologic mesh has been reported to decrease the incidence of hernia recurrence [24]. Biologics should not be used as a bridge because of eventration of the mesh over time. Permanent mesh must be used judiciously, as it may cause erosion of the esophagus.

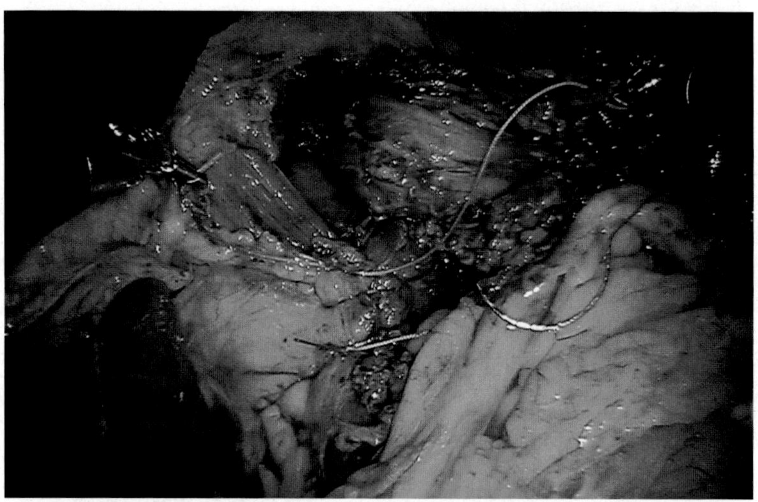
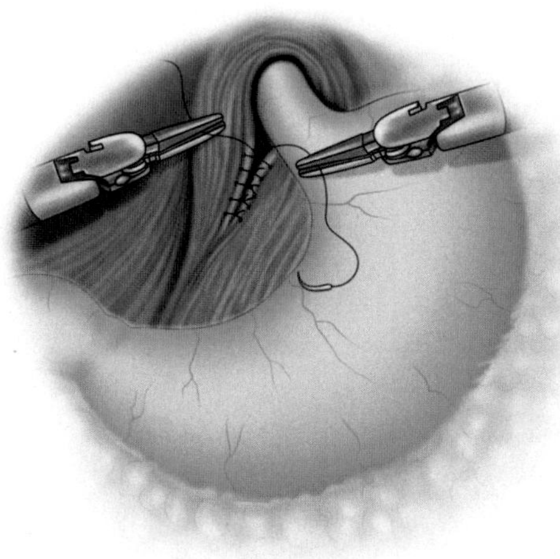

Fig. 33.8 Closure of the diaphragm with figure-of-eight stitches

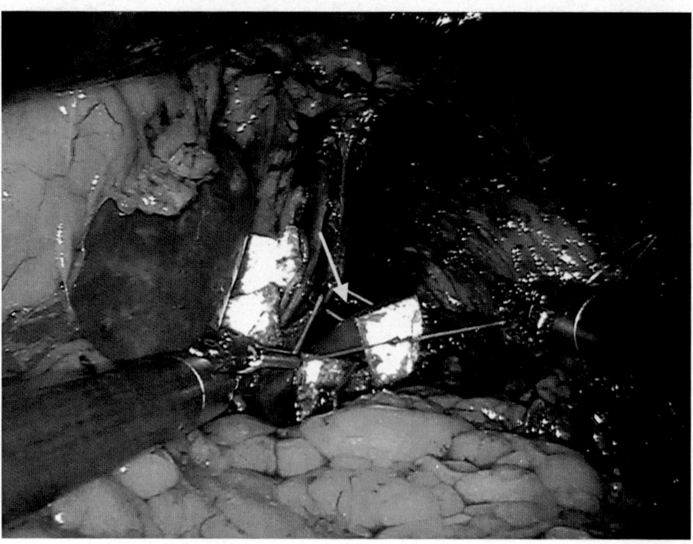
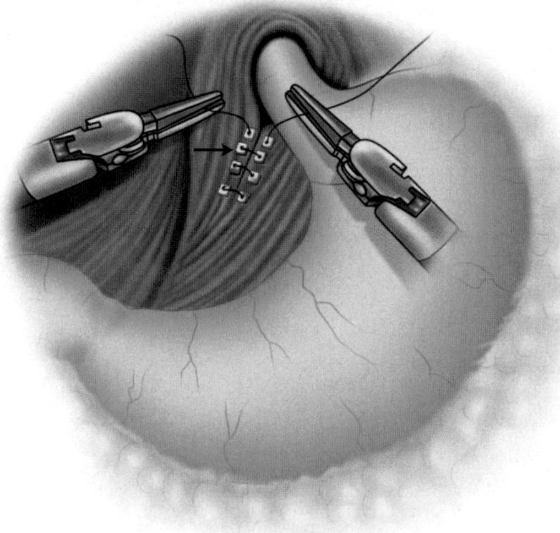

Fig. 33.9 Teflon pledgets and 'U' stitch (*arrow*) to compress the crura together

If the intra-abdominal esophagus appears to be short of the required 3 cm after the maximum length of the esophagus has been obtained by mobilizing the esophagus in the mediastinum, it is prudent to first repair the diaphragm and then determine whether any further length of intra-abdominal esophagus is required. As the diaphragm is dome-shaped, the anterior hiatus is cephalad to the posterior hiatus, and closing the hiatus pushes the esophagus into an anterior position, which in many instances is the 2–3 cm cephalad required. If the esophagus still has no significant length in the abdomen, then a Collis gastroplasty should be performed. Collis gastroplasty for a foreshortened esophagus will decrease the incidence of a recurrent hiatus hernia.

Fundoplication is initiated by placing a clamp behind the esophagus at the diaphragm, followed by passing the fundus to the clamp. Subsequently, the fundus is passed beneath the anterior vagal sling to prevent the wrap from slipping down onto the stomach. The portion of the fundus, which remains on the patient's left side, is grasped and brought up to the fundus from the right side. Stitches are then placed 1 cm apart to make a 3-cm wrap. Every stitch includes left fundus, esophagus, and right fundus. The fundus can then be tacked to the diaphragm in several places to prevent development of a recurrent hernia (Fig. 33.10).

There are several keys to a successful, durable fundoplication:

- Adequate workup to evaluate the patient, to make an accurate diagnosis and exclude contraindications for a Nissen fundoplication
- Mobilization of the esophagus and proximal stomach to have 3 cm of esophagus below the diaphragm without tension
- Removal of the gastroesophageal fat pad
- Adequate closure of the diaphragm over a 50–60 Fr dilator
- Preservation of the anterior and posterior vagus nerves
- Using biological mesh for the closure of the hiatus (if necessary) as an onlay, not as a bridge
- Judicious use of synthetic mesh to repair the hiatus, in order to prevent erosion into the esophagus

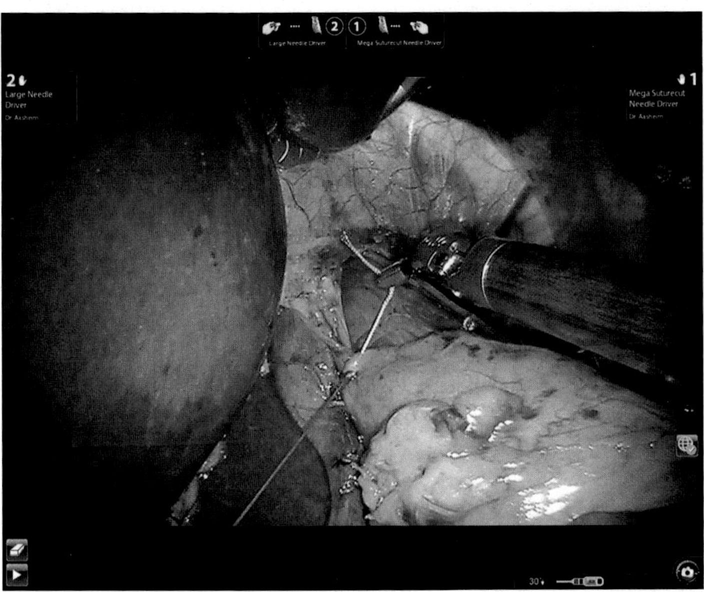

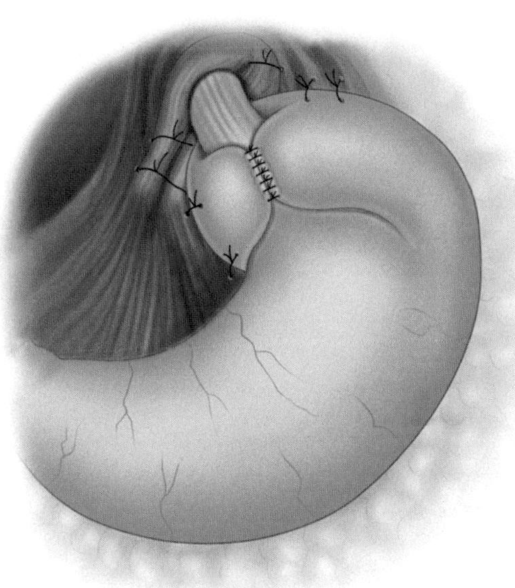

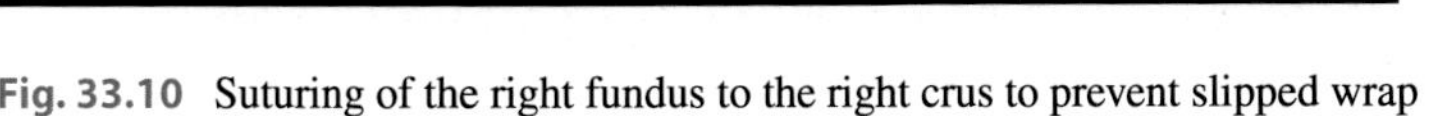

Fig. 33.10 Suturing of the right fundus to the right crus to prevent slipped wrap

Paraesophageal Hiatus Hernia Repair and Nissen Fundoplication

Repair of a paraesophageal hiatus hernia can be challenging, as it is associated with a higher recurrence rate and more complications. Paraesophageal hernias are also usually larger than sliding hernias, and robotic technology has both advantages and disadvantages for repair of large hernias. There have been several classifications of paraesophageal hernias, which are helpful to consider during planning the surgical procedure. That being said, the basic principles of repair of large and small hernias are essentially the same. The entire hernia sac must be taken down from the chest cavity (Fig. 33.11). Mobilization of the esophagus is important. The anterior and posterior vagus nerves must be dissected and preserved. At the beginning of the dissection, the peritoneum at the anterior hiatus is grasped and pulled away from the diaphragm, followed by opening and clearing off of the hiatus. In doing so, a plane is developed between the hernia sac and mediastinal structures such as the pericardium and pleura (Fig. 33.12). If the hernia is very large, the esophagus as well as the apex of the mediastinum can be visualized by pulling down on the peritoneum and bluntly dissecting the hernia sac off the pericardium. By pulling down on the peritoneum, the stomach comes down with the hernia sac. Subsequently, lateral and posterior dissection should be continued in the same plane. Vascular structures on the right crus should be identified in this dissection. Left gastric vessels are

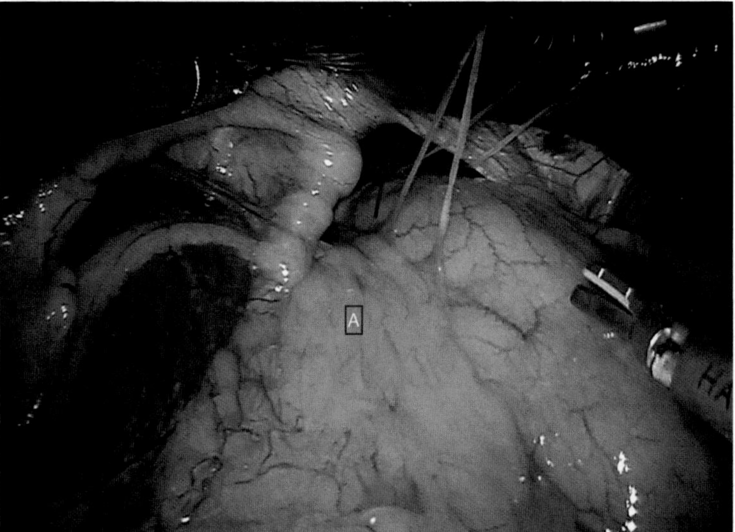

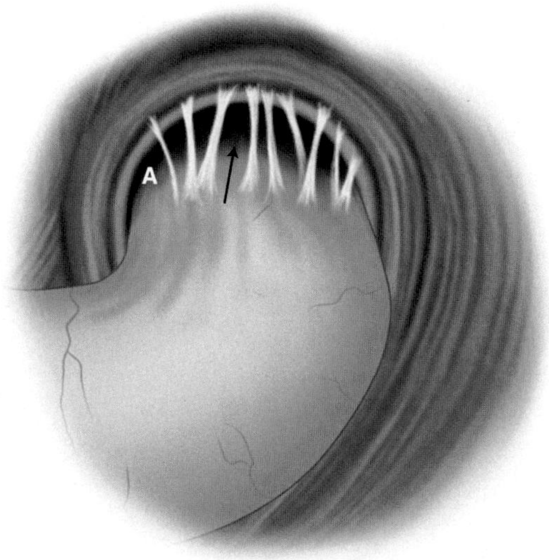

Fig. 33.11 Large paraesophageal hiatus hernia (*arrow*). *A*, Course of left gastric vessels through the hiatus

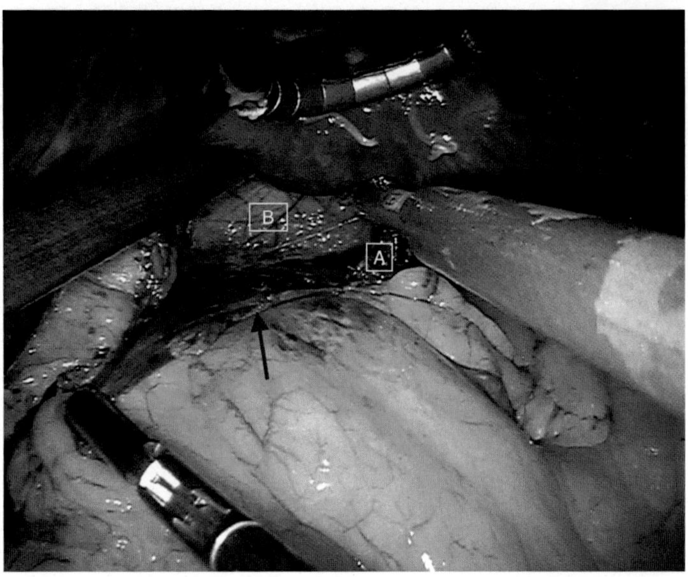

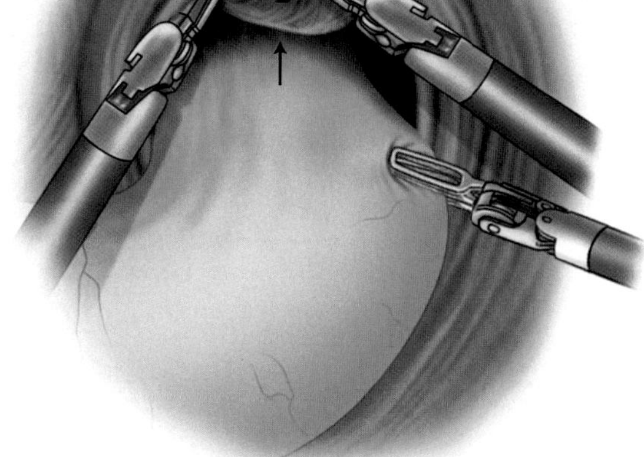

Fig. 33.12 Paraesophageal hernia sac (*arrow*). *A*, Left crus. *B*, Pericardium

usually pulled up into the chest with the stomach (Fig. 33.13). While taking down the hernia sac along the right crus, care must be taken to ensure that the dissection remains in the same plane. If the left gastric artery is erroneously cut, the vessel may retract into the chest, especially if attachments to the hernia sac have not been dissected. A similar error can be made on the left crus, as the short gastric vessels are likewise pulled into the hernia sac.

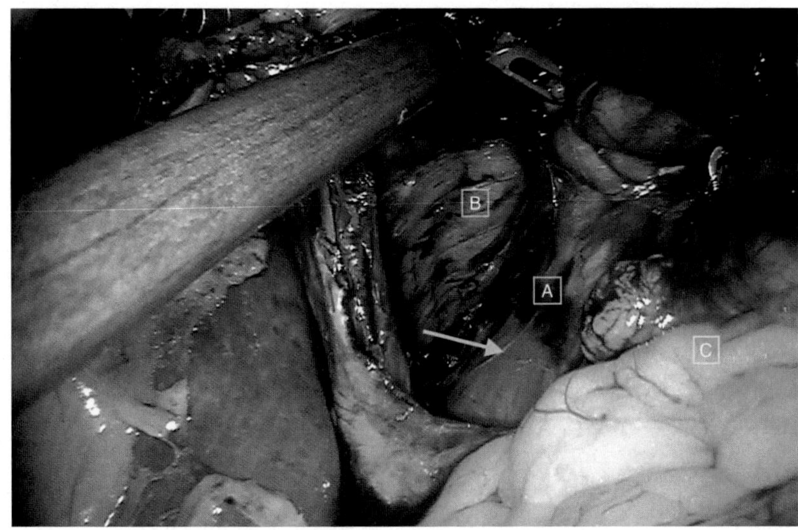

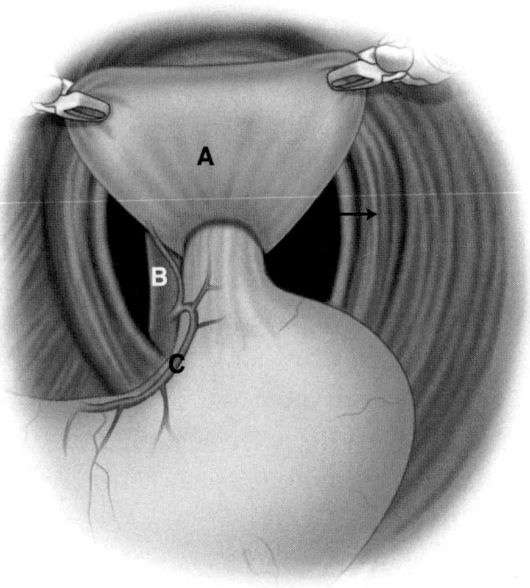

Fig. 33.13 Left crus (*arrow*). *A*, Edge of posterior hernia sac. *B*, Aorta. *C*, Left gastric vessels

Partial Fundoplication: 270-Degree Fundoplication (Toupet Procedure) and Dor Fundoplication (Anterior Partial Fundoplication)

Patients with dysphagia and reflux symptoms require careful evaluation. GERD with resultant Barrett's esophagus increases the risk of adenocarcinoma of the esophagus [25–27]. If a patient with known Barrett's develops dysphagia, the initial diagnosis to be ruled out is esophageal cancer. Other causes of dysphagia in this group of patients are peptic strictures and esophageal dysmotility [28]. Diagnostic endoscopy is important to rule out these diagnoses. Endoscopy can also be therapeutic in patients with stricture, as a dilation can be performed to make a treatment decision regarding improving medical management versus proceeding with surgical management. Once cancer and esophageal stricture have been ruled out, patients should undergo esophageal manometry to determine the presence of esophageal dysmotility. This thorough workup will reduce the likelihood of operating for a GERD diagnosis when a complete evaluation might show dysmotility or achalasia.

Partial fundoplication is indicated in patients with esophageal dysmotility. The Toupet procedure is similar in all respects to a full-wrap Nissen fundoplication, except that the fundus, after being brought around behind the esophagus, is sutured at the 10 o'clock position of the mobilized esophagus with three stitches over a length of 3 cm. Additionally, the left side of the wrapped fundus is sutured to the esophagus at the 2 o'clock position, thereby leaving the anterior esophagus unincorporated in the wrap (Fig. 33.14). The result is reduced pressure on the esophagus at the GE junction and reduced dysphagia, while GERD is still controlled. Several series have reported satisfactory long-term results with the Toupet procedure when compared with a full wrap, even in patients who do not have dysphagia or esophageal dysmotility [11, 29].

A major advantage of the robotic technology is the similarity of suturing ability to an open case. This is true for both Toupet and Dor fundoplication procedures. The Dor fundoplication is most commonly used for patients with achalasia undergoing a Heller esophageal myotomy. The reported incidence of severe reflux with Heller myotomy is 30–50% in peer-reviewed literature [30]. With an anterior fundoplication, the incidence decreases to about 9–14%, and postprocedural reflux is usually relatively easy to control with medications [30]. Published reports indicate promising results with a Dor fundoplication for GERD, with fewer of the severe side effects of a Nissen [31, 32].

Dor fundoplication is an easier procedure than either a full wrap or 270-degree wrap because the short gastric vessels do not need to be divided. After mobilization of the esophagus and closure of the hiatus, the anterior fundus is grasped and stitches are placed through the full-thickness gastric fundus to the anterior esophagus 3–4 cm above the GE junction. Stitches are then placed to cover almost 50% of the anterior esophageal wall. The fundus is not attached to the posterior esophagus.

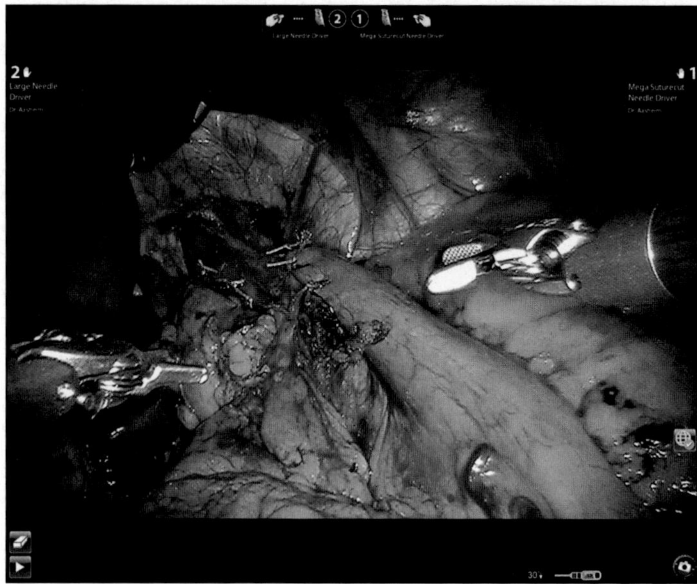

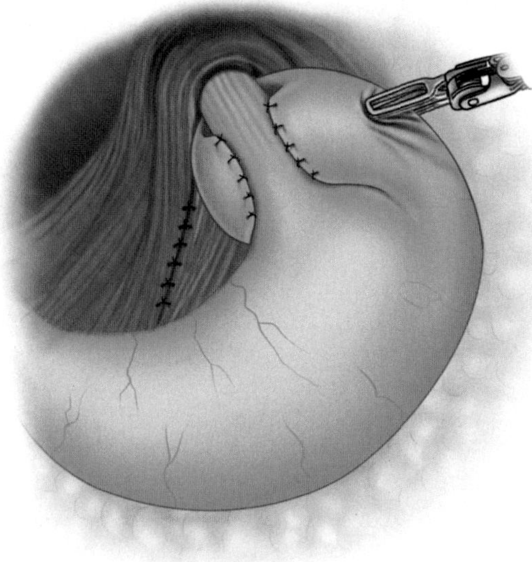

Fig. 33.14 Completed partial fundoplication with sutures at 10 o'clock and 2 o'clock

Collis Gastroplasty

Large paraesophageal hiatus hernias are often associated with a foreshortened esophagus. As a consequence, after hiatus hernia reduction, mobilization of the mediastinal esophagus, removal of the hernia sac, and closure of the hiatus, the esophagus still might not be visible in the abdomen, or it appears only minimally below the diaphragm. In this case, there are two options. One is to perform a gastropexy to hold the stomach in the abdomen. Unfortunately, gastropexy by itself has the potential of worsening GERD. A gastropexy creates an upside-down funnel, which may hold the GE junction open and cause severe reflux. This problem can be prevented by a modified Hill procedure, which imbricates circular fibers of the GE junction at the hiatus, with stitches that include both anterior and posterior cardia. The GE junction is then attached to the diaphragm. The Hill repair is usually not recommended for routine hiatus hernia repairs because of unacceptable recurrent symptoms.

The second option is a Collis gastroplasty. The recurrence rate for repair of large paraesophageal hernias is unacceptably high if the esophagus cannot be brought into the abdomen with at least 3 cm inferior to the diaphragmatic hiatus. If there is sufficient length without tension on the esophagus, a standard Nissen or Toupet can be performed. If <3 cm of esophagus is below the diaphragm, a Collis gastroplasty will reduce the risk of recurrent hernia [33]. Collis gastroplasty is an esophageal lengthening procedure, accomplished by taking a wedge out of the cardia of the stomach on the greater curvature side of the esophagus. Thus, when the fundus is wrapped around esophagus, in reality it is actually being wrapped around the residual cardia. This can be accomplished because only 2–3 cm of the cardia of the stomach is in the wrap, and the peristalsis of the esophagus above the wrapped cardia is carried passively through the wrap.

Collis gastroplasty can be performed robotically with special staplers available for robotic cases. These staplers are very functional and superior to the handheld stapler used by an assistant through a left lateral port. The procedure is similar to the paraesophageal hiatus hernia repair with a Nissen fundoplication, until the closure of the diaphragm. If the esophagus cannot be brought into the abdomen for 3 cm without tension, then a Collis gastroplasty should be considered. At this point, a dilator should be placed into the stomach to prevent narrowing of the "neo-esophagus" (Fig. 33.15). A 45-mm green-load stapler,

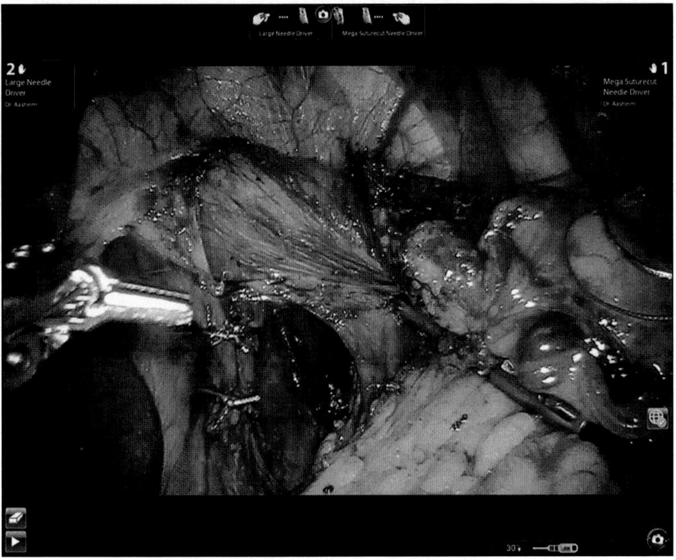

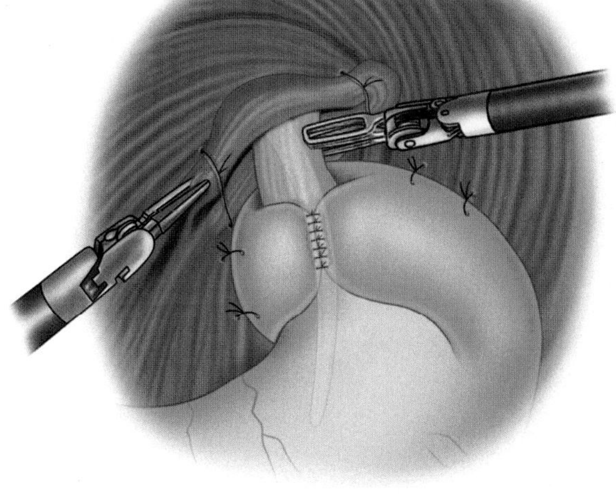

Fig. 33.15 Hiatus closure with dilator in the esophagus

which is easiest to manipulate in the upper abdomen, is brought into the abdomen and placed across the greater curvature near the cardia. The second staple load along the same line as the first load will approach the previously positioned dilator (Fig. 33.16). The third staple load should begin in the "crotch" of the stapled stomach and the dilator (Fig. 33.17).This load is oriented parallel with the dilator and in a cephalad direction. Subsequently, a fourth staple load may be required, which completes the wedge gastric resection (Fig. 33.18). Presently, the fundus is brought around the esophagus with the dilator in the esophagus. Afterward, the left-sided fundus is brought up and sutured to the right fundus with three stitches to complete the wrap (Figs. 33.19 and 33.20).

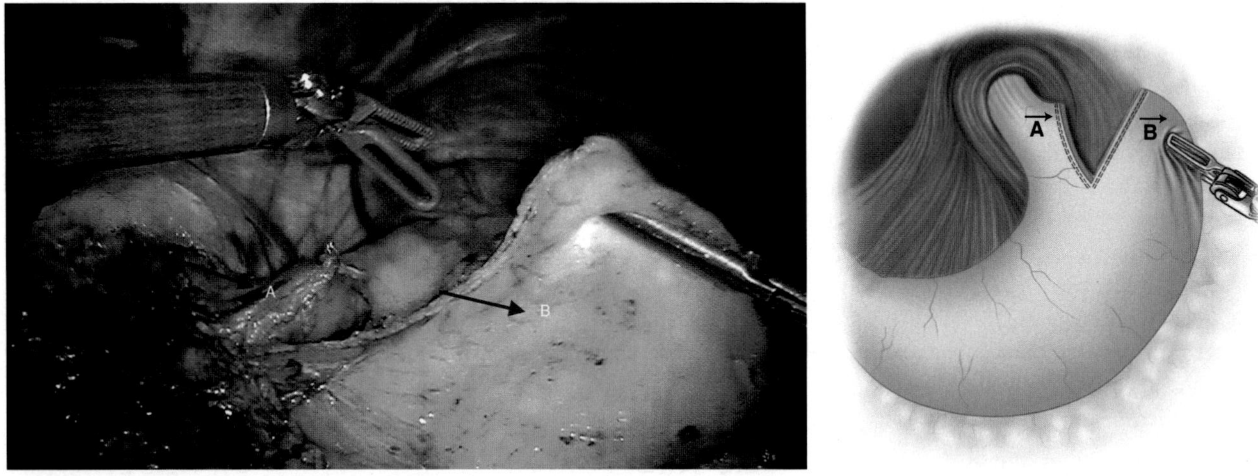

Fig. 33.16 Collis gastroplasty procedure with two staple lines placed with a 45-mm green-load Echelon™ stapler (Ethicon; Somerville, NJ). *A*, Remaining cardia. *B*, Fundus of the stomach

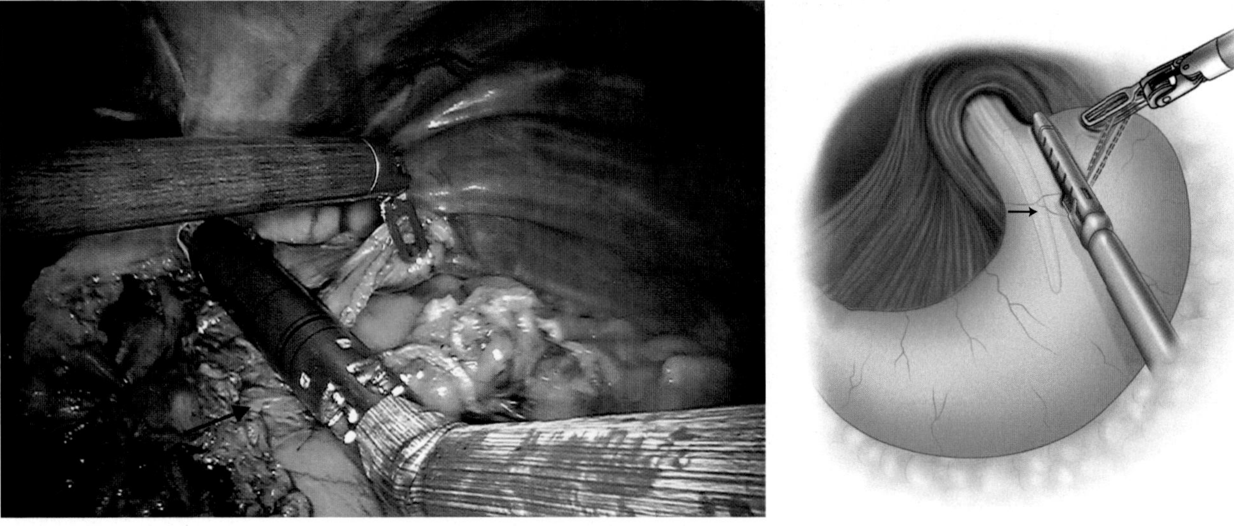

Fig. 33.17 Robotic stapler placed across the cardia parallel to the esophageal dilator (*arrow*)

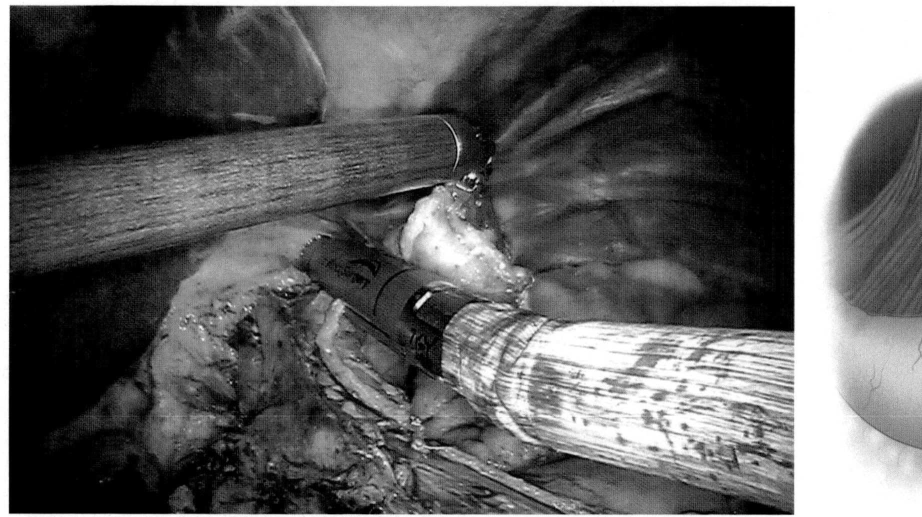

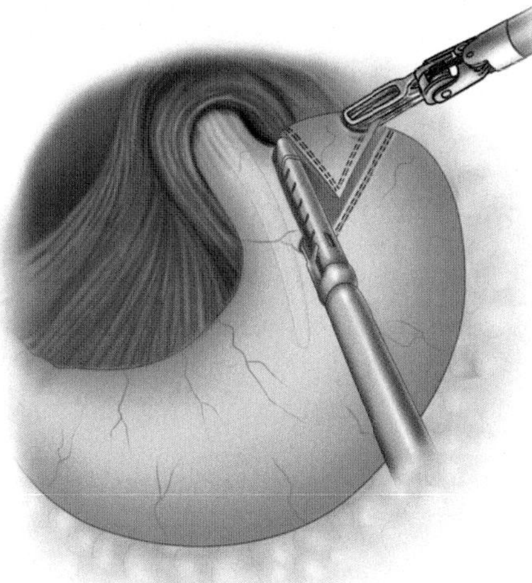

Fig. 33.18 Stapler completes the gastric wedge resection

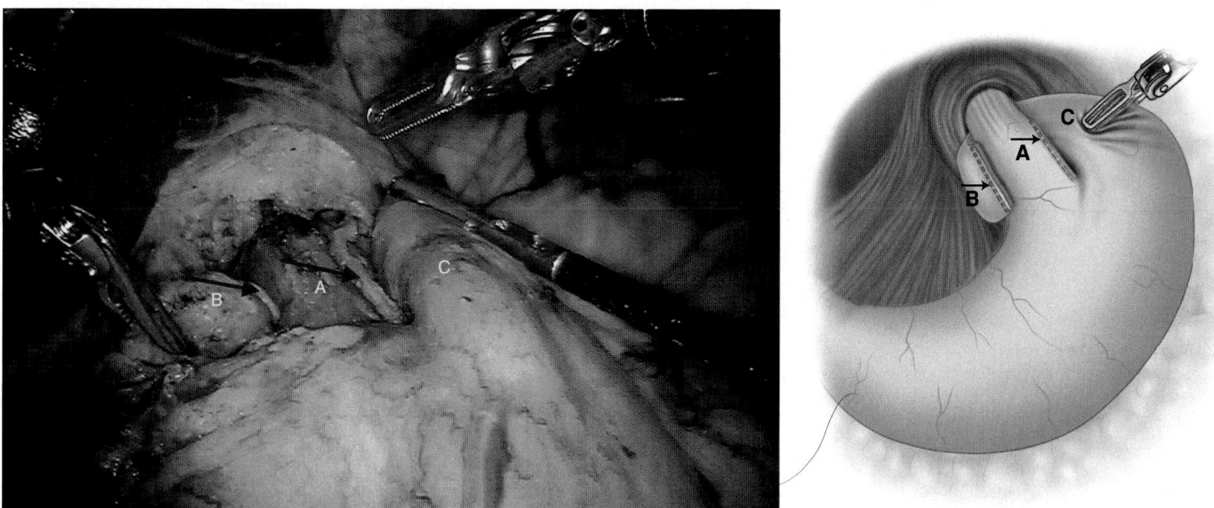

Fig. 33.19 Completion of the Collis gastroplasty wrap. *A*, Staple line on cardioesophageal junction. *B*, Staple line on remaining fundus pulled around behind the esophagus. *C*, Body of the stomach

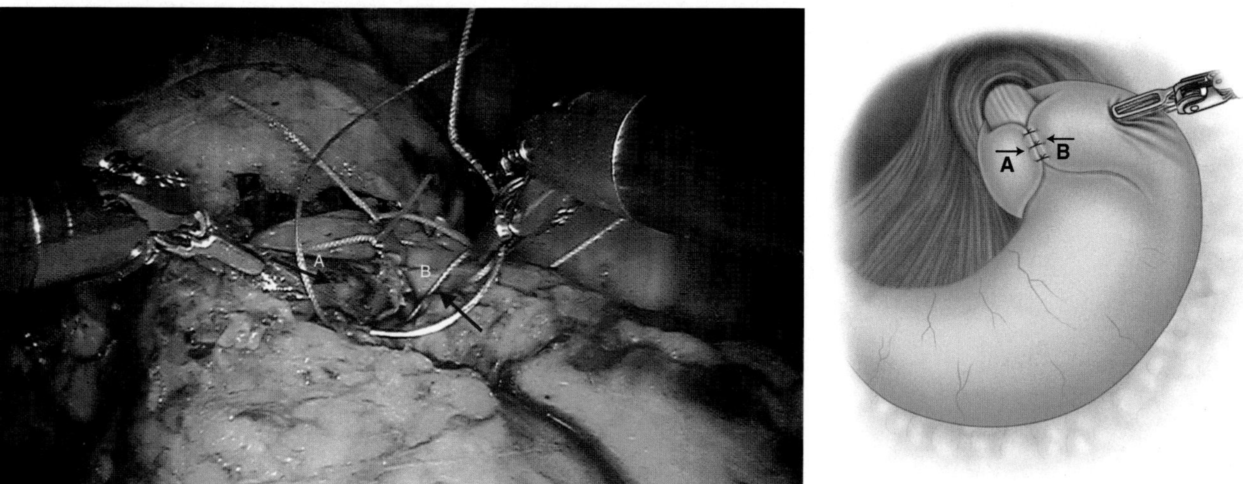

Fig. 33.20 Third stitch of Nissen fundoplication over a Collis gastroplasty. *A*, Right-side fundoplication. *B*, Left-side fundoplication

Robotic Operations for Recurrent Hiatus Hernia and Recurrent GERD and Complications of Hiatus Hernia Repair

Repeat surgical procedures of any kind are usually more difficult and challenging than the initial procedures. Reoperations for esophageal diseases are even more challenging, because exposure of the esophagus can be very difficult (Fig. 33.21). Additionally, an esophageal injury during the surgical procedure in the chest or mediastinum may require a thoracic approach to correct the problem. Recurrent hiatus hernia, in which the stomach or fundoplication are wedged into the hiatus and partially in the chest, demands a careful evaluation with an understanding of the altered anatomy (Figs. 33.22 and 33.23). It is necessary to have a well-thought-out plan and a clear justification for pursuing a laparoscopic, robotic, or open approach (Fig. 33.24). A general surgeon who decides to undertake a thoracic approach must confer with a thoracic surgeon. All possible surgical options must be explored, especially if a thoracic or thoracoscopic approach may be needed (Fig. 33.25).

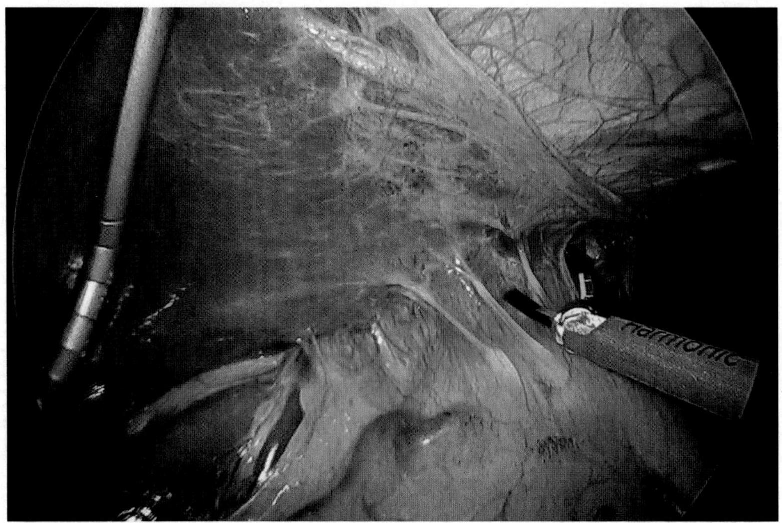

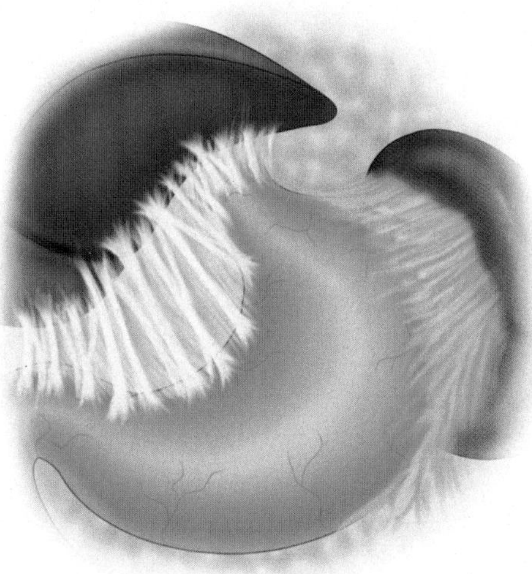

Fig. 33.21 Adhesions covering esophagus and fundoplication

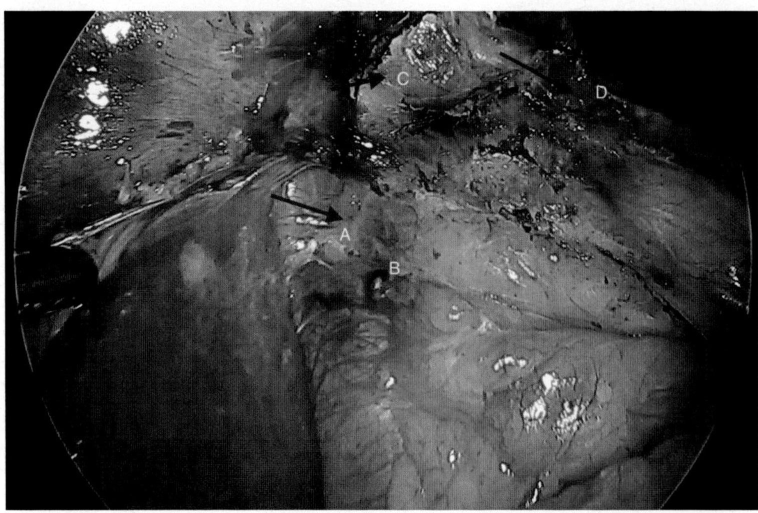

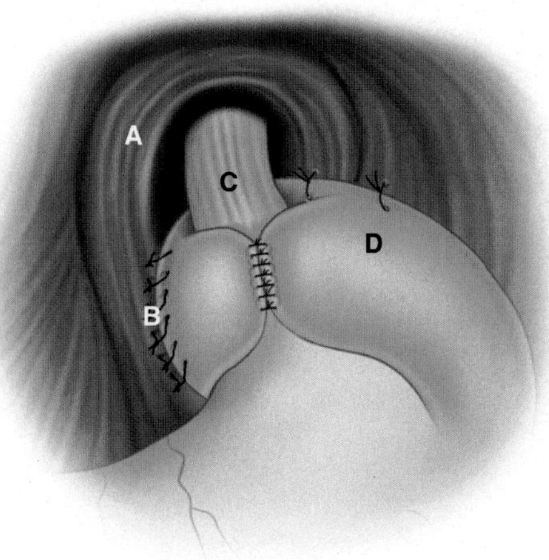

Fig. 33.22 Recurrent hiatal hernia. *A*, Right crus. *B*, Sutures from previous hiatal hernia repair. *C*, Esophagus. *D*, Fundus

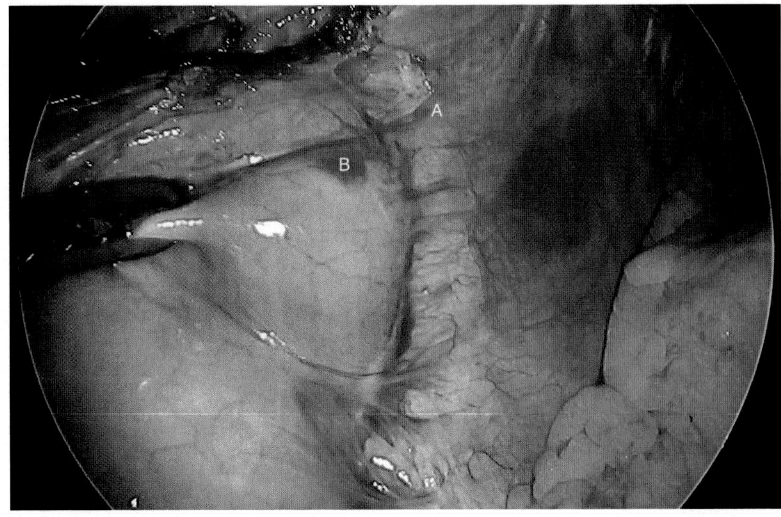

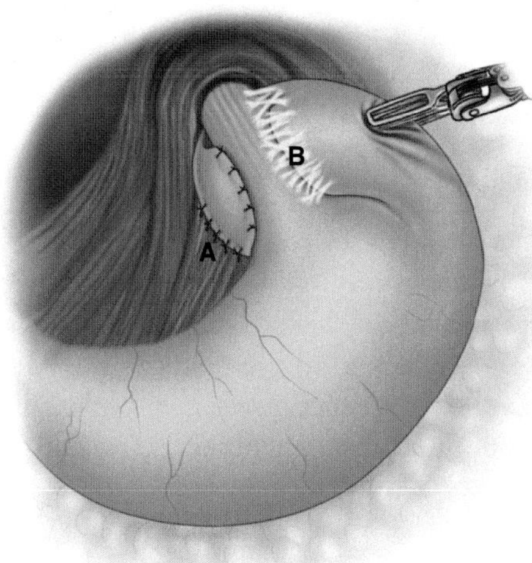

Fig. 33.23 Recurrent hiatal hernia. *A*, Left crus. *B*, Gastric wall with adhesions

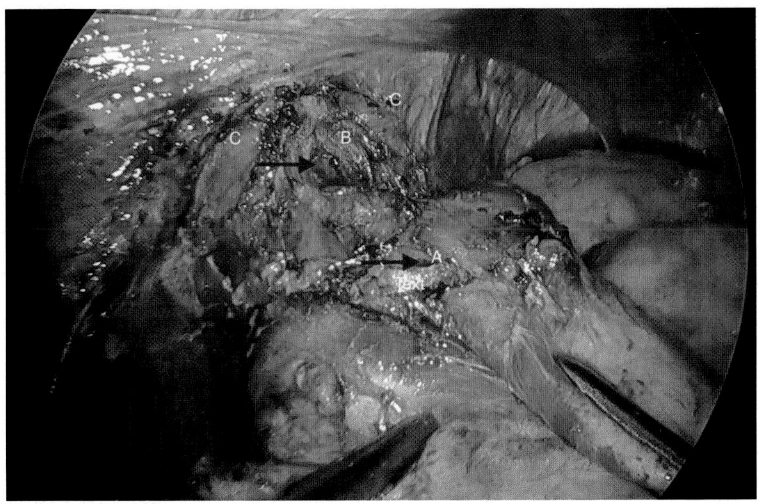

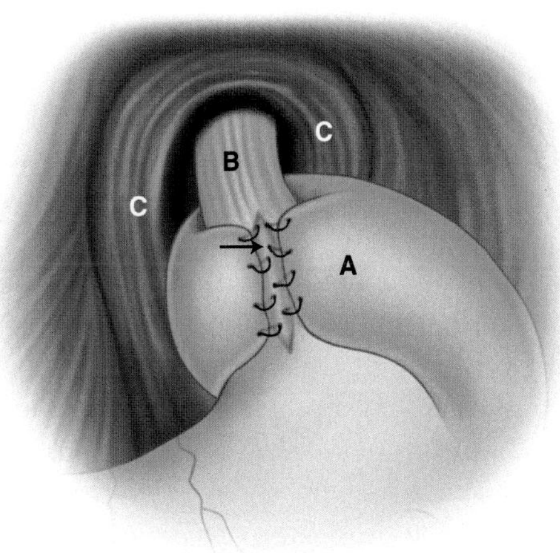

Fig. 33.24 Complications of hiatal hernia repair. *A*, Slipped and separated fundoplication. *B*, Esophagus with myotomy (*arrow*). *C*, Diaphragm

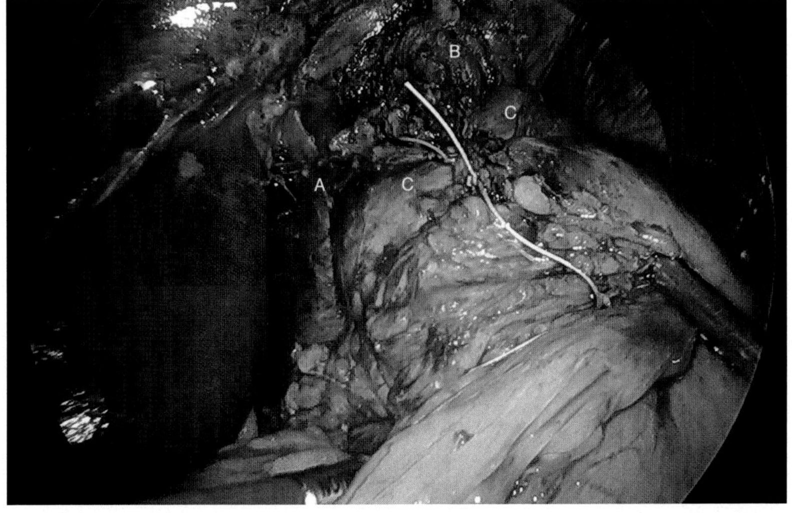

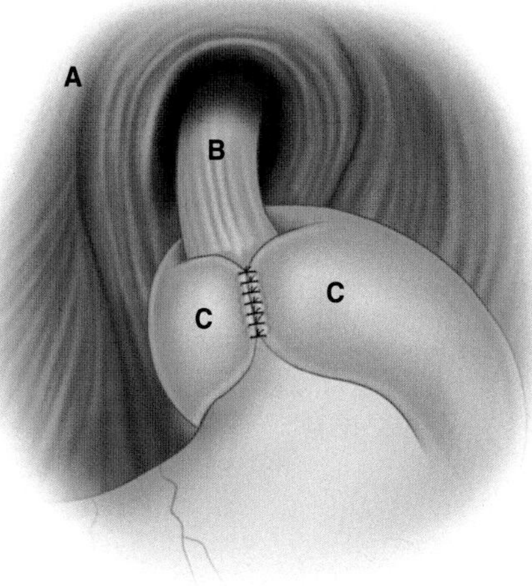

Fig. 33.25 Reapproximation of fundoplication. *A*, Diaphragm. *B*, Esophagus. *C*, Fundoplication

When compared with a laparoscopic approach, a robotic approach presents the advantages of superior visualization and easier suturing. One of the disadvantages with the robotic procedure is lack of tactile sensation and feel for the tissue (haptic sensation). In most cases, dense adhesions are present, and it is relatively easy to tear tissue. Another less obvious disadvantage with the robotic technology is that, despite better local visualization, the view is extremely focused, thereby leading to a lack of a "big picture" view. It may be difficult to know the exact location within the esophagus with such a limited (albeit focused) view during the surgical procedure.

The objective of operations for recurrent GERD or recurrent hiatus hernia with or without obstruction should be reestablishment of normal anatomy. This goal may require reduction of a hernia, reclosing the hiatus, and repeating the fundoplication if the initial repair has slipped or come apart. In turn, an alteration in the planned procedure may be required if there is an injury to the esophagus or stomach. If the repeat surgical procedure is a third or fourth operation and there is an esophageal injury above the fundoplication, with remaining dissection equally challenging, it is recommended to pursue a thoracic approach to repair the esophagus, followed by completion of the fundoplication. An alternative approach might be resection of the distal esophagus above the perforation to bring up the stomach, followed by resection of the cardia and fundus. An anastomosis of the esophagus to the body of the stomach would complete this procedure, but symptom reduction cannot be guaranteed with a repeat procedure and patients may continue having reflux symptoms.

If all surgical options have been exhausted, the surgeon might offer an esophagojejunostomy with Roux-en-Y [34, 35]. This procedure requires a thorough and informative discussion with the patient, followed by obtaining a written informed consent prior to the surgery. It should be considered a last resort after all other options have failed. The anatomy and adhesions are predictably difficult, and the goal should be to eliminate reflux. The esophagojejunostomy accomplishes this. The length of the Roux-en-Y limb should be longer than the usual 40 cm, to ensure that the patient does not continue to reflux.

Conclusion

Robotic surgical procedures have become essential for successful completion of complex, minimally invasive operations, and such technologies have found their place in the operative armamentarium of many more specialties and surgeons. The role of robotic technology for general surgeons is yet to be defined in its entirety, and in this age of limited funds and health-care reform, robotics in surgery is under intense scrutiny by health-care systems and payors. Surgeons with experience in this field must implicitly contribute to the discussions with various stakeholders to ensure that a well-thought-out plan is implemented to provide superior, value-based care to our patients.

Acknowledgments The authors would like to express their gratitude to Gary Edelberg for assisting with procuring images for this chapter and Emily Shoemaker, MPH, for editing the final draft of the manuscript.

References

1. Broeders JA, Mauritz FA, Ahmed Ali U, Draaisma WA, Ruurda JP, Gooszen HG, et al. Systematic review and meta-analysis of laparoscopic Nissen (posterior total) versus Toupet (posterior partial) fundoplication for gastro-oesophageal reflux disease. Br J Surg. 2010;97:1318–30.
2. Anderson JE, Chang DC, Parsons JK, Talamini MA. The first national examination of outcomes and trends in robotic surgery in the United States. J Am Coll Surg. 2012;215:107–14.
3. Niebisch S, Fleming FJ, Galey KM, Wilshire CL, Jones CE, Little VR, et al. Perioperative risk of laparoscopic fundoplication: safer than previously reported--analysis of the American College of Surgeons National Surgical Quality Improvement Program 2005 to 2009. J Am Coll Surg. 2012;215:61–8.
4. Dunn DH, Johnson EM, Morphew JA, Dilworth HP, Krueger JL, Banerji N. Robot-assisted transhiatal esophagectomy: a 3-year single-center experience. Dis Esophagus. 2013;26:159–66.
5. Mi J, Kang Y, Chen X, Wang B, Wang Z. Whether robot-assisted laparoscopic fundoplication is better for gastroesophageal reflux disease in adults: a systematic review and meta-analysis. Surg Endosc. 2010;24:1803–14.
6. Vela MF, Camacho-Lobato L, Srinivasan R, Tutuian R, Katz PO, Castell DO. Simultaneous intraesophageal impedance and pH measurement of acid and nonacid gastroesophageal reflux: effect of omeprazole. Gastroenterology. 2001;120:1599–606.
7. Simorov A, Ranade A, Jones R, Tadaki C, Shostrom V, Boilesen E, et al. Long-term patient outcomes after laparoscopic anti-reflux procedures. J Gastrointest Surg. 2014;18:157–62. discussion 162–3
8. Jianu CS, Fossmark R, Viset T, Qvigstad G, Sørdal O, Mårvik R, et al. Gastric carcinoids after long-term use of a proton pump inhibitor. Aliment Pharmacol Ther. 2012;36:644–9.
9. Jianu CS, Lange OJ, Viset T, Qvigstad G, Martinsen TC, Fougner R, et al. Gastric neuroendocrine carcinoma after long-term use of proton pump inhibitor. Scand J Gastroenterol. 2012;47:64–7.
10. Hafez J, Wrba F, Lenglinger J, Miholic J. Fundoplication for gastroesophageal reflux and factors associated with the outcome 6 to 10 years after the operation: multivariate analysis of prognostic factors using the propensity score. Surg Endosc. 2008;22(8):1763.
11. Shaw JM, Bornman PC, Callanan MD, Beckingham IJ, Metz DC. Long-term outcome of laparoscopic Nissen and laparoscopic Toupet fundoplication for gastroesophageal reflux disease: a prospective, randomized trial. Surg Endosc. 2010;24:924–32.
12. Varin O, Velstra B, De Sutter S, Ceelen W. Total vs partial fundoplication in the treatment of gastroesophageal reflux disease: a meta-analysis. Arch Surg. 2009;144:273–8.
13. Patti MG, Allaix ME, Fisichella PM. Analysis of the causes of failed antireflux surgery and the principles of treatment: a review. JAMA Surg. 2015;150:585–90.

14. Bonavina L, DeMeester TR, Ganz RA. LINX(™) reflux management system: magnetic sphincter augmentation in the treatment of gastroesophageal reflux disease. Expert Rev Gastroenterol Hepatol. 2012;6:667–74.
15. Lipham JC, DeMeester TR, Ganz RA, Bonavina L, Saino G, Dunn DH, et al. The LINX® reflux management system: confirmed safety and efficacy now at 4 years. Surg Endosc. 2012;26:2944–9.
16. Bonavina L, DeMeester T, Fockens P, Dunn D, Saino G, Bona D, et al. Laparoscopic sphincter augmentation device eliminates reflux symptoms and normalizes esophageal acid exposure: one- and 2-year results of a feasibility trial. Ann Surg. 2010;252:857–62.
17. Tolboom RC, Draaisma WA, Broeders IA. Evaluation of conventional laparoscopic versus robot-assisted laparoscopic redo hiatal hernia and antireflux surgery: a cohort study. J Robot Surg. 2016;10:33–9.
18. Broeders IA. Robotics: the next step? Best Pract Res Clin Gastroenterol. 2014;28:225–32.
19. Holloway RW, Ahmad S. Robotic-assisted surgery in the management of endometrial cancer. J Obstet Gynaecol Res. 2012;38:1–8.
20. Gurusamy KS, Samraj K, Fusai G, Davidson BR. Robot assistant for laparoscopic cholecystectomy. Cochrane Database Syst Rev. 2009;1:CD006578.
21. Tamhankar AS, Jatal S, Saklani A. Total robotic radical rectal resection with da Vinci xi system: single docking, single phase technique. Int J Med Robot. 2016;12:642. https://doi.org/10.1002/rcs.1734 [Epub ahead of print].
22. Siesto G, Romano F, Fiamengo B, Vitobello D. Sentinel node mapping using indocyanine green and near-infrared fluorescence imaging technology for uterine malignancies: preliminary experience with the da Vinci xi system. J Minim Invasive Gynecol. 2016;23:470–1.
23. Levine MS, Rubesin SE. Diseases of the esophagus: diagnosis with esophagography. Radiology. 2005;237:414–27.
24. Sutherland J, Banerji N, Morphew J, Johnson E, Dunn D. Postoperative incidence of incarcerated hiatal hernia and its prevention after robotic transhiatal esophagectomy. Surg Endosc. 2011;25:1526–30.
25. Runge TM, Abrams JA, Shaheen NJ. Epidemiology of Barrett's esophagus and esophageal adenocarcinoma. Gastroenterol Clin N Am. 2015;44:203–31.
26. Wang RH. From reflux esophagitis to Barrett's esophagus and esophageal adenocarcinoma. World J Gastroenterol. 2015;21:5210–9.
27. Ishimura N, Okada M, Mikami H, Okimoto E, Fukuda N, Uno G, et al. Pathophysiology of Barrett's esophagus-associated neoplasia: circumferential spatial predilection. Digestion. 2014;89:291–8.
28. Sifrim D, Tutuian R. Oesophageal intraluminal impedance can identify subtle bolus transit abnormalities in patients with mild oesophagitis. Eur J Gastroenterol Hepatol. 2005;17:303–5.
29. Lucenco L, Marincas M, Cirimbei C, Bratucu E, Ionescu S. The 10 years' experience in the laparoscopic treatment of benign pathology of the eso gastric junction. J Med Life. 2012;5:179–84.
30. Stefanidis D, Richardson W, Farrell TM, Kohn GP, Augenstein V, Fanelli RD, Society of American Gastrointestinal and Endoscopic Surgeons. SAGES guidelines for the surgical treatment of esophageal achalasia. Surg Endosc. 2012;26:296–311.
31. Rebecchi F, Giaccone C, Farinella E, Campaci R, Morino M. Randomized controlled trial of laparoscopic Heller myotomy plus dor fundoplication versus Nissen fundoplication for achalasia: long-term results. Ann Surg. 2008;248:1023–30.
32. Cuttitta A, Tancredi A, Andriulli A, De Santo E, Fontana A, Pellegrini F, et al. Fundoplication after Heller myotomy: a retrospective comparison between nissen and dor. Eurasian J Med. 2011;43:133–40.
33. Whitson BA, Hoang CD, Boettcher AK, Dahlberg PS, Andrade RS, Maddaus MA. Wedge gastroplasty and reinforced crural repair: important components of laparoscopic giant or recurrent hiatal hernia repair. J Thorac Cardiovasc Surg. 2006;132:1196–202.
34. Awais O, Luketich JD, Reddy N, Bianco V, Levy RM, Schuchert MJ, et al. Roux-en-Y near esophagojejunostomy for failed antireflux operations: outcomes in more than 100 patients. Ann Thorac Surg. 2014;98:1905–11. discussion 1911–3
35. Wilshire CL, Louie BE, Shultz D, Jutric Z, Farivar AS, Aye RW. Clinical outcomes of reoperation for failed antireflux operations. Ann Thorac Surg. 2016;101:1290–6.

Heller Myotomy

34

Boris Zevin and Kyle A. Perry

Achalasia is the most common primary motility disorder of the esophagus and the second most common functional disorder of the esophagus requiring operative treatment. Diagnosis is made on the basis of symptoms, barium esophagram, esophageal manometry, and esophagogastroduodenoscopy. Treatment options include medical, endoscopic, and surgical modalities. This chapter focuses on the surgical management of achalasia utilizing minimally invasive robotic Heller myotomy with partial fundoplication. Patient outcomes and costs for minimally invasive robotic Heller myotomy with partial fundoplication are discussed in comparison with open and laparoscopic approaches.

Epidemiology, Pathophysiology, and Diagnosis of Achalasia

The annual incidence of achalasia is 1–6 cases per 100,000 individuals. It affects individuals from 25 to 60 years of age, with equal incidence in men and women. The etiology is presumed to be idiopathic, with possible hereditary, degenerative, autoimmune, and infectious components. Microscopically, achalasia is associated with T lymphocyte, eosinophil, and mast cell infiltration in the myenteric plexus of the lower esophagus, with myenteric neural fibrosis, hypertrophy of the circular and longitudinal muscle layers, and hypertrophy of nerve fibers [1]. Interruption of normal vagal cholinergic motor function is thought to lead to aperistalsis of the esophagus, whereas derangement of vagal inhibitory nerves is thought to result in failure of lower esophageal sphincter relaxation.

Classic symptoms of achalasia include progressive dysphagia to solids and liquids, regurgitation, chest pressure, and weight loss. The mean duration of symptoms prior to diagnosis is 4.7 years. Pneumonia, lung abscess, and bronchiectasis can be seen in patients with long-standing symptoms of achalasia. The diagnostic workup includes a barium esophagram, esophageal manometry, and esophagogastroduodenoscopy [1]. A barium esophagram will often show lower esophageal sphincter spasm with a dilated proximal

B. Zevin, MD, PhD
Department of Surgery, Queen's University, Kingston General Hospital, Kingston, ON, Canada

K. A. Perry, MD (✉)
Division of General & Gastrointestinal Surgery, Center for Minimally Invasive Surgery, The Ohio State University, Columbus, OH, USA

Y. Fong et al. (eds.), *The SAGES Atlas of Robotic Surgery*, https://doi.org/10.1007/978-3-319-91045-1_34

esophagus and a classic appearance of a "bird's beak" (Fig. 34.1). A lack of peristaltic waves in the body of the esophagus and failure of relaxation of lower esophageal sphincter are often seen.

Esophagogastroduodenoscopy is performed to evaluate the mucosa for evidence of stasis esophagitis and to rule out malignancy as a cause of pseudoachalasia. Typical findings on endoscopy include a patulous esophagus, a tense lower esophageal sphincter, and the presence of food residue in the distal esophagus.

Esophageal manometry is the gold standard test to diagnose achalasia and to eliminate other potential esophageal motility disorders. High-resolution manometry can be used to define a specific subtype of achalasia based on patterns of esophageal pressurization. Three subtypes have been identified [1]:

- Type I (classic achalasia): impaired lower esophageal sphincter relaxation, absent peristalsis, and normal esophageal pressure.
- Type II: impaired lower esophageal sphincter relaxation, absent peristalsis, and increased panesophageal pressure.
- Type III (spastic achalasia): impaired lower esophageal sphincter relaxation, absent peristalsis, and distal esophageal spastic contractions.

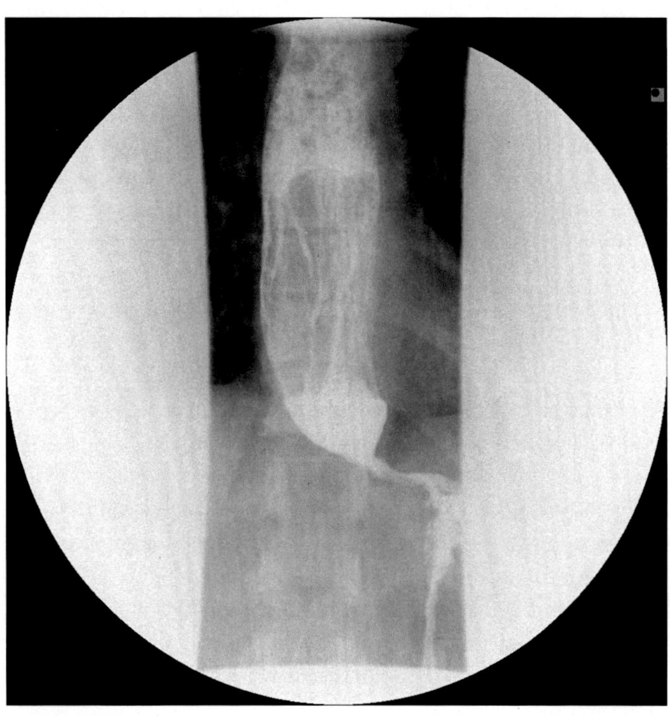

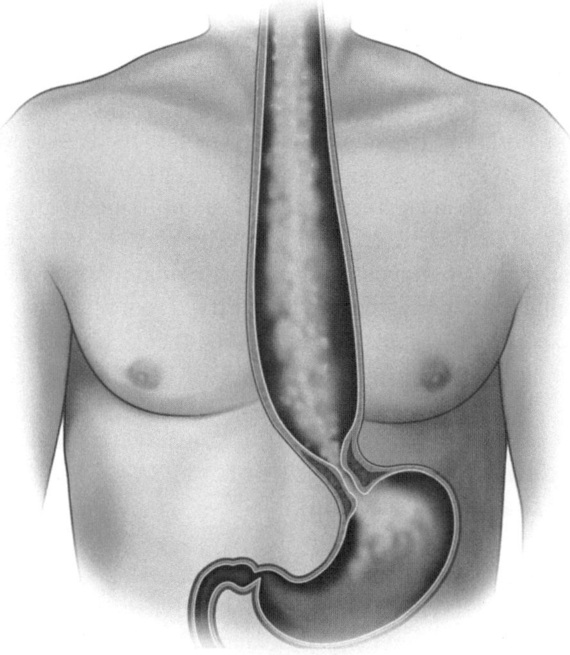

Fig. 34.1 Barium esophagram

Treatment Options for Achalasia

The treatment options for achalasia include medical, endoscopic, and surgical therapies.

Medical Therapy

Medical therapy involves the use of smooth muscle relaxants such as calcium channel blockers and nitrates. This treatment modality is less effective than endoscopic and surgical therapies. It should be considered in individuals who are unwilling or unable to tolerate invasive endoscopic or surgical therapeutic options [2–4]. Calcium channel blockers result in symptomatic improvement in 0–75% of patients, and sublingual nitroglycerine results in symptomatic improvement in 53–87%. Side effects may occur in up to 30% of patients using calcium channel blockers or nitrates. The use of medical therapy is also limited by the development of tachyphylaxis.

Endoscopic Therapy

Endoscopic therapy includes injections of botulinum toxin into the lower esophageal sphincter and pneumatic balloon dilation of the lower esophageal sphincter. Injection of botulinum toxin results in temporary relaxation of the lower esophageal sphincter and symptomatic improvement in dysphagia symptoms. Approximately 50–60% of individuals treated with botulinum toxin injection will require repeat treatment in 6–12 months [1]. Pneumatic dilation of the lower esophageal sphincter physically weakens the sphincter by tearing the circular muscle fibers. The initial success rate for relief of dysphagia is as high as 85% at 1 month [5]. Unfortunately, the efficacy of pneumatic dilation decreases over time, with nearly one third of patients reporting symptom relapse and requiring retreatment over 4–6 years [6].

Surgical Therapy

Surgical therapy includes a surgical esophageal myotomy with partial fundoplication and can be performed using open, laparoscopic, or robotic technique. Dr. Ernest Heller first described a longitudinal esophageal myotomy in 1913 [7]. The first laparoscopic Heller myotomy with partial fundoplication was described in the early 1990s [8]. The robotic minimally invasive Heller myotomy with partial fundoplication was first described by Melvin and colleagues at the Ohio State University in 2001 [9]. The results of Heller myotomy with partial fundoplication are excellent, with symptomatic relief of dysphagia in 85% of patients at 10 years and 65% of patients at 20 years [10].

The minimally invasive surgical approach to achalasia, by laparoscopic or robotic technique, has clear advantages over the open approach, including decreased morbidity, decreased length of hospital stay, and decreased postoperative pain [11]. A large retrospective comparative analysis of 2683 patients with achalasia managed by an open Heller myotomy with partial fundoplication (418 patients), a laparoscopic Heller myotomy with partial fundoplication (2116 patients), and a robotic Heller myotomy with partial fundoplication (149 patients) demonstrated decreased in-hospital morbidity (9.1% vs. 5.2% vs. 4.0%), decreased hospital length of stay (4.42 ± 5.25 vs. 2.70 ± 3.87 vs. 2.42 ± 2.69 days), and decreased ICU admission rate (14.0% vs. 6.6% vs. 3.4%) for laparoscopic and robotic technique as compared with the open technique [11].

The advantages of the robotic platform over traditional laparoscopic technique for Heller myotomy with partial fundoplication include improvements in fine motor control of the instruments, elimination of tremor, increased freedom of movement, three-dimensional magnification, and motion scaling [12]. The disadvantages of the robotic platform include increased operational costs, increased setup and operating times, and a requirement for additional training of the entire operative team [12]. The outcomes and costs of robotic and laparoscopic Heller myotomy with partial fundoplication have been compared in several studies. Horgan and colleagues carried out a retrospective review of a prospectively collected database and identified 121 patients who underwent 59 robotic and 62 laparoscopic Heller myotomies with partial fundoplication for achalasia at three different institutions [13]. Good or excellent symptomatic relief of dysphagia was reported in 92% of patients in the robotic surgery group and 90% of patients in the laparoscopic surgery group. Similarly, postoperative gastroesophageal reflux was reported by 17% of patients in the robotic surgery group and by 16% of patients in the laparoscopic surgery group. Operative times were significantly longer in the robotic surgery group versus the laparoscopic surgery group (141 ± 49 min vs. 122 ± 44 min; $p = 0.03$). But more importantly, the rate of intraoperative esophageal perforation was significantly lower in the robotic surgery group than in the laparoscopic surgery group (0% vs. 16%; $p < 0.01$). The authors postulated that the decrease in the esophageal perforation rate can be explained by the improved vision, freedom of instrument movement, and elimination of tremor offered by the robotic platform.

Perry and colleagues conducted a retrospective cohort study comparing 56 patients who underwent robotic Heller myotomy with partial fundoplication and 19 patients who underwent laparoscopic Heller myotomy with partial fundoplication between 1995 and 2006 at a tertiary academic center [14]. The primary outcome measure was durable relief of dysphagia symptoms without the need for further intervention. Secondary outcomes were presence of gastroesophageal reflux symptoms, disease-specific quality of life, and patient satisfaction with their operation. The median follow-up interval was 9 years. Reported results demonstrate similar duration of surgery for the robotic and the laparoscopic group (133 ± 29 min vs. 121 ± 22 min; $p = 0.14$), shorter length of hospital stay for the robotic group (1 (1–3) vs. 2 (1–9) days, $p < 0.01$), and lower rate of esophageal perforation in the robotic group (0% vs. 16%; $p = 0.01$). The rates of dysphagia, presence of gastroesophageal reflux, and proton pump inhibitor use were equivalent between the groups. Over 90% of the patients in each group reported being satisfied with their operation.

Two other studies replicated the finding of decreased esophageal perforation rates for the robotic Heller myotomy with partial fundoplication as compared with laparoscopic Heller myotomy with partial fundoplication [12, 15]. Huffman and colleagues analyzed the outcomes of 24 consecutive patients undergoing robotic Heller myotomy with partial fundoplication and 37 consecutive patients undergoing laparoscopic Heller myotomy with partial fundoplication by a single surgeon at a single institution between 2000 and 2006 [15]. There were no esophageal perforations reported in the robotic group and three (8%) esophageal perforations reported in the laparoscopic group. Another group reported no esophageal perforations in 104 patients who underwent a robotic Heller myotomy with partial fundoplication at three academic institutions between 2000 and 2004 [12].

The per-case cost of open, laparoscopic, and robotic Heller myotomy with partial fundoplication for treatment of achalasia was compared in a multicenter, retrospective analysis of 2683 patients from 2007 to 2011 [11]. The estimated per-case cost in US dollars was $9802 ± 10,111 for an open approach, $7441 ± 7897 for a laparoscopic approach, and $9515 ± 5515 for a robotic approach. The laparoscopic Heller myotomy with partial fundoplication was significantly cheaper than the open and the robotic operations.

Operative Technique for Robotic Heller Myotomy with Partial Fundoplication

Patient Preparation

Clinical symptoms and the results of barium esophagram, esophageal manometry, and esophagogastroduodenoscopy must confirm the diagnosis of achalasia prior to operative treatment. Once the diagnosis is established and operative treatment is decided upon, patients are kept on clear liquid diet for 48 h prior to surgery, to minimize the risk of aspiration during the induction of general anesthesia in the operating room. *Candida* esophagitis should be treated preoperatively with antifungal medications.

Patient Positioning and Operating Room Setup

The general setup of the operating room is illustrated in Fig. 34.2. The patient is positioned in split-leg or lithotomy position, and general anesthesia is induced. Prophylactic antibiotics and venous thromboembolism prophylaxis are administered. An orogastric tube is introduced to decompress the distal esophagus and stomach. The abdomen and the lower chest are prepped and draped in the usual sterile fashion. The assistant surgeon is positioned on the left side of the patient, and the scrub technician can be positioned on either the right or the left.

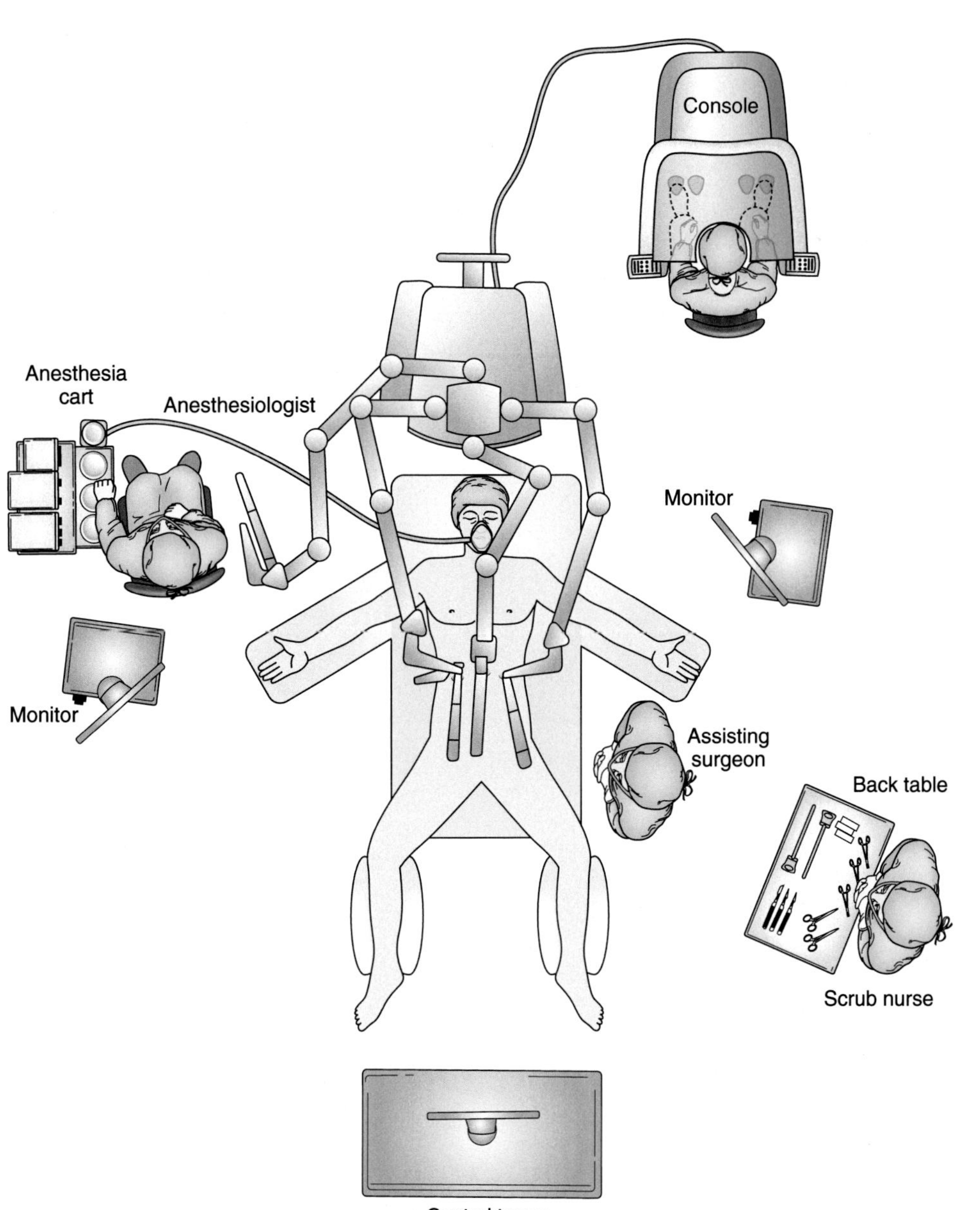

Fig. 34.2 Operating room setup

Operative Steps

Access to the peritoneal cavity is gained with a Veress needle placed in the left upper quadrant. Carbon dioxide pneumoperitoneum (15 mm Hg) is established. A five-port technique is utilized (Fig. 34.3). The robotic camera port is placed in the supraumbilical position to the left of the midline. Two additional ports are placed in the left upper quadrant, and one in the right upper quadrant. A triangle or fan liver retractor is placed via a right lower quadrant abdominal port to retract the left lobe of the liver. The patient is positioned in steep reverse Trendelenburg, and the robotic platform is docked over the patient's head or left shoulder.

Dissection is begun by dividing the pars flaccida of the lesser omentum to identify the right crus of the diaphragm. Blunt dissection is used to mobilize the right crus from the esophagus. Attention is then turned to the greater curvature of the stomach. The short gastric vessels are divided, and the left crus of the diaphragm is identified and mobilized from the esophagus. Circumferential dissection around the esoph-

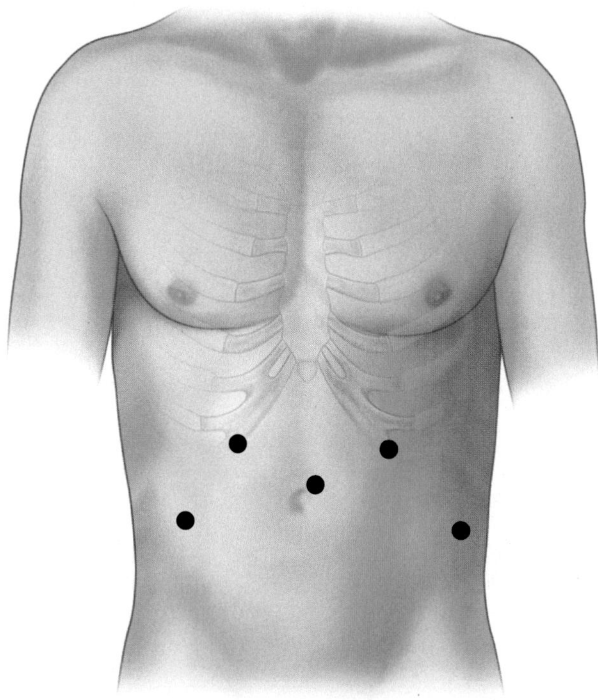

Fig. 34.3 Port placement

agus is carried out, and a Penrose drain is placed around the distal esophagus (Fig. 34.4). The esophagus is then mobilized for 8–10 cm into the mediastinum, using a combination of inferior traction on the Penrose drain and blunt dissection in the avascular plane around the esophagus. The anterior vagus nerve is identified and protected during the dissection. The gastroesophageal fat pad is bivalved to expose the anterior wall of the esophagus and stomach.

An anterior longitudinal myotomy is created using hook electrocautery, with special attention paid to keep the heel of the instrument parallel to the esophageal wall. Once the submucosal tunnel is created, the myotomy is carried for 8–10 cm proximally on the esophagus and 2–3 cm distally onto the stomach (Fig. 34.5). If deemed necessary, a posterior cruroplasty is performed using interrupted 0 braided nonabsorbable sutures (Fig. 34.6).

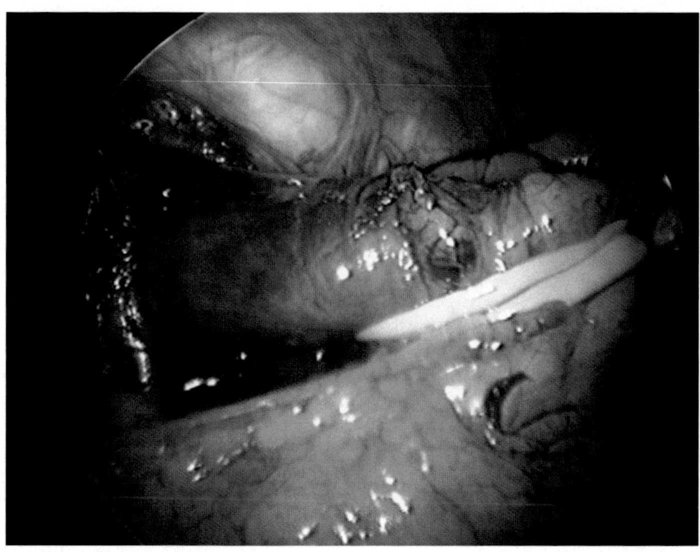
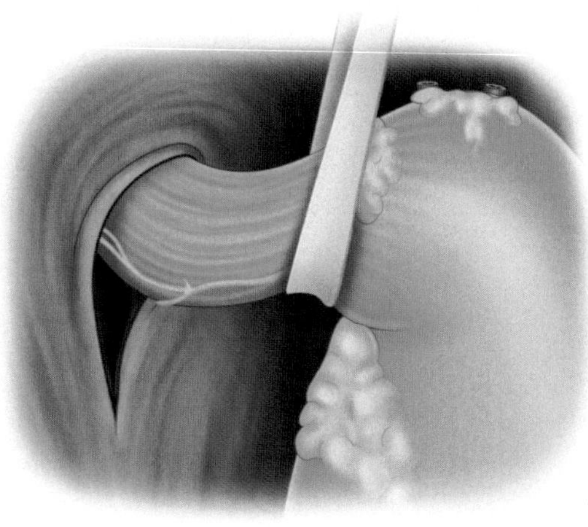

Fig. 34.4 Diaphragmatic hiatus

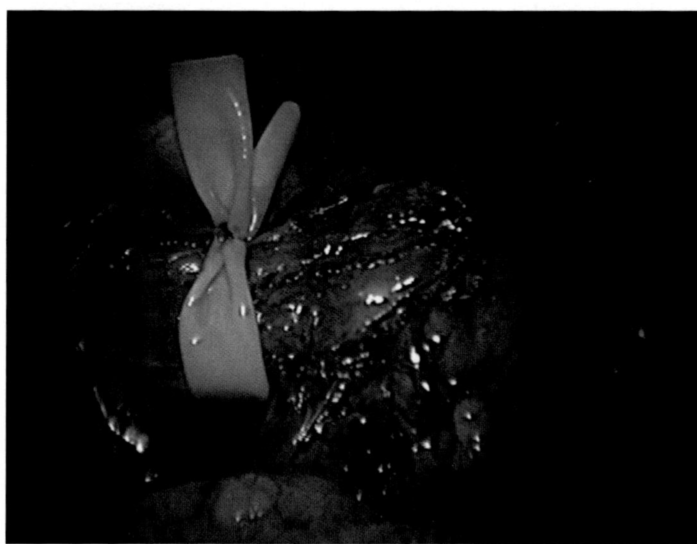
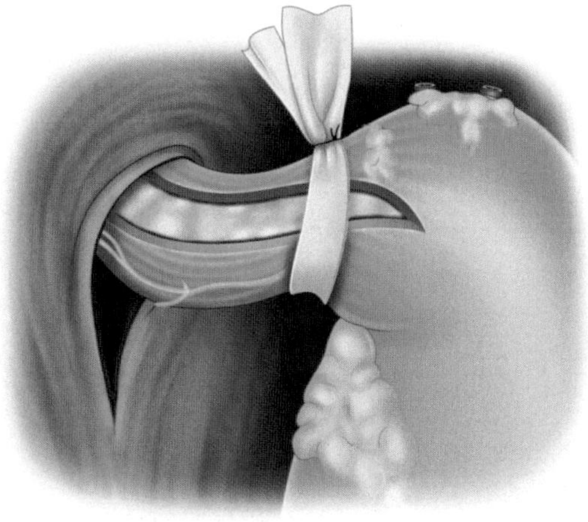

Fig. 34.5 Esophageal myotomy

Intraoperative esophagogastroduodenoscopy is performed to confirm complete lower esophageal myotomy with adequate extension onto the stomach and to rule out a mucosal perforation. If mucosal perforation is identified, it should be repaired primarily with 3–0 absorbable suture. The Penrose drain is then removed, and an anterior (Dor) or posterior (Toupet) partial fundoplication is performed. At our institution, we perform a Dor fundoplication by passing the fundus of the stomach anterior to the esophagus and suturing it to the left and right crus of the diaphragm with interrupted 0 nonabsorbable braided sutures (Fig. 34.7).

Hemostasis is confirmed and the robotic platform is disengaged. The ports are removed, and fascia of port sites larger than 10 mm is closed under direct vision.

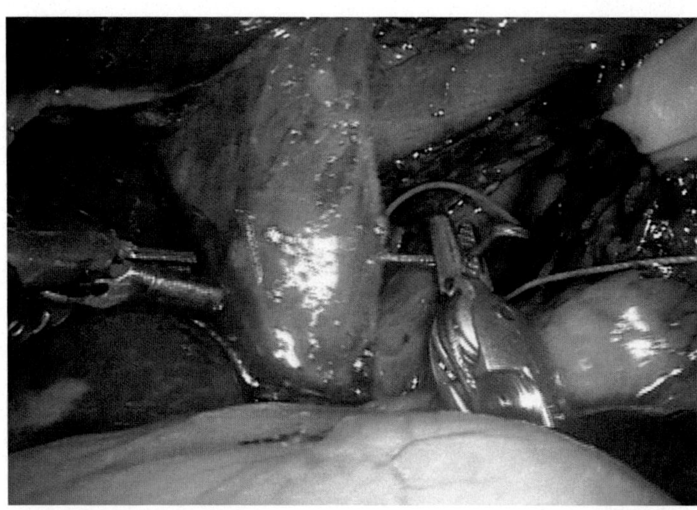

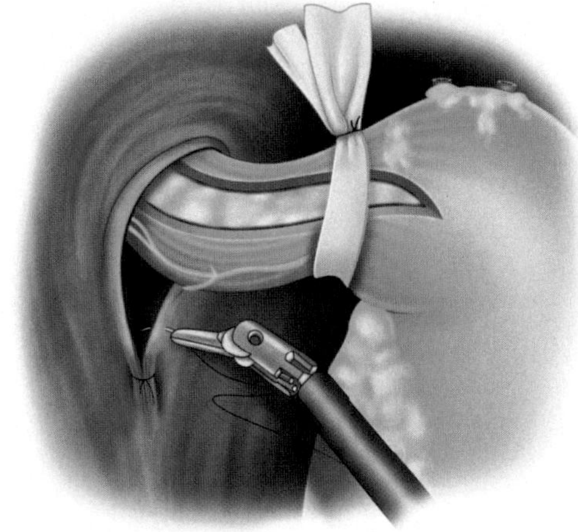

Fig. 34.6 Posterior cruroplasty

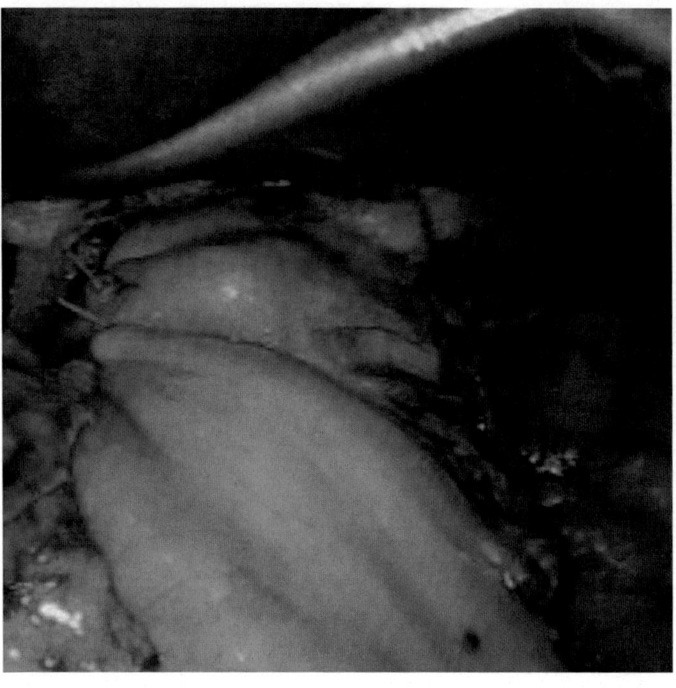

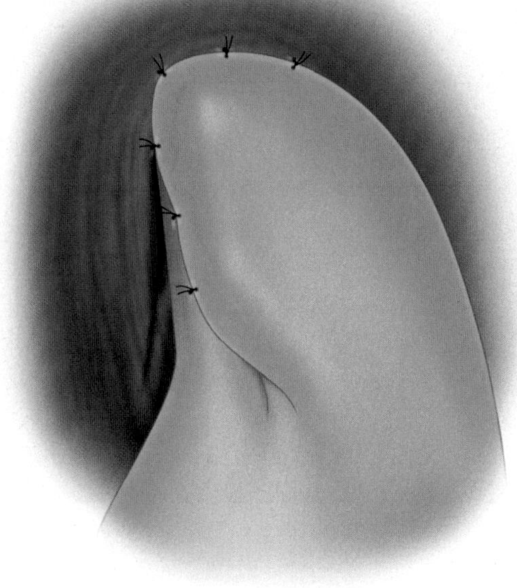

Fig. 34.7 Dor fundoplication

Postoperative Care

Patients are started on clear fluids on the day of surgery and are transitioned to a soft diet on the first postoperative day. Patients are usually discharged home on postoperative day #1 and are instructed to remain on a soft diet for 2 weeks postoperatively.

Postoperative Complications

Esophageal Perforation

An esophageal perforation may present within 24–48 h. It is usually a result of delayed perforation from a thermal injury to the esophageal mucosa. Characteristic signs and symptoms include fever, tachycardia, chest pain, abdominal pain, and pleural effusion on the chest x-ray. The diagnosis of an esophageal perforation is confirmed with a dilute barium esophagram. Treatment includes appropriate intravenous resuscitation, initiation of broad spectrum antibiotics, maintenance of nil per os, and wide drainage of the perforation with or without primary repair. Early leaks that present within 24–48 h of surgery are best managed with primary repair and drainage in the operating room. Persistent leaks may require an esophagectomy.

Hemorrhage

Postoperative hemorrhage is a rare complication of Heller myotomy with partial fundoplication, occurring in less than 0.5% of cases [16]. The site of hemorrhage is often the short gastric vessels. Treatment consists of resuscitation and operative exploration for control of the hemorrhage.

Pneumothorax

Pneumothorax (capnothorax) can occur intraoperatively if the parietal pleura is violated during the mediastinal dissection. Clinical presentation ranges from no symptoms to hemodynamic instability. Initial treatment involves the release of pneumoperitoneum and Valsalva maneuvers. Placement of a chest tube is rarely necessary. Carbon dioxide will be reabsorbed from the thoracic cavity within 24 h. This situation demands clear and concise communication with members of the anesthesia team.

Dysphagia

Dysphagia may be persistent or recurrent. Persistent dysphagia is usually a result of incomplete myotomy or incorrect configuration of the partial fundoplication. Recurrent dysphagia after a symptom-free interval is likely a result of scarring in the distal portion of the myotomy, esophageal stricture from gastroesophageal reflux, or slipped partial fundoplication. The rate of recurrent dysphagia is reported to be approximately 20% at a median follow-up of 9 years [14]. Recurrent dysphagia mandates a complete workup with barium esophagram, esophageal manometry, and esophagogastroduodenoscopy to determine the underlying cause. Treatment should be individualized based on the specific findings from these investigations. Endoscopic pneumatic dilation or reoperation may be indicated.

Gastroesophageal Reflux

Approximately 10–20% of patients will develop moderate-to-severe gastroesophageal reflux disease after robotic Heller myotomy with partial fundoplication [14]. Reflux symptoms respond well to acid-reducing medications.

References

1. Pandolfino JE, Gawron AJ. Achalasia: a systematic review. JAMA. 2015;313:1841–52.
2. Gelfond M, Rozen P, Gilat T. Isosorbide dinitrate and nifedipine treatment of achalasia: a clinical, manometric and radionuclide evaluation. Gastroenterology. 1982;83:963–9.
3. Coccia G, Bortolotti M, Michetti P, Dodero M. Prospective clinical and manometric study comparing pneumatic dilatation and sublingual nifedipine in the treatment of oesophageal achalasia. Gut. 1991;32(6):604.
4. Bassotti G, Annese V. Review article: pharmacological options in achalasia. Aliment Pharmacol Ther. 1999;13:1391–6.
5. Boeckxstaens GE, Annese V, des Varannes SB, Chaussade S, Costantini M, Cuttitta A, et al. Pneumatic dilation versus laparoscopic Heller's myotomy for idiopathic achalasia. N Engl J Med. 2011;364:1807–16.
6. Vela MF, Richter JE, Khandwala F, Blackstone EH, Wachsberger D, Baker ME, Rice TW. The long-term efficacy of pneumatic dilatation and Heller myotomy for the treatment of achalasia. Clin Gastroenterol Hepatol. 2006;4:580–7.
7. Brewer LA. History of surgery of the esophagus. Am J Surg. 1980;139:730–43.
8. Ancona E, Peracchia A, Zaninotto G, Rossi M, Bonavina L, Segalin A. Heller laparoscopic cardiomyotomy with antireflux anterior fundoplication (dor) in the treatment of esophageal achalasia. Surg Endosc. 1993;7:459–61.

9. Melvin WS, Needleman BJ, Krause KR, Wolf RK, Michler RE, Ellison EC. Computer-assisted robotic Heller myotomy: initial case report. J Laparoendosc Adv Surg Tech A. 2001;11:251–3.
10. Reavis KM, Renton DR, Melvin WS. Robotic telesurgery for achalasia. J Robot Surg. 2007;1:25–30.
11. Shaligram A, Unnirevi J, Simorov A, Kothari VM, Oleynikov D. How does the robot affect outcomes? A retrospective review of open, laparoscopic, and robotic Heller myotomy for achalasia. Surg Endosc. 2012;26:1047–50.
12. Melvin WS, Dundon JM, Talamini M, Horgan S. Computer-enhanced robotic telesurgery minimizes esophageal perforation during Heller myotomy. Surgery. 2005;138:553–8.
13. Horgan S, Galvani C, Gorodner MV, Omelanczuck P, Elli F, Moser F, et al. Robotic-assisted Heller myotomy versus laparoscopic Heller myotomy for the treatment of esophageal achalasia: multicenter study. J Gastrointest Surg. 2005;9:1020–9.
14. Perry KA, Kanji A, Drosdeck JM, Linn JG, Chan A, Muscarella P, et al. Efficacy and durability of robotic Heller myotomy for achalasia: patient symptoms and satisfaction at long-term follow-up. Surg Endosc. 2014;28:3162–7.
15. Huffman LC, Pandalai PK, Boulton BJ, James L, Starnes SL, Reed MF, et al. Robotic Heller myotomy: a safe operation with higher postoperative quality-of-life indices. Surgery. 2007;142:613–8.
16. Ross SW, Oommen B, Wormer BA, Walters AL, Matthews BD, Heniford BT, et al. National outcomes of laparoscopic Heller myotomy: operative complications and risk factors for adverse events. Surg Endosc. 2015;29:3097–105.

Part V

Thoracic Procedures

35 Robotically-Assisted Minimally Invasive Esophagectomy (RAMIE): The Ivor Lewis Approach

Fernando M. Safdie, Nicholas R. Hess, and Inderpal S. Sarkaria

Introduction

The incidence of esophageal cancer has increased exponentially over the past three decades, particularly in the United States and other western countries, with rates of esophageal adenocarcinoma rising faster than rates for any other solid organ tumor [1, 2]. According to the Surveillance, Epidemiology, and End Results Program (SEER) database, an estimated 16,910 newly diagnosed cases and 15,690 deaths due to esophageal malignancy were expected in the United States in 2016. These estimates place esophageal cancer as the sixth most lethal cancer in both the United States and the rest of the world [3].

In appropriate patients, surgical resection achieving complete removal of the tumor en bloc with all periesophageal lymph node-bearing tissues with adequate margins remains the cornerstone of multimodality therapy for optimal locoregional control and to maximize long-term survival [4–7]. Complete en bloc resection of local lymph node-bearing tissues has correlated with improved cancer recurrence and survival profiles [8, 9]. In patients with advanced-stage cancers, the implementation of neoadjuvant chemotherapy with or without combined radiotherapy improves overall survival and may improve local control and the likelihood of achieving a complete surgical resection [10].

F. M. Safdie, MD
Department of Cardiothoracic Surgery, University of Pittsburgh Medical Center, Pittsburgh, PA, USA
e-mail: safidefm@upmc.edu

N. R. Hess, BS
University of Pittsburgh School of Medicine, Pittsburgh, PA, USA

I. S. Sarkaria, MD (✉)
Department of Cardiothoracic Surgery, University of Pittsburgh Medical Center, Pittsburgh, PA, USA

The choice of surgical approach is determined largely by surgeon preference, experience, and prior training, as well as tumor location, patient body habitus, history of prior operation, and patient comorbidities. The Ivor Lewis approach is the preferred approach at the University of Pittsburgh for tumors of the gastroesophageal junction and most tumors of the lower and mid-esophagus. In experienced centers with high patient volume, the operation can be safely performed with acceptable mortality rates as low as 1%. In low-volume centers, this mortality rate may reach 10–20% [11–16]. Minimally invasive esophagectomy (MIE) has emerged with the aims of reducing surgical trauma, morbidity, and mortality. Multiple reports have demonstrated significantly reduced pulmonary morbidity, blood loss, time to recovery, and decreased hospital stay while maintaining oncologic outcomes equivalent to those with open operations [13, 14, 16–18]. The utilization of minimally invasive practices may add additional technical complexity to the operation, however, requiring additional experience to perform the operation safely. It is likely that the learning curve for MIE is long, so its use has been limited to a relatively small but growing number of centers.

In more recent years, the pre-existing techniques of MIE have been adapted to incorporate the use of robotically assisted operating platforms. The introduction of robotically-assisted surgery may offer specific advantages to facilitate complex minimally invasive procedures, such as an enlarged, three-dimensional field of view, operator control of the camera, and articulated instrumentation within the abdominal and thoracic cavities. Additionally, several robotic platforms support the use of near-infrared fluorescence imaging technology for real-time organ perfusion evaluation and intraoperative assessment of key vascular structures [19, 20]. Though robotically-assisted minimally invasive esophagectomy (RAMIE) is still in its early stages of development and dissemination into surgical practice, early short-term out-

Y. Fong et al. (eds.), *The SAGES Atlas of Robotic Surgery*, https://doi.org/10.1007/978-3-319-91045-1_35

comes have been comparable to other MIE approaches [21–23]. In this chapter, we present our total robotically-assisted Ivor Lewis approach to MIE.

Surgical Technique

Preoperative Planning

In all potential surgical candidates, tissue diagnosis of esophageal cancer is required. Patients commonly present to our clinic with a diagnosis made via endoscopy with multiple site biopsies. If referred from an outside healthcare system, these biopsies are routinely reviewed by our own pathologists in order to confirm the diagnosis. Repeat endoscopy and biopsy may be considered if tissue is not available for review by our own institution. Potential surgical candidates also undergo an extensive clinical staging workup, including endoscopic ultrasound and CT scans, combined with 18-fluorodeoxyglucose positron-emission tomography (PET) scanning of the chest, abdomen, and pelvis. Patients with early-stage lesions confined to the mucosa (T1a or less) are referred for endoscopic mucosal resection. Patients with clinically early-stage lesions (T1b or T2 with no evidence of local lymph node metastases) are referred for surgery. Patients with clinically advanced local-regional disease (T3 and/or any N) are referred for induction chemotherapy and radiation, followed by reevaluation for surgical resection, ideally 4–6 weeks after completion of treatment.

In addition to cancer diagnosis and staging, potential surgical candidates are assessed for their health, fitness, and ability to tolerate surgery and single-lung ventilation. Such assessment begins with careful review of health records and medical comorbidities. Patients with a long-standing history of smoking and/or chronic pulmonary obstructive disease undergo pulmonary function testing. An echocardiogram and routine blood metabolic panel are also typically obtained. All patients scheduled for surgery are placed on a full liquid diet 72 h prior to their operative date. At 24 h prior to surgery, their diet is reduced to clear liquids, and they undergo bowel preparation with an oral solution of polyethylene glycol and electrolytes.

Preparation and Patient Positioning

On the day of surgery, antibiotics and prophylactic subcutaneous heparin are given prior to general anesthesia induction. A double-lumen endotracheal tube is placed, and the bronchial cuff is deflated during the abdominal portion of the procedure, minimizing the risk of left main stem ischemic injury. Extension tubing is added to the anesthesia circuit to allow for bed movement during the procedure. Endoscopy is routinely performed to evaluate the current tumor size, location, and potential extension into the stomach, as these factors may dictate the operative approach and suitability of the stomach for conduit creation.

The robotic cart is set up on the patient's right side, with the tower on the left (Fig. 35.1). At our institution, we use a four-arm robotic platform with two operating consoles. One console is designated for the primary surgeon and the other for the surgical trainee.

For the abdominal phase, patients are placed supine on the operative table. The arms are abducted 45° on arm rests, and the patient is shifted to the right side of the bed to facilitate the use of the liver retractor. Alternatively, to minimize interaction with the robotic assistant arm, the left arm may be tucked. A footboard is placed under the feet. To ensure that the patient has been properly secured to the operating table, we routinely place the bed in steep reverse Trendelenburg to check for signs of patient movement or slippage prior to prepping and draping.

For the thoracic phase, the patient is placed in standard left lateral decubitus position, with flexion of the operating table at the level of the patient's costal margin/iliac crest to facilitate expansion of the intercostal spaces.

Surgical Access and Port Placement

For the abdominal phase, the robotic cart and arms are centered directly over the midline of the patient (Fig. 35.1). Port placement is shown in Fig. 35.2. A point 1–2 cm above the xiphoid process is marked in the midline. This represents the hiatus and is the highest point of dissection during the abdominal phase. All instruments must reach this point. A midline 12-mm incision is marked, preferably just above the umbilicus but no more than 23 cm from the supraxiphoid reference point. This port site will be utilized by the robotic camera. A left lateral subcostal 5-mm incision is marked for use by the robotic atraumatic grasper. A midclavicular 8-mm incision no more than 13–15 cm from the supraxiphoid reference point is marked in the left mid-

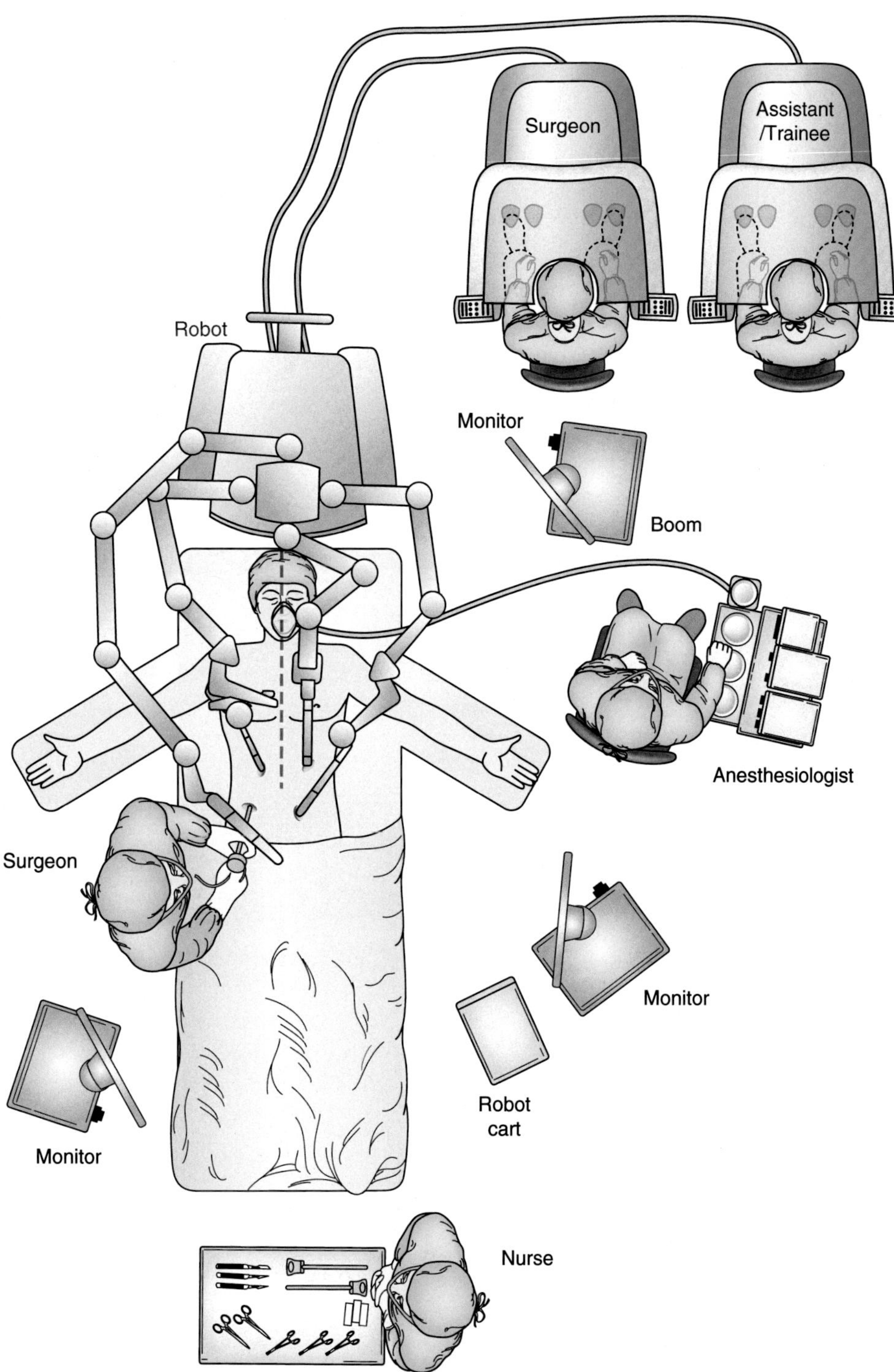

Fig. 35.1 Intraoperative setup and robotic cart and console placement during robotically-assisted minimally invasive esophagectomy (RAMIE). (**a**) The patient is placed in supine and steep reverse Trendelenburg positioning for the abdominal phase. The robotic cart may or may not be placed directly over the midline, depending on the robotic surgical platform used. (**b**) The patient is placed in left lateral decubitus position for the thoracic phase of the operation

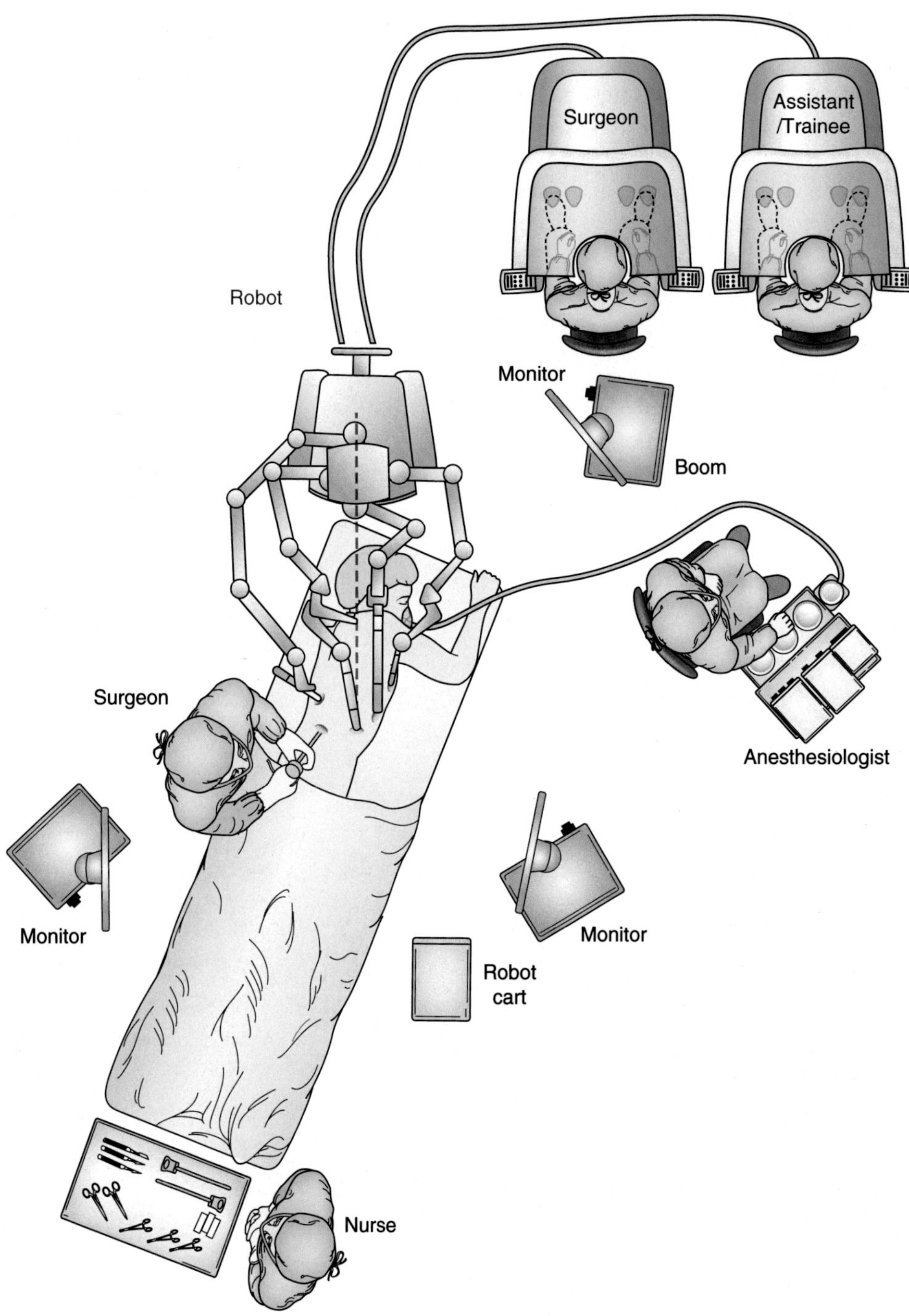

Fig. 35.1 (continued)

abdomen. This port will be used for the ultrasonic shears (Harmonic® scalpel, Ethicon Inc.), which has a shorter operative length than most other instruments on the current robotic platform. An additional right lateral 5-mm subcostal port for placement of the liver retractor is marked, as well as an additional 8-mm right midclavicular and midabdominal port for use with the bipolar atraumatic grasper. A 12-mm port is marked between the umbilical and the right midclavicular ports and is used by the bedside assistant for both suctioning and additional retraction. During later phases of the operation, this port may be expanded to 15 mm to allow entry of larger stapler sizes during gastric conduit formation, if needed. This assistant port can also be used as an alternative camera entry site to improve visualization along the greater curve of the stomach, if necessary, during mobilization of the omentum and gastroepiploic arcade.

The patient is prepped and draped, and the 12-mm camera is placed above the umbilicus using a direct Hassan cutdown technique. Pressurized CO_2 pneumoperitoneum is established to 15 mm Hg. A standard 5- or 10-mm 30° laparoscope is used for the initial inspection of the peritoneal cavity and for identification of any metastatic disease, as well as for port placement. The robotic camera may be used as well. The patient is placed in steep reverse Trendelenburg position while the robotic cart is simultaneously positioned. Trendelenburg positioning facilitates the caudal movement of bowel and other abdominal viscera, allowing for better exposure of the diaphragmatic hiatus. Importantly, once the ports are docked to the robotic arms, further positioning of the patient cannot occur without first undocking the arms.

For the thoracic phase, an insufflation needle with a saline-filled open syringe is placed into the chest, with water entry confirming intrapleural position. CO_2 insufflation is instituted at a pressure of 8 mm Hg. A standard laparoscopic 10-mm camera is placed into the obturator of the camera port, which is introduced into the chest in the eighth intercostal space in the mid-to-posterior axillary line under direct video guidance. The remaining ports are placed under direct intrathoracic visualization (Fig. 35.2). A 5-mm robotic port is placed in the third intercostal space in the mid-to-posterior axillary line, and an 8-mm robotic port is placed in the fifth intercostal space. An additional 8-mm port is placed laterally in approximately the eighth or ninth interspace, roughly in line with the scapular tip. A 12-mm assistant port is placed at the diaphragmatic insertion. To avoid collisions with the bedside assistant, this port should lie midway between the camera port and the lateral 8-mm robotic port. The robotic arms are docked to the ports, and the robotic camera is placed within the chest at a 30° downward orientation.

Robotic arm collisions are minimized by maintaining a minimum distance of 7–10 cm between robotic ports. An experienced bedside assistant can perform simple intraoperative adjustments to the arms as needed.

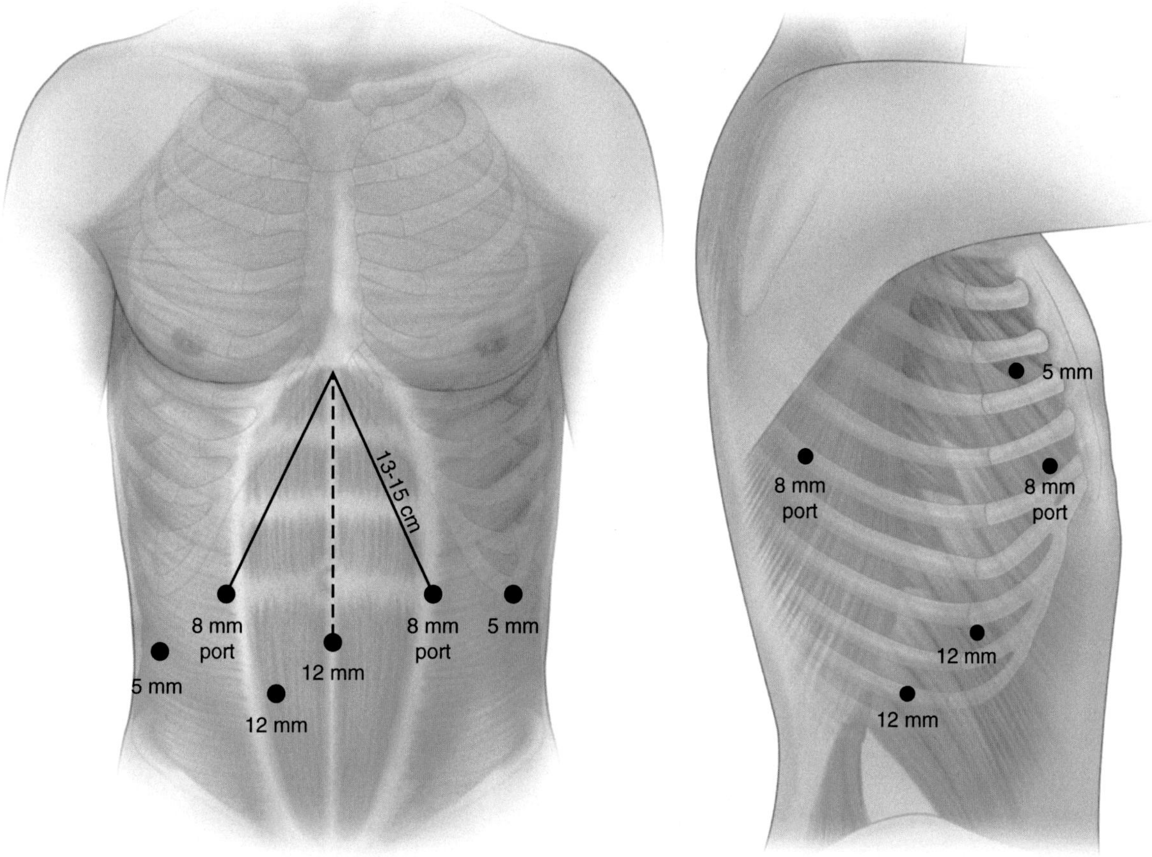

Fig. 35.2 Robotic port size and location for the abdominal phase (*top*) and the thoracic phase (*bottom*) of RAMIE

Surgical Procedure: Abdominal Phase

Step One: Hiatal Dissection

Initial dissection begins by opening the lesser sac (Fig. 35.3). If a replaced left hepatic artery is encountered, it is clipped temporarily; the left liver lobe is assessed after a period of time, and the artery is often sacrificed if no vascular compromise to the liver is identified. Dissection is carried along the left gastric vessels. Complete lymph node dissection is also performed. The right and left crus are identified, and the peritoneal lining is preserved. Initial circumferential esophageal dissection is performed bilaterally along the crural pillars and pleurae, anteriorly along the pericardium, and posteriorly along the aorta and vertebral column. For lower esophageal tumors, portions of the right or left crus are removed en bloc with the esophagus if tumor involvement is identified or suspected. It is preferable to avoid pleural violation during the abdominal phase, to prevent loss of intraperitoneal CO_2 insufflation and potential hemodynamic instability. Should this occur, an expedient temporizing measure is to stop insufflation while applying suction directly through the pleural defect within the operative field, while placing a pleural catheter.

Step Two: Retrogastric Dissection

The retrogastric space is entered through the lesser curve, and the robotic assistant arm is used to gently retract the stomach anteriorly (Fig. 35.3). This retraction exposes the left gastric vascular pedicle, and additional retraction by the bedside assistant provides optimal visualization. Complete celiac and retrogastric lymphadenectomy is performed along the superior border of the pancreas and splenic artery, posteriorly to the retroperitoneal planes, cephalad to the hiatus, and medially along the initial part of the common hepatic artery. Thus, all retrogastric lymph nodes are dissected free circumferentially around the left gastric vascular pedicle. During this dissection, the celiac axis is assessed for bulky adenopathy with persistent disease, the presence of which may preclude resection. We prefer to skeletonize the proximal vascular pedicle, thus lifting all node-bearing tissue en bloc toward the lesser gastric curve, to be removed with the surgical specimen. The vascular pedicle of the left gastric artery is divided with an endovascular stapler introduced through the assistant port. Gentle retraction of the stomach by the robotic assistant arm allows for exposure and additional dissection of the left crus from the lesser gastric curve.

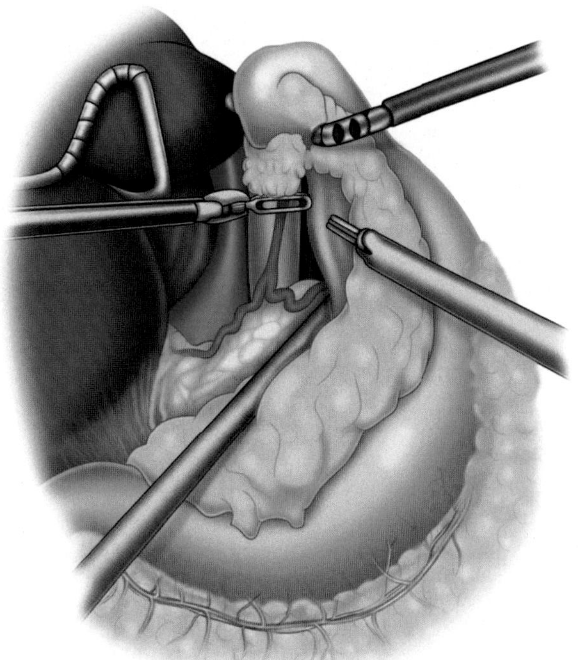

Fig. 35.3 Hiatal dissection. Upon entry into the lesser sac, the esophagus is mobilized from the left and right crus. The proximal left gastric artery is skeletonized and divided. All celiac, splenic, and retrogastric lymph node tissue is removed en bloc with the specimen

Step Three: Gastric Mobilization

Attention is next turned to the greater curve of the stomach, and the termination of the gastroepiploic arcade is identified. Near-infrared fluorescence imaging with indocyanine green may be used to more clearly identify the course of the vascular arcade [20]. The short gastric arteries are divided using the ultrasonic shears, with careful dissection of the gastrosplenic attachments and completion of the left crural mobilization (Fig. 35.4). The lesser sac is entered through the greater omentum, and the gastric mobilization is completed to the level of the pylorus, lysing any remaining retrogastric attachments and taking great care to visualize and preserve the gastroepiploic arcade at all times. To better visualize the gastroepiploic vasculature, the left lateral robotic assistant arm can be used to gently retract the greater curve of the stomach medially and superiorly.

In the event of prior induction chemoradiotherapy, a pedicled omental flap, based off two or more robust omental perforating arteries, is created along the greater curve of the stomach. This flap will later be interposed between the conduit and airway and around the future anastomosis.

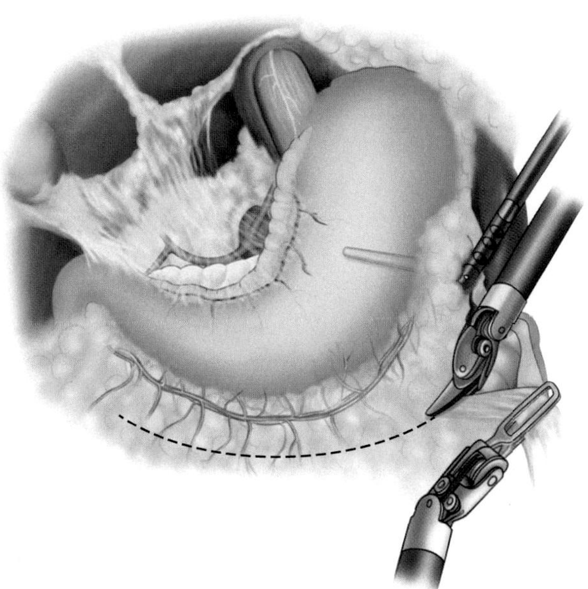

Fig. 35.4 Gastric mobilization. The greater omentum and short gastric arteries are divided from the greater curve. Care is taken to visualize and preserve the gastroepiploic arcade at all points during the dissection

Step Four: Pyloroplasty

The thickened muscle of the pyloric sphincter is identified; this may be done by gently sweeping a handheld grasper or the suction device along the stomach antrum toward the duodenum to delineate the pyloric muscle. The left lateral robotic assistant arm is used to gently grasp the antrum of the stomach and retract it laterally to the left (Fig. 35.5). Retraction stitches are placed at the 12 o'clock and 6 o'clock positions. Orientation of the pylorus is maintained by gentle traction on the stitches by both the right robotic arm and the bedside

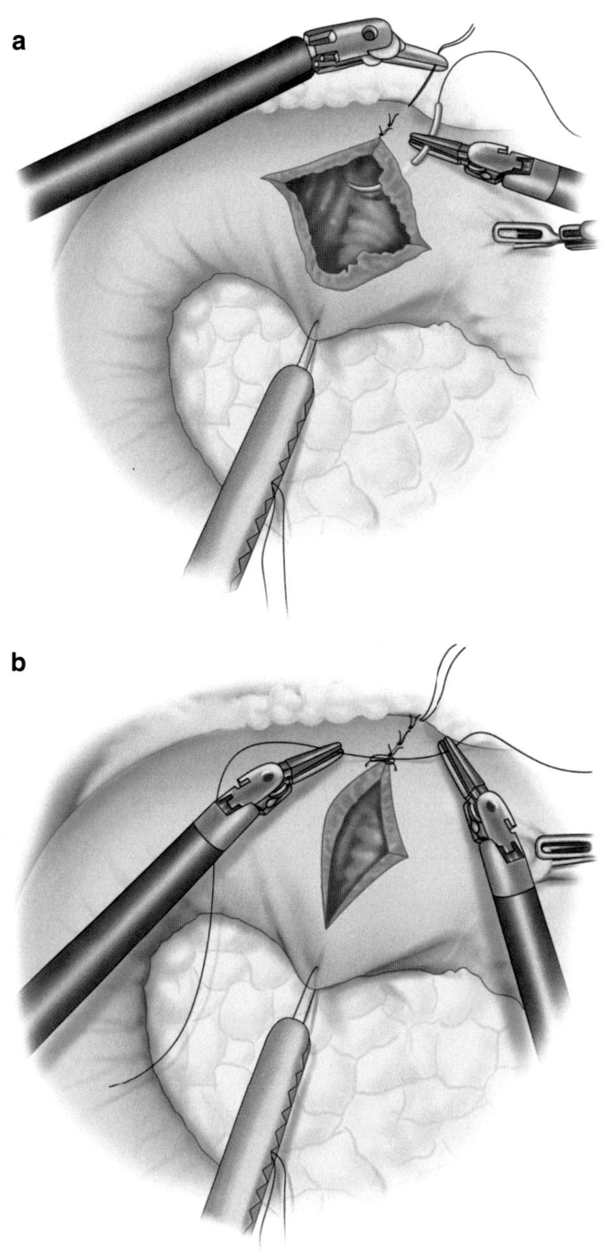

Fig. 35.5 Pyloroplasty. A longitudinal pyloromyotomy is created, followed by transverse closure using a Heineke-Mikulicz technique

assistant. The pylorus is opened across its full width with the ultrasonic shears, and it is closed transversely with 2–0 permanent braided suture on an SH needle. Proper retraction is crucial to ensure a perpendicular incision while creating the pyloromyotomy and to prevent transluminal injury. Typically, five stitches are required for the transverse closure. The closure is reinforced with patch of omentum.

Step Five: Gastric Conduit Formation

In preparation for gastric tubularization, the left lateral robotic assistant arm is used to retract the most mobile portion of the gastric fundus toward the left upper quadrant (Fig. 35.6). If a nasogastric tube is in place, it must be withdrawn into the esophagus. An endovascular stapler is used to divide the lesser curve vasculature at a point approximating the incisura. The gastric tube is constructed with multiple fires of the endo-gastrointestinal stapler, introduced through the 12-mm assistant port. Care is taken to maintain proper orientation of the evolving conduit at all times, with lateral visualization of the short gastric line in order to prevent spiraling. The staple line is extended parallel to the greater curve of the stomach, and a conduit width of approximately 4 cm is maintained. A final stapler fire divides the conduit from the specimen. A "no touch" technique is employed during conduit creation, with care to avoid grasping any portion of the usable conduit. Grasping of the lesser curve/specimen is generally sufficient to manipulate the conduit as needed. The conduit is reapproximated to the specimen with a broad-based, horizontal mattress suture to allow for proper orientation as it is advanced through the hiatus and into the chest during the thoracoscopic phase of the operation. If an omental flap is to be used, it is also secured to the tip of the conduit. The abdominal phase concludes with placement of a standard laparoscopic feeding jejunostomy.

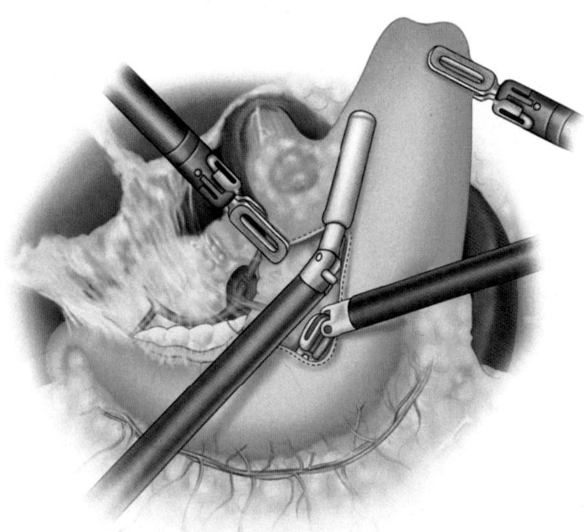

Fig. 35.6 Conduit formation. The stomach is retracted, employing a "no touch" technique with respect to the future neo-esophagus. The conduit is created with multiple applications of the linear stapler

Surgical Procedure: Thoracic Phase

Step Six: En Bloc Esophageal Mobilization

Initial Pericardial and Hiatal Dissection

Using the 5-mm robotic assistant arm, the lower lobe of the lung is retracted superiorly, and the inferior ligament is divided to the level of the inferior pulmonary vein. The initial en bloc dissection is begun along the pericardium adjacent to the inferior vena cava. A combination of gentle blunt and sharp dissection readily allows the surgeon to completely mobilize the esophageal hiatus down to the contralateral pleura.

Subcarinal Dissection

Dissection is continued cephalad by first opening the mediastinal pleura along the hilum, with the lung retracted anteriorly. Great care is taken to identify the airway early in this dissection. This is imperative during dissection of the subcarinal lymph nodes to avoid injury to the membranous airway, leading to potential fistulous complications. The surgeon must be careful to maintain distance between the dissection plane and the airway when using the ultrasonic shears (Fig. 35.7). Use of alternative energy sources for dissection, such as the robotic bipolar Maryland forceps, is highly recommended during this portion of the

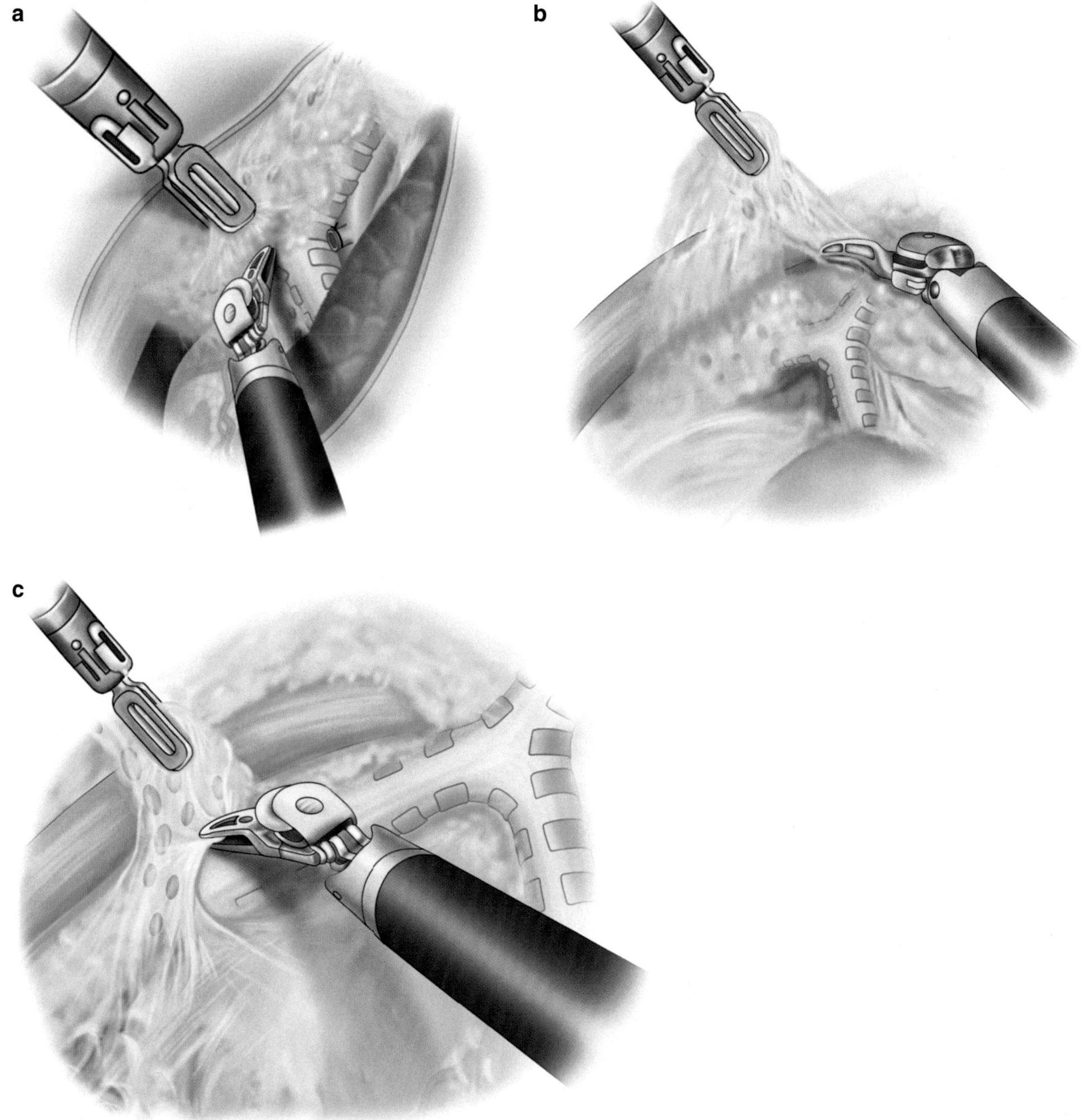

Fig. 35.7 Subcarinal dissection. The level 7 nodal packet is removed, taking care to avoid thermal injury to the membranous trachea and left main stem bronchus

procedure. At all times, the bedside assistant's use of thoracoscopic suction to maintain a clear surgical field aids in this dissection.

Superior Mediastinal and Para-Aortic Dissection

Dissection is continued en bloc up to the level of the azygos vein, which is divided with an endovascular stapler. The vagus nerve is also divided at this level to avoid traction injury to the recurrent laryngeal nerve. The dissection is continued superiorly along the esophagus 3–4 cm above the azygos vein. The posterior mediastinal pleura is divided anterior to the thoracic duct, and the posterior dissection is completed along the aorta to the level of the hiatus. During this para-aortic dissection, surgical clips placed through the assistant port are used liberally to ligate perforating aorto-esophageal arteries and lymphatics prior to division with the ultrasonic shears. The thoracic duct is not routinely resected.

Conduit Advancement and Deep Mediastinal Dissection

The conduit is carefully brought into the chest in proper orientation, with the longitudinal staple line facing laterally. The specimen and conduit are separated, and the conduit is reattached to the diaphragm to prevent retraction into the abdomen during the remainder of the dissection. The specimen is retracted laterally and superiorly with the assistant robotic grasper, and the deep dissection along the contralateral pleura and left main stem bronchus is completed. Thus, all node-bearing tissues along the pericardium, airway, contralateral pleura, and aorta are removed en bloc with the specimen.

The nasogastric tube is withdrawn proximally, and the esophagus is divided above the azygos vein. The posterior 8-mm robotic port is extended to a mini access incision 4 cm in length, and a wound-protector device is placed. The specimen is removed and the surgical margins are assessed grossly and by frozen section.

Step Seven: Creation of Circular-Stapled Anastomosis

Securing the Stapler Anvil

The orifice of the open esophagus is gently retracted and held open by the bedside assistant with the aid of the atraumatic robotic grasper. With the orifice retracted open, a running baseball purse-string suture (2–0 permanent monofilament on SH needle) is placed along the circumference of the opening (Fig. 35.8). Care should be taken to incorporate the muscular and mucosal layers within each stitch and to maintain an even and relatively shallow depth of approximately 5 mm or less to each bite. This helps prevent "rose-budding" and excessive bundling of tissue within the housing of the end anastomotic stapler. Next, the anvil of the end anastomotic stapler is grasped with the robotic forceps

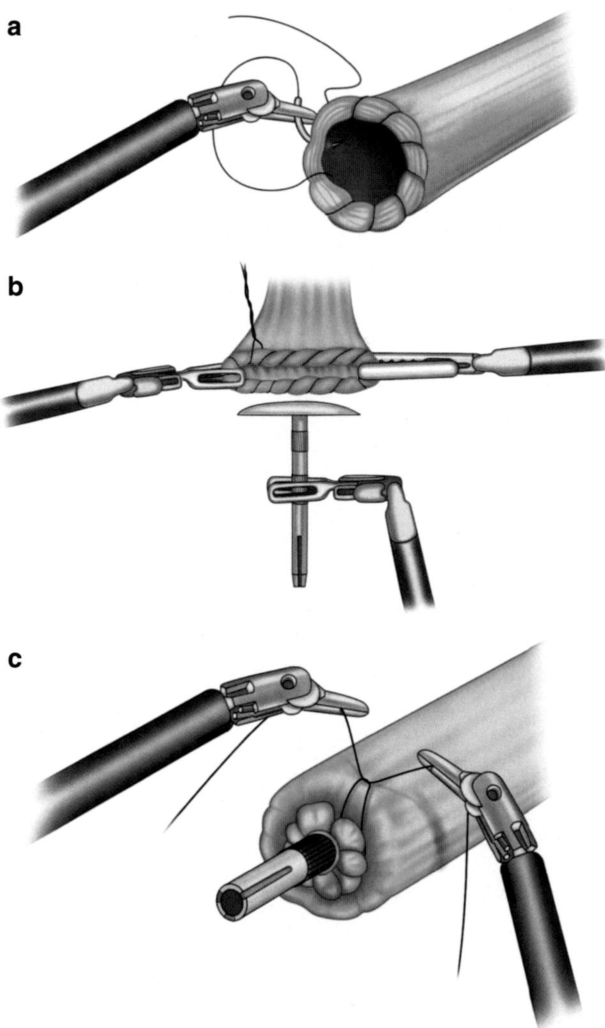

Fig. 35.8 Anvil insertion into the proximal esophagus. The proximal esophagus is retracted open, and a purse-string suture is placed circumferentially. The anvil is placed within the open proximal esophagus and secured with a second purse-string suture

and introduced into the esophagus, and the purse-string is tied. A second running purse-string suture is placed to reinforce and secure any additional tissue or areas of concern.

Stapler Insertion and Firing

The conduit is brought gently into the chest, maintaining proper orientation with the longitudinal staple line facing laterally. A gastrotomy is created at the most proximal portion of the conduit and carefully held open with the assistance of robotic retraction and by the bedside assistant. The end anastomotic stapler is introduced through the mini access incision and placed through the gastrotomy and into the proximal conduit. The conduit-stapler pair is carefully advanced into the chest and positioned, and the stapler spike is deployed along the greater curve in close apposition to the gastroepiploic arcade (Fig. 35.9). Some authors have advocated visualization of the conduit with near-infrared imaging to assess perfusion at this time, although the current authors have not found this routinely necessary if deployment of the spike can be performed close to the gastroepiploic vascular supply [24]. The spike and anvil are married, and the stapler is fired. Once the anastomosis has been created, the stapler is removed from the chest and examined to ensure complete anastomotic esophageal and gastric tissue "rings." The nasogastric tube is advanced into the gastric conduit under direct vision. The proximal redundant conduit is resected with the endo-gastrointestinal stapler. Care is taken to allow a distance of 2 cm between the anastomotic and gastrotomy closure staple lines. If an omental flap was created, this flap is then wrapped around the anastomotic area. The chest cavity is irrigated and a retro-anastomotic Jackson-Pratt drain is placed to a suction-free bile bag. A single 28-French chest tube is also placed in the right hemithorax. Patients are routinely extubated in the operating room.

Postoperative Care

Early ambulation on the first postoperative day is routine. Tube feeding is initiated and slowly advanced on postoperative day two. Nasogastric tubes are left in place for 3–5 days. An esophagram is performed upon removal of the nasogastric tubes to assess for leak. If no leak (or only a small, asymptomatic, and contained leak) is identified, a liquid diet can be started. Patients are typically discharged home between postoperative days 6–8 and return to the clinic in approximately 3 weeks. At that time, the peri-anastomotic drain is removed. If the patient is able to tolerate a soft diet and maintain adequate oral caloric intake, the feeding jejunostomy tube is removed during this visit.

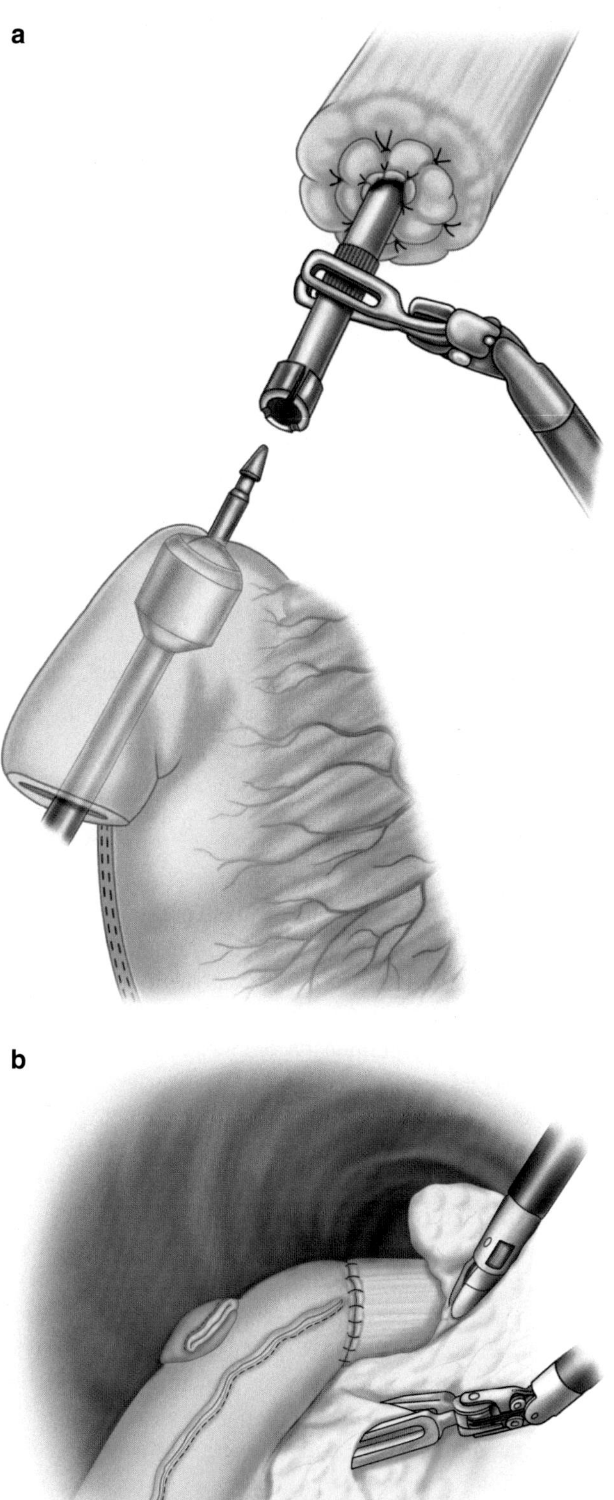

Fig. 35.9 Stapler preparation and anastomosis. Gastrotomy is made in the distal aspect of the conduit, where the end-to-end anastomotic stapler is inserted. The stapler spike is deployed and met with the anvil, and anastomosis is created

Clinical Results in the Literature

Although it is growing, the current experience with RAMIE is still in its early stages, and the literature remains limited. Table 35.1 provides a summary of the current worldwide experience with RAMIE.

In 2002, Melvin et al. [25] published the first description of RAMIE as part of an early institutional experience with robotic surgery for upper gastrointestinal operations. Giulianotti et al. [26] included a series of five esophagectomies with robotically-assisted thoracoscopy featuring three-hole resection as part of their overall experience with robotic surgery. Additional small case series include reports by Bodner et al. [27] and Dapri et al. [28].

In 2004, Kernstine et al. [29] reported the first case of a total thoraco-laparoscopic robotic approach to three-hole esophagectomy. The operative time was 660 min, but the authors noted that more than half of the operating room time was nonsurgical in nature, highlighting the need to develop an experienced team.

Larger series of three-hole esophagectomy with robotic assistance during the thoracoscopic phase vary widely in reported outcomes. Ruurda et al. [30] and van Hillegersberg et al. [31] reported on the same cohort of more than 20 patients. The overall morbidity was 64%, with a predominance of pulmonary complications. One death (5%) was reported, due to tracheal-esophageal fistula. The median operative time was 451 min, and the median estimated blood loss was 950 mL (range, 250–5300 mL). Boone et al. [32] updated this institutional series in 2009 with a total of 47 patients. Reported morbidity remained high, with 47% of patients experiencing pulmonary complications. Anastomotic leaks developed in 21% of patients, and mortality was reported to be 6%.

Puntambekar et al. [33] reported a thoracoscopic-assisted approach with the patient in prone position. Kernstine et al. [34] documented the first case series of completely robotic three-hole esophagectomy in a subset of eight patients. One patient died from respiratory failure, and one suffered bilateral vocal cord paralysis requiring a tracheostomy. One patient suffered intraoperative airway injury, which was repaired robotically. In a follow-up report from the same institution, Anderson et al. [35] reported an additional 25 cases operated on after the initial report, 22 of whom underwent total robotic three-hole esophagectomy. In this series, operative time decreased to a median of 480 min, and there was no operative mortality.

In 2003, Horgan et al. [36] described a transhiatal approach to RAMIE in a detailed case report of a patient with early-stage distal adenocarcinoma. Espat et al. [37], in a later publication from the same institution, reported a series of 15 patients with high-grade dysplasia or early-stage cancer who underwent transhiatal RAMIE. The operative time was 274 min (range 180–360); minimal blood loss and no postoperative mortality were reported. The overall complication rate was 50%, and reported anastomotic leak and stricture rates were 33% each. The mean operative time decreased to 210 min for the last five cases. Average lymph node retrieval was 14 (range, 7–27). Although the initial gastric mobilization was performed with standard laparoscopy, the authors considered the robotic approach to be greatly beneficial during the mediastinal dissection.

In 2013, Cerfolio et al. [38] reported the first series of cases with a robotically-assisted hand-sewn, double-layer intrathoracic anastomosis. Twenty-two patients underwent Ivor Lewis resection with robotic thoracoscopic assistance. The abdominal portion was completed by standard laparoscopy. Among the initial six patients undergoing a posterior stapled and anterior hand-sewn anastomosis, the authors noted significant morbidity, with anastomotic leak, gastric conduit leak, and five reoperations during the hospital stay. Among the remaining 16 patients, who underwent robotically hand-sewn two-layer anastomosis, there was a significant decrease in morbidity, leading the authors to advocate for intrathoracic robotic approaches to this anastomosis.

The senior author of this chapter (I.S.S.) reported on an initial 21 patients undergoing RAMIE at Memorial Sloan Kettering Cancer Center, including a first description of total robotically-assisted laparo-thoracoscopic Ivor Lewis RAMIE in 17 patients; 4 other patients underwent total RAMIE with a three-hole approach [39]. Intrathoracic anastomoses were performed with standard circular anastomotic staplers, as described above. Anastomotic leaks occurred in three patients. Of concern, three patients in this early experience developed airway fistulas (a complication associated with minimally invasive esophageal resections), accounting for the single mortality from respiratory failure at 70 days in this report. The authors caution that these injuries are likely caused by the use of rigid thermal devices such as the ultrasonic shears and fixed tangential instrument angles. These features, combined with a lack of haptic feedback offered by robotic systems, may increase the risk of thermal insult to the airway, which is not immediately apparent at the time of initial injury. The authors advise selective use of wristed bipolar energy dissectors during the subcarinal dissection.

In a follow-up experience of 100 sequential RAMIE cases, no such additional injuries were identified with adjustment of technique as described [22]. Between the first and second half of the experience, there were significant decreases in conversion to open surgery (8 vs. 2%, $p = 0.003$), median operative time (448 vs. 356 min, $p < 0.001$), estimated blood loss (300 vs. 200 mL), and complications ($p = 0.05$). There was a non-statistically significant rise in median lymph node count (22 vs. 25). The anastomotic leak

Table 35.1 Summary of experience in robotically-assisted esophagectomy

Study	Year	Surgical approach	Robotic phase	Patients, *n*	Morbidity, %	Mortality, %	Operative time, *min* (range)	Estimated blood loss, *mL* (range)	Length of stay, *days* (range)	Lymph nodes harvested, *n*
Melvin et al. [25]	2002	Ivor Lewis	NR	1	NR	NR	462	NR	12	NR
Horgan et al. [36]	2003	Transhiatal	Abdominal	1	NR	NR	246	50	7	NR
Guilianotti et al. [26]	2003	McKeown	Thoracic only	5	NR	20	490 (420–540)	NR	NR	NR
Kernstine et al. [29]	2004	McKeown	Abdominal and thoracic	1	0	0	660	900	8	NR
Bodner et al. [27]	2004	McKeown	Thoracic	4	0	NR	173 (171–190)	NR	NR	NR
Espat et al. [37]	2005	Transhiatal	Abdominal	15	NR	0	274 (180–360)	NR	NR	NR
Ruurda et al. [30]	2005	McKeown	Thoracic	22	64	5	180 (120–240)	NR	NR	NR
Van Hillegersberg et al. [31]	2006	McKeown	Thoracic	21	NR	5	451 (370–550)	950 (250–5300)	18 (11–82)	20 (9–30)
Dapri et al. [28]	2006	McKeown	Thoracic	2	0	0	NR	NR	7, 12	18, 21
Kernstine et al. [34]	2007	McKeown	Thoracic only	6	29	7	NR	NR	22 (8–72)	18 (10–32)
			Thoracic and abdominal	8			672 (570–780)	275 (50–950)		
Anderson et al. [35]	2007	McKeown	Thoracic and abdominal	22	32	0	480 (391–646)	350 (100–1600)	11 (5–64)	22 (10–49)
Cerfolio et al. [38]	2013	Ivor Lewis	Thoracic only	22	23	0	367 (290–453)	75 (40–800)	7 (6–32)	18 (15–28)
de la Fuente et al. [40]	2013	Ivor Lewis	Abdominal and thoracic (approximately half, rest with conventional laparoscopy and HALS)	50	28	NR	445, mean (NR)	146, mean (NR)	9 (6–35)	19 (8–63)
Sarkaria et al. [39]	2013	Ivor Lewis	Thoracic and abdominal	17	24	5	556 (395–626)	300, mean	10 (7–70)	20 (10–49)
		McKeown	Thoracic and abdominal	4						
Trugeda Carrera et al. [42]	2015	Ivor Lewis	Thoracic only	21	28	3	218 (190–285) console time only	170 (40–255)	12 (8–50)	16 (2–23)
		McKeown	Thoracic only	11						
Hodari et al. [19]	2015	Ivor Lewis	Thoracic only	54	90	2	362 (280–516)	74.4, average	12.9 (7–37)	16.2 (3–35)
Van der Sluis et al. [42]	2015	McKeown	Abdominal and thoracic	108 (20 converted to open)	66	5	381 (264–636)	NR	16 (9–123)	26(5–53)
Sarkaria et al. [22]	2017	Ivor Lewis	Thoracic and abdominal	100	26	1	379 (275–807)	250 (20–700)	9 (5–70)	24 (10–56)

NR not reported

rate was 6%, and there was no additional surgical mortality (0% 30-day and 1% 90-day mortality).

Other significant institutional series have also been reported. A report from de la Fuente et al. [40] covered a series of 50 RAMIE cases with intrathoracic anastomosis, approximately half of which underwent total robotic Ivor Lewis procedures. Anastomoses were created using a transoral 25-mm end anastomotic stapler. The authors reported no 30-day mortality, a 2% anastomotic leak rate, and a median lymph node retrieval of 19 (range, 8–63).

Trugeda Carrera et al. [41] reported on their case series of 32 patients, 20 of whom underwent Ivor Lewis operations; 11 had McKeown operations with robotic assistance for the thoracic portion. They reported a morbidity of 28% and a mortality of 3%. Console time ranged from 190 to 285 min (218 average), the average hospital length of stay was 12 days, and an average of 16 lymph nodes were retrieved. Similarly, Hodari et al. [19] reported their experience in a retrospective review of 54 patients who underwent RAMIE with a robotically-assisted thoracic phase and a standard laparoscopic approach for the abdominal portion. The most common complication in this series was cardiac arrhythmia (25%). They also reported a 6.8% leak rate and 2% 30-day mortality.

Van der Sluis et al. [42] reported a prospective study of 108 patients undergoing robotically-assisted laparoscopic and/or thoracoscopic esophagectomy with two-field lymphadenectomy and hand-sewn cervical anastomosis. Twenty patients were converted to an open approach (11 transthoracic and 9 transhiatal). Three patients required a conversion to open laparotomy for uncontrolled bleeding, advanced tumor requiring a total gastrectomy with colonic interposition, or unusual anatomic features. There was a significant decrease in the rate of conversions between the two sequential cohorts of 54 patients. The total median procedure time was 381 min (range, 264–550). Similarly, the authors reported a learning curve effect, with a significant decrease in the thoracoscopic operative time between the first and second cohort of patients (199 vs. 166 min; $p < 0.001$). Postoperative complications included pneumonia (36 [33%]), esophagogastric leak (20 [19%]) chylothorax (19 [18%]), and vocal cord paralysis (10 [9%]), with a permanent paralysis in 2% of the individuals. The median lymph node harvest was 26 nodes (range, 5–57), and the hospital length of stay was 16 days (range, 9–123). In-hospital mortality was 5%. 30-day and 90-day mortalities were not reported. R0 resection was achieved in 95% of patients, and median disease-free survival was 21 months.

Summary

Robotically-assisted MIE is still in relatively early stages of development, dissemination, and adoption within the surgical field. Early institutional series have suggested that RAMIE is a feasible and reasonable alternative to standard MIE or open esophagectomy. Care must be taken during the learning phase of these operations to avoid known pitfalls leading to significant morbidity and potential mortality. High-volume single-center series have reported operative and oncologic outcomes comparable with other minimally invasive and open approaches, although more long-term cancer survival data are necessary. There is a paucity of prospective trials directly comparing RAMIE with these procedures. A prospective trial comparing quality of life and operative outcomes in RAMIE versus open esophagectomy at Memorial Sloan Kettering Cancer Center has completed accrual. Short-term outcomes are expected to be reported in the near future. The first randomized, controlled trial comparing RAMIE versus open approaches (ROBOT trial) also is expected to be nearing completion soon. Early experiences are promising, but further study into the cost-effectiveness, short-term and long-term oncologic outcomes, and patient quality of life is warranted to better identify the comparative utility of RAMIE in esophageal cancer.

References

1. Blot WJ, McLaughlin JK. The changing epidemiology of esophageal cancer. Semin Oncol. 1999;26(5 Suppl 15):2–8.
2. Pohl H, Welch HG. The role of overdiagnosis and reclassification in the marked increase of esophageal adenocarcinoma incidence. J Natl Cancer Inst. 2005;97:142–6.
3. Howlader N, Noone AM, Krapcho M, Miller D, Bishop K, Altekruse SF, et al.. SEER cancer statistics review, 1975–2013. Bethesda, MD: National Cancer Institute. http://seer.cancer.gov/csr/1975_2013/, based on November 2015 SEER data submission, posted to the SEER web site. Accessed Feb 2017.
4. Bosset JF, Gignoux M, Triboulet JP, Tiret E, Mantion G, Elias D, et al. Chemoradiotherapy followed by surgery compared with surgery alone in squamous-cell cancer of the esophagus. N Engl J Med. 1997;337:161–7.
5. Turner GG. Excision of the thoracic esophagus for carcinoma with construction of an extra-thoracic gullet. Lancet. 1933;222:1315–6. https://doi.org/10.1016/S0140-6736(01)18863-X.
6. Denk W. Zur Radikaloperation des Osophaguskarfzentralbl. Chirurg. 1913;40:1065–8.
7. Walsh TN, Noonan N, Hollywood D, Kelly A, Keeling N, Hennessy TP. A comparison of multimodal therapy and surgery for esophageal adenocarcinoma. N Engl J Med. 1996;335(7):462.
8. Rizk N, Venkatraman E, Park B, Flores R, Bains MS, Rusch V. The prognostic importance of the number of involved lymph nodes in esophageal cancer: implications for revisions of the American Joint Committee on Cancer staging system. J Thorac Cardiovasc Surg. 2006;132:1374–81.

9. Rizk NP, Ishwaran H, Rice TW, Chen LQ, Schipper PH, Kesler KA, et al. Optimum lymphadenectomy for esophageal cancer. Ann Surg. 2010;251:46–50.
10. van Hagen P, Hulshof MC, van Lanschot JJ, Steyerberg EW, van Berge Henegouwen MI, Wijnhoven BP, et al. Preoperative chemoradiotherapy for esophageal or junctional cancer. N Engl J Med. 2012;366:2074–84.
11. Boone J, Livestro DP, Elias SG, Borel Rinkes IH, van Hillegersberg R. International survey on esophageal cancer: part I surgical techniques. Dis Esophagus. 2009;22:195–202.
12. Hulscher JB, van Sandick JW, de Boer AG, Wijnhoven BP, Tijssen JG, Fockens P, et al. Extended transthoracic resection compared with limited transhiatal resection for adenocarcinoma of the esophagus. N Engl J Med. 2002;347:1662–9.
13. Luketich JD, Alvelo-Rivera M, Buenaventura PO, Christie NA, McCaughan JS, Litle VR, et al. Minimally invasive esophagectomy: outcomes in 222 patients. Ann Surg. 2003;238:486–94; discussion 494–5
14. Luketich JD, Schauer PR, Christie NA, Weigel TL, Raja S, Fernando HC, et al. Minimally invasive esophagectomy. Ann Thorac Surg. 2000;70:906–11. discussion 911–2
15. McCulloch P, Ward J, Tekkis PP, ASCOT Group of Surgeons, British Oesophago-Gastric Cancer Group. Mortality and morbidity in gastro-oesophageal cancer surgery: initial results of ASCOT multicentre prospective cohort study. BMJ. 2003;327:1192–7.
16. Luketich JD, Pennathur A, Awais O, Levy RM, Keeley S, Shende M, et al. Outcomes after minimally invasive esophagectomy: review of over 1000 patients. Ann Surg. 2012;256:95–103.
17. Singh RK, Pham TH, Diggs BS, Perkins S, Hunter JG. Minimally invasive esophagectomy provides equivalent oncologic outcomes to open esophagectomy for locally advanced (stage II or III) esophageal carcinoma. Arch Surg. 2011;146:711–4.
18. Verhage RJ, Hazebroek EJ, Boone J, Van Hillegersberg R. Minimally invasive surgery compared to open procedures in esophagectomy for cancer: a systematic review of the literature. Minerva Chir. 2009;64:135–46.
19. Hodari A, Park KU, Lace B, Tsiouris A, Hammoud Z. Robot-assisted minimally invasive Ivor Lewis esophagectomy with real-time perfusion assessment. Ann Thorac Surg. 2015;100:947–52.
20. Sarkaria IS, Bains MS, Finley DJ, Adusumilli PS, Huang J, Rusch VW, et al. Intraoperative near-infrared fluorescence imaging as an adjunct to robotic-assisted minimally invasive esophagectomy. Innovations. 2014;9:391–3.
21. Sarkaria IS, Rizk NP. Robotic-assisted minimally invasive esophagectomy: the Ivor Lewis approach. Thorac Surg Clin. 2014;24(2):211–22, vii
22. Sarkaria IS, Rizk NP, Grosser R, Goldman D, Finley DJ, Ghanie A, et al. Attaining proficiency in robotic-assisted minimally invasive esophagectomy while maximizing safety during procedure development. Innovations. 2016;11(4):268–73.
23. Weksler B, Sharma P, Moudgill N, Chojnacki KA, Rosato EL. Robot-assisted minimally invasive esophagectomy is equivalent to thoracoscopic minimally invasive esophagectomy. Dis Esophagus. 2012;25:403–9.
24. Campbell C, Reames MK, Robinson M, Symanowski J, Salo JC. Conduit vascular evaluation is associated with reduction in anastomotic leak after esophagectomy. J Gastrointest Surg. 2015;19(5):806–12.
25. Melvin WS, Needleman BJ, Krause KR, Schneider C, Wolf RK, Michler RE, et al. Computer-enhanced robotic telesurgery. Initial experience in foregut surgery. Surg Endosc. 2002;16:1790–2.
26. Giulianotti PC, Coratti A, Angelini M, Sbrana F, Cecconi S, Balestracci T, et al. Robotics in general surgery: personal experience in a large community hospital. Arch Surg. 2003;138:777–84.
27. Bodner J, Wykypiel H, Wetscher G, Schmid T. First experiences with the da Vinci operating robot in thoracic surgery. Eur J Cardiothorac Surg. 2004;25:844–51.
28. Dapri G, Himpens J, Cadiere GB. Robot-assisted thoracoscopic esophagectomy with the patient in the prone position. J Laparoendosc Adv Surg Tech A. 2006;16:278–85.
29. Kernstine KH, DeArmond DT, Karimi M, Van Natta TL, Campos JH, Yoder MR, et al. The robotic, 2-stage, 3-field esophagolymphadenectomy. J Thorac Cardiovasc Surg. 2004;127:1847–9.
30. Ruurda JP, Draaisma WA, van Hillegersberg R, Borel Rinkes IH, Gooszen HG, Janssen LW, et al. Robot-assisted endoscopic surgery: a four-year single-center experience. Dig Surg. 2005;22:313–20.
31. van Hillegersberg R, Boone J, Draaisma WA, Broeders IA, Giezeman MJ, Borel Rinkes IH. First experience with robot-assisted thoracoscopic esophagolymphadenectomy for esophageal cancer. Surg Endosc. 2006;20(9):1435.
32. Boone J, Schipper ME, Moojen WA, Borel Rinkes IH, Cromheecke GJ, van Hillegersberg R. Robot-assisted thoracoscopic oesophagectomy for cancer. Br J Surg. 2009;96:878–86.
33. Puntambekar SP, Rayate N, Joshi S, Agarwal G. Robotic transthoracic esophagectomy in the prone position: experience with 32 patients with esophageal cancer. J Thorac Cardiovasc Surg. 2011;142:1283–4.
34. Kernstine KH, DeArmond DT, Shamoun DM, Campos JH. The first series of completely robotic esophagectomies with three-field lymphadenectomy: initial experience. Surg Endosc. 2007;21:2285–92.
35. Anderson C, Hellan M, Kernstine K, Ellenhorn J, Lai L, Trisal V, et al. Robotic surgery for gastrointestinal malignancies. Int J Med Robot. 2007;3:297–300.
36. Horgan S, Berger RA, Elli EF, Espat NJ. Robotic-assisted minimally invasive transhiatal esophagectomy. Am Surg. 2003;69:624–6.
37. Espat NJ, Jacobsen G, Horgan S, Donahue P. Minimally invasive treatment of esophageal cancer: laparoscopic staging to robotic esophagectomy. Cancer J. 2005;11:10–7.
38. Cerfolio RJ, Bryant AS, Hawn MT. Technical aspects and early results of robotic esophagectomy with chest anastomosis. J Thorac Cardiovasc Surg. 2013;145:90–6.
39. Sarkaria IS, Rizk NP, Finley DJ, Bains MS, Adusumilli PS, Huang J, et al. Combined thoracoscopic and laparoscopic robotic-assisted minimally invasive esophagectomy using a four-arm platform: experience, technique and cautions during early procedure development. Eur J Cardiothorac Surg. 2013;43:e107–15.
40. de la Fuente SG, Weber J, Hoffe SE, Shridhar R, Karl R, Meredith KL. Initial experience from a large referral center with robotic-assisted Ivor Lewis esophagogastrectomy for oncologic purposes. Surg Endosc. 2013;27:3339–47.
41. Trugeda Carrera MS, Fernandez-Diaz MJ, Rodriguez-Sanjuan JC, Manuel-Palazuelos JC, de Diego Garcia EM, Gomez-Fleitas M. Initial results of robotic esophagectomy for esophageal cancer. Cir Esp. 2015;93:396–402.
42. van der Sluis PC, Ruurda JP, Verhage RJ, van der Horst S, Haverkamp L, Siersema PD, et al. Oncologic long-term results of robot-assisted minimally invasive thoraco-laparoscopic esophagectomy with two-field lymphadenectomy for esophageal cancer. Ann Surg Oncol. 2015;22(Suppl 3):S1350–6.

36 Robotic Pulmonary Resections

Jae Y. Kim

Introduction

Minimally invasive pulmonary resection has been shown to have multiple advantages over open lung resection, including fewer complications, decreased length of stay, decreased pain, improved quality of life, and improved compliance with adjuvant chemotherapy [1–3]. Although oncologic outcomes appear equivalent, the majority of pulmonary resections for lung cancer are still performed via thoracotomy. The robotic platform offers unique advantages over traditional thoracoscopic lung resection and may overcome some barriers to wider adoption of minimally invasive lung surgery.

Indications and Patient Selection

In our practice, more than 80% of lobectomies are performed robotically. With experience, larger tumors, T3 tumors, and postinduction tumors may all be approached robotically. Bronchial sleeve resections may also be performed safely in experienced hands. As in traditional thoracoscopic lobectomy, earlier in the learning curve, it is best to select patients with smaller, more peripheral tumors. Patients with large, calcified lymph nodes may also pose a challenge. Because tactile feedback is lacking with the robot, we generally do not perform nonanatomic wedge resections robotically. However, in some cases, we have performed localization of a nodule using navigational bronchoscopy. Injection of dye allows for identification of small nodules that may not be palpated thoracoscopically.

J. Y. Kim, MD
Division of Thoracic Surgery, Department of Surgery, City of Hope National Medical Center, Duarte, CA, USA
e-mail: jaekim@coh.org

Y. Fong et al. (eds.), *The SAGES Atlas of Robotic Surgery*, https://doi.org/10.1007/978-3-319-91045-1_36

Positioning and Preparation

After performing bronchoscopy and placing a double-lumen endotracheal tube, the patient is placed in the lateral decubitus position. We typically use bolsters, but a bean bag may also be used for positioning. If using an Si robot model, the operating table is rotated away from the anesthesia station, and the robot is docked over the patient's head at an angle approximately 15° anterior to the axis of the patient (Fig. 36.1). When using an Xi robot, the table does not need to be rotated. The boom is brought at an angle roughly perpendicular to the patient. It may come in either anteriorly or posteriorly. The axis of the boom should again be approximately 15° anterior to the axis of the patient.

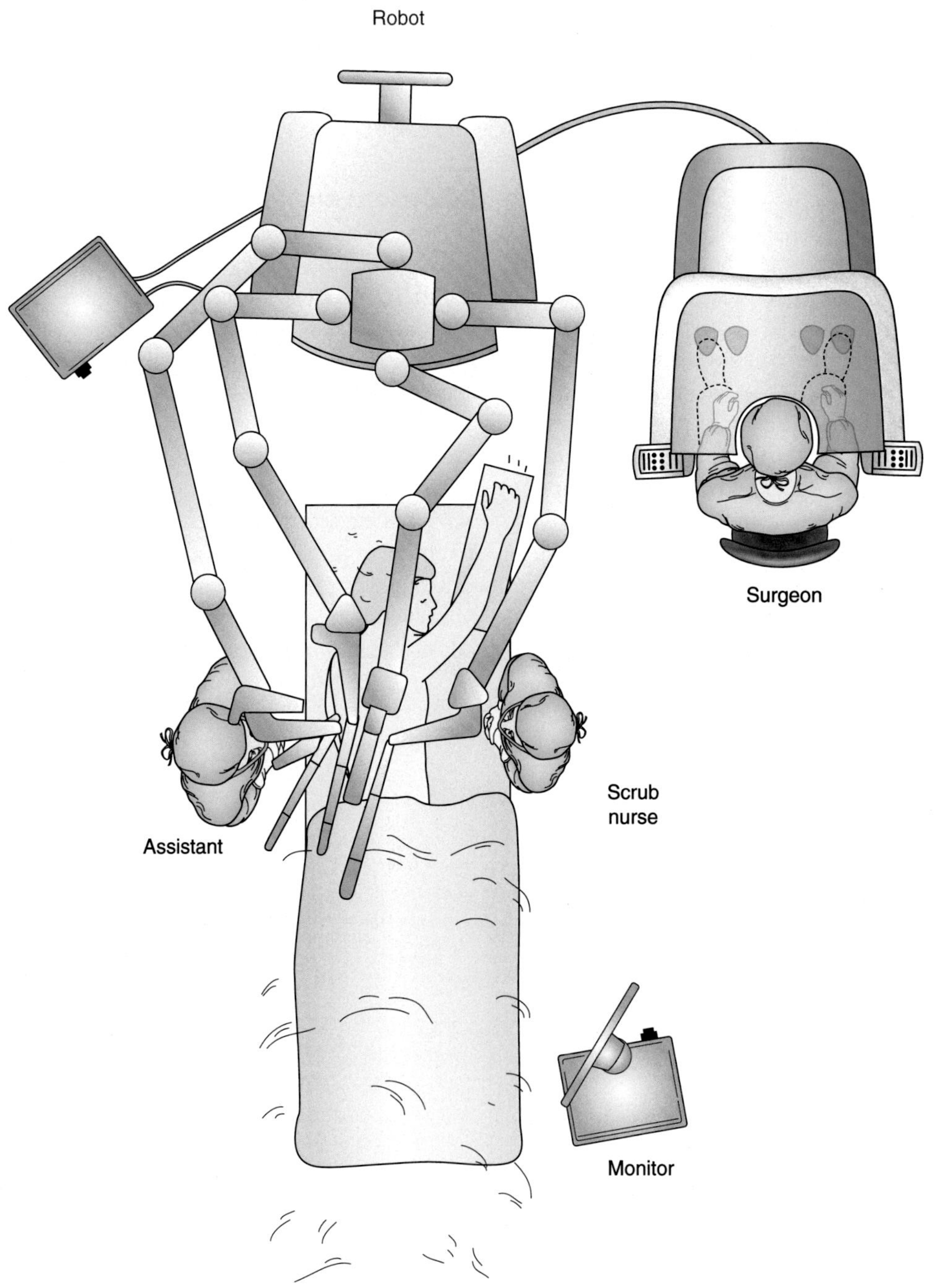

Fig. 36.1 Operative positioning for right-sided lobectomy using the Si robot

Port Placement

The most anterior port is placed first in the seventh intercostal space just posterior to the costal margin. If stapling from this port, it should be placed as far anteriorly as possible within this interspace or the eighth interspace. The chest is slowly insufflated to a pressure of 8 mm Hg. Transient hypotension may occur with initial insufflation, which will resolve with release of pressure from the chest. Insufflating the chest aids in collapsing the ipsilateral lung and pushing the diaphragm down, creating more working space within the chest. It also facilitates the mediastinal lymph node dissection.

The remaining ports are placed under direct vision overlying the major fissure. This is often in the same interspace as the initial anterior port. The camera port is placed at roughly the midpoint of the fissure. The posterior operating port is placed 8 cm posterior to the camera port, again overlying the fissure. The most posterior port, which is the retracting port, is placed in the same interspace, 2 cm lateral to the edge of the spine. When using the Si robot, the most posterior port is 5 mm and the camera port is 12 mm. For the Xi, all ports are 8 mm. An assistant port is placed adjacent to the costal margin in the tenth interspace, just above the diaphragm. In most cases, all stapling can be performed through this port, which is eventually enlarged to accommodate removal of the specimen (Fig. 36.2).

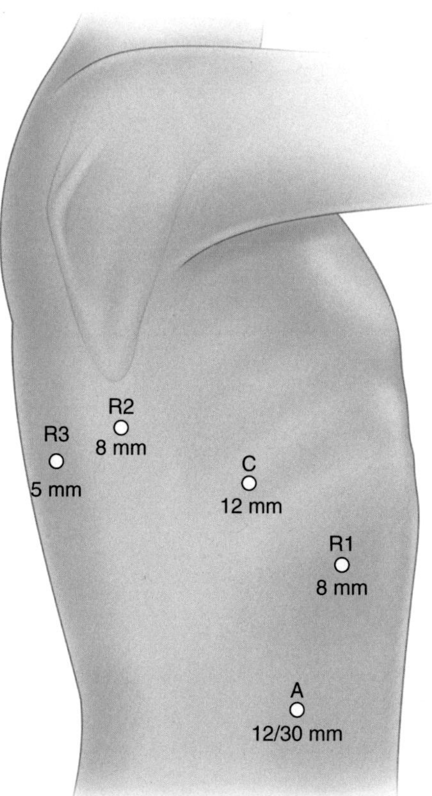

Fig. 36.2 Port placement for right-sided robotic lobectomy using the Si robot

General Considerations

We have found that complete lymph node removal is easier to perform with robotic assistance compared to traditional thoracoscopic resection. In general, exposure and dissection of the hilar structures are enhanced by removing the station 11 and 12 lymph nodes. We prefer to use the most posterior port to retract, and there is seldom any need for additional retraction by the bedside assistant. As a rule, passive retraction should be used without grasping the lung tissue, which can easily be traumatized by robotic instruments. Either a thoracic grasper or a small grasping retractor may be used to retract the lung. Monopolar scissors or a cautery spatula can be used to perform dissection; however, for the most part we prefer to use bipolar dissecting instruments that have less lateral spread of thermal energy to sensitive structures such as the pulmonary artery and membranous airway. The surgeon uses the bipolar dissector in his or her dominant hand. Cadiere forceps or fenestrated bipolar forceps are used in the nondominant hand. We usually pass a soft, silastic vessel loop around structures prior to passing the stapler. The following descriptions use standard thoracoscopic techniques, with division of the fissure after the hilar dissection. However, one advantage of robotic lobectomy is the relative ease of dissecting within the fissure first, which may be preferred depending on the surgeon's experience and patient anatomy. The surgeon and the entire operating team should have an established plan for conversion to thoracotomy if the need arises. In nearly all cases, including pulmonary artery injuries, intraoperative complications can be stabilized with minimal pressure, and the operation can be converted to an open procedure in a controlled fashion.

Right Upper Lobectomy

We typically perform right upper lobectomy using a fissure-last technique, similar to that of thoracoscopic lobectomy. A 0° scope or 30° down scope is used. The lung is retracted posteriorly, and the upper lobe pulmonary vein is divided using a vascular staple load (Fig. 36.3). This allows for exposure of the truncus anterior branch of the pulmonary artery, which is next divided with a vascular staple load (Fig. 36.4). Depending on the size of the posterior ascending branch of the pulmonary artery, it may be divided between clips, with an energy device or with another vascular staple load (Fig. 36.5). A thick tissue stapler is used to clamp the upper lobe bronchus. Unlike a typical thoracoscopic lobectomy,

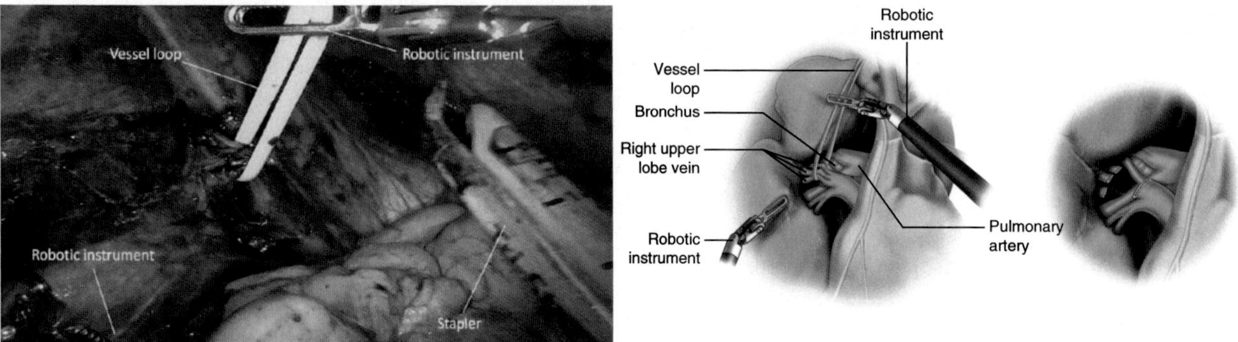

Fig. 36.3 Dissection of the right upper lobe vein. The upper lobe vein is encircled with a vessel loop, and the lung is retracted with Cadiere forceps

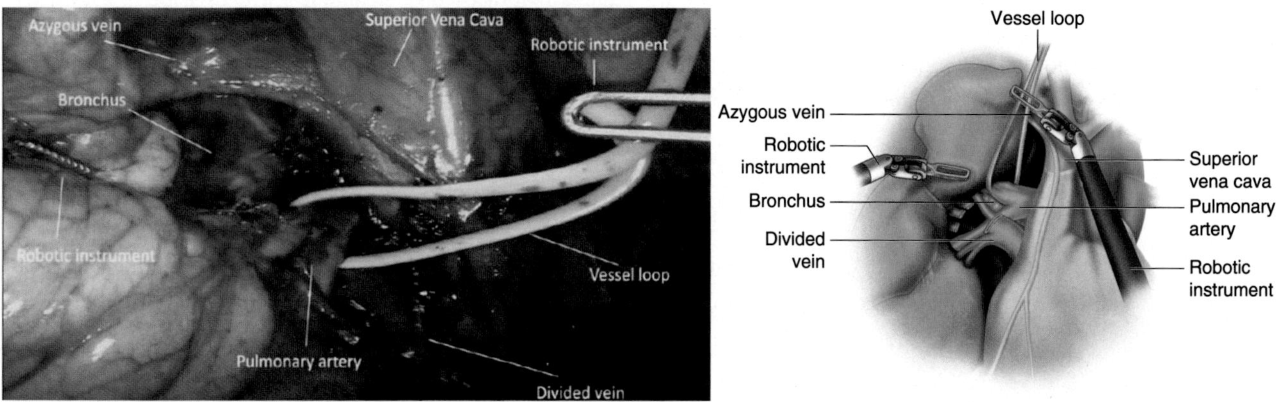

Fig. 36.4 After division of the right upper lobe vein, the truncus anterior branch of the pulmonary artery is encircled with a vessel loop

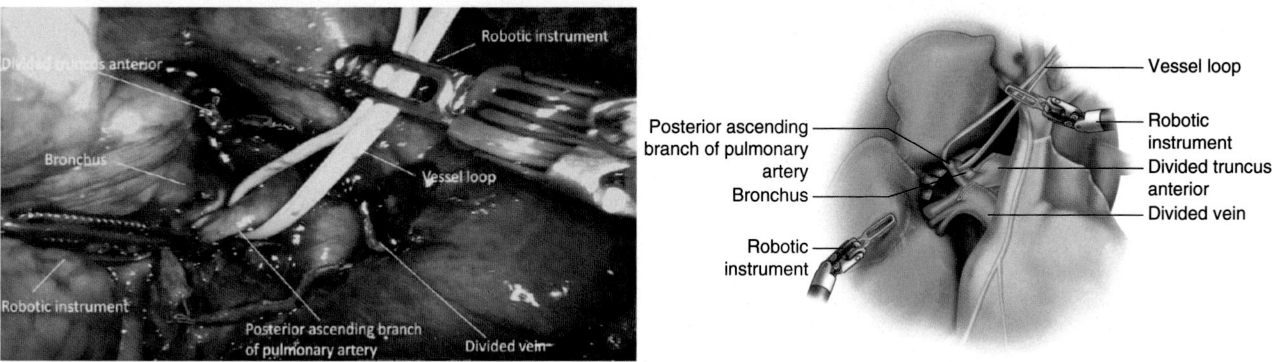

Fig. 36.5 Division of the truncus anterior exposes the posterior ascending branch of the pulmonary artery. The artery is dissected away from the bronchus and may be divided with a vascular stapler, between clips, or with an energy device

when encircling the right upper lobe bronchus for robotic lobectomy, the stapler is usually passed from posterior to anterior (Fig. 36.6). After ensuring adequate inflation of the remaining lung, the stapler is fired and the bronchus is divided. The minor fissure and the posterior aspect of the major fissure are then completed with thick tissue staple loads. The specimen is placed in a bag and removed through the assistant port site, which is enlarged to accommodate it. The mediastinal lymph node dissection may be performed either before or after the lobectomy, depending on the surgeon's preference. Local anesthetic is injected adjacent to the intercostal nerves. After testing the bronchial stump and ensuring good hemostasis, a chest tube is directed apically and the incisions are closed.

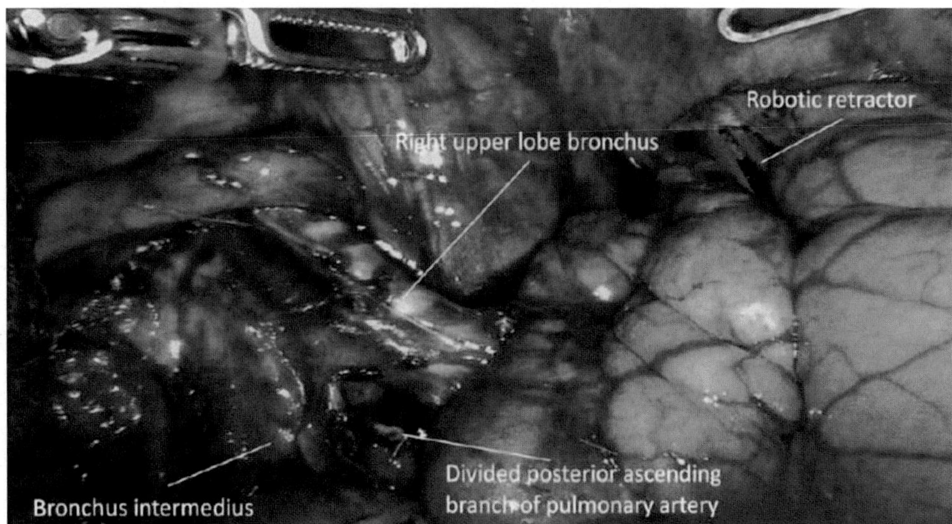

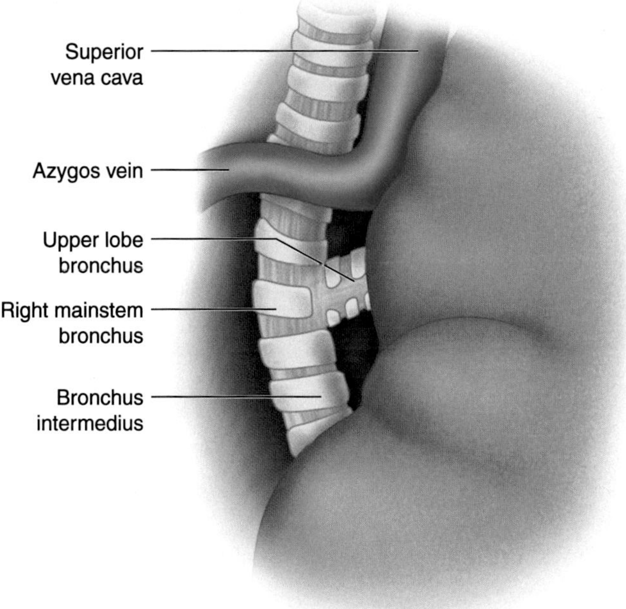

Fig. 36.6 Posterior view of the bronchus with the upper lobe retracted anteriorly after division of vascular structures

Left Upper Lobectomy

Left upper lobectomy is also best performed using a fissure-last technique. After ensuring there is a separate lower lobe vein, the upper lobe vein is divided with a vascular staple load. Next, the most apical branch of the pulmonary artery is divided with a vascular staple load. The upper lobe bronchus is then clamped with a thick tissue staple load. After ensuring adequate inflation of the lower lobe, the bronchus is divided with the stapler. The remaining upper lobe and lingular branches of the pulmonary artery are divided with vascular staple loads, and the fissure is completed with thick tissue staple loads.

Right Lower Lobectomy

A 30° down scope is used for lower lobectomies. After dividing the inferior pulmonary ligament, the lung is retracted cephalad, and the lower lobe vein is divided with a vascular staple load (Fig. 36.7). This allows exposure of the bronchus from an inferior approach. After dissecting the bronchus away from the artery, which lies just cephalad to the bronchus, the bronchus is divided with a thick tissue staple load (Fig. 36.8). The lower lobe artery branch is then divided with a vascular staple load (Fig. 36.9). Often it is easier to divide the lower lobe superior segmental branch separately from the

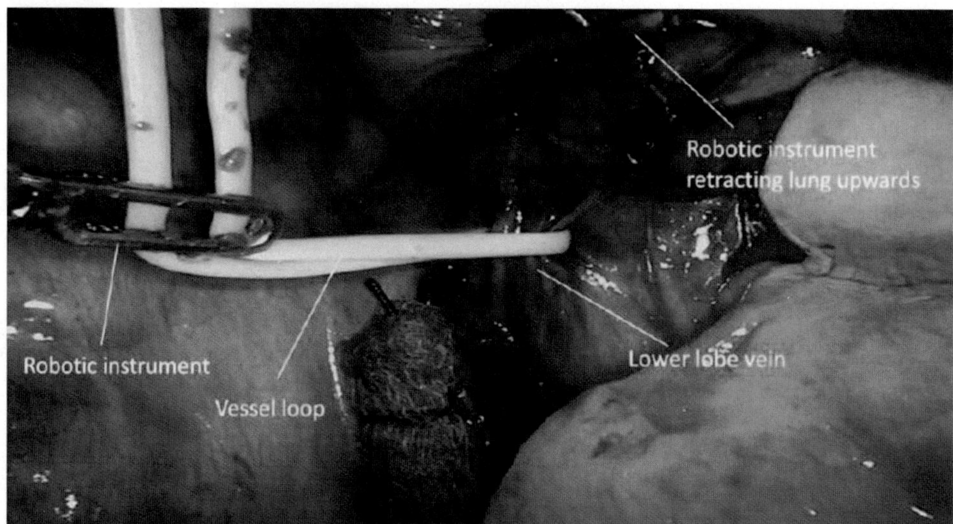

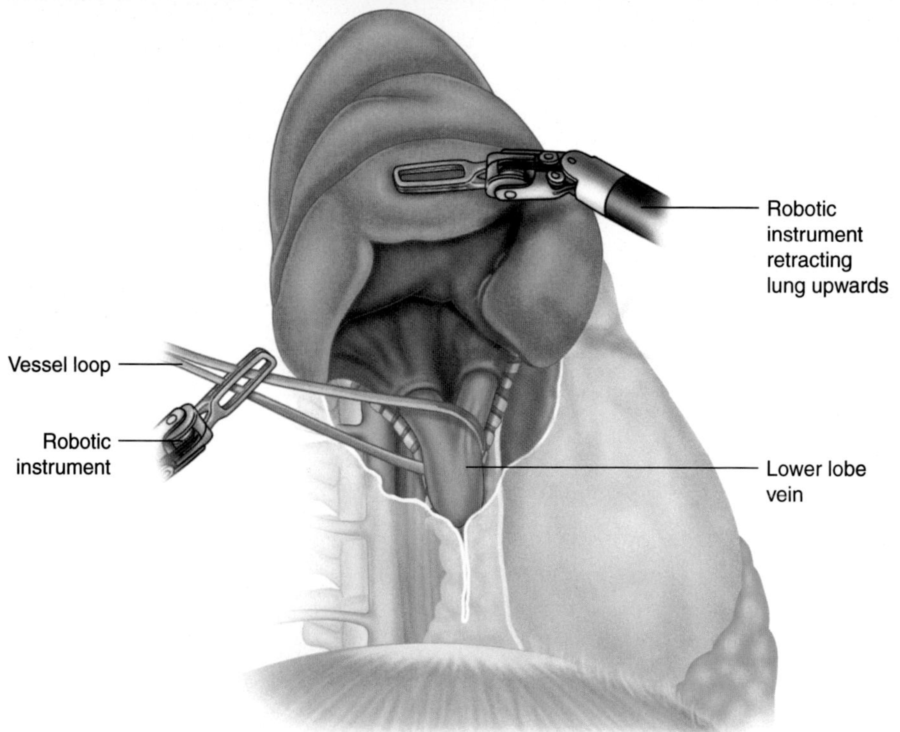

Fig. 36.7 The lung is retracted cephalad, and the lower lobe vein is encircled with a vessel loop

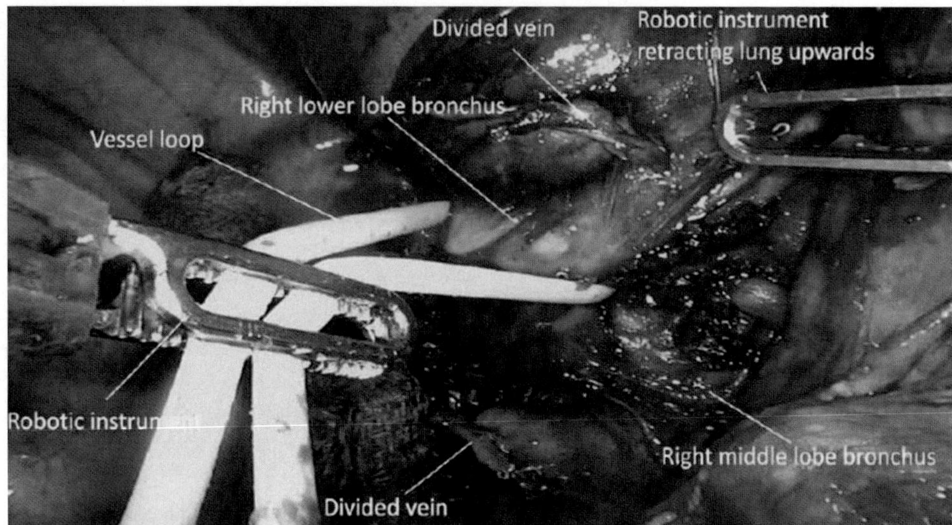

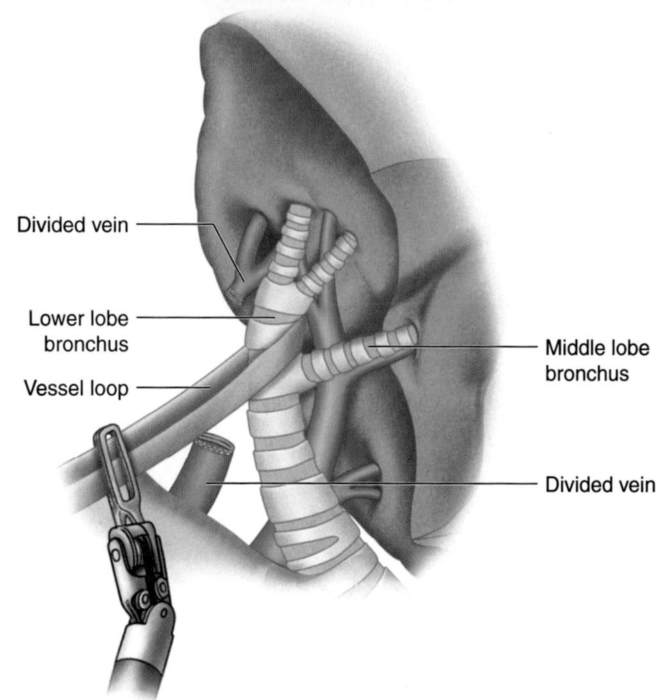

Fig. 36.8 Division of the right lower lobe vein exposes the right lower lobe and middle lobe bronchi

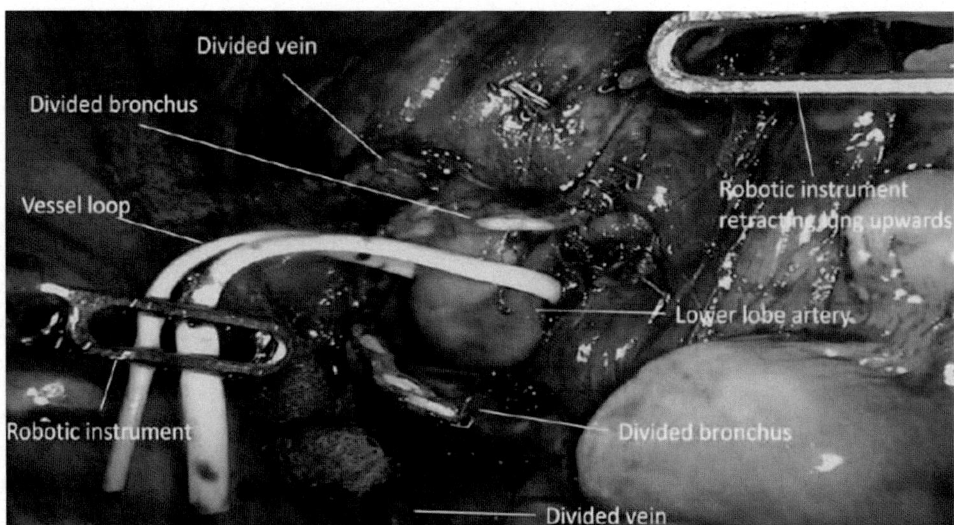

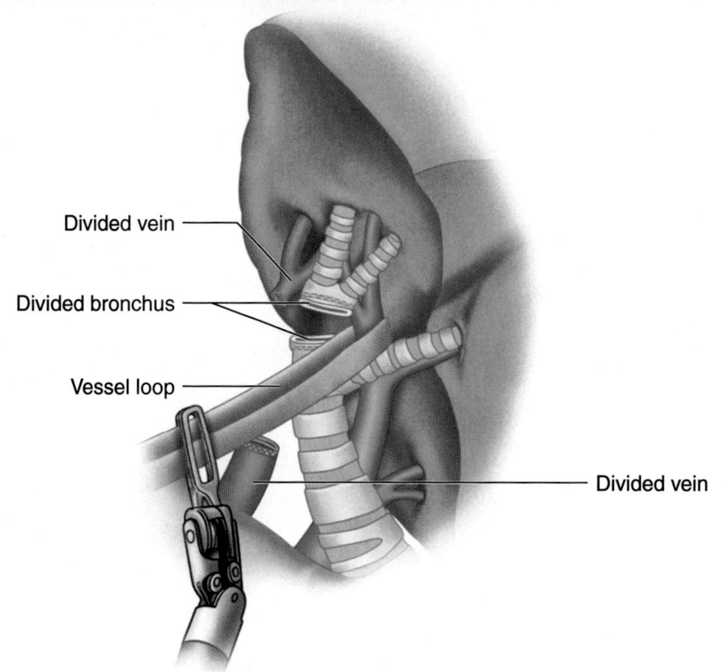

Fig. 36.9 Division of the lower lobe bronchus exposes the lower lobe artery, which is oriented vertically when the lung is retracted cephalad

main basilar branch. The major fissure is then completed with thick tissue staple loads. Alternatively, in patients with a well-developed fissure, it may be easier to complete the fissure and then divide the artery branches prior to dividing the bronchus. For surgeons making the transition from open lung resection to the robotic technique, the anatomy may be more familiar when the fissure is completed first.

Left Lower Lobectomy

The left lower lobectomy is performed in the same fashion as the right lower lobectomy. If dividing the fissure last, it is important to preserve any lingular pulmonary artery branches. By retracting the lower lobe cephalad and upward, these lingular branches can be recognized as branches that appear to travel more laterally or anteriorly. We usually divide the superior segment branch of the pulmonary artery separately from the basilar branches, which often facilitates identification of the lingular branches.

Right Middle Lobectomy

The lung is retracted posteriorly, and the middle lobe vein is divided with a vascular staple load. This exposes the bronchus, which is then divided with a thick tissue staple load. There are usually two middle lobe arterial branches that are then exposed. These may be divided together or separately. The fissure is completed with thick tissue staple loads.

Segmentectomy

Virtually any anatomic segmentectomy may be performed with the robot in a fashion similar to open segmentectomy. Just as in open resection, this is done for patients who require more resection than a simple wedge resection but who do not require or cannot tolerate a lobectomy. We have performed the following segmentectomies robotically: lower lobe superior segmentectomy, basilar segmentectomy (superior segment preserving lower lobectomy), lingulectomy, lingular preserving left upper lobectomy, right upper lobe apical segmentectomy, and right upper lobe posterior segmentectomy.

Lower lobe superior segmentectomies are performed in a fashion similar to that of the open technique. The major fissure is completed first. The superior segmental branch of the pulmonary artery is divided. The superior segmental branch of the lower lobe vein is then divided, followed by the bronchus. The parenchyma is divided with thick tissue staple loads, often after inflating the lung to demarcate the border of the segment.

When performing basilar segmentectomies, we usually divide the basilar vein tributary first, followed by the bronchus and then the artery. The major fissure is completed, and then the lung parenchyma is divided with thick tissue staple loads.

When performing a lingulectomy, we divide the lingular vein first, which exposes the bronchus behind it. After dividing the bronchus, the lingular artery branches are divided. The major fissure is completed, and last the lung parenchyma is divided with thick tissue staple loads. For a lingular preserving upper lobectomy, the upper lobe vein is again divided first, preserving the lingular vein. The anterior pulmonary artery branch is divided next, followed by the bronchus. The remaining upper lobe artery branches are then divided followed by the lung parenchyma.

Right upper lobe apical segmentectomy is performed by dividing the apical branch of the truncus anterior first, followed by the apical segmental bronchus. The lung parenchyma along with the venous drainage is then divided with thick tissue staple loads. If necessary, the apical vein tributary may be divided separately. The right upper lobe posterior segmentectomy is most easily performed by completing the major fissure first, followed by division of the posterior segmental bronchus. The posterior ascending branch of the pulmonary artery is divided between clips or with a vascular staple load, and the lung parenchyma and the venous drainage are divided with thick tissue staple loads.

Sleeve Resection

Bronchial sleeve resections, particularly for carcinoid tumors, may be performed robotically in much the same way as open resections. For right upper lobe sleeve resections, we find that it is often easier to divide the bronchus before completing the minor fissure, just as in the standard robotic right upper lobectomy. For all other lobes, we typically divide the vascular structures and complete the fissures, leaving the bronchus to divide last. The bronchial anastomosis can then be done with 4–0 braided absorbable sutures. It may be easier to run the back row of the anastomosis. The anterior row of sutures should be interrupted. The interrupted sutures may all be placed before tying the sutures. A pedicled, pericardial fat flap may be mobilized in just a few minutes robotically and may be placed over the bronchial anastomosis.

References

1. Teh E, Abah U, Church D, Saka W, Talbot D, Belcher E, et al. What is the extent of the advantage of video-assisted thoracoscopic surgical resection over thoracotomy in terms of delivery of adjuvant chemotherapy following non-small-cell lung cancer resection? Interact Cardiovasc Thorac Surg. 2014;19:656–60.
2. Whitson BA, Andrade RS, Boettcher A, Bardales R, Kratzke RA, Dahlberg PS, et al. Video-assisted thoracoscopic surgery is more favorable than thoracotomy for resection of clinical stage I non-small cell lung cancer. Ann Thorac Surg. 2007;83:1965–70.
3. Whitson BA, Groth SS, Duval SJ, Swanson SJ, Maddaus MA. Surgery for early-stage non-small cell lung cancer: a systematic review of the video-assisted thoracoscopic surgery versus thoracotomy approaches to lobectomy. Ann Thorac Surg. 2008;86:2008–16; discussion 16–18.

37 Robotic Mediastinal Surgery

Boris D. Hristov, Prasad S. Adusumilli, and Bernard J. Park

The mediastinum lies within the thorax and is bordered by the lungs laterally on both sides, the sternum anteriorly, and the spine posteriorly. It extends from the thoracic inlet superiorly to the diaphragm inferiorly. It is divided into anterior, middle, and posterior compartments. The anterior compartment contains the thymus, and the middle compartment contains the heart, tracheal bifurcation, ascending aorta, and pulmonary trunk. The posterior compartment contains the esophagus, descending thoracic aorta, thoracic duct, and the azygos veins [1]. Thymic procedures are the most common surgeries performed in the anterior compartment. Cardiac procedures are most common in the middle compartment, while neurogenic lesion excisions are the most performed surgeries in the posterior compartment.

Traditional open approaches to the mediastinum include a median sternotomy or thoracotomy, depending on which compartment needs to be entered. These approaches require large incisions and may result in morbidity and a longer hospitalization [2]. More recently, minimally invasive approaches, such as video-assisted thoracic surgery (VATS) and robotics, have become more common and have demonstrated improved patient recovery and decreased length of hospital stay. Telerobotic surgery utilizing the da Vinci® Surgical System (Intuitive Surgical, Sunnyvale, CA) has added additional technological advantages for minimally invasive approaches because it affords an increased range of motion and ease of manipulation compared with standard VATS instrumentation [3]. The added flexibility is accomplished using an extra articulating wrist joint that is not available in standard VATS instrumentation. These advantages are beneficial in the anterior mediastinum because the operative field is constrained by the confines of the chest wall and surrounding organs, which greatly limits surgical maneuverability. The first thoracic applications of robotic surgery were demonstrated in 1998 by Falk and colleagues in a series of eight successful mitral valve repairs [4]. Since then, a large number of successful robotic mediastinal procedures have been documented in the literature, the majority being thymectomies [5–8]. These studies indicate that robotic approaches are safe and effective while maximizing the amount of dissection that can be done through minimal incisions. There is also a potential theoretical advantage of reduced postoperative adhesion formation. The benefits conferred on patients include improved cosmesis, reduced postoperative pain, and shorter recovery times [9]. This is of particular importance to patients with myasthenia gravis (MG), who often have impaired healing and respiratory function due to immunosuppressive medications [10].

Indications for Surgery

Anterior Mediastinal Lesions

The vast majority of mediastinal masses are anterior, and most of these lesions are of thymic origin. The indications for thymectomy include thymic neoplasms such as thymoma (with and without MG), thymic carcinoid tumors, thymic carcinoma [11], and other encapsulated lesions of the thymus such as thymic cysts, mediastinal germ cell tumors, and teratomas. Other conditions that may require anterior mediastinal surgery include other cystic lesions (bronchogenic or pericardial), ectopic parathyroid adenomas, substernal goiter, and lymphoma.

Myasthenia Gravis Without Thymoma

In generalized MG without thymoma, there is evidence that thymectomy is beneficial in certain patient populations [12] and can lead to complete remission, depending on the extent of dissection. The decision to pursue thymectomy for

B. D. Hristov, MD · P. S. Adusumilli, MD (✉) · B. J. Park, MD
Thoracic Service, Department of Surgery, Memorial Sloan Kettering Cancer Center, New York, NY, USA

Y. Fong et al. (eds.), *The SAGES Atlas of Robotic Surgery*, https://doi.org/10.1007/978-3-319-91045-1_37

treatment of MG should be a mutual one among the surgeon, the neurologist, and the patient. When the decision has been made to proceed with thymectomy for patients with active MG, they must be medically treated for optimal results prior to surgery, often with preoperative plasmapheresis [11]. The goal of any thymectomy should be radical resection because of the high incidence of ectopic thymic tissue and because as little as 3 g of residual thymic tissue is associated with persistence or recurrence of MG following surgical resection [11].

Indications for Posterior Mediastinal Resections

On the other hand, posterior mediastinal masses requiring surgery are less frequent and are usually neurogenic tumors. Common posterior mediastinal masses include neuroblastomas, nerve sheath tumors, and sarcomas. Surgical resection is recommended for benign and malignant schwannomas, Askin tumors, ganglioneuromas, ganglioneuroblastomas, and low-grade neuroblastomas. High-grade neuroblastomas are usually treated solely with chemoradiation.

Robotic Surgical Approach Considerations

In general, all masses that are candidates for thoracoscopic surgical resection are amenable to robotically assisted resections. Tumor invasion of surrounding structures does not preclude robotic resection [10]; however, the approach must be chosen carefully in order to optimize exposure. In general, tumors that are larger than 3 cm should be resected by more experienced robotic surgeons [10]. For masses significantly larger than 3 cm, an open approach may be more suitable because a larger incision will be necessary to remove the mass and intramediastinal space for safe mobilization becomes too limited.

Anesthesia

The standard approach for robotic thymectomy utilizes general anesthesia with single-lung ventilation contralateral from the surgical approach side. This can be achieved with either double-lumen intubation or bronchial blockers. In patients with MG, it is especially important to avoid depolarizing agents on induction to minimize the risk of myasthenic crisis. If absolutely necessary, however, single doses of either depolarizing or nondepolarizing agents can be used [9].

Patient Positioning

Anterior Mediastinal Surgery

For anterior mediastinal mass resections, patients are routinely positioned in a supine position with the ipsilateral arm left at the side on an arm board. The ipsilateral chest is elevated for better exposure of the lateral chest wall (Fig. 37.1). The complete chest wall should be exposed. Patients are prepped and draped in the usual sterile fashion with prepping of the complete chest in case a contralateral trocar insertion is needed or conversion to an open procedure is necessary. The sternal notch, angle of Louis, and xiphoid process should be marked at the midline for reference [9].

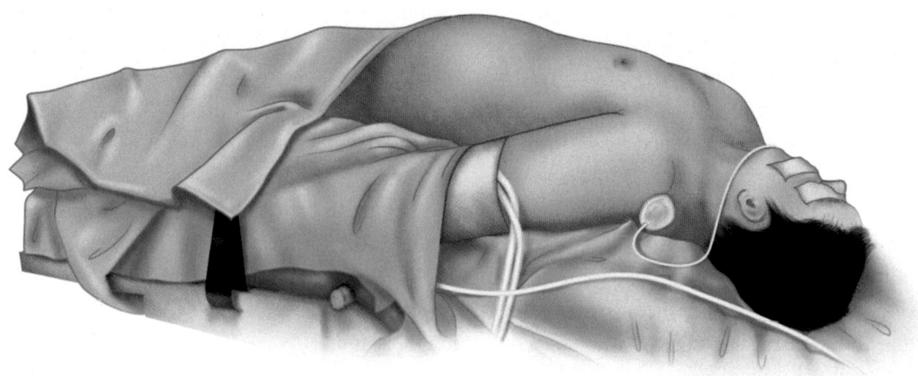

Fig. 37.1 Patient position for anterior mediastinal surgery

Approach Options for Thymectomy

The left-sided thoracoscopic approach is usually preferred for a thymectomy because the left phrenic nerve is frequently mobilized during the excision and it is more safely approached from the ipsilateral side. Dissection and mobilization around the right phrenic nerve occur less often because there is rarely any thymic tissue in its vicinity. Additionally, the left side of the thymus is usually larger and is the more likely site of cancer [9]. If the right phrenic nerve cannot be visualized appropriately through the left side of the chest or there is aberrant thymic tissue obscuring the view, a 5-mm camera can be placed on the right side to ensure an appropriate resection.

Posterior Mediastinal Surgery

For posterior mediastinal masses, the patient is positioned in the lateral decubitus position with the ipsilateral chest up (Fig. 37.2). The table may be flexed in order to maximize spacing between the ribs for optimal access. This also minimizes interference from the patient's hip [13]. It is often helpful to place the patient slightly toward the prone position. This helps displace the lung medially, reducing the need for active retraction.

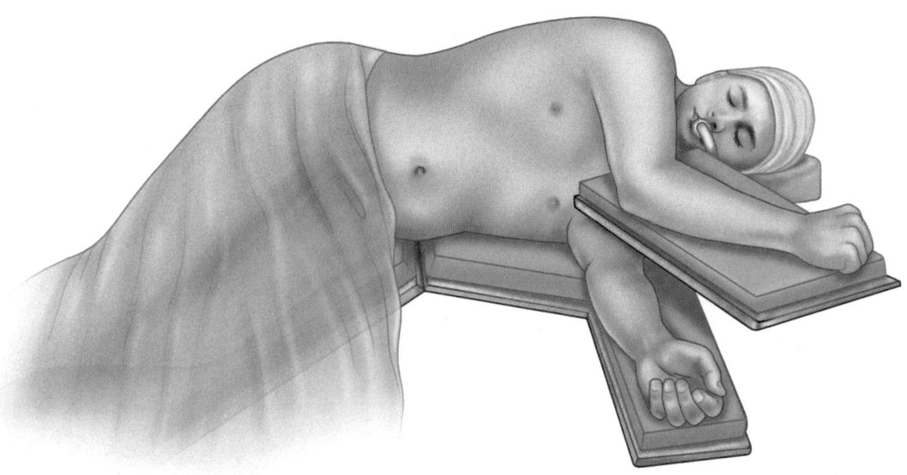

Fig. 37.2 Patient position for posterior mediastinal surgery

Trocar Placement

Anterior Mediastinal Mass Resection

The first port is a 12-mm trocar placed in the anterior axillary line in the fifth intercostal space for the 10-mm 30° camera. Once 8 mm Hg of pneumothorax is created with insufflated CO_2 in the left side of the chest, the operative field should be inspected with the camera and optimum positioning for the 8-mm trocars identified. The cephalad trocar is usually introduced in the third intercostal space between the anterior and middle axillary lines, whereas the caudal trocar is introduced in the fifth intercostal space at the midclavicular line (Fig. 37.3) [9]. The robot can be docked at this time with the monopolar electrocautery in the cephalad port and the fenestrated bipolar forceps in the caudal trocar.

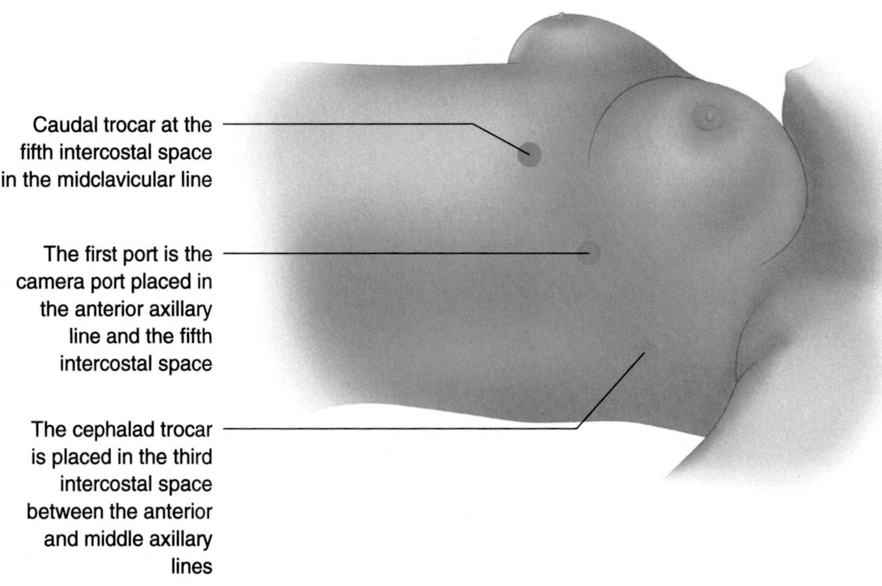

Fig. 37.3 Trocar placement for anterior mediastinal surgery

Posterior Mediastinal Mass Resection

The first incision is made in the ipsilateral posterior axillary line to place a 12-mm trocar, which is used to insert the camera and inspect the operative field. The next two 8-mm trocars are placed in the seventh intercostal space between the posterior axillary line and the infrascapular line as well as in the fourth intercostal space between the anterior axillary line and the midclavicular line on the ipsilateral side (Fig. 37.4) [13].

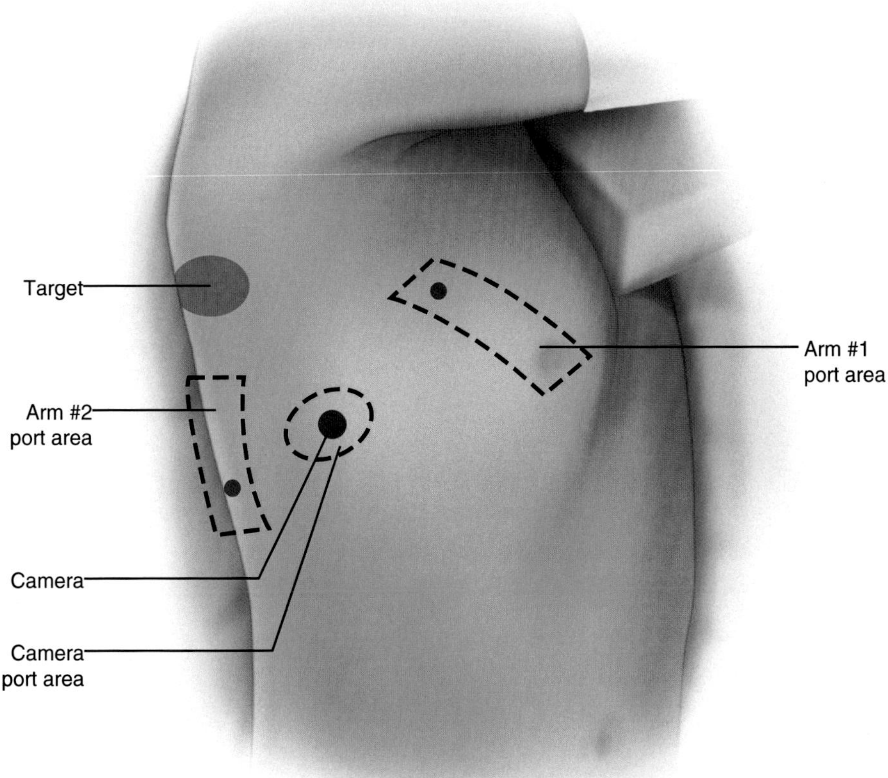

Fig. 37.4 Trocar placement for posterior mediastinal surgery

Thymectomy Technique

Step 1: Dissection of the thymic gland starts by mobilizing the gland and pericardial fat away from the ipsilateral phrenic nerve. For radical thymectomy and in cases of MG, every effort should be made to mobilize all tissue from the diaphragmatic surface to the neck. As the dissection approaches the neck, the innominate vein should be identified (Fig. 37.5).

Step 2: The next step is to mobilize the superior horns of the thymus from the neck. The thyrothymic ligaments and the horns can be divided following the application of clips or by the use of energy (harmonic scalpel or vessel sealer). The horns can then be dissected away from the anterior surface of the innominate vein (Fig. 37.6).

Step 3: The thymic veins draining into the undersurface of the innominate vein should be identified. These can be

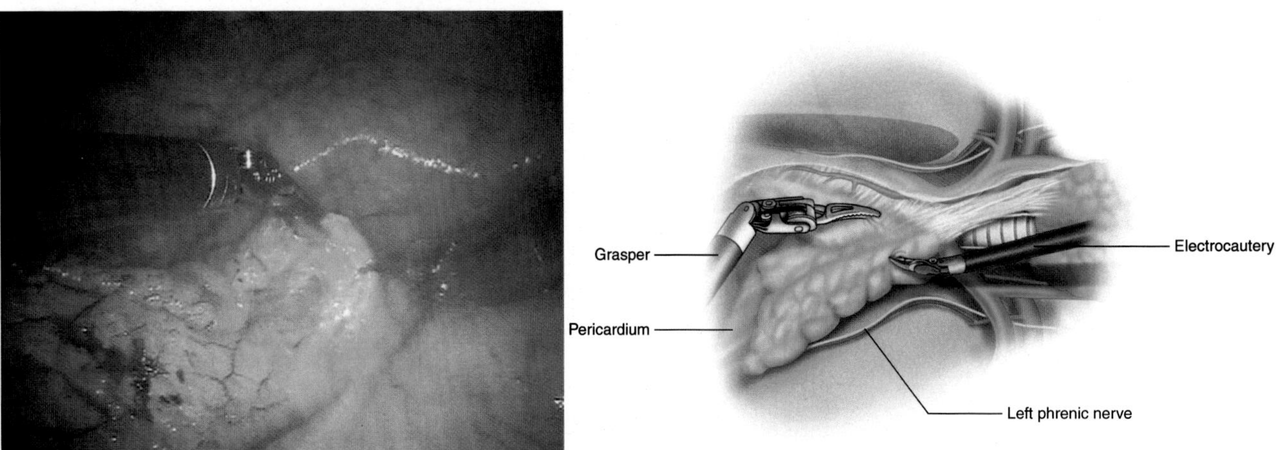

Fig. 37.5 Initial mobilization medial to ipsilateral phrenic nerve

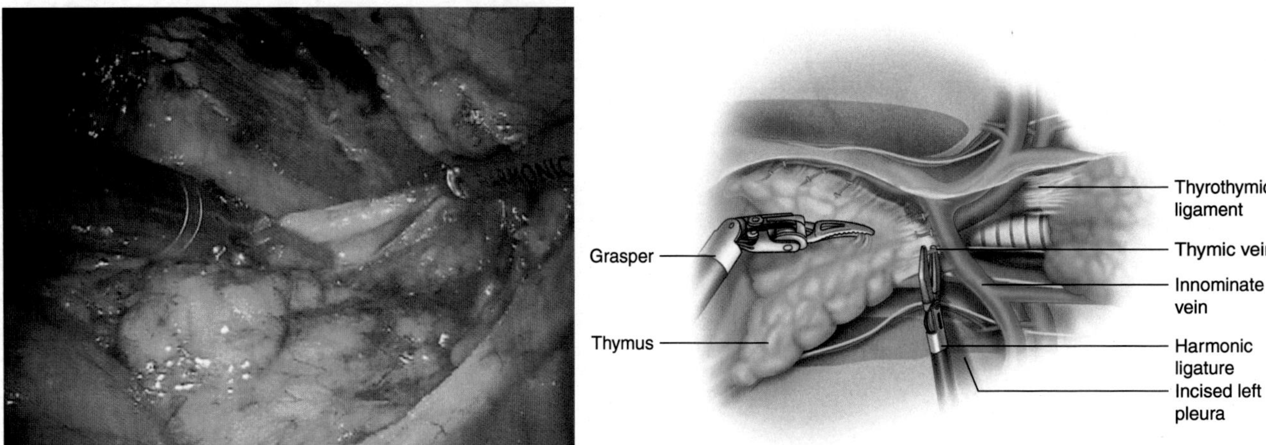

Fig. 37.6 Mobilization of superior poles

serially clipped and divided (Fig. 37.7) or, once again, mobilized with an energy source. When using the latter, it is advisable to keep a safe distance from the innominate vein. On occasion a significant amount of thymic tissue may be located posterior to the innominate vein, and this portion of the gland should be resected rather than left in situ.

Step 4: Once the ipsilateral and bilateral superior horns have been mobilized, the remainder of the gland can be freed from the pericardium and posterior sternal table using a combination of cautery and blunt dissection. For encapsulated lesions and MG, the thymic tissue is easily separated in a relatively avascular plane.

Step 5: Once the whole median retrosternal tissue portion has been mobilized, the contralateral portion of the gland may be dissected. This typically includes a portion of the pericardial fat extending to the level of the contralateral phrenic nerve (Fig. 37.8). This is facilitated by opening the contralateral pleura widely. A 30° scope, with the angle pointing downward, aids in identifying the contralateral phrenic nerve. Another useful strategy includes placement of a second thoracoscope to help visualize the nerve. Care should also be taken to avoid the right internal thoracic vein, which often enters the innominate vein near the right border of the thymus.

Step 6: Once the specimen is fully mobilized, one of the access incisions is enlarged in order to introduce a retrieval

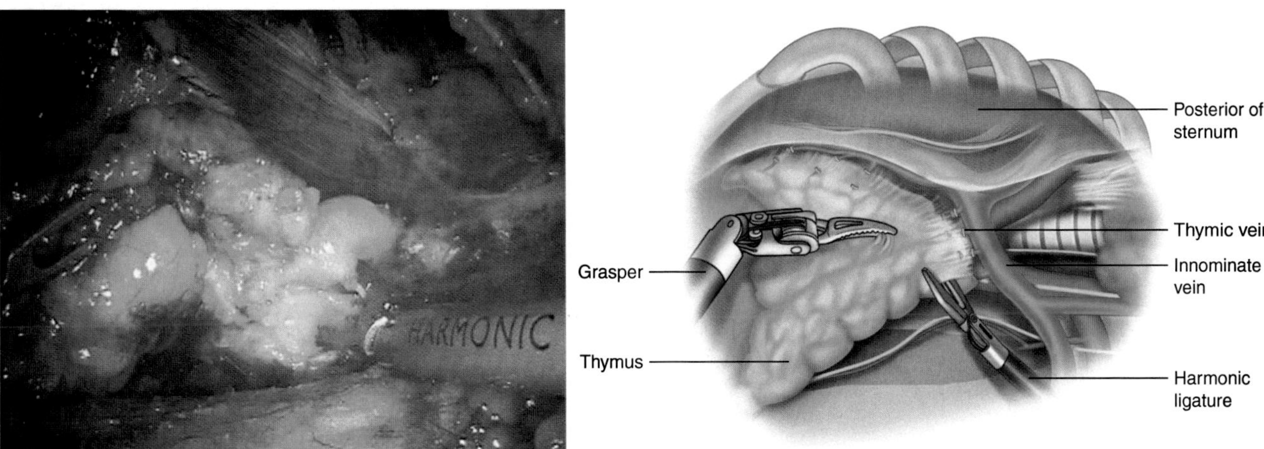

Fig. 37.7 Division of thymic veins

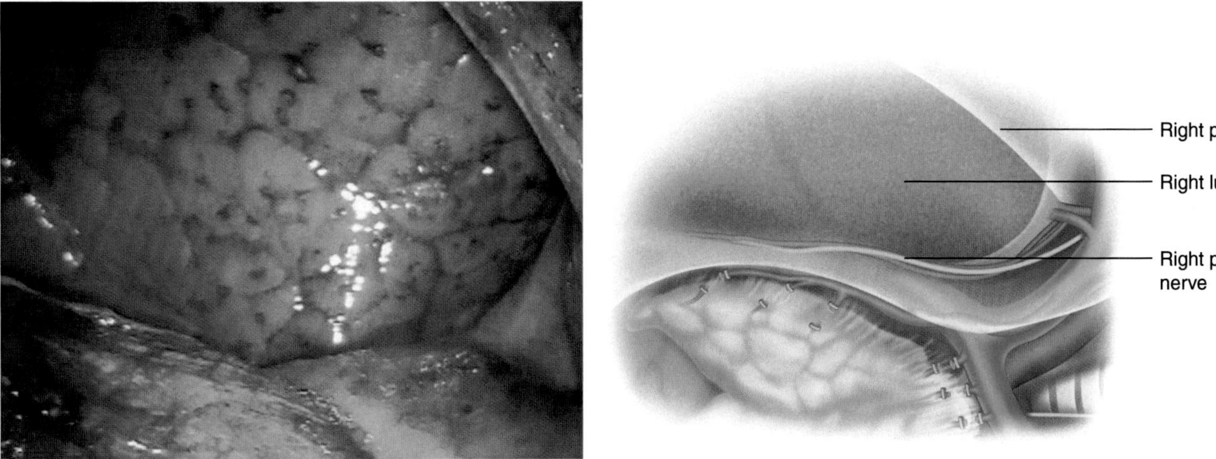

Fig. 37.8 Right lung with right phrenic nerve

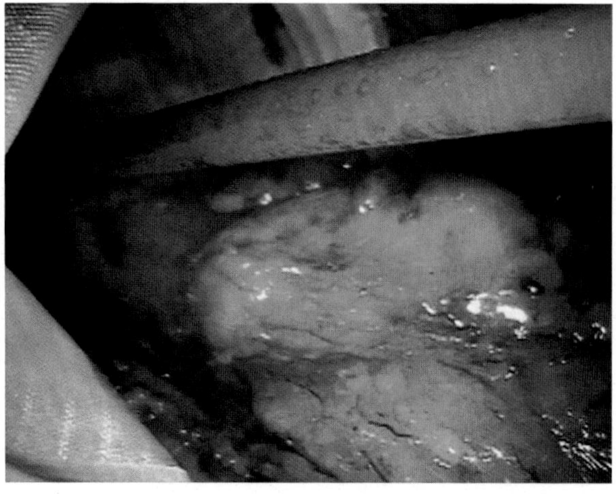

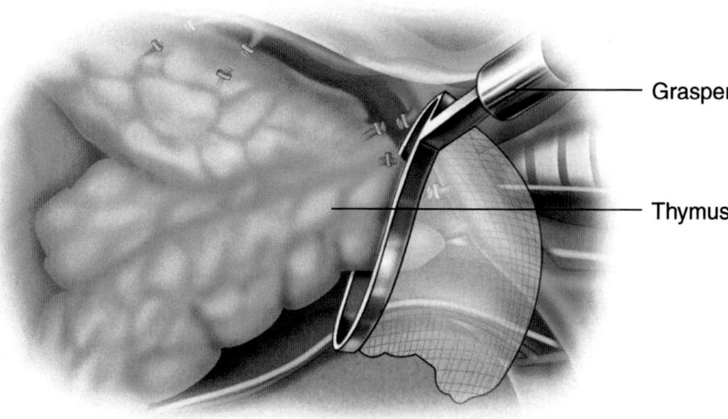

Fig. 37.9 Placement of specimen in Endobag

bag (Fig. 37.9). We favor the most anterior caudal incision because the rib space is largest in this region. The operative field is subsequently thoroughly inspected for residual tissue and hemostasis. Finally, a chest tube is placed in the left anterior pleural cavity under thoracoscopic guidance. Both lungs are subsequently reinflated and the trocar incisions are closed.

Postoperative Care

Postoperatively, patients are extubated in the operating room and should be observed in a monitored setting. The chest tube can be removed once full lung expansion has been documented, and patients are usually discharged once pain control is adequate and there are no signs of complications. This is typically on postoperative day one or two with a follow-up visit in 2 weeks [10]. Patients with MG should be monitored for at least 24 h for signs of crisis and should continue to follow up with their neurologist after discharge [9].

References

1. Netter FH. Atlas of human anatomy. 5th ed. Philadelphia, PA: Saunders Elsevier; 2011.
2. Ferguson MK. Difficult decisions in thoracic surgery. 3rd ed. London: Springer-Verlag; 2014.
3. Kumar A, Asaf BB. Robotic thoracic surgery: the state of the art. J Minim Access Surg. 2015;11:60–7.
4. Falk V, Walther T, Autschbach R, Diegeler A, Battellini R, Mohr FW. Robot-assisted minimally invasive solo mitral valve operation. J Thorac Cardiovasc Surg. 1998;115:470–1.
5. Freeman RK, Ascioti AJ, Van Woerkom JM, Vyverberg A, Robison RJ. Long-term follow-up after robotic thymectomy for nonthymomatous myasthenia gravis. Ann Thorac Surg. 2011;92:1018–22; discussion 22–3
6. Schneiter D, Tomaszek S, Kestenholz P, Hillinger S, Opitz I, Inci I, et al. Minimally invasive resection of thymomas with the da Vinci(R) surgical system. Eur J Cardiothorac Surg. 2013;43:288–92.
7. Rueckert J, Swierzy M, Badakhshi H, Meisel A, Ismail M. Robotic-assisted thymectomy: surgical procedure and results. Thorac Cardiovasc Surg. 2015;63:194–200.
8. Ding R, Tong X, Xu S, Zhang D, Gao X, Teng H, et al. A comparative study of Da Vinci robot system with video-assisted thoracoscopy in the surgical treatment of mediastinal lesions. Chin J Lung Cancer. 2014;17:557–62.
9. Ismail M, Swierzy M, Ruckert RI, Ruckert JC. Robotic thymectomy for myasthenia gravis. Thorac Surg Clin. 2014;24:189–95, vi–vii
10. Schwartz GS, Yang SC. Robotic thymectomy for thymic neoplasms. Thorac Surg Clin. 2014;24:197–201, vii
11. Givel J-C. Surgery of the thymus. 5th ed. In: Givel J-C, Merlini M, Clarke DB, Dusmet M, editors. Berlin, Heidelberg: Springer-Verlag; 1990. p. 245–6.
12. Skeie GO, Apostolski S, Evoli A, Gilhus NE, Illa I, Harms L, et al. Guidelines for treatment of autoimmune neuromuscular transmission disorders. Eur J Neurol. 2010;17:893–902.
13. Xu S, Ding R, Liu B, Meng H, Wang T, Wang S. Technical highlights of robotic-assisted mediastinal tumor resection. Ann Transl Med. 2015;3:84.

Part VI

Other Procedures

Transoral Robotic Surgery

38

Robert Kang, Thomas Gernon, and Ellie Maghami

Transoral robotic surgery (TORS) refers to surgery that is performed on the upper aerodigestive tract through the mouth, assisted by robotic instruments. The arms of the robot can reach previously inaccessible areas of the pharynx and larynx through the mouth, allowing for a minimally invasive approach through the natural oral cavity orifice. Prior to the advent of robotic technology, open techniques requiring mandible splitting often were necessary to surgically access cancers in these anatomic areas, and radiation with or without chemotherapy was often relied upon to treat these tumors, in order to avoid this morbid type of approach. Therefore, TORS has enabled the head and neck surgeon to surgically remove tumors that not only were difficult to access but also were often treated nonsurgically.

Introduction

Squamous cell carcinoma (SCC) of the head and neck is diagnosed in approximately 62,000 people yearly in the United States and is responsible for approximately 13,000 deaths [1]. Various sites of the upper aerodigestive tract can be affected, from the oral cavity down to the larynx. It is traditionally a disease of older patients, related to alcohol and tobacco use. The steady decline in the use of tobacco over the past few decades has been accompanied by a decrease in SCC incidence in some head and neck subsites such as the oral cavity [2].

The incidence of SCC of the oropharynx has risen dramatically [3]. The primary subsites of the oropharynx involved are the palatine tonsils and the base of the tongue (BOT). The underlying etiology in this setting is related to infection with the human papillomavirus (HPV) [4]. This patient population is younger and often lacks a history of significant tobacco or alcohol use [5].

R. Kang, MD (✉) · T. Gernon, MD · E. Maghami, MD
Division of Otolaryngology/Head & Neck Surgery, Department of Surgery, City of Hope, Duarte, CA, USA
e-mail: rkang@coh.org

HPV is a sexually transmitted infection (STI) that is often eradicated by the immune system without the development of any signs or symptoms. There are over 100 types of HPV, but 90% of HPV-related oropharyngeal cancers are related to the high-risk types, HPV-16 and HPV-18, which are also implicated in cervical and other anogenital cancers [6]. HPV is thought to settle into the deep, immune-privileged crypts of the tonsillar tissue in the palatine and lingual tonsils, causing cellular transformation that leads to carcinoma after many years of residence in these tissues.

Traditional, HPV-negative, oropharyngeal SCC has carried a guarded prognosis similar to other sites of head and neck SCC, but HPV-positive oropharyngeal SCC has demonstrated a significantly improved prognosis [7]. As a result of the improved outcomes, treatment de-escalation has been the goal of many ongoing multicenter trials, with lower doses of radiation, sparing use of adjuvant chemotherapy, and single-modality treatments for select tumors. For the most part, single-modality surgical management was not a good option for oropharyngeal tumors owing to access, as well as the need for multimodality treatment anyway, in the form of chemoradiation. Transoral robotic surgery has allowed the head and neck surgeon to reach the oropharynx and beyond for careful dissection using high-definition, 3-D video; robotic telescopes; and small, articulated robotic instruments. As a result, select patients have been able to avoid the long-term effects of chemotherapy and radiation and have had improved functional outcomes.

Indications

For the treatment of head and neck SCC, transoral robot use has been safe and effective for all T stages, from the oropharynx down to the larynx. At this time, however, FDA indications for the da Vinci® Si System (Intuitive Surgical; Sunnyvale, CA) are restricted to benign and malignant tumors classified as T1 and T2 and for benign base-of-tongue resection procedures.

Y. Fong et al. (eds.), *The SAGES Atlas of Robotic Surgery*, https://doi.org/10.1007/978-3-319-91045-1_38

Other oncologic considerations in patient selection include anticipated adjuvant therapies. If a tumor cannot be adequately resected with clear margins, or if cervical nodal disease involves multiple nodes or appears to demonstrate extracapsular extension on the preoperative exam, adjuvant chemotherapy and radiation may be necessary. In this scenario, adding the third treatment modality of surgery, particularly in the HPV-positive setting, may not afford any additional benefit to the patient.

Preoperative Preparation

The preoperative history should quantify alcohol and tobacco consumption. Sexual history may give indication to the likelihood of HPV positivity, but a biopsy specimen from the primary tumor or an involved cervical lymph node should be tested for the presence of HPV regardless. Even in the presence of HPV, oropharyngeal tumors carry poorer prognoses when associated with an extensive smoking history.

The physical examination should demonstrate mobility of the tonsil. Immobility suggests invasion through deep fascia, masticator muscles, or the skull base, precluding transoral surgical resection with adequate margins. Fixation of cervical nodes to deep fascia and muscles also suggests significant extracapsular extension, warranting adjuvant chemoradiation and thereby also precluding transoral surgery, as a third treatment modality would produce additional morbidity without additional benefit. The ability to achieve adequate transoral exposure to the oropharynx must also be assessed preoperatively. Occasionally a patient will be brought to the operating room for a thorough examination under general anesthesia specifically to evaluate the tumor's transoral robotic resectability.

The staging workup includes imaging of the neck with either a contrast CT or MRI. An MRI may better delineate the extent of the tumor in the soft tissues of the pharynx and tongue base, particularly when the tumor is more endophytic. Bilateral tongue base involvement is a contraindication to surgical resection, as this may compromise the viability and function of the entire tongue. Cervical lymph nodes are evaluated on imaging to determine the number and size of the nodes, their laterality, and the potential for extracapsular extension. In addition, the relationship of the tumor to branches of the carotid artery and other larger vessels in the pharynx is closely examined and noted.

Surgical Technique

Patient and Robot Positioning

The patient is positioned on the operating table in reversed fashion, with the head at the foot of the bed and vice versa, in order to allow more room below the head of the bed for the base of the robot (Figs. 38.1 and 38.2). The patient is intubated with a wire-reinforced endotracheal tube, which is secured to the contralateral buccal and retromolar trigone mucosa with a 2–0 silk suture. The eyes are protected with an adherent mask eye cover. The table is turned 90° counterclockwise, and manual palpation of the tonsil or tongue base tumor is performed to reassess its mobility, location, and extent.

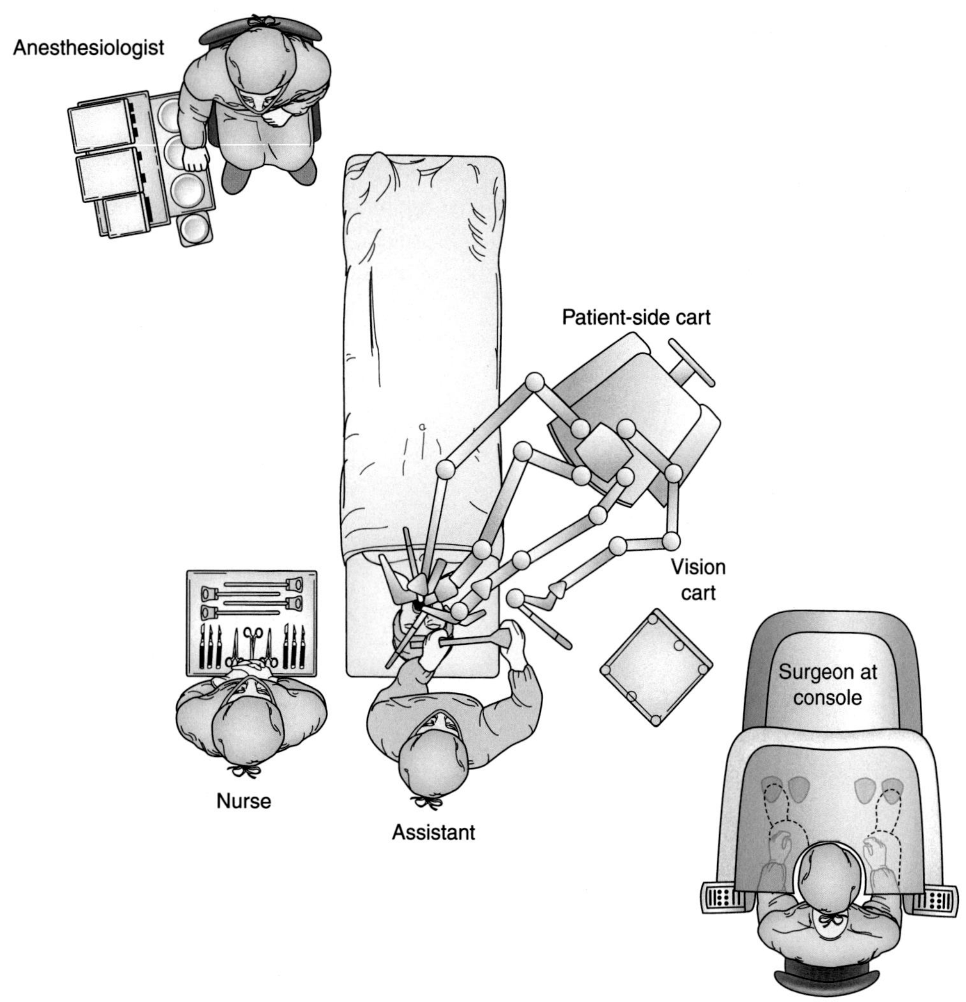

Fig. 38.1 Patient positioning with docked robot

A variety of tongue retractors are available within several different size options (Fig. 38.3). We generally apply the Crowe-Davis mouth gag with a size 2.5, 3, or 3.5 Davis-Meyer tongue blade. These tongue blades feature integrated suction tubing for smoke evacuation. The gag and tongue blade are applied until the correct size and positioning provides optimal visualization of the tumor, while retracting the tongue anterolaterally using a 2–0 silk suture placed through near the tip of the tongue in horizontal mattress fashion. FK-WO retractors can also be placed if visualization is limited with the Crowe-Davis. Additional tongue blades are available with this system, with cutouts on the left or right of the retractor tip, allowing protrusion of tongue base tissue if necessary for exposure, depending on the side of the tumor. The entire apparatus is then suspended on a suspension arm attached to the operating table.

The draped da Vinci® system patient cart is then carefully driven into position, with care to clear the space around the head of the bed to avoid collision. The robot arms are optimally aligned into the oral cavity when the angle created between the axis of the robot patient cart and the operating table is 30°. Once the robot is well positioned, the trocars are placed in the instrument ports. A 0° or 30° scope is placed in the middle arm. Depending on the sidedness and location of the tumor, a Maryland dissector is placed into one of the lateral arms, and a 5-mm monopolar spatula is placed in the other. For a right-sided tonsil tumor, for example, the dissector is placed in the left instrument port to allow medial retraction of tissue, whereas the monopolar spatula is placed in the right instrument port.

Other nonrobotic surgical tools are prepared at the head of the bed for the assistant. These include two Yankauer suctions, Metzenbaum scissors, long-toothed forceps, a long bayonet bipolar cautery, suction monopolar cautery, headlight, needle driver, curved Allis clamp, tonsil clamp, and a box of nonsterile gloves.

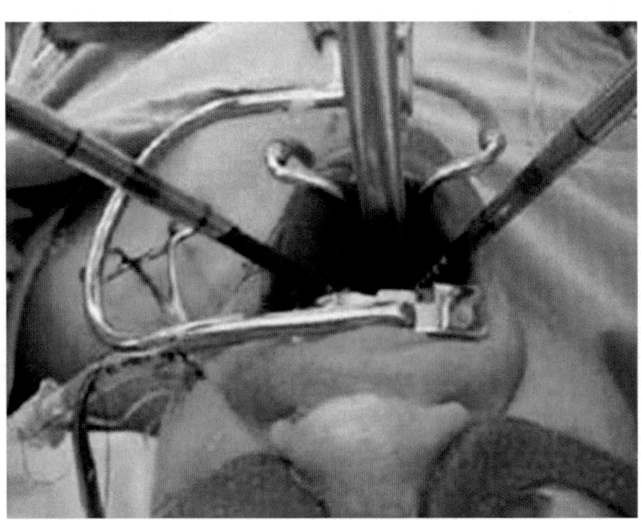

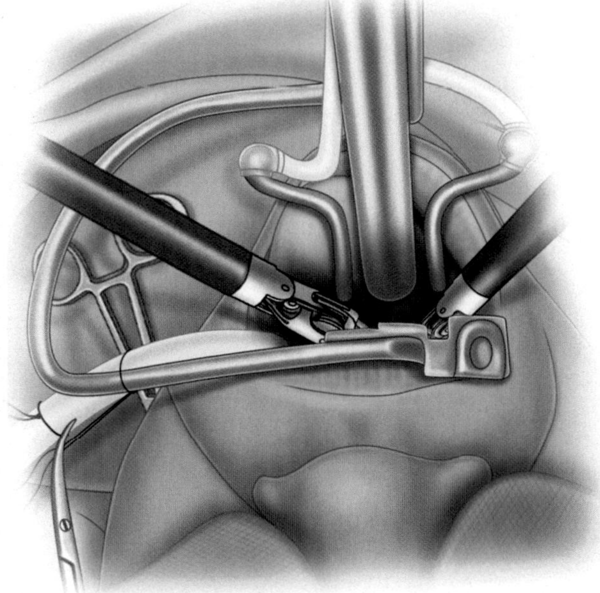

Fig. 38.2 Assistant's intraoral view from the head of bed

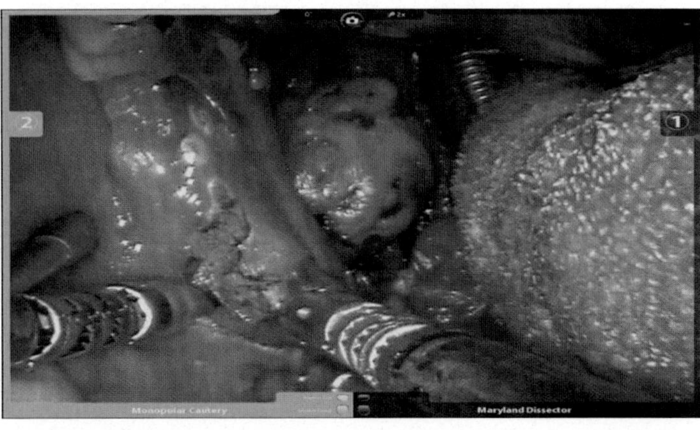

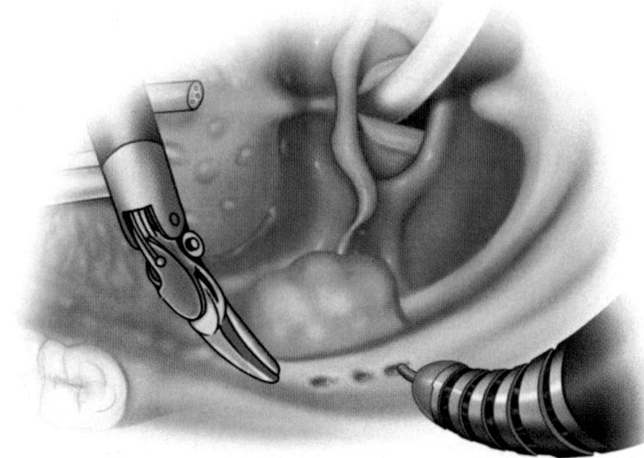

Fig. 38.3 Intraoral view from robotic endoscope

Transoral Robotic Radical Tonsillectomy

An incision is first made in the buccal mucosa along the pterygomandibular raphe. The pharyngeal constrictor muscles are identified and retracted medially, and a plane is developed between the constrictor medially and pterygoid muscles laterally (Figs. 38.4 and 38.5). The intervening fat is left laterally with the pterygoid muscles to provide cover for the underlying pharyngeal vessels. Dissection proceeds down to the styloglossus and stylopharyngeus muscles.

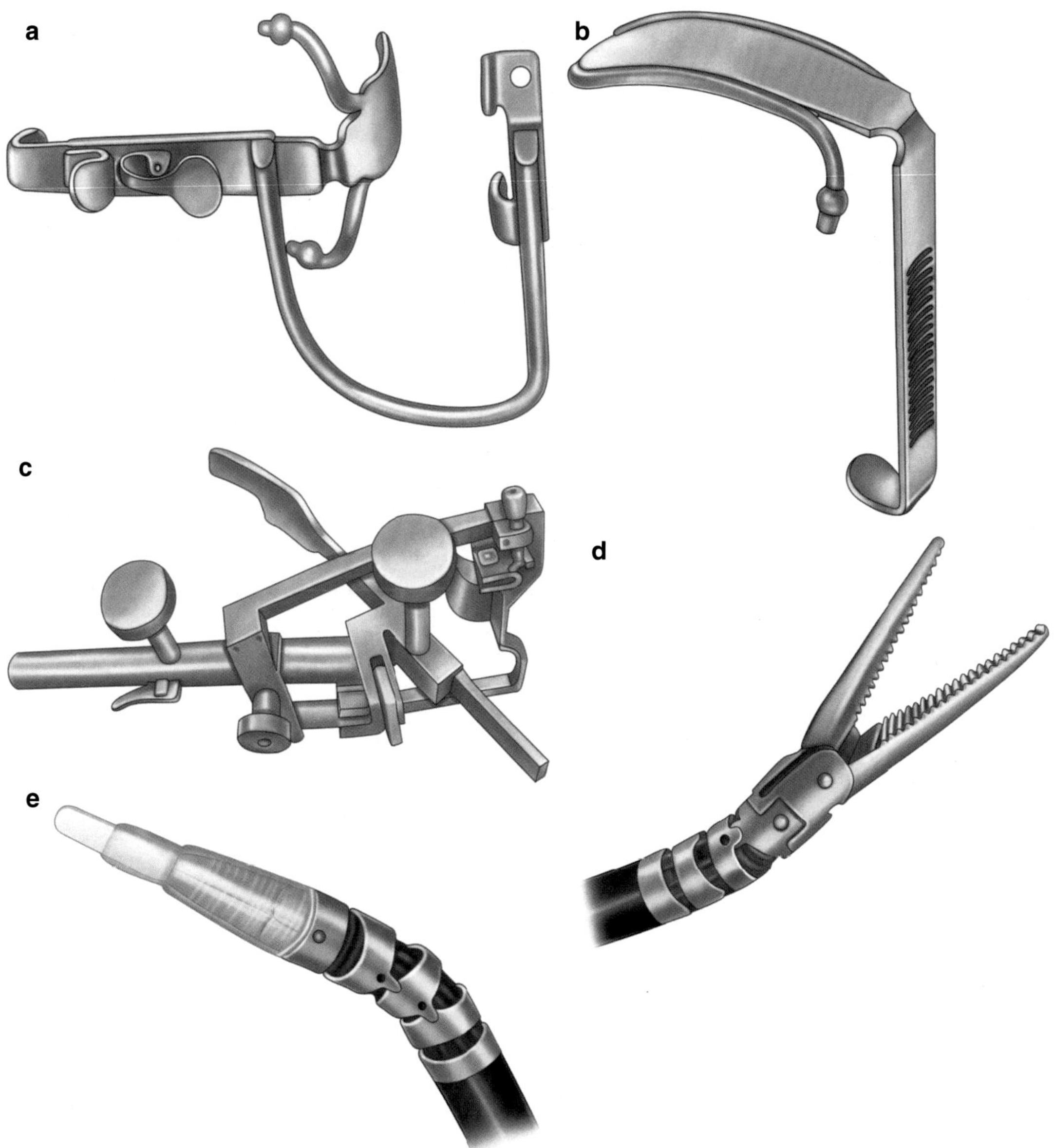

Fig. 38.4 Surgical instruments. (**a**) Crowe-Davis mouth gag. (**b**) Davis-Meyer tongue blade. (**c**) Feyh-Kastenbauer (FK) retractor. (**d**) 5-mm EndoWrist® Maryland dissector. (**e**) 5-mm EndoWrist® monopolar cautery

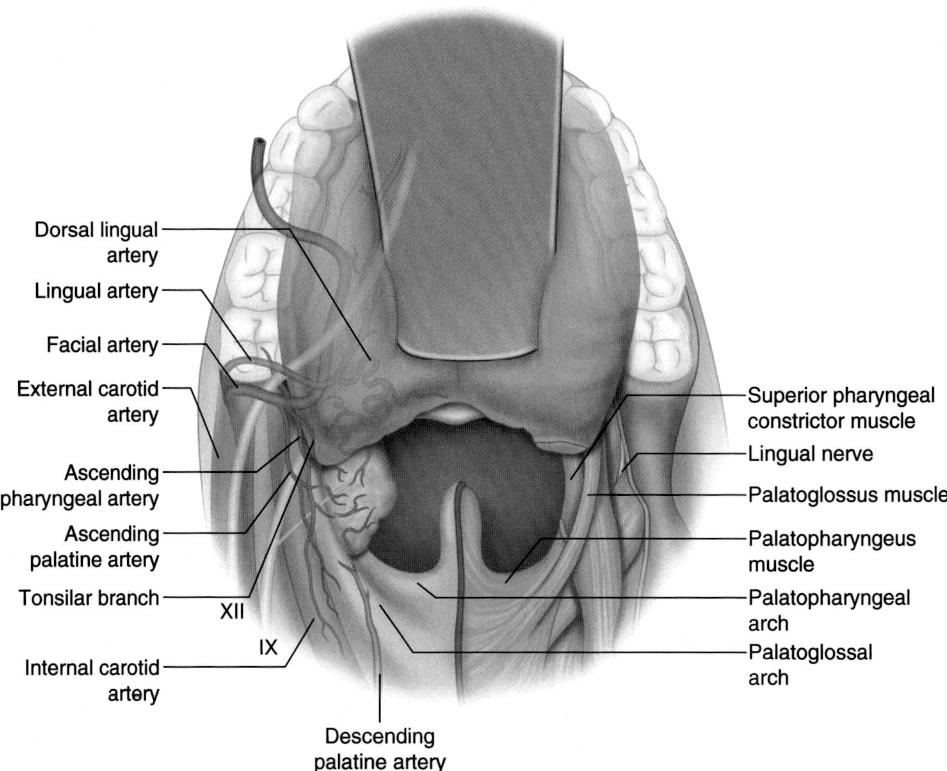

Fig. 38.5 Robotic tonsillectomy anatomy

The superior aspect of the dissection is addressed next by completing a curvilinear incision through the ipsilateral soft palate, until the palate is transected just lateral to the uvula. The medial aspect of the dissection is defined with a vertical incision through the posterior oropharyngeal mucosa, leaving a margin of tissue around the tonsil and connecting this to the palatal incision superiorly. The palatal incision is deepened through the palatal musculature until the prevertebral fascia is encountered. The constrictor muscles are then bluntly dissected off of this fascia from superior to inferior. Small vessels must be clipped carefully with at least three clips on the patient side of vessel ligation. The carotid artery may course medially by the deep aspect of the dissection, so careful attention must be paid to the preoperative imaging to prepare for this encounter. Pulsations from the carotid artery can be visualized through the lateral fat and muscles. The stylopharyngeus and styloglossus muscles are defined and transected carefully, as vessels will be encountered deep to these muscles.

The tongue base resection is performed in rectangular fashion with a longitudinal incision made through the midline and a transverse incision in the tongue base as far anteriorly as needed to establish a clear margin from tumor in the inferior tonsil. The longitudinal incision is connected to the midline posterior pharyngeal wall incision, and the transverse incision is made, taking care to bevel the monopolar spatula anteriorly in order to prevent an inadvertently thin cut of the tongue base. The tongue base incision may extend deep into the vallecula as margins necessitate. As the final cuts are made in the inferolateral aspect of the tongue base, the lingual artery and nerve must be carefully avoided. Branches of the glossopharyngeal nerve may be encountered and safely ligated.

Palatopharyngoplasty can be performed to aid in closure of the palatal defect to minimize the risk of permanent velopharyngeal insufficiency (VPI). Though many patients develop a degree of VPI initially following surgery, it usually resolves spontaneously after months of scarring. 3–0 Vicryl sutures are used to approximate the nasal mucosal surface of the palatal defect to the mucosal edge of the posterior oropharyngeal incision, with knots buried on the nasal surface of the closure.

The wound is inspected for exposed vessels, which are carefully clipped if necessary. Bipolar cautery is used with a headlight at the bedside to maintain strict hemostasis. Surgiflo® (Johnson & Johnson; New Brunswick, NJ) or Floseal (Baxter; Bloomington, IN) is applied to the defect (Fig. 38.5). The larynx and epiglottis are inspected, and if there are no significant concerns for airway obstruction due to edema, the patient may be extubated in the operating room. A nasogastric feeding tube may be placed in the operating room under direct visualization in order to prevent agitation of the wound.

Postoperative Management

Patients who have significant edema of the larynx or a particular risk for bleeding may be kept intubated and observed in the ICU on intravenous steroids until they can be safely extubated over the first few days of the postoperative period. Other patients may be immediately extubated and recovered on a surgical floor. Steroids may be administered to prevent excessive edema, nausea, and immediate inflammatory pain. A standard clean/contaminated perioperative prophylactic antibiotic protocol is followed. Patients may begin ingesting clear liquids if their pain permits. Tube feeding is initiated on the first postoperative day and advanced while patients recover their swallow function. If they are not able to manage enough PO intake for hydration by the time of discharge, they are discharged with a feeding tube until they have been sufficiently rehabilitated, generally by the first postoperative clinic appointment. The speech pathologist is vital in aiding in a safe and rapid swallow recovery. Patients without complications are discharged in 4 days, with or without a nasogastric feeding tube.

Outcomes

Treatment of the oropharynx traditionally has involved primary chemoradiation because of the surgical inaccessibility of the anatomy. Surgery would involve a mandibulotomy with incisions made through the entire floor of the mouth to access the oropharynx. Because of the morbidity of such an approach, surgery was often left for salvage settings. With the ability of the robotic arms to access the back of the throat, and the high-definition optics of the robotic endoscopes, surgery has become the mainstay for early-stage cancers of the tonsil and base of the tongue. Surgery alone provided high local control and low surgical morbidity in low-risk oropharyngeal SCC [8]. Disease control, survival, and safety outcomes commensurate with standard treatments have also been demonstrated in later-stage cancers, with lower rates of gastrostomy dependency [9]. Disease control was also observed with TORS as a primary surgical modality (followed by adjuvant treatments as indicated) for both HPV-negative and HPV-positive patients [10]. A large multi-institutional study also supports the role of TORS as a tool in the multidisciplinary treatment of head and neck cancer, especially for patients with oropharyngeal SCC [11].

The Future of Transoral Robotic Surgery

Though the advent of the da Vinci® Si System has revolutionized the treatment of oropharyngeal SCC, it is a tool adopted from other surgical specialties and created without specific consideration of the unique anatomy of the head and neck. As TORS became more commonplace, attention has been drawn to the need for a single-port system to access the oropharynx, and this device is now in use for the head and neck. The three bulky robot arms that pass instruments through the mouth inevitably will be abandoned once the single-port system becomes widely available.

HPV-positive oropharyngeal cancer has been shown to be more responsive to treatment, with improved outcomes. Ongoing trials are aimed at de-escalating treatment in this setting. The intent is to improve functional outcomes such as speech and swallow with less morbid doses of radiation and chemotherapy and narrower indications following TORS resection.

Conclusion

TORS is an effective tool that has changed the treatment paradigm of head and neck SCC, particularly of the oropharynx. The growing understanding of the effect of HPV on oropharyngeal cancer has evolved hand in hand with the use of transoral robotic technology. With future studies aimed at de-escalation of adjuvant treatments, patients face the potential of improved functional and disease outcomes, with diminished morbidity and treatment recovery time. As robotic devices become fine-tuned for head and neck anatomy and the prevalence of both technology and trained surgeons continues to increase across institutions, more patients with oropharyngeal SCC will have access to this minimally invasive technique.

References

1. Siegel RL, Miller KD, Jemal A. Cancer statistics, 2016. CA Cancer J Clin. 2016;66:7–30.
2. Chaturvedi AK, Engels EA, Anderson WF, Gillison ML. Incidence trends for human papillomavirus-related and -unrelated oral squamous cell carcinomas in the United States. J Clin Oncol. 2008;26:612–9.
3. Chaturvedi AK, Engels EA, Pfeiffer RM, Hernandez BY, Xiao W, Kim E, et al. Human papillomavirus and rising oropharyngeal cancer incidence in the United States. J Clin Oncol. 2011;29:4294–301.
4. Gillison ML, Koch WM, Capone RB, Spafford M, Westra WH, Wu L, et al. Evidence for a causal association between human papillomavirus and a subset of head and neck cancers. J Natl Cancer Inst. 2000;92:709–20.

5. Gillison ML, D'Souza G, Westra W, Sugar E, Xiao W, Begum S, Viscidi R. Distinct risk factor profiles for human papillomavirus type 16-positive and human papillomavirus type 16-negative head and neck cancers. J Natl Cancer Inst. 2008;100:407–20.
6. Dayyani F, Etzel CJ, Liu M, Ho CH, Lippman SM, Tsao AS. Meta-analysis of the impact of human papillomavirus (HPV) on cancer risk and overall survival in head and neck squamous cell carcinomas (HNSCC). Head Neck Oncol. 2010;2:15.
7. Fakhry C, Westra WH, Li S, Cmelak A, Ridge JA, Pinto H, et al. Improved survival of patients with human papillomavirus-positive head and neck squamous cell carcinoma in a prospective clinical trial. J Natl Cancer Inst. 2008;100:261–9.
8. Weinstein GS, Quon H, Newman HJ, Chalian JA, Malloy K, Lin A, et al. Transoral robotic surgery alone for oropharyngeal cancer: an analysis of local control. Arch Otolaryngol Head Neck Surg. 2012;138:628–34.
9. Weinstein GS, O'Malley BW Jr, Cohen MA, Quon H. Transoral robotic surgery for advanced oropharyngeal carcinoma. Arch Otolaryngol Head Neck Surg. 2010;136:1079–85.
10. Cohen MA, Weinstein GS, O'Malley BW Jr, Feldman M, Quon H. Transoral robotic surgery and human papillomavirus status: oncologic results. Head Neck. 2011;33:573–80.
11. de Almeida JR, Li R, Magnuson JS, Smith RV, Moore E, Lawson G, et al. Oncologic outcomes after transoral robotic surgery: a multi-institutional study. JAMA Otolaryngol Head Neck Surg. 2015;141:1043–51.

Robotically-assisted Ventral Hernia Repair

39

Ioannis Konstantinidis and Byrne Lee

Introduction

Since the introduction of laparoscopic ventral hernia repair in the early 1990s [1], the benefits of the procedure—decreased postoperative pain, faster recovery with less wound, and overall complication rates, while maintaining recurrence rates equal or less to those of open ventral hernia repair—have led to its widespread adoption. Laparoscopy, however, has its own limitations. The lack of articulation limits the degrees of motion of laparoscopic instruments, and visualization is also limited to two dimensions. As a result, technically demanding maneuvers such as intracorporeal closure of hernia defect or minimally invasive myofascial release have not been widely adopted. This can compromise the outcome of the repair, leading to increased mesh bulging, hernia recurrences, seroma formation, and patient dissatisfaction [2]. Additionally, the tackers and transabdominal sutures used to secure the mesh have been implicated in the occurrence of increased pain and postoperative adhesions.

Robotic surgery continues to evolve in general surgical procedures. Robotically-assisted herniorrhaphy [3] maintains the benefits of faster recovery and decreased morbidity associated with minimally invasive surgery while addressing the limitations of laparoscopy by providing superior three-dimensional imaging and improved ergonomics with 7° of motion. Consequently, it is particularly useful in closing the hernia defects intracorporeally; it facilitates suturing of the mesh to the fascia, thus eliminating the need for tackers and transabdominal sutures; and it provides an opportunity for minimally invasive myofascial release and complex repairs [4].

The experience with robotically-assisted ventral hernia repairs, albeit in an early phase, demonstrates perioperative outcomes comparable to the existing published data on open and laparoscopic repairs [5], whereas the ease of fascial defect closure might be associated with decreased recurrence rates [6].

Indications

In general, ventral hernias should be repaired in good operative candidates even if they are not symptomatic due to concern for incarceration. Robotically-assisted ventral hernia repair cannot be utilized in patients unable to tolerate pneumoperitoneum.

Step 1. Patient Positioning and Theater Setup

The procedure is performed under general anesthesia. Preoperative systemic antibiotic for wound infection prophylaxis is given within 30 min of skin incision. In all cases, sequential compression devices, a Foley catheter, and an orogastric tube for stomach decompression are placed with the patient in supine position and the abdomen covered with iodine-impregnated dressing.

I. Konstantinidis · B. Lee (✉)
Department of Surgery, City of Hope National Medical Center, Duarte, CA, USA
e-mail: ikonstantinidis@coh.org

Y. Fong et al. (eds.), *The SAGES Atlas of Robotic Surgery*, https://doi.org/10.1007/978-3-319-91045-1_39

When utilizing the Si system, the robot is docked either at the left or the right side of the patient. Entry into the peritoneal cavity is performed with a Veress needle and an OPTIVIEW trocar (or alternatively using an open technique). Pneumoperitoneum with a maximum pressure of 15 mmHg is established. After the insertion of a 12-mm trocar (for the 10-mm 30° robotic camera), two 8-mm operating arm trocars are then placed under direct visualization, 8 cm lateral to the first trocar (Fig. 39.1). The trocars are placed as far lateral as possible to maximize distance away from the fascial defect. If no adhesions are present, or there is sufficient distance to safely visualize the arms and perform adhesiolysis, the robot is subsequently docked.

Step 2. Adhesiolysis, Hernia Reduction

Adhesions are lysed using the robotic shears for sharp dissection and blunt dissection as needed. Special care must be taken to avoid bowel injury, and we typically limit the use of energy devices during this step, especially while working in proximity to the bowel.

The hernia sac contents are subsequently reduced using a combination of blunt and sharp dissection. The peritoneal sac is removed, particularly easily in its entirety, with the use of the robot, and this can lead to decreased seroma formation (Fig. 39.2). The hernia defect is measured and an appropriately sized prosthetic mesh overlapping the defect by 5 cm in all directions is prepared.

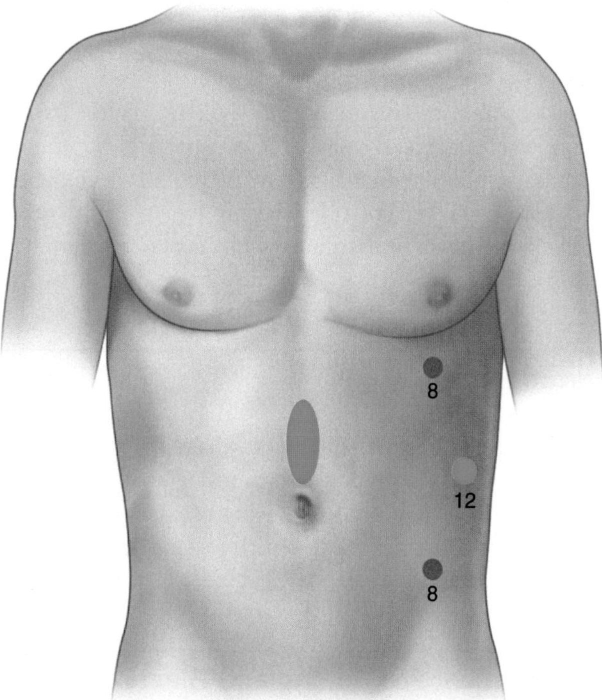

Fig. 39.1 Port configuration for the Si robotic system

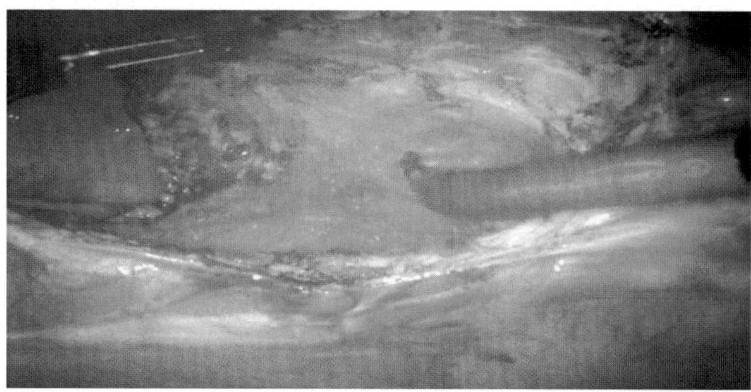

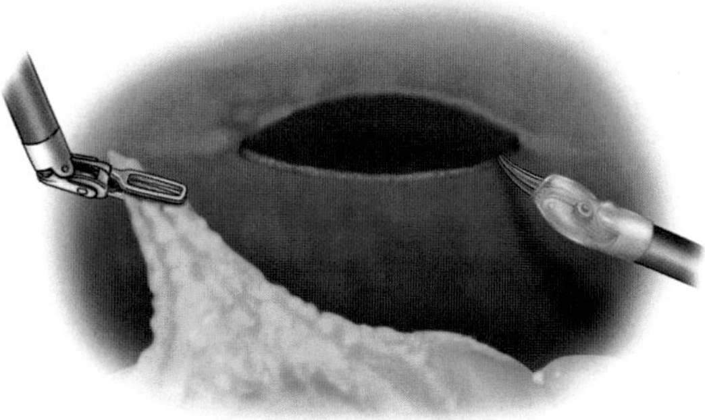

Fig. 39.2 Articulating instruments facilitate complete excision of the peritoneal sac even from large ventral hernias

Step 3. Facial Defect Closure, Mesh Fixation

The fascial defect is closed with a 0-absorbable self-fixating suture in a running fashion (Fig. 39.3). This allows greater overlap of the mesh. We typically lower the intra-abdominal pressure to 7 mmHg during this step of the procedure, as this decreases tension and facilitates the fascial closure.

Fixation of the mesh to the posterior fascia is performed around the circumference of the mesh with a nonabsorbable self-fixating suture in a running fashion (interrupted sutures at regular 1-cm intervals and a in a figure-eight configuration can be alternatively used). No transabdominal sutures or tacks are needed, and this reduces the postoperative pain (Fig. 39.4). No surgical drain is needed. The 12-mm trocar site is closed with absorbable suture using a Carter-Thomasson suture passer.

Complex Abdominal Wall Reconstructions

The use of the robotic platform greatly facilitates the performance of complex repairs such as myofascial advancement flaps (component separation). If myofascial release is required to allow closure of the hernia defect with no tension, we typically use unilateral or bilateral posterior rectus sheath release. The posterior rectus sheath is incised, and the retrorectal space is created and extended along the entire rectus sheath and lateral as far as the linea semilunaris (Fig. 39.5). The mesh is placed in a retromuscular rather than intraperitoneal space. If bilateral posterior rectus sheath release is needed, this will require dual-sided docking. Additional myofascial release can be achieved with release of the transversus abdominis muscle if needed.

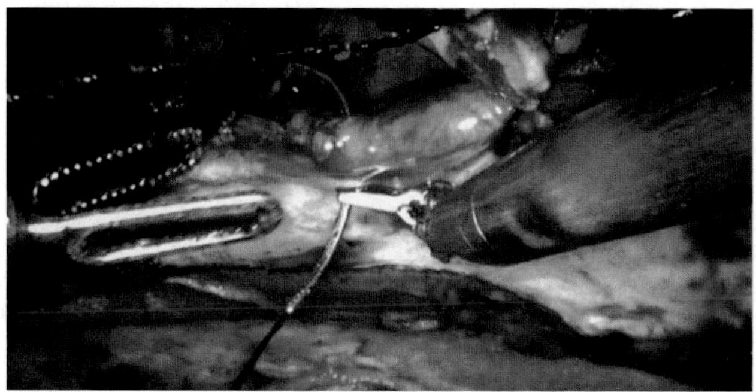

Fig. 39.3 Intracorporeal closure of the hernia defect

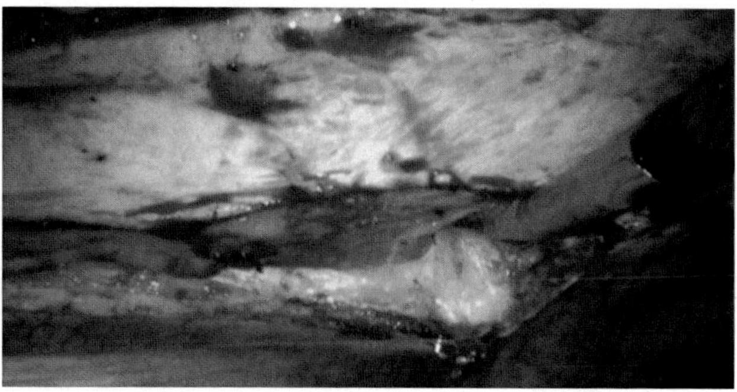

Fig. 39.5 Robotic complex abdominal wall reconstructions. Component separation. Incision of the rectus sheath and development of the retrorectal space

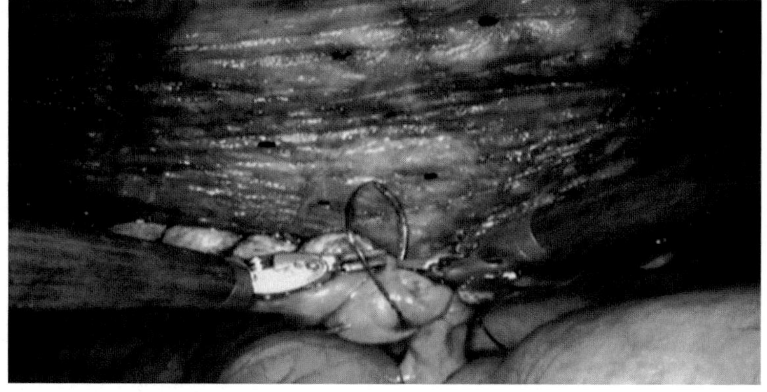

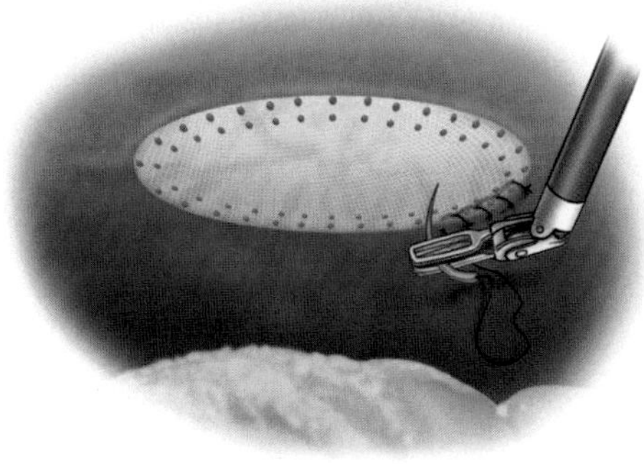

Fig. 39.4 Mesh fixation with circumferential suturing avoiding transabdominal sutures and tackers

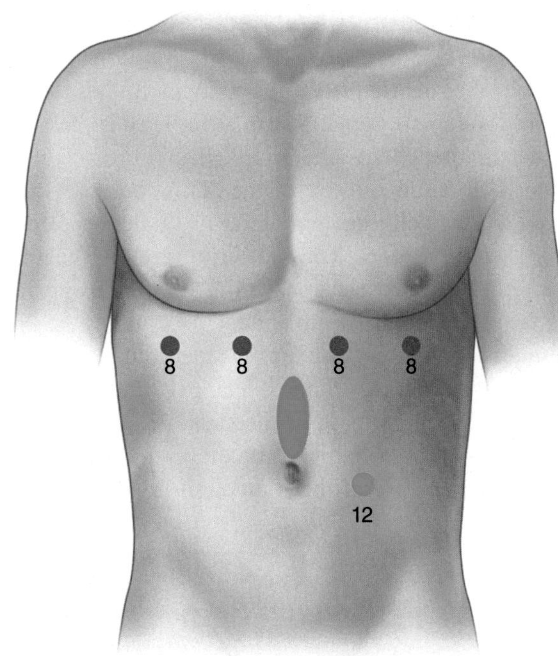

Fig. 39.6 Port configuration for the Xi Robotic system

Xi Differences

When utilizing the Xi robotic platform, we typically place our ports in a transverse line in the upper abdomen with an assistant port at the lateral abdomen. We typically use all four robotic arms and reduce the distance between them to 5 cm when the Xi is used (Fig. 39.6). In this position, release of components can be achieved without repositioning or re-docking the robot. Additionally, suture fixation of the mesh is aided by the ability to swap the camera port. This allows for the use of different arm configurations to ensure proper positioning for suturing.

Tricks of the Master

The lack of tactile feedback with the current robotic platforms means that the surgeon should be very cautious and rely on the improved visualization to estimate the amount of tension placed on tissues. This is especially important, along with the careful use of energy devices, in order to avoid a bowel injury.

Lowering the intra-abdominal pressure during the hernia defect closure will allow less tension on the repair. Closing the hernia defect provides greater mesh overlap of the defect with the mesh and equally distributes tension; it is therefore our favored approach.

Postoperative Care

In general, postoperative pain control requires a one-night hospitalization even though many patients are being discharged the day of surgery. Postoperative ileus is not uncommon, especially when extensive adhesiolysis is needed. Wound seromas are also common and should not be drained unless they become symptomatic or signs of infection appear. The possibility of occult bowel injury should be entertained in patients who do not recover appropriately and/or demonstrate signs of peritonitis, which should lead to prompt imaging and re-exploration.

Conclusion

The introduction of the robotic platform for ventral hernia repair maintains the benefits of faster recovery and decreased morbidity associated with minimally invasive surgery. It overcomes limitations of traditional laparoscopy as it greatly facilitates the intracorporeal closure of the hernia defect. Suturing the hernia mesh to the posterior fascia avoids the use of transabdominal sutures and tackers. These technical benefits of the robotic platform render complex abdominal wall reconstructions quite feasible in a minimally invasive fashion and will likely lead to increased adoption by the next generation of surgeons.

References

1. LeBlanc KA, Booth WV. Laparoscopic repair of incisional abdominal hernias using expanded polytetrafluoroethylene: preliminary findings. Surg Laparosc Endosc. 1993;3(1):39–41.
2. Nguyen DH, Nguyen MT, Askenasy EP, Kao LS, Liang MK. Primary fascial closure with laparoscopic ventral hernia repair: systematic review. World J Surg. 2014;38(12):3097–104.
3. Schluender S, Conrad J, Divino CM, Gurland B. Robotic-assisted laparoscopic repair of ventral hernia with intracorporeal suturing. Surg Endosc. 2003;17(9):1391–5.
4. Warren JA, Cobb WS, Ewing JA, Carbonell AM. Standard laparoscopic versus robotic retromuscular ventral hernia repair. Surg Endosc. 2017;31(1):324–32.
5. Gonzalez A, Escobar E, Romero R, Walker G, Mejias J, Gallas M, et al. Robotic-assisted ventral hernia repair: a multicenter evaluation of clinical outcomes. Surg Endosc. 2017;31(3):1342–9.
6. Gonzalez AM, Romero RJ, Seetharamaiah R, Gallas M, Lamoureux J, Rabaza JR. Laparoscopic ventral hernia repair with primary closure versus no primary closure of the defect: potential benefits of the robotic technology. Int J Med Robot. 2015;11(2):120–5.

40 Inguinal Hernia Repair

Kamaljot S. Kaler, Simone L. Vernez, and Thomas E. Ahlering

Inguinal hernia (IH) is a well-known complication of radical prostatectomy. The prevalence of groin hernias, including inguinal and femoral, is between 5 and 10% in the United States, with inguinal hernias (IHs) making up the vast majority [1]. In general, risk factors for hernia development include a history of hernia or hernia repair, older age, male gender, Caucasian race, chronic cough or constipation, abdominal wall injury, smoking, and family history [2]. IH also occurs as a complication of radical prostatectomy. In 1996, Regan and coworkers were the first to show a significantly higher incidence of IH following radical prostatectomy when compared to the general population [3]. Indeed, up to 20% of patients develop IHs postoperatively [4–7]. Further, studies have shown that patients who have undergone radical prostatectomy for the treatment of prostate cancer have a higher incidence of IH than prostate cancer patients who do not undergo surgery [8, 9]. Additionally, patients are more likely to suffer from IH after combined radical prostatectomy with lymph node dissection than just lymph node dissection alone [10]. Risk for IH extends beyond the immediate postoperative period and may be observed as a long-term complication [11]. Importantly, patients undergoing minimally invasive radical prostatectomy are at increased risk of requiring hernia repair compared to open prostatectomy patients [12].

A number of risk factors have been identified in patients who experience IH after radical prostatectomy, including prior hernia repair, wound infection, advanced age, or a history of cigarette smoking [5, 7, 8]. In a 2001 study, a majority of patients with prior hernia repair experienced reherniation following surgery [10]. This has since been substantiated in several studies. In our experience, nearly 30% of patients who underwent herniorrhaphies at the time of robotically-assisted radical prostatectomy (RARP) had a previous history of hernia repair [13, 14]. Further, cigarette smoking is commonly accepted as a risk factor for IH because incidences of IH are higher in smoking populations than nonsmoking populations [15]. It has been proposed that tissue hypoxia and reduced production of collagen in smokers may explain this [16, 17]. However, smoking history has not been found to be a statistically significant predictor of herniation after radical prostatectomy [7]. Additionally, in our experience, smoking history was not significant between those who required IH repair at the time of RARP and controls [13, 14]. Interestingly, Ichioka suggested that a body mass index of less than 23 kg/m^2 may predispose to hernia after radical prostatectomy [8]. However, this finding has not been substantiated and the mechanism by which a low body mass index may increase the risk of IH is not clear.

Moreover, it is not uncommon to discover an IH during laparoscopy. In one study, Watson found that in 100 patients undergoing laparoscopy, the incidence rate of asymptomatic IH approached 13% [18]. In fact, incidental IHs are found in 20–30% of patients undergoing radical prostatectomy. Fukuta found evidence of IH in the preoperative CT scans of 20.4% of patients undergoing prostatectomy upon a retrospective review [2]. In a prospective study, Neilson and Walsh discovered that nearly 33% of patients had visible evidence of a dilated inguinal ring or the presence of an existing hernia at the time of radical prostatectomy [19]. In our experience, only 52.5% of patients requiring IH repair at the time of RARP had IH on their preoperative examination; the remainder were asymptomatic, and the IH was discovered incidentally at the time of surgery [14]. Given the patient population, predominantly men over the age of 60, it is not at all surprising that we should discover the presence of IH upon closer examination. However, the significance of these increased rates in patients undergoing radical prostatectomy is not yet known.

Regardless of pre- and postoperative risk factors, radical prostatectomy alone with a lower midline incision seems to be an independent risk factor for clinically relevant IH following surgery. Lepor and Robins assert that the high incidence of IH following prostatectomy may be accounted for

K. S. Kaler, MD · S. L. Vernez, BA · T. E. Ahlering, MD (✉)
Department of Urology, University of California, Orange, CA, USA
e-mail: kkaler@uci.edu

Y. Fong et al. (eds.), *The SAGES Atlas of Robotic Surgery*, https://doi.org/10.1007/978-3-319-91045-1_40

by failure to diagnose IHs preoperatively [20]. Fukuta [5] showed that of the 20.4% patients found to have subclinical IHs prior to surgery, 55% went on to develop clinically significant hernias postoperatively, an estimated risk of 60.6%. Postoperative IHs are most often indirect, protruding through a defect in the area of the deep inguinal ring lateral to the inferior epigastric vessels [6, 10]. Normally the tensile strength of the transversalis fascia produces a "shutter mechanism" at the myopectineal orifice [21]. Disrupting the normal shutter mechanism may lead to compromised integrity of the internal inguinal ring, resulting in a predisposition to herniation [22, 23]. In a patient with an inguinal ring that is already weak, further disruption of the tensile strength of the abdominal wall may prove to be the final insult.

In 1949, McDonald and Huggins performed the first combined open prostatectomy and hernia repair through two incisions [24]. In 1989, Schlegel and Walsh reported simultaneous inguinal hernia repair during surgery on the bladder and prostate [25]. Several studies have examined the safety and feasibility of simultaneous IH repair with standard laparoscopic extraperitoneal, transperitoneal, or combined prostatectomy [19, 26–30]. However, few studies have examined combined herniorrhaphy with RARP [14, 19, 31]. Our experience shows that hernia repair at the time of RARP is quick (adds less than 15 min to the procedure), causes no change in postoperative pain or the use of pain killers, results in no significant change in length of hospital stay, and causes very few complications [13, 14]. Recent smaller studies have shown similar results [31–33].

Why Repair?

Inguinal herniation is a serious and common complication that has significant impact on morbidity and use of healthcare resources following radical prostatectomy. Symptomatic hernias are generally treated by open or laparoscopic repair. Mean operative times for a subsequent hernia repair, either laparoscopic or open, range from 45 to 111 min [34], while repair during radical prostatectomy adds approximately 15 min to the procedure. An additional surgical procedure is not without attendant risks, not to mention disruption of the patient quality of life and productivity. Moreover, untreated IHs may lead to complications such as bowel obstruction and/or strangulation requiring emergent open surgery. Moreover, scarring in the preperitoneal space after radical prostatectomy may render a subsequent hernia repair difficult. Some have even argued that prophylactic measures should be taken to reduce the risk of this complication even in the absence of visible herniation at the time of surgery. Stranne performed a modified hernia repair on patients with evidence of herniation at the time of prostatectomy, using a figure-of-eight suture placed between the transversus arch and the iliopubic tract to narrow the opening of the internal ring. This prophylactic measure decreased the incidence of IH by 62% [35].

The main argument against hernia repair at the time of radical prostatectomy is the risk of mesh infection. This concern arises from the possibility that the mesh may come into contact with urine in the presence of a vesicourethral anastomotic leak. Peritoneal integrity cannot be restored after the bladder is dropped from the abdominal wall during laparoscopic transperitoneal prostatectomy. However, a review of 2500 consecutive laparoscopic transperitoneal inguinal herniorrhaphies using mesh found no incidences of mesh infection [36]. Additionally, a meta-analysis comparing eight randomized-controlled trials showed fewer wound infections and no significant difference in wound infections requiring mesh removal in laparoscopic versus open hernia repairs [37]. Even in clean contaminated or contaminated fields, the incidence of mesh infection is low [38]. While performing combined extraperitoneal laparoscopic radical prostatectomy and intraperitoneal inguinal hernia repair with mesh presents a method by which contamination may be avoided [26], there is no evidence that such complexity is warranted. Studies examining simultaneous IH repair with mesh and radical retropubic prostatectomy have shown no incidence of mesh infection [24, 27, 29, 39]. Moreover, urine may be sterilized prior to undergoing radical prostatectomy with appropriate antibiotic treatment in patients with positive urine cultures, further safeguarding against mesh infection.

The risk of bowel adhesions with the use of prosthetic mesh is another concern. However, there are two methods by which this may be reduced. First, reperitonealization may be safely achieved during the time of prostatectomy to avoid contact of mesh with intraperitoneal structures. Using adhesion-resistant coated mesh is another solution that reduces the risk of adhesion formation while avoiding related postoperative complications. We have not observed any mesh-related complications in patients undergoing simultaneous RARP and IH repair with mesh [13, 14].

Inguinal Hernia Repair during Robotically-assisted Radical Prostatectomy

The robotic approach offers several advantages. First as opposed to standard laparoscopy, the da Vinci Surgical System robot (Intuitive Surgical, Sunnyvale, CA) provides three-dimensional, ten times magnification, facilitating visualization and hernia reduction. It also offers the surgeon better ergonomics and improved maneuverability. Furthermore, use of the robot is intuitive, allowing for adoption of simultaneous IH repair early in the learning curve of RARP [13].

After completion of transperitoneal RARP and pelvic node lymph node dissection, the myopectineal orifice should be inspected for the presence of a hernia. It is our practice to use a transperitoneal approach followed by a modified Rives-Stoppa technique [40]. Following dissection of the hernia sac to free the area of the abdominal wall containing the defect, the mesh of choice should be secured to the abdominal wall. For direct hernias, a cone-shaped mesh or an appropriately sized flat mesh sheet may be secured to the Cooper ligament inferiorly and then along the superolateral borders to the rectus sheath. A 5-mm laparoscopic ProTrack (Baylis Medical Co., Mississauga, Ontario) may be used through the right lower quadrant port to secure the flat mesh along the pubic bone. However, interrupted sutures placed along the superolateral portions of the mesh will suffice without the need for the stapling device. For indirect hernias, mesh should be sutured between the iliopubic tract and the transverse arch lateral to the inferior epigastric vessels (Figs. 40.1, 40.2, 40.3, 40.4, 40.5, 40.6 and 40.7).

Although reperitonealization may reduce the risk of mesh adhesion to bowel, risks of more dangerous complications may outweigh these concerns. Reperitonealization may be achieved by fixing the peritoneal edge near the epigastric vessels while the midline incision is closed to avoid stretching the vesicourethral anastomosis. In our study, a postoperative urine leak occurred after reperitonealization despite ensuring that the vesicourethral anastomosis was watertight. Therefore, we have since avoided reperitonealization and have used coated mesh, Proceed mesh (Ethicon Inc., Somerville, NJ), to avoid adherence [13]. As such, it is our recommendation that coated mesh be used to minimize the risk of adhesion. In a smaller cohort of just four, Joshi reported oversewing mesh with peritoneum with no complications, arguing that this technique prevents fistula and adhesion formation [31].

An extraperitoneal approach has been well described for laparoscopic hernia repair [27, 39, 41]. In this approach, the spermatic cord vessels and vas deferens are isolated and removed from the hernia sac and peritoneum. This creates a space from the pubic symphysis to the anterior superior iliac spine, over which mesh may be positioned. This approach allows for the use of standard polypropylene mesh without the need for fixation with staples or sutures.

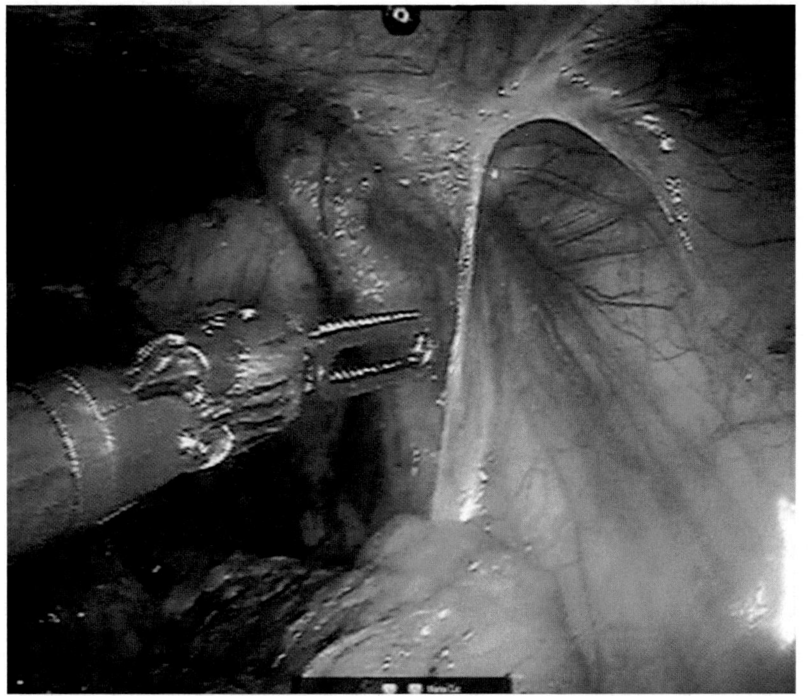

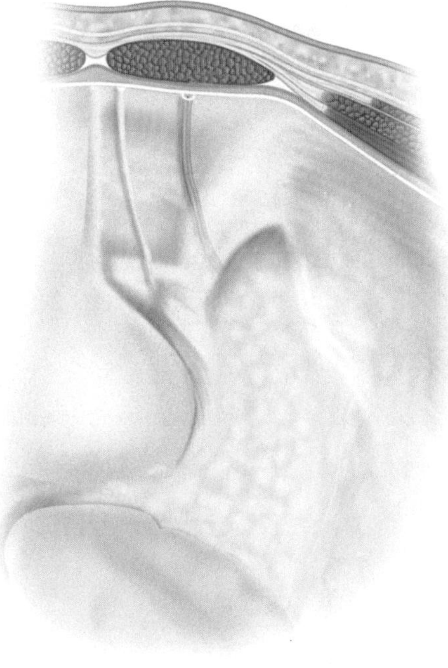

Fig. 40.1 Area right inguinal canal containing hernia prior to dissection

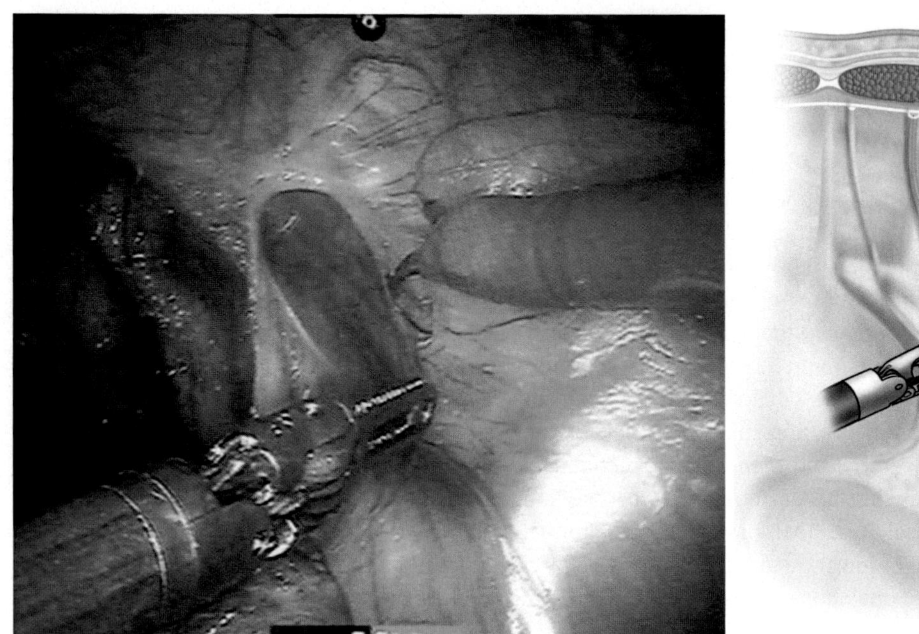
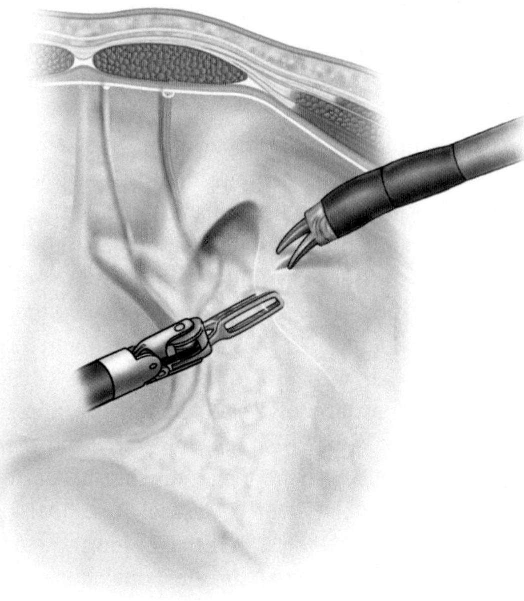

Fig. 40.2 Start of lateral dissection

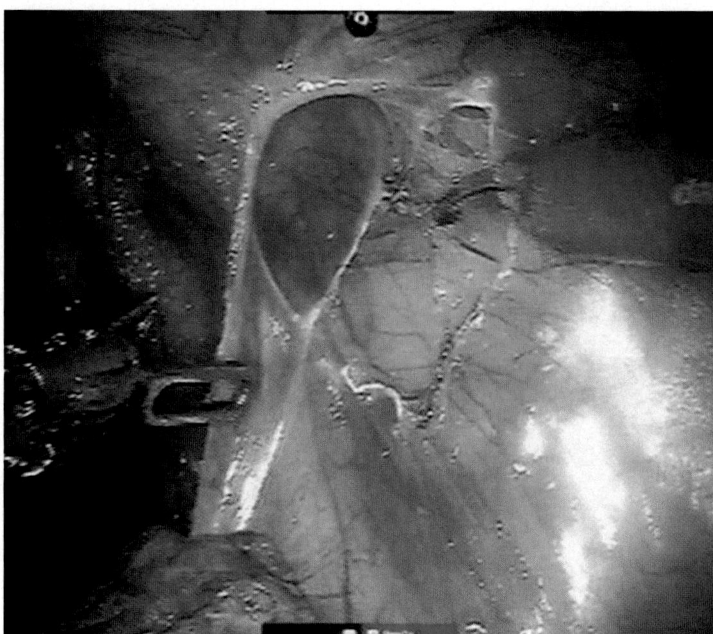
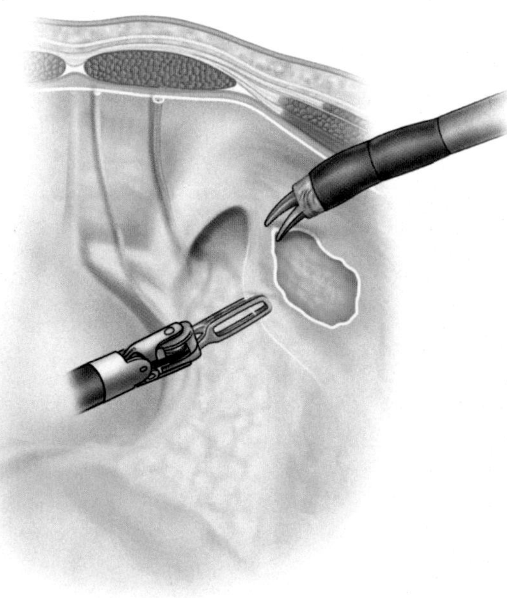

Fig. 40.3 Lateral dissection complete

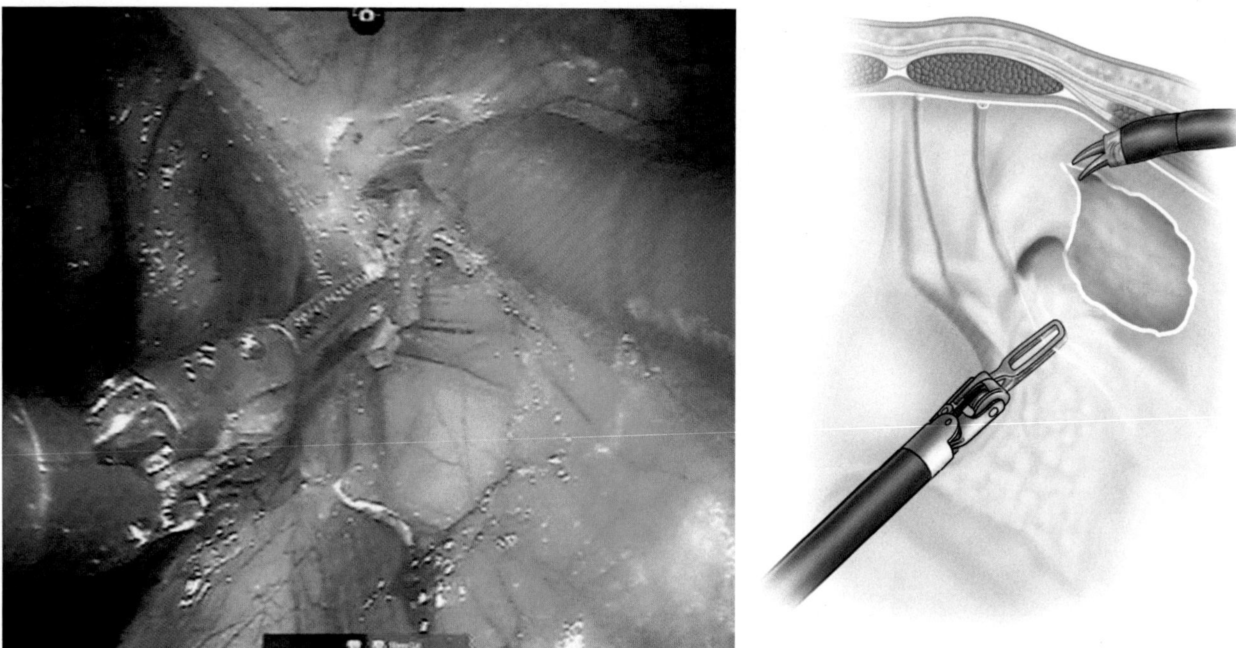

Fig. 40.4 Anterior dissection around the hernia

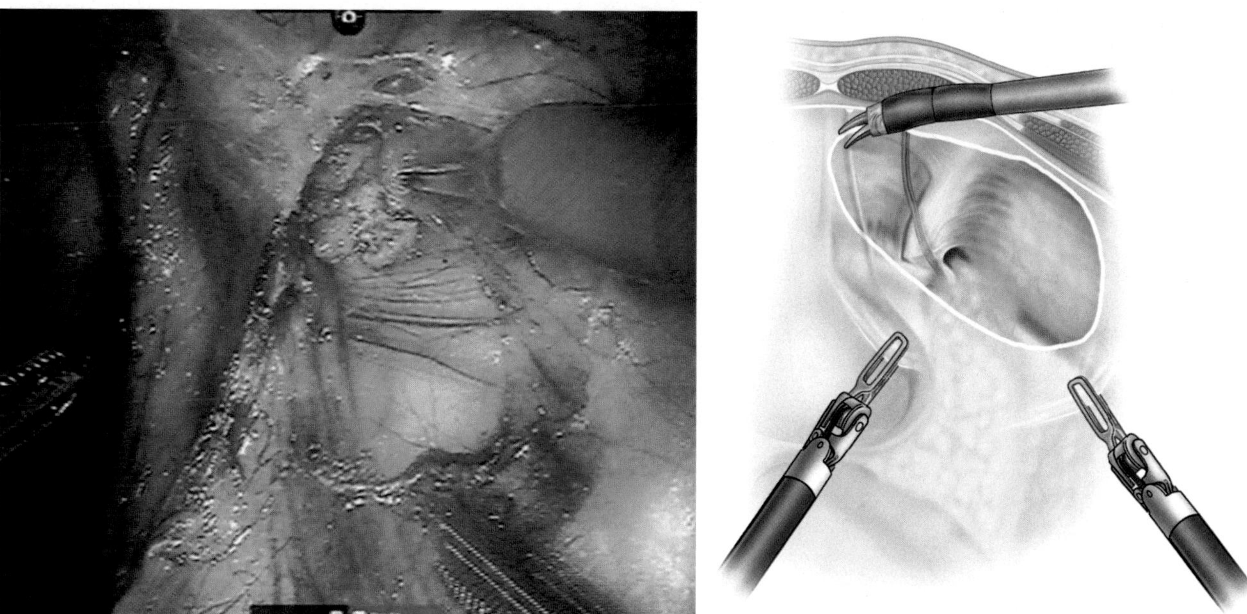

Fig. 40.5 Circumferential hernia dissection complete

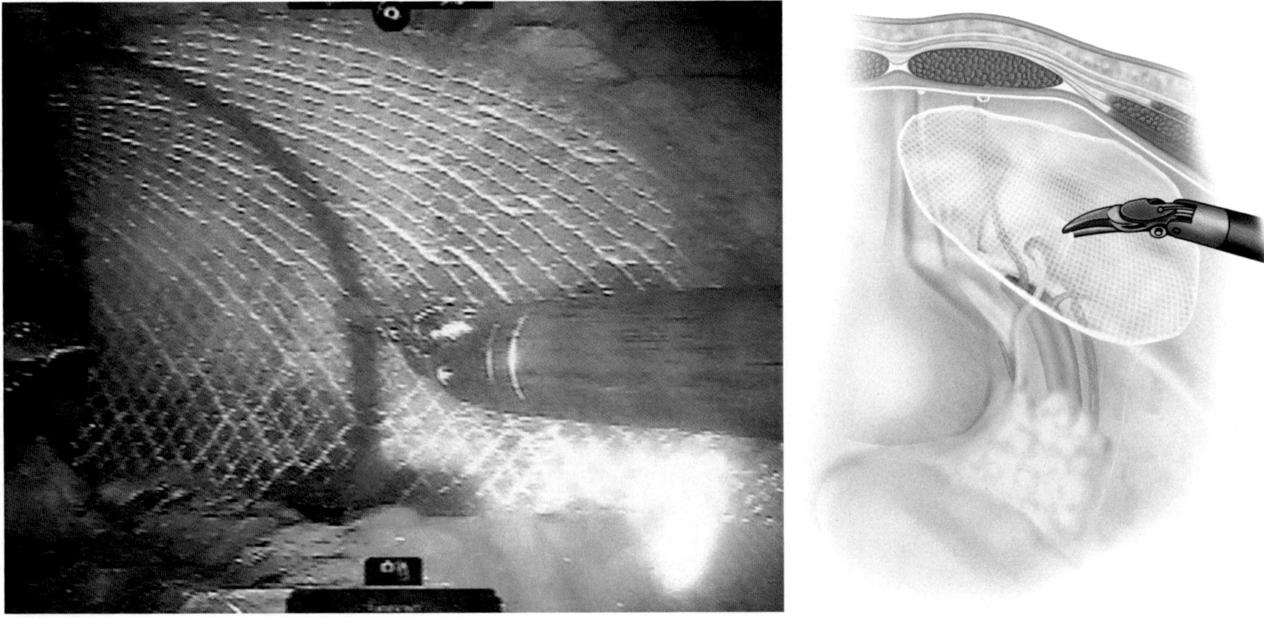

Fig. 40.6 Application of appropriately sized flat mesh over inguinal hernia

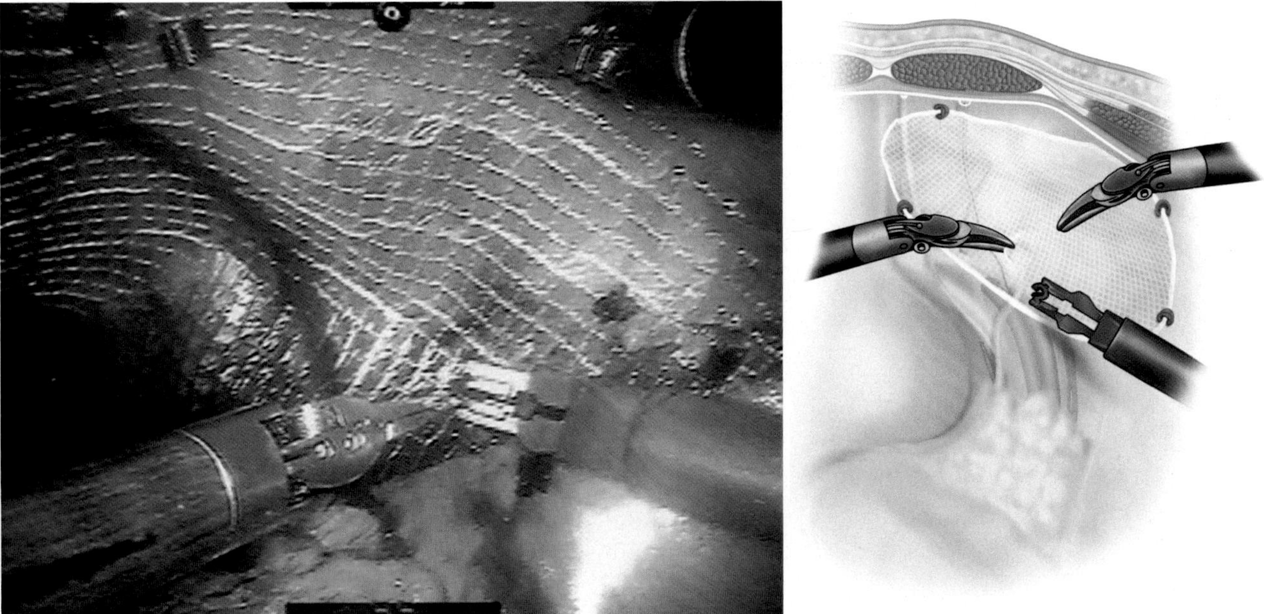

Fig. 40.7 Inguinal hernia with applied flat mesh, secured to Cooper ligament inferiorly and along the superolateral borders to the rectus sheath

Operative Variables and Complications

In our experience, operative times were not significantly increased with concomitant hernia repair. In four patients, Joshi reported additional operating time for hernia repair from 15 to 40 min [31]. Ludwig reported a mean of an additional 32 min [33]. All other operative and postoperative variables, including estimated blood loss and length of stay, were unchanged among patients undergoing RARP and herniorrhaphy. While we have found no significant difference in analgesic use, Teber found that patients undergoing laparoscopic radical prostatectomy with laparoscopic hernia repair had increased analgesic requirements. In their study, pain medication requirements were especially higher among patients who underwent transperitoneal rather than extraperitoneal procedures [27, 39].

In our previous studies with short-term follow-up (average 12.5 months), patients who underwent simultaneous RARP and robotic hernia repair reported no inguinal, scrotal, or testicular pain or paresthesias. As described earlier, we observed one incidence of postoperative urine leakage following reperitonealization during transperitoneal hernia repair [13, 14]. The leak occurred as a consequence of reperitonealization, and hence we stopped this technique in 2003, thereby resolving the issue. Smaller, more recent studies have reported no herniorrhaphy or mesh-related complications with a mean follow-up time of 33 months [31]. In a cohort of 26 patients, Ludwig reported one anterior mesh seroma that resolved by itself [33]. Similarly, among cohorts undergoing laparoscopic radical prostatectomy and hernia repair, no complications related to hernia repair have been observed [26, 27, 29, 42].

Rates of Recurrence After Repair

There is conflicting evidence regarding rates of recurrence after laparoscopic hernia repair. It has been previously reported that rates of recurrence are higher in laparoscopic than in open hernia repair [30]. Yet others have reported fewer complications and lower recurrence rates in patients undergoing laparoscopic repair compared with those undergoing open repair [43]. A meta-analysis comparing eight randomized-controlled trials showed no significant difference in recurrence rates [34].

We have observed one recurrence after IH repair concurrent with RARP in a patient who underwent hernia repair with placement of an umbrella mesh. This recurrence occurred 4 months into our combined IH repair with RARP. The mesh was noted to have migrated upon subsequent open repair [14]. Since this incident, we discontinued the use of umbrella mesh and have seen no further recurrences using flat Proceed mesh sutured over the hernia defect at multiple points. These findings are similar to recurrence rates in three other studies to date, documenting combined RARP and herniorrhaphy as well as after combined open or laparoscopic prostatectomy and hernia repair [26, 27, 29, 31, 33, 42].

Preoperative physical examination and abdominal computed tomography may be used to identify inguinal hernias with a 42.5 and 96.3% sensitivity rate, respectively [20]. Systematic detection and repair of IHs during radical prostatectomy reduces the risk of subsequent inguinal herniation. Initial studies indicate that concomitant herniorrhaphy at the time of RARP is safe and feasible.

References

1. Ruhl CE, Everhart JE. Risk factors for inguinal hernia among adults in the US population. Am J Epidemiol. 2007;165:1154–61.
2. Everhart JE. Abdominal wall hernia. In: Everhart JE, editor. Digestive diseases in the United States: epidemiology and impact. Bethesda, MD: National Institute of Diabetes and Digestive and Kidney Diseases; 1994. p. 471–507.
3. Regan TC, Mordkin RM, Constantinople NL, Spence IJ, Dejter SW Jr. Incidence of inguinal hernias following radical retropubic prostatectomy. Urology. 1996;47:536–7.
4. Stranne J, Hugosson J, Lodding P. Post-radical retropubic prostatectomy inguinal hernia: an analysis of risk factors with special reference to preoperative inguinal hernia morbidity and pelvic lymph node dissection. J Urol. 2006;176:2072.
5. Fukuta F, Hisasue S, Yanase M, Kobayashi K, Miyamoto S, Kato S, et al. Preoperative computed tomography finding predicts for postoperative inguinal hernia: new perspective for radical prostatectomy-related inguinal hernia. Urology. 2006;68:267.
6. Abe T, Shinohara N, Harabayashi T, Sazawa A, Suzuki S, Kawarada Y, Nonomura K. Postoperative inguinal hernia after radical prostatectomy for prostate cancer. Urology. 2007;69:326.
7. Twu CM, Ou YC, Yang CR, Cheng CL, Ho HC. Predicting risk factors for inguinal hernia after radical retropubic prostatectomy. Urology. 2005;66:814.
8. Ichioka K, Yoshimura K, Utsunomiya N, Ueda N, Matsui Y, Terai A, et al. High incidence of inguinal hernia after radical retropubic prostatectomy. Urology. 2004;63:278.
9. Stranne J, Hugosson J, Iversen P, Morris T, Lodding P. Inguinal hernia in stage M0 prostate cancer: a comparison of incidence in men treated with and without radical retropubic prostatectomy—an analysis of 1105 patients. Urology. 2005;65:847.
10. Lodding P, Bergdahl C, Nyberg M, Pileblad E, Stranne J, Hugosson J. Inguinal hernia after radical retropubic prostatectomy for prostate cancer: a study of incidence and risk factors in comparison to no operation and lymphadenectomy. J Urol. 2001;166:964.
11. Stranne J, Lodding P. Inguinal hernia after radical retropubic prostatectomy: risk factors and prevention. Nat Rev Urol. 2011;8:267.
12. Carlsson SV, Ehdaie B, Atoria CL, Elkin EB, Eastham JA. Risk of incisional hernia after minimally invasive and open radical prostatectomy. J Urol. 2013;190:1757–62.
13. Finley DS, Rodriguez E, Ahlering TE. Combined inguinal hernia repair with prosthetic mesh during transperitoneal robot assisted laparoscopic radical prostatectomy: a 4-year experience. Urology. 2007;178:1296–300.

14. Finley DS, Savatta D, Rodriguez E, Kopelan A, Ahlering TE. Transperitoneal robotic-assisted laparoscopic radical prostatectomy and inguinal herniorrhaphy. J Robot Surg. 2008;1:269–72.
15. Bielecki K, Puawaksi R. Is cigarette smoking a causative factor in the development of inguinal hernia? Pol Tyg Lek. 1988;43:974.
16. Jensen JA, Goodson WH, Hopf HW, Hunt TK. Cigarette smoking decreases tissue oxygen. Arch Surg. 1991;126:1131.
17. Jorgensen LN, Kallehave F, Christensen E, Siana JE, Gottrup F. Less collagen production in smokers. Surgery. 1998;123:450–5.
18. Watson DS, Sharp KW, Vasquez JM, Richards WO. Incidence of inguinal hernias diagnosed during laparoscopy. South Med J. 1994;87:23–5.
19. Nielsen ME, Walsh PC. Systematic detection and repair of subclinical inguinal hernias at radical retropubic prostatectomy. Urology. 2005;66:1034.
20. Lepor H, Robbins D. Inguinal hernias in men undergoing open radical retropubic prostatectomy. Urology. 2007;70:961–4.
21. Nyhus LM, Condon RE. Inguinal hernia. In: Nyhus LM, editor. Condon's hernia. 3rd ed. Philadelphia: Lippincott Williams & Wilkins; 1989. p. 74–7.
22. Sekita N, Suzuki H, Kamijima S, Chin K, Fujimora M, Mikami K, Ichikawa T. Incidence of inguinal hernia after prostate surgery: open radical retropubic prostatectomy versus open simple prostatectomy versus transurethral resection of the prostate. Int J Urol. 2009;16:110.
23. Koie T, Yoneyama T, Kamimura N, Imai A, Okamoto A, Ohyama C. Frequency of postoperative inguinal hernia after endoscope-assisted mini-laparotomy and conventional retropubic radical prostatectomies. Int J Urol. 2008;15:226.
24. McDonald DF, Huggins C. Simultaneous prostatectomy and inguinal herniorrhaphy. Surg Gynecol Obstet. 1949;89:621.
25. Schlegel PN, Walsh PC. The use of the preperitoneal approach for the simultaneous repair of inguinal hernia during surgery on the bladder and prostate. World J Surg. 1989;13:555–9.
26. Ghavamian R, Knoll A, Teixeira JA. Simultaneous extraperitoneal laparoscopic radical prostatectomy and intraperitoneal inguinal hernia repair with mesh. JSLS. 2005;9:231.
27. Stolzenburg JU, Rabenalt R, Dietel A, Do M, Pfeiffer H, Schwalbe S, et al. Hernia repair during endoscopic (laparoscopic) radical prostatectomy. J Laparoendosc Adv Surg Tech A. 2003;13:27.
28. Manoharan M, Vyas S, Araki M, Nieder AM, Soloway MS. Concurrent radical retropubic prostatectomy and Lichtenstein inguinal hernia repair through a single modified Pfannenstiel incision: a 3-year experience. BJU Int. 2006;98:341.
29. Antunes A, Dall'Oglio M, Crippa A, Srougi M. Inguinal hernia repair with polypropylene mesh during radical retropubic prostatectomy: an easy and practical approach. BJU Int. 2005;96:330.
30. Neumayer L, Giobbie-Hurder A, Jonasson O, Fitzgibbons R, Dunlop D, Giggs J, et al. Open mesh versus laparoscopic mesh repair of inguinal hernia. N Engl J Med. 2004;350:1819.
31. Joshi AR, Spivak J, Ruback E, Goldberg G, DeNoto G. Concurrent robotic trans-abdominal pre-peritoneal (TAP) herniorrhaphy during robotic-assisted radical prostatectomy. Int J Med Robot. 2010;6:311–4.
32. Fan JKM, Tam PC, Law WL. Synchronous trans-abdominal preperitoneal (TAPP) hernioplasty in a patient with robotic-assisted prostatectomy for carcinoma of prostate. Surg Pract. 2010; 14:32.
33. Ludwig WW, Spoko NA, Azoury SC, Dhanasopon A, Mettee L, Dwarakanath A, et al. Inguinal hernia repair during extraperitoneal robot-assisted laparoscopic radical prostatectomy. J Endourol. 2016;30(2):208–11.
34. Forbes SS, Eskicioglu C, McLeod RS, Okrainec A. Meta-analysis of randomized controlled trials comparing open and laparoscopic ventral and incisional hernia repair with mesh. Br J Surg. 2009;96:851–8.
35. Stranne J, Aus G, Bergdahl DJE, Hugosson J, Khatami A, Lodding P. Post-radical prostatectomy inguinal hernia: a simple surgical intervention can substantially reduce the incidence-- results from a prospective randomized trial. J Urol. 2010;184:984–9.
36. Schultz C, Baca I, Gotzen V. Laparoscopic inguinal hernia repair. Surg Endosc. 2001;15:582.
37. Schmedt CG, Sauerland S, Bittner R. Comparison of endoscopic procedures vs Lichtenstein and other open mesh techniques for inguinal hernia repair: a meta-analysis of randomized controlled trials. Surg Endosc. 2005;19:188–99.
38. Kelly ME, Behrman SW. The safety and efficacy of prosthetic hernia repair in clean-contaminated and contaminated wounds. Am Surg. 2002;68:524–8; discussion, 528–9
39. Teber D, Erdogru T, Zukosky D, Frede T, Rassweiler J. Prosthetic mesh hernioplasty during laparoscopic radical prostatectomy. Urology. 2005;65:1173–8.
40. Stoppa RE, Rives JL, Warlaumont CR, Palot JP, Verhaeghe PJ, Delattre JF. The use of Dacron in the repair of hernias of the groin. Surg Clin North Am. 1984;64:269.
41. Rassweiler J, Deglmann W, Renner C, Frede T, Seeman O. Results of the laparoscopic extraperitoneal hernioplasty in comparison to open surgery. Aktuelle Urol. 2000;31:229–37.
42. Lee BC, Rodin DM, Shah KK, Dahl DM. Laparoscopic inguinal hernia repair during laparoscopic radical prostatectomy. BJU Int. 2007;99:637.
43. Lomanto D, Iyer SG, Shabbir A, Cheah WK. Laparoscopic versus open ventral hernia mesh repair: a prospective study. Surg Endosc. 2006;20:1030–5.

Robotic Transaxillary Thyroidectomy: A Modified Protocol for the Western Medical Community

41

Sang-Wook Kang, Emad Kandil, and Woong Youn Chung

Robotic transaxillary thyroidectomy is currently of great interest, particularly in Asia, Europe, and North and South America. Considerable research has shown that it is safe and that its outcome is at least equivalent, if not superior, to open thyroidectomy. It has been slow to gain widespread acceptance in clinical practice, however, perhaps because of reservations about its general applicability to all patient populations, uncertainty about the instruments involved, and questions about the willingness of insurance companies to fund the procedure. This chapter provides detailed information on the method and summarizes important modifications that may pave the way for its widespread adoption.

Robotic surgery has advanced greatly over the past decade, although its implementation has not kept pace, perhaps because of the limited availability of the technology or the hesitation of surgeons to adopt it. Another consideration is that coverage of the costs by patients' insurance companies is uncertain and varies according to the type and complexity of the procedure [1–3]. This general scenario describes the current state of robotic thyroidectomies, the topic of this chapter.

The thyroid gland is surrounded by critical nerves, organs, and vessels, so it is of primary importance to remove the thyroid without damage to the adjacent structures. Traditionally, removal has been accomplished with an open method that requires an incision in the skin of the neck that is approximately 4–6 cm long. The drawbacks of this method are a conspicuous scar and discomfort.

In recent years, minimally invasive approaches to thyroidectomies, including video-assisted surgery and a variety of endoscopic methods using remote site incisions, have been adopted in order to avoid the unsightly neck scars [4–8]. In 2007, these extracervical endoscopic thyroidectomies were successfully combined with dexterous robotic surgical systems. The facilitation of these surgeries with robotics was safe, and the surgical outcomes were comparable or even superior to those of conventional surgery. The results also had excellent cosmesis [9–11].

Transaxillary thyroidectomy, one of the endoscopic thyroidectomy methods that adopts an extracervical approach, is the focus of attention in this chapter. This method employs a lateral approach to the thyroid gland, and the operation view is quite similar to the open method. Consequently, it is easy for the surgeon to locate and preserve the recurrent laryngeal nerve (RLN) and parathyroid gland, to divide the superior thyroidal vessels securely, and to perform complete central compartment neck lymph node dissection, should there be a malignancy [8, 9, 11–17]. Since the first robotic thyroidectomy, numerous studies have shown that transaxillary robotic thyroidectomies are safe and practical and have outcomes that compare well with those of the conventional open method [9–17].

Transaxillary thyroidectomy requires incision of the skin of the armpit area and an additional subcutaneous tunnel to the thyroid gland, a wide dissection that cannot be considered minimally invasive. Nonetheless, many researchers conclude that it is superior to the open procedure with respect to many postoperative factors: patients experience less discomfort, less modification of their voices and sensory functions, and better cosmesis. An additional consideration is that the transaxillary procedure offers excellent ergonomics to the surgeon [18, 19].

This chapter introduces a detailed method for transaxillary robotic thyroidectomy, including some minor modifications that should enhance its applicability to Western medicine.

Surgical Indications for Transaxillary Robotic Thyroidectomy

Candidates for transaxillary robotic thyroidectomy should be diagnosed with surgical disease. The diagnosis should be histologically confirmed by ultrasonography-guided fine-needle aspiration biopsy. Staging neck ultrasonography and a neck CT scan can be used to evaluate preoperative clinical stages.

S.-W. Kang, MD (✉) · W. Y. Chung
Department of Surgery, Yonsei University College of Medicine, Seoul, South Korea
e-mail: oralvanco@yuhs.ac

E. Kandil
Department of Endocrine Surgery, Tulane University School of Medicine, New Orleans, LA, USA

Y. Fong et al. (eds.), *The SAGES Atlas of Robotic Surgery*, https://doi.org/10.1007/978-3-319-91045-1_41

Transaxillary thyroidectomy can limit the surgeon's working field. There is no preformed space for working on the neck area, and the newly developed access route to the thyroid gland can be a major space restriction. Hence, the volume of thyroid gland, the tumor size, and the tumor location should be evaluated and considered before the surgery is planned. Patients with conditions that result in an enlarged thyroid, including multinodular goiter, thyroiditis, and Graves' disease, are not good candidates for the surgery, as the enlarged gland can limit the working space and result in easy tearing of the tissue and bleeding.

The ideal candidate for transaxillary robotic thyroidectomy is one who has a follicular neoplasm with a tumor no larger than 5 cm. When the tumor is malignant, it is safest to limit the procedure to cases with well-differentiated thyroid carcinomas composed of tumors of 2 cm or less that have no definite extrathyroidal tumor invasion (T1 lesions). Finally, patients with malignant lesions in the dorsal thyroid, especially adjacent to the tracheoesophageal groove, are at risk for injury to the trachea, esophagus, or RLN during surgery and are not good candidates.

As robotic surgical experience accumulates, it seems likely that it will be possible to employ the technique in most cases, including advanced ones.

The following criteria for transaxillary robotic thyroidectomy are currently used for thyroid malignancy in high-volume centers:

- Surgery is *indicated* only when the thyroid carcinoma is well-differentiated.
- Surgery is *indicated* usually when the primary tumor is less than 4 cm.
- Surgery is *acceptable* when there is minimal invasion by the tumor into the anterior thyroid capsule and strap muscle.
- Surgery is *contraindicated* when there is definite tumor invasion to an adjacent organ such as the RLN, esophagus, major vessels, or trachea.
- Surgery is *contraindicated* when any coexisting substernal or retropharyngeal lymph node is involved by the cancer.
- Surgery is *contraindicated* when there is any evidence for perinodal infiltration of the lymph node to an adjacent organ: the internal jugular vein, common carotid artery, vagus nerve, or RLN.

Table 41.1 Special equipment needed for robotic thyroidectomy

Procedure	Instruments or materials
Patient position	Arm board Soft pillow
Creation of skin flap	Electrocautery with regular and extended-sized tip Vascular Debakey or Russian forceps (extended length) Army-navy retractor × 2 Breast lighted retractor × 2
Maintenance of working space	Chung's external retractor system (Fig. 41.2a) Or Modified retractor system (Fig. 41.2b)
Robotic procedure	5-mm Maryland dissector 8-mm ProGrasp™ forceps 5-mm harmonic® curved shears Dual-channel 30° endoscope Endoscopic rolled gauzes Endoscopic suction irrigator

Preparations

Special Instruments

The patient's arm on the lesion side will be fixed over the patient's head with an arm board that can be attached to the operating table. The neck will be extended with a soft pillow. As listed on Table 41.1, several devices will be needed during the creation of working space: electrocautery that has both a regular and a long tip, a vascular Debakey or Russian extended length forceps, two Army-Navy retractors, and breast lighted retractors (Fig. 41.1). The working space will be maintained with an external retractor system consisting of Chung's retractors or another modified type of retractor for robotic thyroidectomy (Fig. 41.2). For the robotic procedures, either the da Vinci® S or Si system (Intuitive Surgical, Sunnyvale, CA, USA) should be acquired, as well as three other robotic instruments: a 5-mm Maryland dissector, an 8-mm ProGrasp™ forceps (Intuitive Surgical), and 5-mm Harmonic® curved shears (Intuitive Surgical). A dual-channel camera (30°, used in the down view position) also will be needed. Harmonic® curved shears are the preferred energy device.

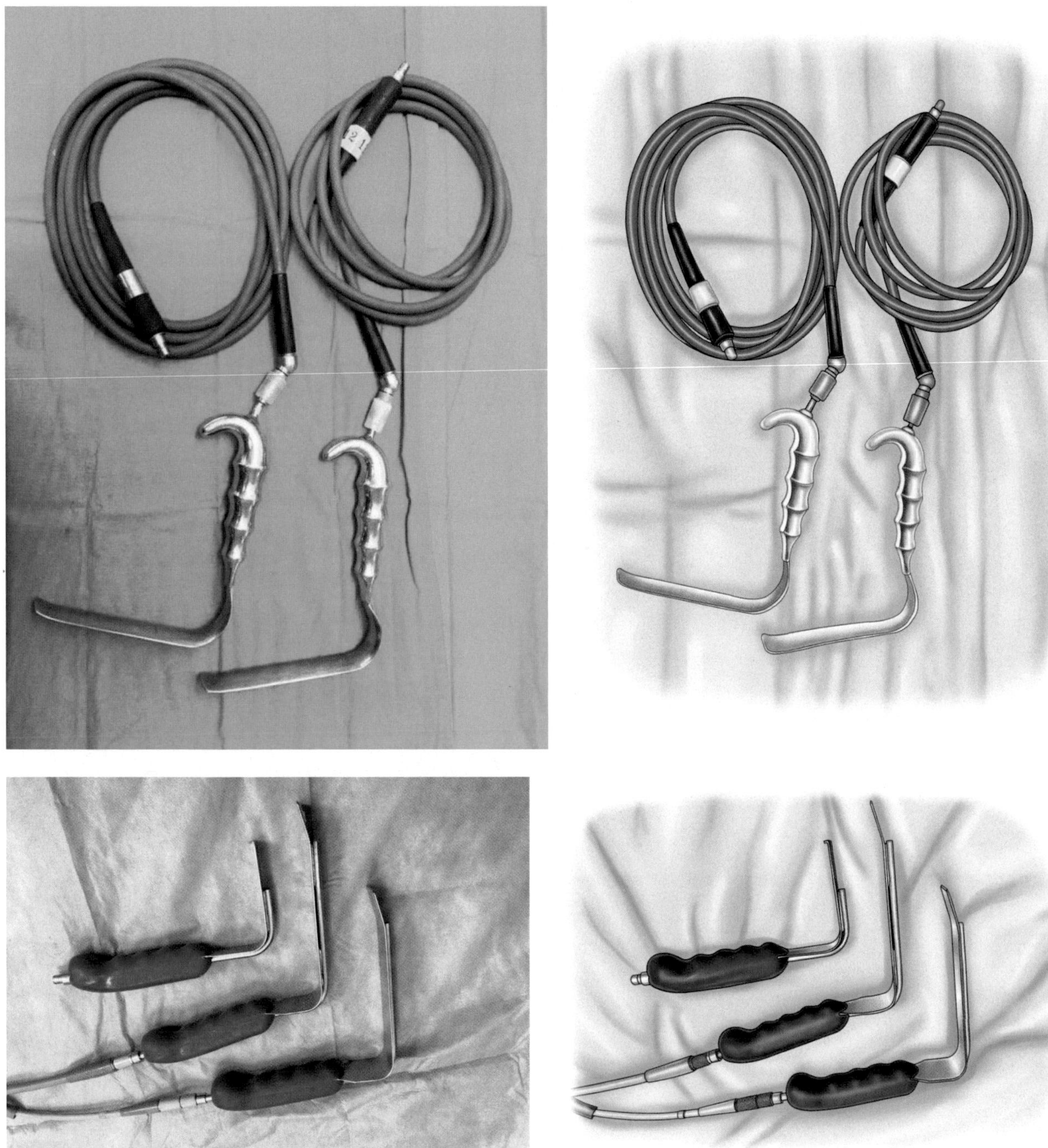

Fig. 41.1 Breast lighted retractor

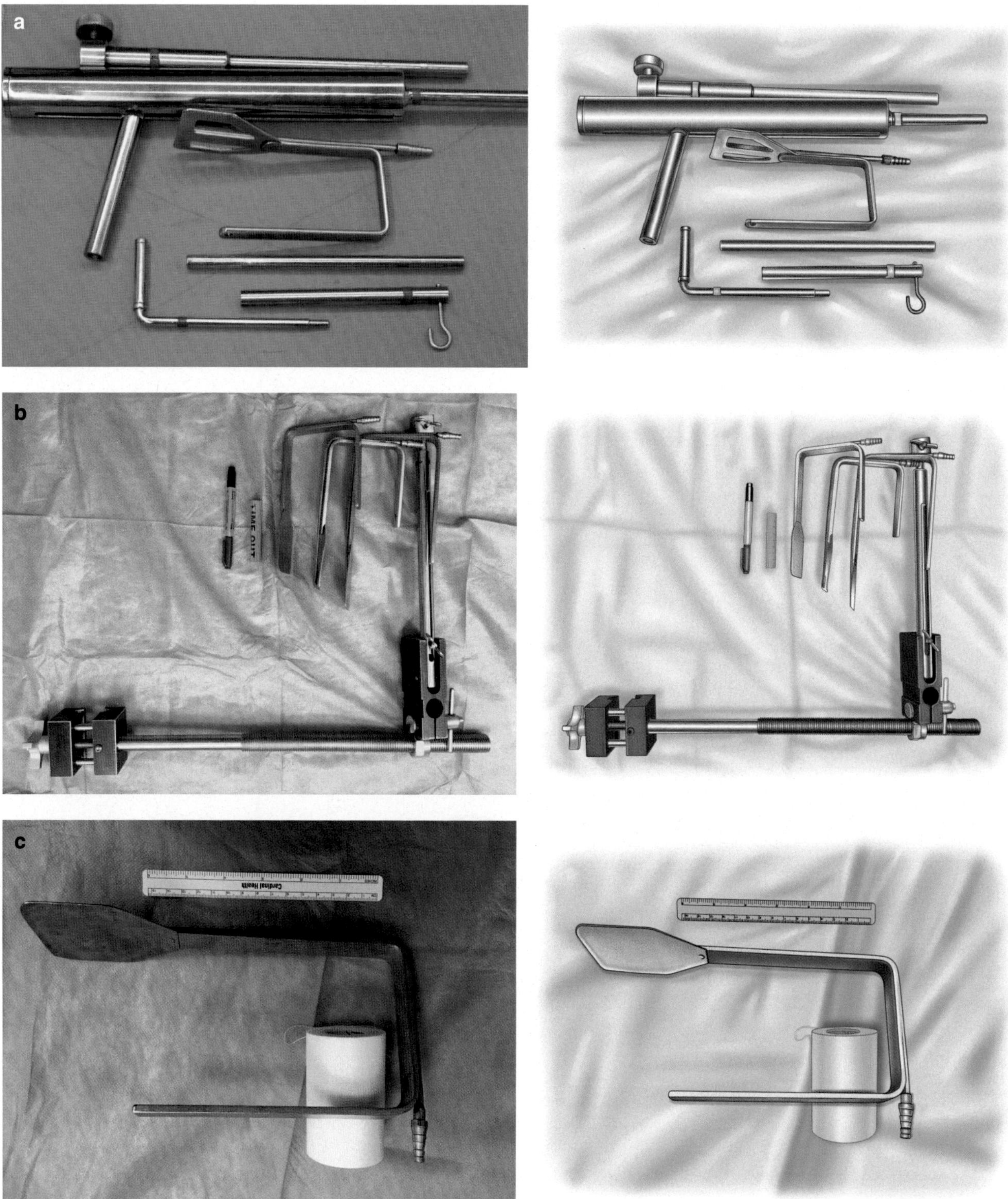

Fig. 41.2 External retractor system. (**a**) Original Chung's retractor (BR Holdings, Seoul, Korea). Modified special retractor set (**b**) and blade (**c**) for big and obese patients (Marina Medical, Sunrise, FL, USA)

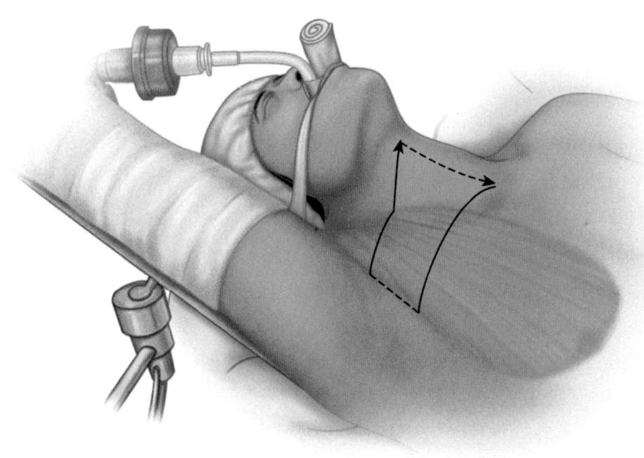

Fig. 41.3 Original patient positioning

Patient Position

The patient is placed in a supine position under general anesthesia, with the neck slightly extended with a soft pillow inserted under the shoulder. The lesion-side arm is raised and fixed to provide the shortest distance from the axilla to the anterior neck, shown in Fig. 41.3. If the patient is obese or has limited shoulder motion, the arm position is slightly modified (Fig. 41.4) by raising the lesion-side arm, bending it at the elbow, and placing the forearm just over the forehead without straightening the elbow. In this position, the arm can be placed and fixed using the soft pillow and pads without arm boards. This position also carries a low risk of stretching injury to the brachial plexus.

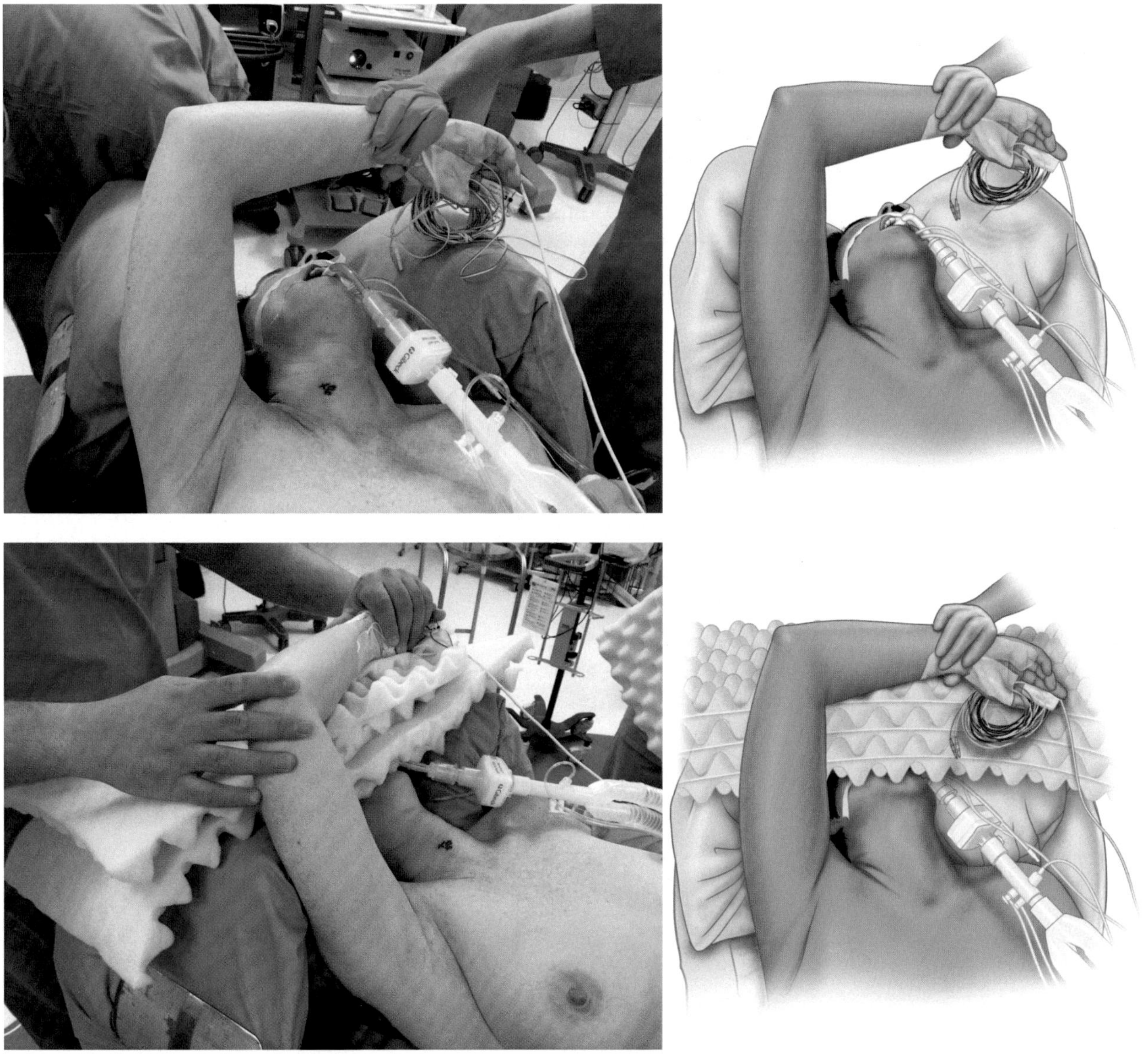

Fig. 41.4 Modified patient position for obese patients or patients with stiff shoulder joints

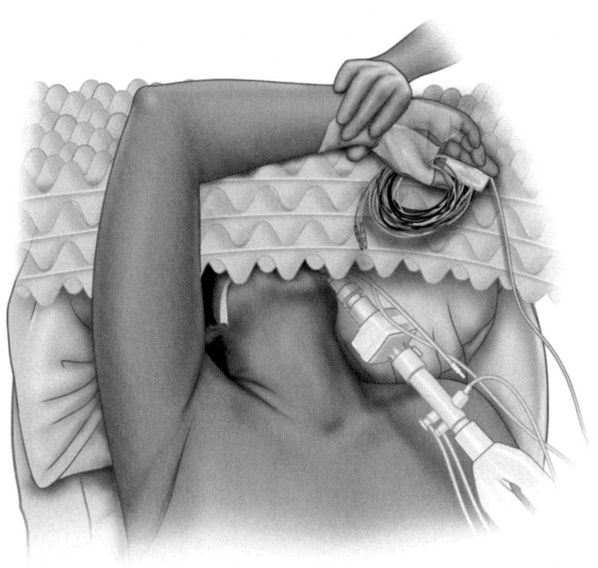

Fig. 41.4 (continued)

Surgical Techniques

Protocol for Development of Working Space

A curvilinear skin incision about 5–6 cm in length is made in the axilla along the anterior axillary fold. A subcutaneous skin flap is made over the anterior surface of the pectoralis major muscle from the axilla to the clavicle and the sternal notch. After crossing the clavicle, an adequate subplatysmal skin flap is created. It is recommended that an adequate extent of subplatysmal flap should also be made in the posterior neck area. The flap is dissected medially to the medial border of the sternocleidomastoid (SCM) muscle under direct vision. At this point, the dissection continues through the avascular space between the sternal and clavicular heads of the SCM muscle. The breast lighted retractor is the best choice for viewing the inside of the flap; some of the other tools are too short. Upon opening the avascular space between the heads of the SCM muscle, the superior belly of the omohyoid muscle and the internal jugular vein (IJV) usually can be identified. These are carefully detached from the lateral aspect of the thyroid gland, exposing the full lateral aspect of the gland. The strap muscle is detached from the anterior surface of the thyroid gland and lifted until the contralateral lobe of the thyroid gland is exposed (Fig. 41.5). Next, the blades of the external retractor system are inserted through the skin incision in the axilla and maneuvered to lift up the skin flap, the sternal head of the SCM muscle, and the strap muscles together, serving to maintain the working field for the robotic procedure (Fig. 41.6).

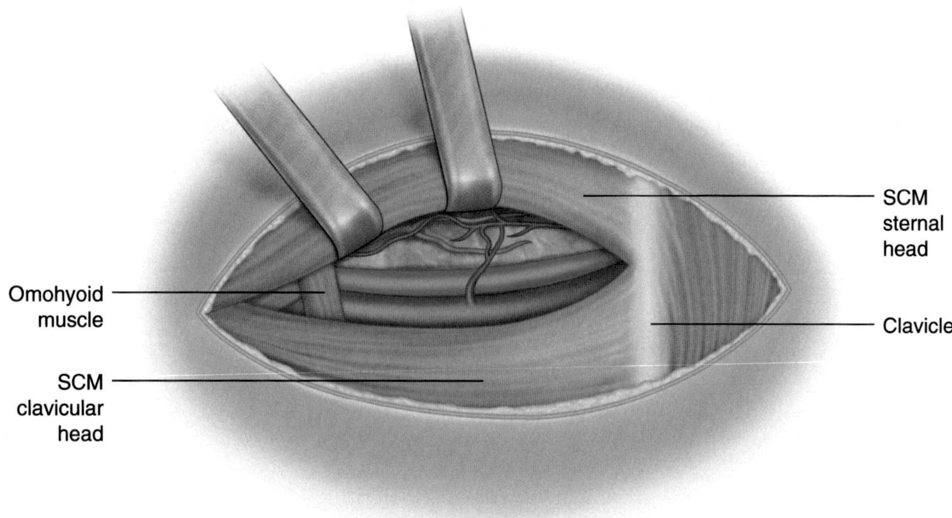

Fig. 41.5 The route of transaxillary approach (the space between two branches of sternocleidomastoid [SCM] muscle)

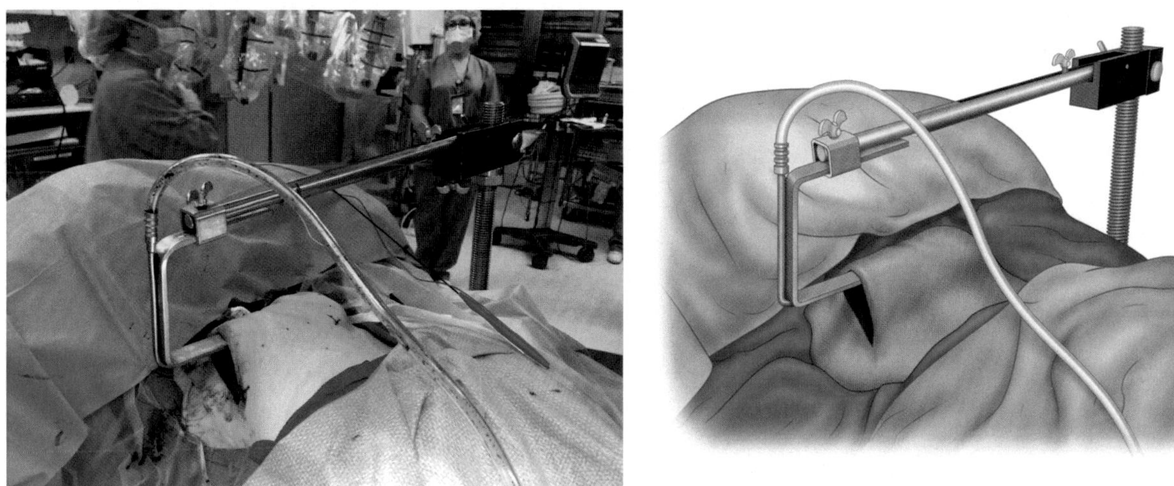

Fig. 41.6 The blades of the external retractor system elevate the skin flap, sternal head of the SCM muscle, and strap muscles together to maintain the working field for the robotic procedure

Protocol for Docking and Instrumentation

All the robotic arms are inserted through the axillary incision. Interference between the robotic arms can be a problem, and the guidelines in this protocol should prevent this interference. The critical issues are correct placement of the ProGrasp™ forceps, the ideal angles of the robotic arms, and maintenance of the correct interarm distances.

The patient cart is placed on the lateral aspect of the patient, opposite to the route of approach. The robotic column is located near the operating table so that the robotic camera is in a straight line with the axis of the external retractor (Fig. 41.7). For an approach from the right side, a 12-mm trocar for the camera and a 30° dual-channel endoscope are located in the center of the axillary incision. The camera is inserted in the upward direction: its external third joint is in the lowest part

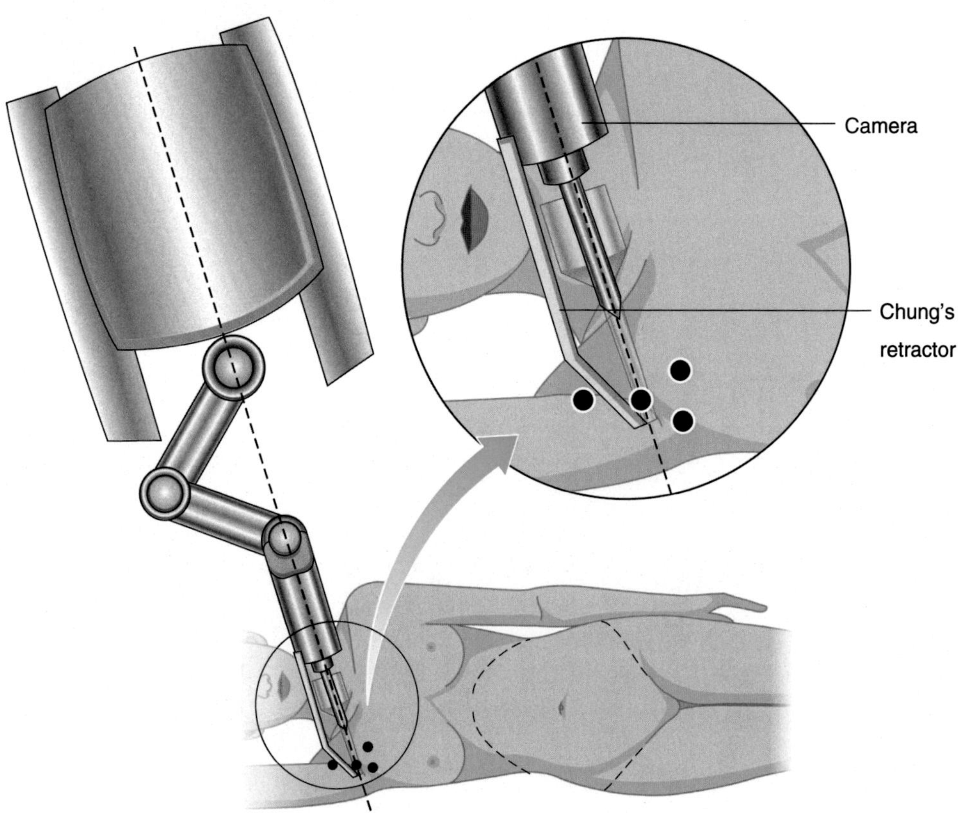

Fig. 41.7 Adjustment of the operating table for optimum efficiency. The robotic camera should be in a straight line between the robotic column and the surgical approach route (the direction of retractor insertion)

(floor) of the incision entrance, with its tip directed upward. An 8-mm trocar for the ProGrasp™ forceps is then positioned to the right of the camera, parallel with the suction tube of the retractor blade. At this point, the ProGrasp™ forceps are located as close as possible to the ceiling of the working space (the retractor blade). The 5-mm trocar of a Maryland dissector is then positioned on the left of the camera, also at the left edge of the incision, and the 5-mm trocar for the Harmonic® curved shears at the right side of the camera, at the right edge of the incision. Instruments should be as far apart as possible and inserted upward, in the same direction that the camera is inserted (Fig. 41.8).

Protocol for Robotic Total Thyroidectomy with Central Compartment Neck Dissection

The Harmonic® curved shears are used for ligations of vessels and hemostasis. With traction of the upper pole of the thyroid gland in the medio-inferior direction by the ProGrasp™ forceps, the superior thyroid artery and veins are individually divided (Fig. 41.9). The upper pole of the thyroid gland is pulled steadily for countertraction with the ProGrasp™ forceps. Frequent repositioning allows optimal exposure of the superior parathyroid gland and Zuckerkandl's tubercle of the thyroid gland. The thyroid

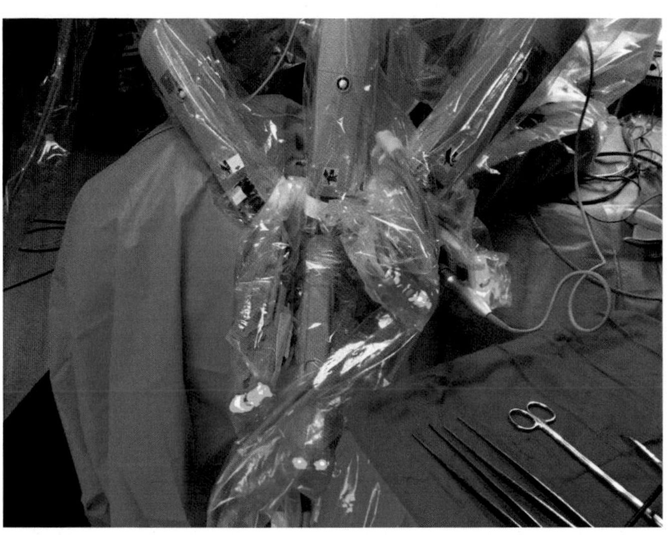

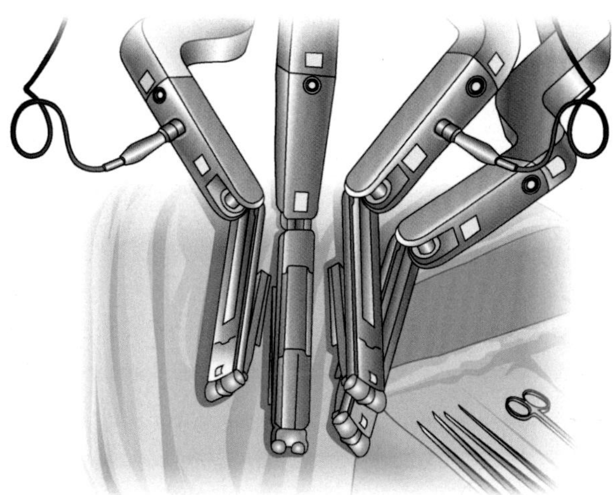

Fig. 41.8 Placement of robotic instruments. The camera should be placed down in the center of the skin incision in an advanced upward direction. Two instruments should be introduced through the caudal side, with the camera as the center. The ProGrasp™ forceps should be inserted and secured to the highest part of the working space, close to the retractor blade (caudal side of the retractor). The Maryland dissector and Harmonic® curved shears should be located on both ends of the skin incision, as far apart as possible

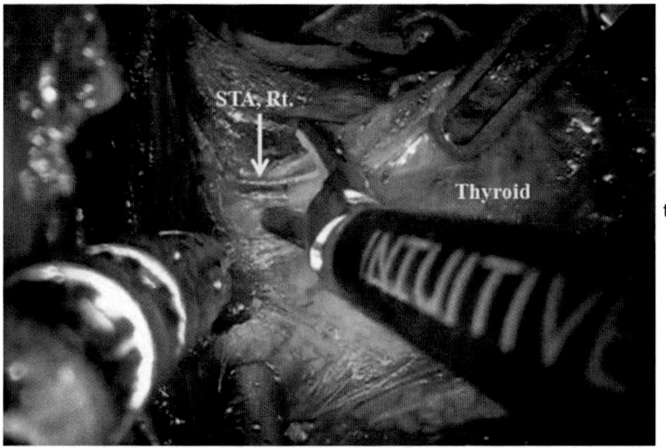

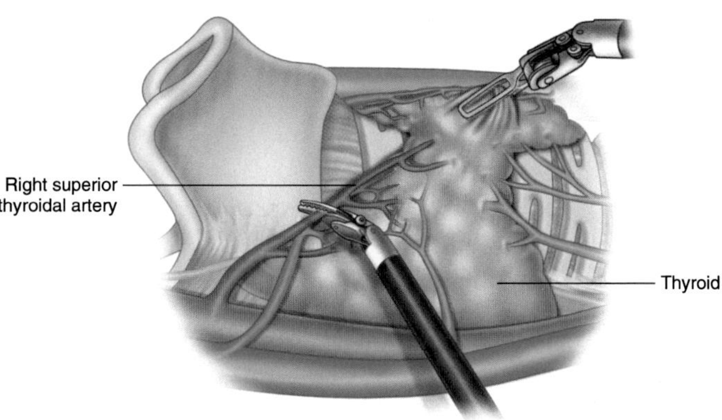

Fig. 41.9 The ligation of superior thyroidal vessels. With medio-inferior traction of the thyroid gland, the pedicles of superior thyroidal vessels are exposed and can be individually divided

gland is peeled from the cricothyroid muscle; this method allows the identification and preservation of the superior parathyroid gland (Fig. 41.10). The upper pole dissection is continued until the superior part of Zuckerkandl's tubercle is exposed, using great care around the RLN insertion site. The next step follows upper pole mobilization but is not attempted until the RLN is identified and traced along its whole path (Fig. 41.11). After this, the central compartment lymph node is dissected, preserving the critical structures. This step involves complete detachment of the thyroid gland and central lymph nodes from the trachea. In the Berry ligament region, great caution is required to prevent direct or indirect thermal injury to the RLN by the Harmonic® curved shears. After right lobectomy of the thyroid gland, contralateral lobectomy of the thyroid is performed by subcapsular dissection, taking care to preserve

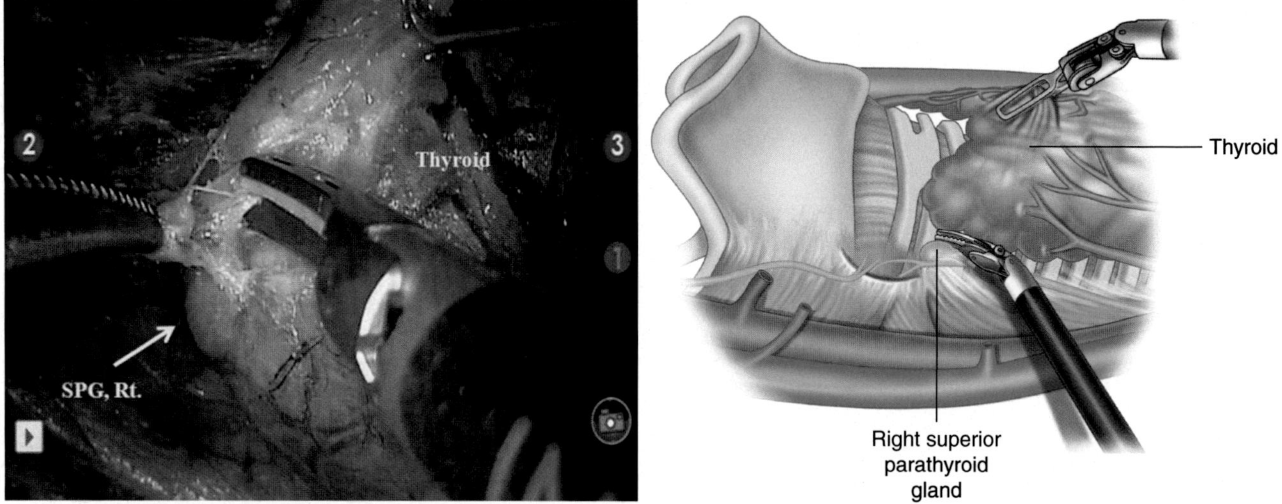

Fig. 41.10 Identification of the superior parathyroid gland. The superior parathyroid gland is identified and preserved by detaching the thyroid gland from the cricothyroid muscle

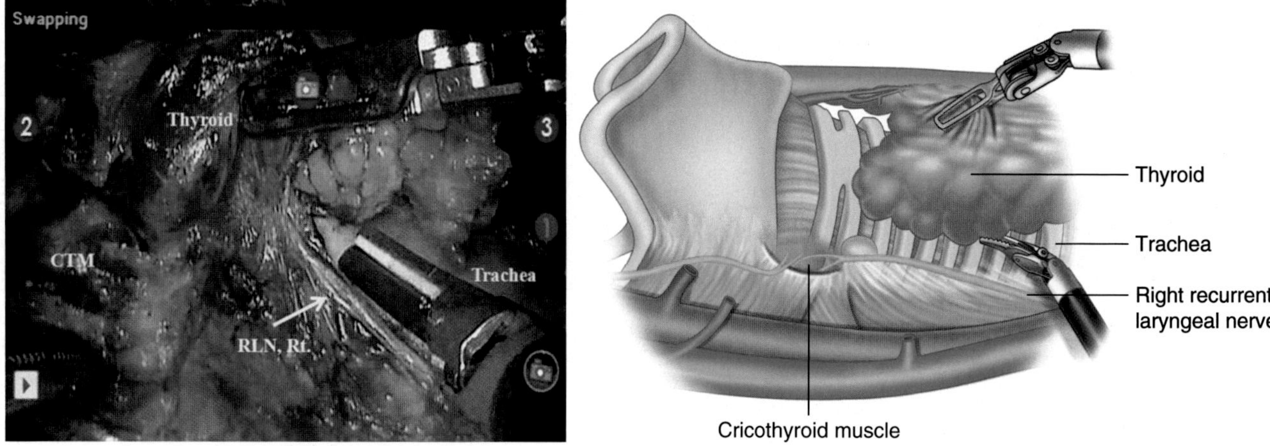

Fig. 41.11 Ipsilateral recurrent laryngeal nerve (RLN) identification. After tracing the whole running course of the RLN, the thyroid can be detached from the trachea completely

the parathyroid glands and the RLN (Figs. 41.12 and 41.13). In some cases (e.g., a male patient or one with a prominent trachea), it is possible to achieve better exposure of the contralateral tracheoesophageal groove by tilting the operating table to 10–15°, left side up.

After extraction of the specimen, irrigation is performed to clean the operative fields. Finally, a 3-mm closed-suction drain is inserted through a separate skin incision below the axillary skin incision, and the wound is closed cosmetically (Fig. 41.14).

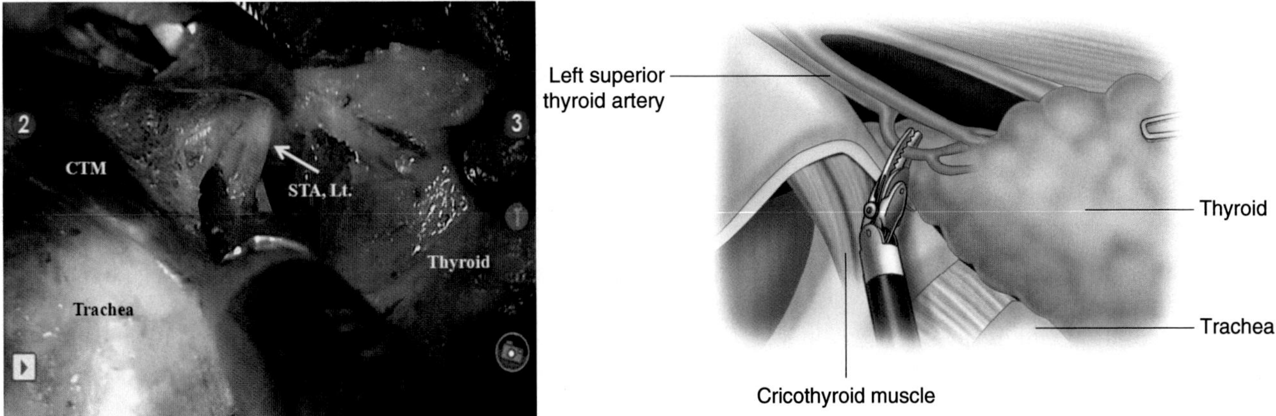

Fig. 41.12 Ligation of contralateral superior thyroidal vessels. With the inferolateral traction of the contralateral thyroid gland, the space of Reeves can be identified and the superior thyroidal vessels can be safely divided

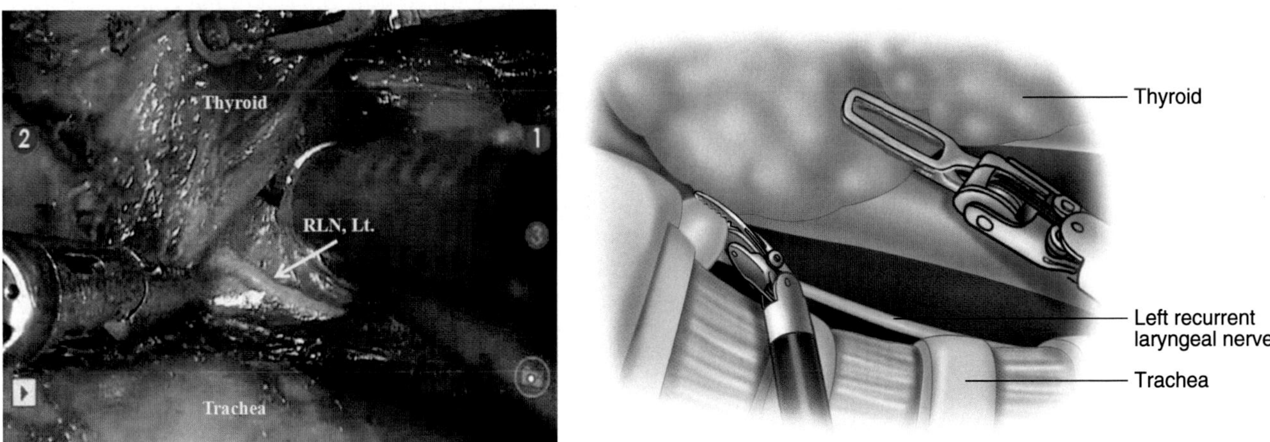

Fig. 41.13 Identification of the contralateral RLN. Contralateral thyroidectomy usually proceeds with the subcapsular dissection to preserve the parathyroid gland and RLN

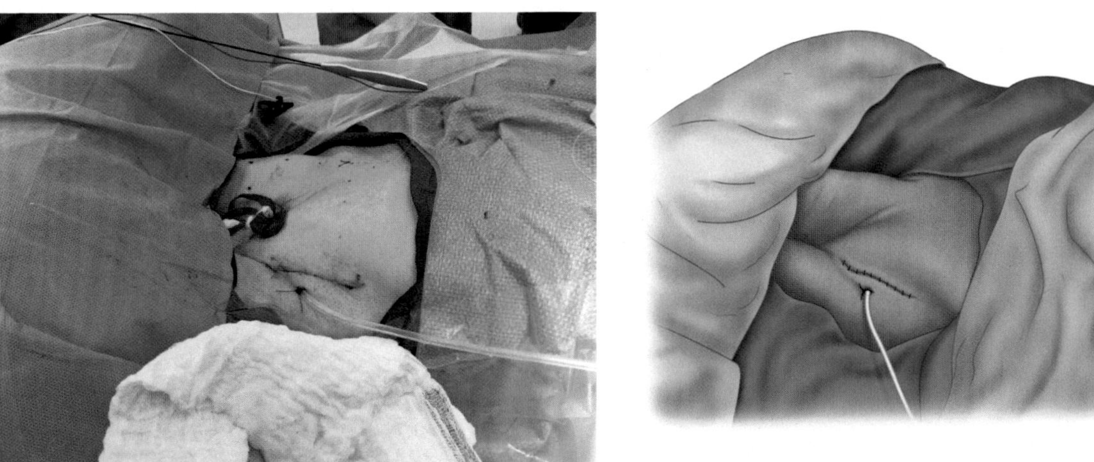

Fig. 41.14 Postoperative wound after drain insertion and skin closure

Postoperative Management

Postoperative pain can be controlled with the usual postoperative medication regimen. The period of drain placement after the operation usually depends on the patient's age, medication, and underlying disease; it can be safely removed without the risk of postoperative seroma if there is less than 50 mL of drainage per day. Discharge and the outpatient follow-up plan should be based on the surgeon's experience and preference.

Complications

The typical complications of any thyroidectomy, regardless of the surgical methods, are transient or permanent hypoparathyroidism, injury to the RLN or the superior laryngeal nerve, hemorrhage, seroma, and wound infection. The robotic approach carries some specific risk of complications such as injury to the skin flap (either thermal or from penetration), injury to the IJV or trachea, and ipsilateral arm paralysis. The injury to the skin flap or IJV may occur during the creation of the skin flap and is most likely when the surgeon is inexperienced with the approach. Tracheal injury is possible due to the lateral approach of this method and the possible reduction of the surgeon's tactile sensation by the robotic instruments. Injury to the tracheal wall is particularly likely around the Berry ligament if the operational field is not properly maintained and appropriate caution is not taken.

Transient ipsilateral arm paralysis can result from incorrect patient positioning, usually overtraction or overrotation of the shoulder joint, which can eventually overstretch the brachial plexus. This paralysis is usually transient, and arm movement will be recovered within several weeks. To avoid this inconvenient complication, especially for patients who have stiff joints, the surgeon can use an intraoperative neural monitoring system for real-time checking of the median and ulnar nerve (Fig. 41.15). This system also carries the benefit of allowing the surgeon to identify and avoid damage to the RLN and superior laryngeal nerve simultaneously by adding a nerve integrity monitor (NIM) endotracheal tube (Medtronic Xomed; Jacksonville, FL, USA).

Remaining Problems and the Future of Robotic Thyroidectomy

Despite its promise for cosmesis and postoperative outcome, robotic thyroidectomy has some limitations that must be overcome. Specifically, robotic transaxillary thyroidectomy is more invasive than the open conventional method because of the wide dissection from the axilla to the anterior neck, and it is also more time-consuming. The one-sided approach is a complicated avenue to the contralateral upper pole of the thyroid gland, particularly for the inexperienced surgeon. In contralateral upper pole dissection, all the instruments should cross over the trachea and approach the deep, narrow area as the trachea is depressed. Depression can be difficult in male patients with prominent trachea. Furthermore, the use of the non-articulating Harmonic® curved shears makes some areas of the deep and narrow working spaces inaccessible.

Although these limitations must be acknowledged, mechanical technology often evolves rapidly, and these limitations may soon be overcome. It seems likely that robotic instruments will become smaller and multifunctional in the near future, permitting precise and delicate procedures to be performed. Also on the horizon is the possibility of image-guided surgery, such as fusion of preoperative imaging techniques with the high-definition, three-dimensional images of the surgical field. For thyroid surgery, these techniques may permit surgeons to preserve important structures like the RLN and parathyroid glands with confidence and ease.

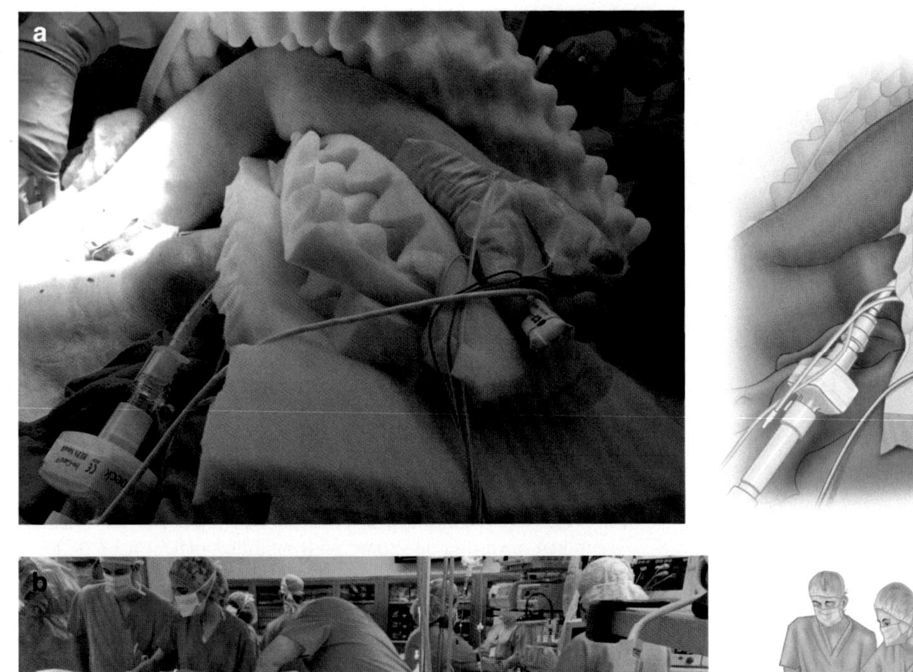

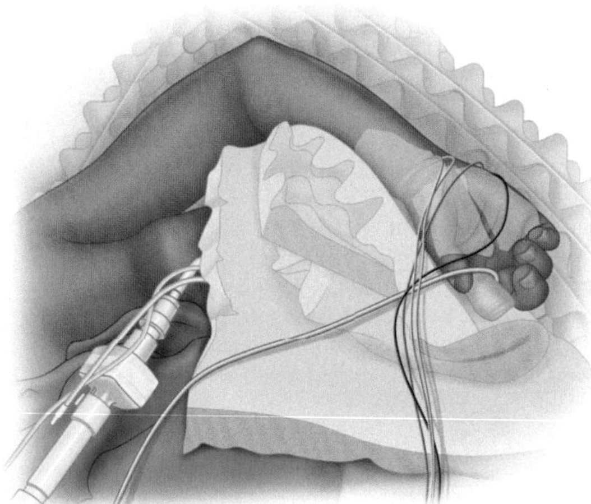

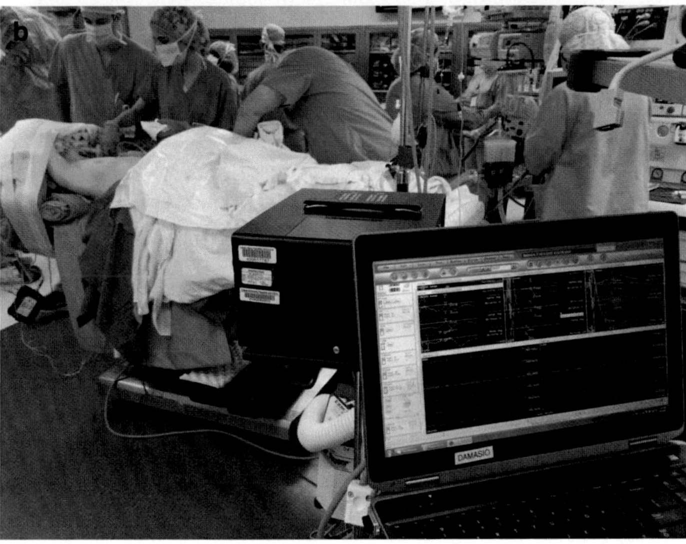

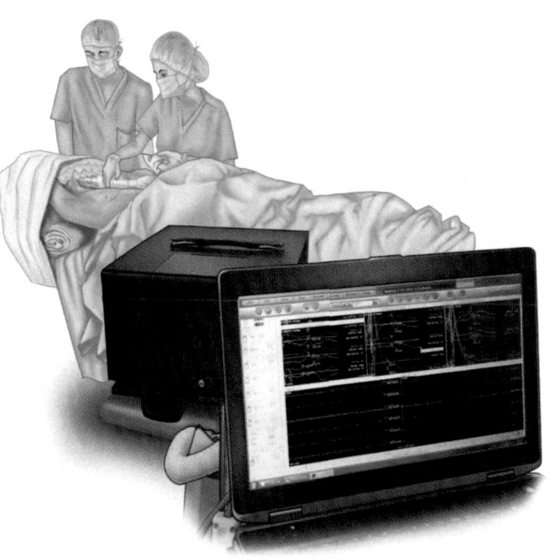

Fig. 41.15 (**a** and **b**) Real-time monitoring of median and ulnar nerves using somatosensory evoked potentials (SSEP) (Biotronic; Ann Arbor, MI, USA)

Conclusion

The application of robotic technology in the treatment of thyroid disease has been shown to be postoperatively superior to the conventional open procedure and to have acceptable surgical outcomes. We hope that the information in this chapter will serve to overcome some of the major obstacles to the adoption of robotic thyroidectomy in Western medicine.

The robotics instruments currently in use were not originally designed for thyroidectomies, and some are unsuitable for thyroid surgery. With the advance of robotic mechanics, more stabilized procedures of robotic thyroidectomy can be developed with improved safety and surgical outcome.

References

1. Rencuzogullari A, Gorgun E. Robotic rectal surgery. J Surg Oncol. 2015;112:326–31.
2. O'Malley DM, Smith B, Fowler JM. The role of robotic surgery in endometrial cancer. J Surg Oncol. 2015;112(7):761–8. https://doi.org/10.1002/jso.23988.
3. Ramirez D, Zargar H, Caputo P, Kaouk JH. Robotic-assisted laparoscopic prostatectomy: an update on functional and oncologic outcomes, techniques, and advancements in technology. J Surg Oncol. 2015;112(7):746–52. https://doi.org/10.1002/jso.24040.
4. Hüscher CS, Chiodini S, Napolitano C, Recher A. Endoscopic right thyroid lobectomy. Surg Endosc. 1997;11:877.
5. Ohgami M, Ishii S, Arisawa Y, Ohmori T, Noga K, Furukawa T, Kitajima M. Scarless endoscopic thyroidectomy: breast approach for better cosmesis. Surg Laparosc Endosc Percutan Tech. 2000;10:1–4.

6. Miccoli P, Berti P, Raffaelli M, Conte M, Materazzi G, Galleri D. Minimally invasive video-assisted thyroidectomy. Am J Surg. 2001;181:567–70.
7. Inabnet WB 3rd, Jacob BP, Gagner M. Minimally invasive endoscopic thyroidectomy by a cervical approach. Surg Endosc. 2003;17(11):1808.
8. Yoon JH, Park CH, Chung WY. Gasless endoscopic thyroidectomy via an axillary approach: experience of 30 cases. Surg Laparosc Endosc Percutan Tech. 2006;16:226–31.
9. Kang SW, Jeong JJ, Yun JS, Sung TY, Lee SC, Lee YS, et al. Robot-assisted endoscopic surgery for thyroid cancer: experience with the first 100 patients. Surg Endosc. 2009;23:2399–406.
10. Lee KE, Rao J, Youn YK. Endoscopic thyroidectomy with the da Vinci robot system using the bilateral axillary breast approach (BABA) technique; our initial experience. Surg Laparosc Endosc Percutan Tech. 2009;19:e71–5.
11. Kang SW, Lee SC, Lee SH, Lee KY, Jeong JJ, Lee YS, et al. Robotic thyroid surgery using a gasless, transaxillary approach and the da Vinci S system: the operative outcomes of 338 consecutive patients. Surgery. 2009;146:1048–55.
12. Kuppersmith RB, Salem A, Holsinger FC. Advanced approaches for thyroid surgery. Otolaryngol Head Neck Surg. 2009;141:340–2.
13. Lewis CM, Chung WY, Holsinger FC. Feasibility and surgical approach of transaxillary approach robotic thyroidectomy without CO_2 insufflation. Head Neck. 2010;32:121–6.
14. Holsinger FC, Sweeney AD, Jantharapattana K, Salem A, Weber RS, Chung WY, et al. The emergence of endoscopic head and neck surgery. Curr Oncol Rep. 2010;12:216–22.
15. Landry CS, Grubbs EG, Morris GS, Turner NS, Holsinger FC, Lee JE, Perrier ND. Robot assisted transaxillary surgery (RATS) for the removal of thyroid and parathyroid glands. Surgery. 2011;149:549–55.
16. Lee J, Chung WY. Robotic surgery for thyroid disease. Eur Thyroid J. 2013;2:93–101.
17. Kang SW, Lee SH, Ryu HR, Lee KY, Jeong JJ, Nam KH, et al. Initial experiences of robot-assisted modified radical neck dissection for the management of thyroid carcinoma with lateral neck node metastasis. Surgery. 2010;148:1214–21.
18. Lee J, Chung WY. Robotic thyroidectomy and neck dissection: past, present, and future. Cancer J. 2013;19:151–61.
19. Lee J, Kwon IS, Bae EH, Chung WY. Comparative analysis of oncological outcomes and quality of life after robotic versus conventional open thyroidectomy with modified radical neck dissection in patients with papillary thyroid carcinoma and lateral neck node metastases. J Clin Endocrinol Metab. 2013;98:2701–8.

Thyroidectomy: Robotic Facelift Approach

42

Jonathan H. Dell, William S. Duke, and David J. Terris

Robotic technology has led to advances in many surgical fields and has recently been utilized to perform remote access thyroid surgery. This allows for personalized thyroid surgery in which the operation can be performed without a visible anterior neck scar. The robotic facelift thyroidectomy (RFT), which hides the incision in the postauricular region, is especially tailored for North American patients and has been increasingly adopted in many practices that perform robotic thyroid surgery. Proper exposure and pocket development are critical for successful robotic facelift thyroidectomy. A flap is dissected from the posterior auricular incision site to the clavicle. The sternocleidomastoid muscle is retracted, and the omohyoid and strap muscles are elevated to reveal the superior pole of the thyroid. The robot is docked with the patient. The superior vascular pedicle is ligated, and the superior parathyroid gland is identified and saved. The recurrent laryngeal nerve is then identified and preserved. With the recurrent laryngeal nerve in view, the remaining attachments and blood supply to the thyroid lobe are transected, the inferior parathyroid gland is dissected inferolaterally, and the lobe is removed. Unlike other remote access approaches, patients undergoing RFT are discharged on the day of surgery without a drain [1, 2].

J. H. Dell, DO
Department of Otolaryngology-Head and Neck Surgery, Augusta University, Augusta, GA, USA

W. S. Duke, MD (✉)
Department of Otolaryngology, MultiCare Health System, Tacoma, WA, USA

D. J. Terris, MD
Department of Otolaryngology-Head and Neck Surgery, Augusta University Thyroid and Parathyroid Center, Augusta University, Augusta, GA, USA

Introduction

Recent advances in technology have allowed safe thyroid surgery to be performed through increasingly smaller incisions [3]. While the basic tenets of the operation have not changed, incision lengths have decreased from 10 to 12 cm to as little as 2 cm in some minimally invasive approaches. This scar, however, remains conspicuous on the visible portion of the anterior neck. For some patients and in some cultures [4], this can be a significant burden, and the desire to further improve the cosmetic outcomes of thyroid surgery has been the driving force behind the development of remote access thyroidectomy techniques. Remote access techniques initially utilized incisions placed in the chest wall or axilla [5–8]. A more recent development, the remote access robotic facelift thyroidectomy (RFT) approach, utilizes an incision that is concealed behind the occipital hairline. This approach requires less dissection than the axillary techniques [1] and involves anatomy that is familiar to head and neck surgeons.

Anatomy

Surgeons performing RFT should be familiar with the cervical anatomy from the postauricular sulcus to the thyroid bed. An incision is made behind the ear and carried into the occipital hairline. A soft-tissue flap is developed deep to the platysma and carried down along the sternocleidomastoid muscle (SCM) to the clavicle. The first major landmark encountered during this dissection is the great auricular nerve (GAN). Its anterior extent is usually identified 4 cm inferior to the apex of the incision, while its posterior extent is 8 cm inferior to that landmark [9]. The nerve is preserved along the anterolateral aspect of the SCM. The next structure encountered is the external jugular vein. This vessel lies 2–3 cm anteromedial to the GAN and is preserved on the anterior surface of the SCM or divided if necessary [9].

Once the SCM is dissected down to the clavicle, it is retracted posterolaterally, and the omohyoid muscle is

Y. Fong et al. (eds.), *The SAGES Atlas of Robotic Surgery*, https://doi.org/10.1007/978-3-319-91045-1_42

identified deep to the SCM approximately 11 cm from the incision apex [9]. The omohyoid muscle is reflected ventrally, exposing the sternohyoid and sternothyroid muscles. The upper pole of the thyroid is immediately deep to these strap muscles and is exposed by reflecting them anteromedially.

The inferior constrictor muscle (ICM) is a crucial landmark in thyroid surgery and is located medial to the superior pole of the thyroid. The external branch of the superior laryngeal nerve is often visualized traversing the ICM. The ICM is also used to identify the recurrent laryngeal nerve (RLN) as it passes under the muscle to enter the larynx. While the superior parathyroid gland is deep to the RLN, it may appear to be anterior as a result of the ventral retraction of the thyroid.

The middle thyroid vein is found anterior to the RLN. The inferior parathyroid gland and inferior vascular pedicle are located on the inferior aspect of the thyroid gland. The ligament of Berry serves to anchor the medial aspect of the thyroid and the isthmus to the trachea.

Indications

Remote access RFT is indicated for patients who are highly motivated to avoid a visible neck scar. The purely cosmetic benefits of the procedure should be discussed with the patient, along with the need for increased dissection, longer surgical time, and transient auricular hypesthesia. The patient should also be counseled that conversion to an anterior cervical approach, although unlikely, may be necessary. The patient should be relatively healthy (American Society of Anesthesiologists class 1 or 2) and have had no prior neck surgery or radiation and no history of thyroiditis.

The disease should ideally be unilateral, although a staged bilateral RFT can be performed on selected candidates. The dominant nodule should be smaller than 4 cm with no concern for extrathyroidal spread or substernal extension. There should also be no suspicious lymphadenopathy (Table 42.1) [10].

Patient Marking

Successful completion of the surgery begins in the preoperative holding area. While conversion to an anterior approach is unlikely, a low anterior cervical incision is still marked in a natural skin crease with the patient seated upright. The facelift incision is then drawn starting near the inferior aspect of the earlobe just adjacent to the postauricular crease. This line is carried superiorly along the crease and gently curved posteriorly into the occipital hairline about 1 cm within the edge of the hairline (Fig. 42.1). This ensures that the scar will be concealed once the hair has regrown. The incision parallels the natural hairline for about 6 cm.

Table 42.1 Selection criteria for robotic facelift thyroidectomy

Robotic facelift thyroidectomy selection criteria	
Patient factors	Disease factors
• Highly motivated to avoid cervical scar • American Society of Anesthesiologists class 1 or 2 • No prior neck surgery or radiation • Body mass index <40	• Extent of disease appropriate for unilateral surgery • Largest nodule ≤4 cm • No thyroiditis • No substernal extension • No extrathyroidal extension • No pathologic lymphadenopathy

(*Adapted from* Terris et al. [10]; with permission)

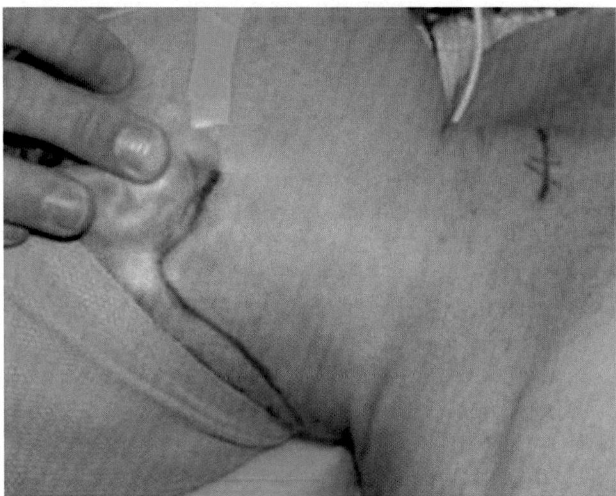

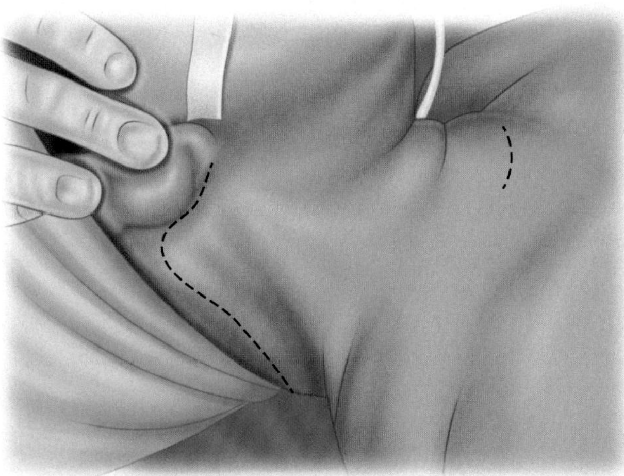

Fig. 42.1 The RFT incision begins in the postauricular crease and crosses over to the occipital hairline concealed behind the ear. The incision is placed approximately 1 cm within the hairline to ensure that it is invisible (*Reprinted with permission from* Terris et al. [10])

Equipment

Open Dissection

- No. 15 blade
- Double-pronged skin hooks (two)
- Terris malleable nerve suction (Integra, York, PA)
- Electrosurgical handpiece with extension and Teflon-tipped guarded blade
- Terris thyroid retractors (two) (Integra, York, PA)
- Medium malleable retractor
- Renal vein retractor
- Long DeBakey forceps
- 2–0 Silk suture (Ethicon, Somerville, NJ)

Robotic Dissection

- Da Vinci Si® Surgical robotic system (Intuitive Surgical Inc., Sunnyvale, CA) with the following three arms:
  - Camera arm with 30° down endoscope
  - Harmonic® device (Ethicon Endosurgery Inc., Cincinnati, OH)
  - Maryland grasper
- Terris long malleable suction (Integra, York, PA)
- Modified Chung retractor and fixed retractor system (Marina Medical, Sunrise, FL)
- Singer hook (Integra, York, PA) with adjustable Greenberg retractor arm (Codman & Shurtleff Inc., Raynham, MA)

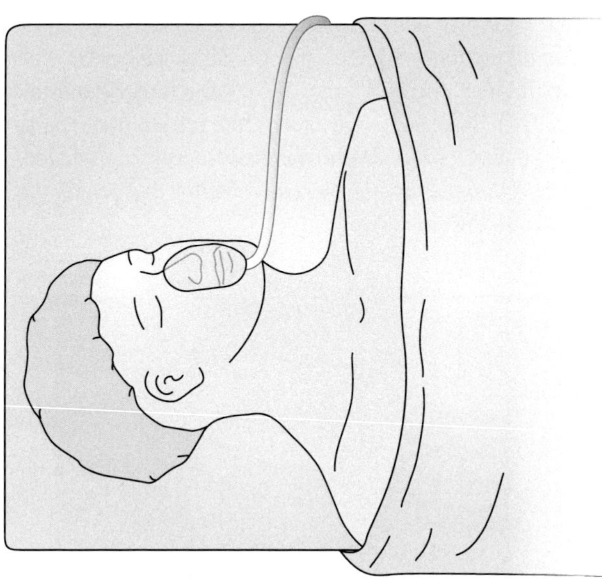

Fig. 42.2 Patient position on table (*Redrawn with permission from* White et al. [11])

Position

The patient is placed supine and slightly off-center toward the side to be operated on. The head is rotated 20–30° away from the side of surgery and supported with a soft towel to prevent over-rotation (Fig. 42.2). The arms are tucked on both sides. The bed is rotated 180° from the anesthesia with the anesthesia circuit taped to the operative table in a manner that avoids tension. This avoids rotation or migration of the laryngeal electromyographic tube.

Operative Steps

Muscle Flap

The marked incision site is infiltrated with 0.25% bupivacaine and 1:200,000 epinephrine. The area is prepped and draped in sterile fashion. The incision is made with a number 15 blade, and electrocautery is then used to elevate a subplatysmal flap (Table 42.2). The patient is placed in the reverse Trendelenburg position and rotated away from the surgeon to improve the angle of approach. The SCM is identified and

Table 42.2 Operative steps and important landmarks

1. Open dissection (a) A modified facelift incision is made (b) A subplatysmal musculocutaneous flap is raised (c) The SCM is skeletonized. The external jugular vein and GAN are identified (d) The muscular triangle defined by the omohyoid, sternohyoid, and SCM is identified (e) The thyroid gland is exposed by ventral reflection of the omohyoid muscle and anterior and medial reflections of the sternohyoid and sternothyroid muscles (f) The modified Chung retractor and Singer hook retractor are positioned to maintain operative working space
2. Robotic deployment (a) The robotic pedestal is angled approximately 30° from the operating table (b) A 30° down endoscope is positioned in the center arm, a Maryland grasper is positioned in the nondominant instrument arm, and a harmonic shears device is positioned in the dominant instrument arm
3. Robotic dissection (a) The superior vascular pedicle is divided, and the superior thyroid pole mobilized. The external branch of the superior laryngeal nerve is preserved (b) The superior parathyroid gland is identified and preserved (c) The recurrent laryngeal nerve is identified proximal to its entrance into the larynx as it passes underneath the inferior constrictor muscle and is dissected inferiorly to expose the ligament of Berry (d) The ligament of Berry is divided with the recurrent laryngeal nerve under visualization (e) The isthmus is transected (f) The middle thyroid vein is identified and divided (g) The inferior parathyroid gland is identified and preserved (h) The remaining tissue attachments between the thyroid gland and anterior trachea are divided
4. Closure (a) The robot is undocked and the fixed retractors are removed (b) The subcutaneous tissues and superficial skin layer are closed

followed anteriorly and inferiorly until the GAN is identified. The dissection continues superficial to the nerve. The external jugular vein is the next structure identified (Fig. 42.3). It is usually preserved and reflected dorsally, although it may be divided to facilitate access as needed. Dissection continues along the anteromedial border of the SCM down to the clavicle.

Muscular Triangle

The SCM is retracted laterally, and the omohyoid muscle is identified. The muscular triangle bounded by the anterior border of the SCM, the superior border of the omohyoid muscle, and the posterior border of the sternohyoid muscle is then defined (Fig. 42.4).

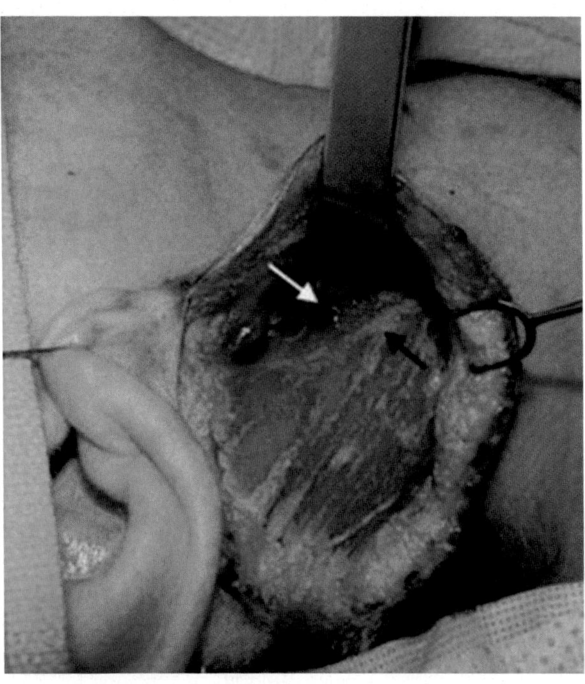

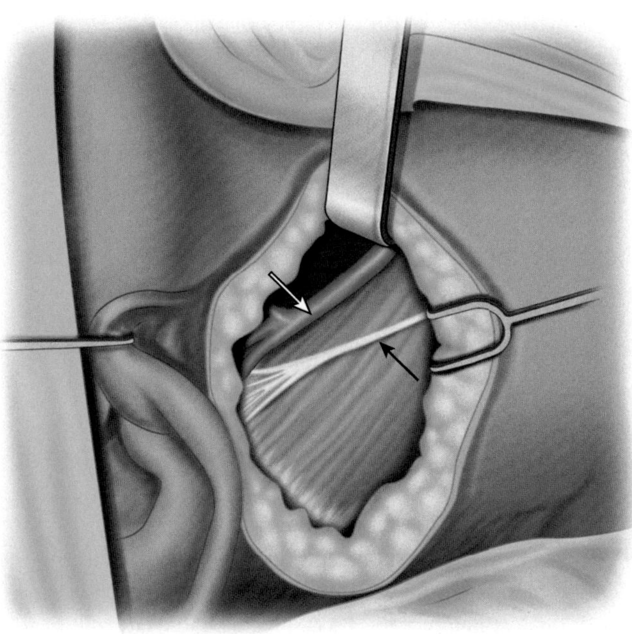

Fig. 42.3 The great auricular nerve (*black arrow*) and external jugular vein (*white arrow*) are identified and preserved on the surface of the SCM (*Reprinted with permission from* Duke et al. [12])

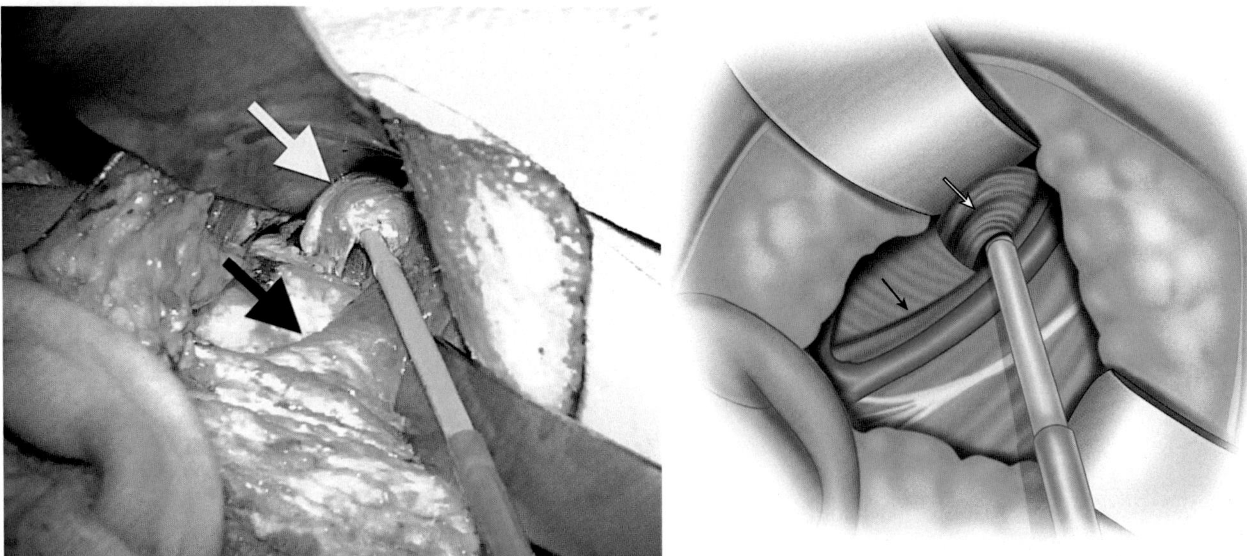

Fig. 42.4 The muscular triangle bordered by the anterior surface of the SCM (black arrow), the superior border of the omohyoid muscle (white arrow), and the posterior border of the sternohyoid muscle (*Reprinted with permission from* Duke et al. [12])

Exposing Superior Pole

The omohyoid, sternohyoid, and sternothyroid muscles are then retracted anteriorly, exposing the superior pole of the thyroid gland (Fig. 42.5). Careful and thorough open dissection helps facilitate the robotic dissection.

Retractor Placement

The modified Chung retractor is placed under the omohyoid and other strap muscles and retracted ventrally. The retractor system is then anchored to the frame of the operating table on the contralateral side. A Singer hook is placed on the SCM and used to retract it laterally and dorsally (Fig. 42.6). It is secured to the ipsilateral frame of the bed.

Robot Deployment

One critical aspect of the procedure is correctly positioning and docking the robotic console with the patient, which ensures that the instruments and camera have maximum maneuverability. The robotic console is placed near the top

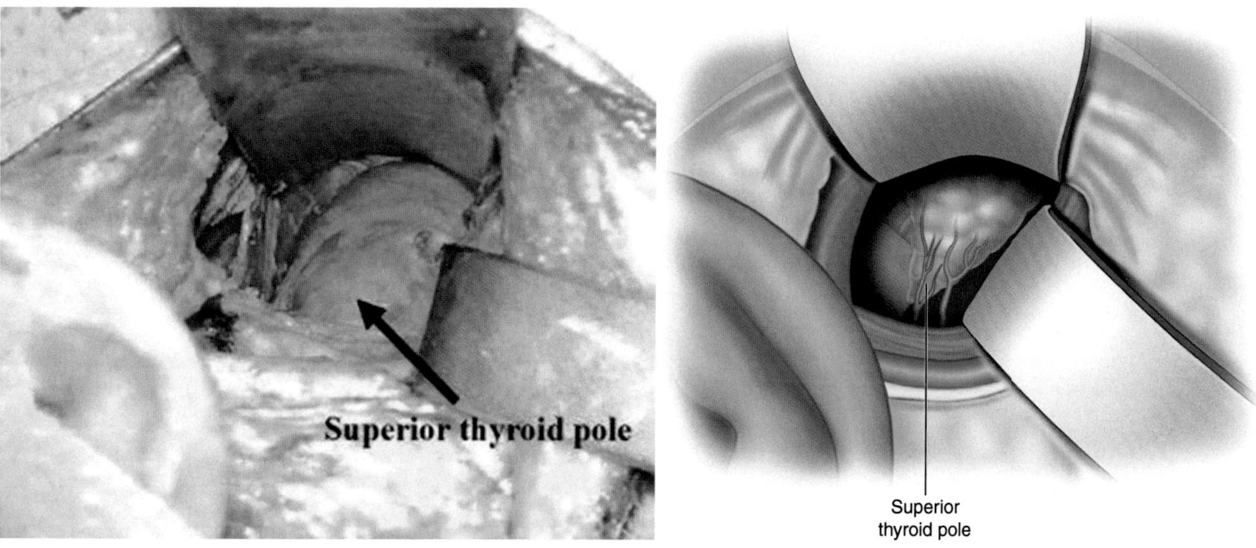

Fig. 42.5 The strap muscles are retracted ventrally, exposing the superior pole of the thyroid gland (*arrow*) (*Reprinted with permission from* Terris et al. [1])

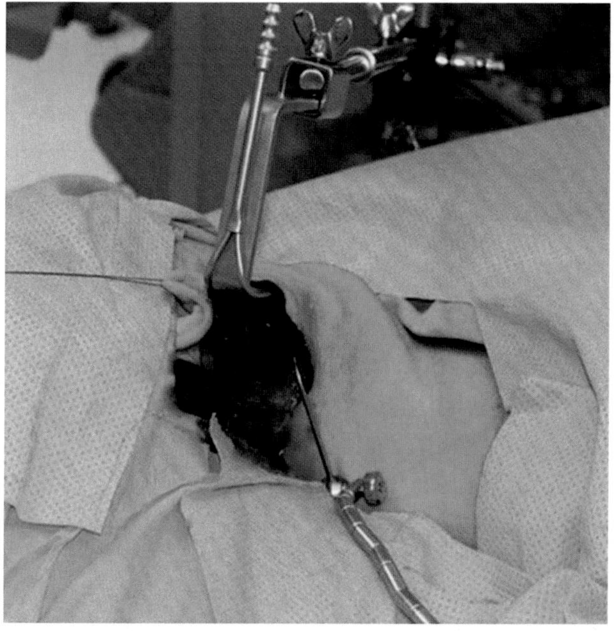

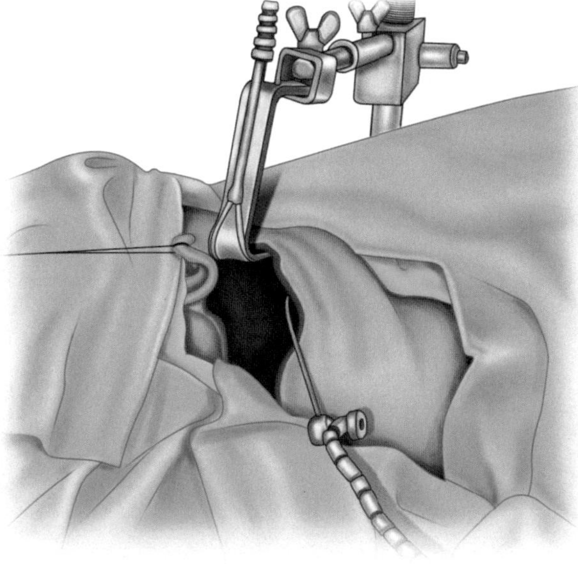

Fig. 42.6 The operative pocket with retractors in place (*Redrawn with permission from* Duke et al. [13])

of the bed opposite the side of dissection. The pedestal is angled 30° away from the table.

The camera arm is placed first. The 30° scope is faced downward and advanced just beneath and parallel to the long axis of the Chung retractor. The camera arm should be almost fully extended so that the elbow joints of the arm do not interfere with the movement of the two instrument arms. A Harmonic shears device is placed in the dominant arm, and a Maryland grasper is placed in the nondominant arm (Figs. 42.7 and 42.8). The instruments are positioned so that they will not collide or cross one another during the operation.

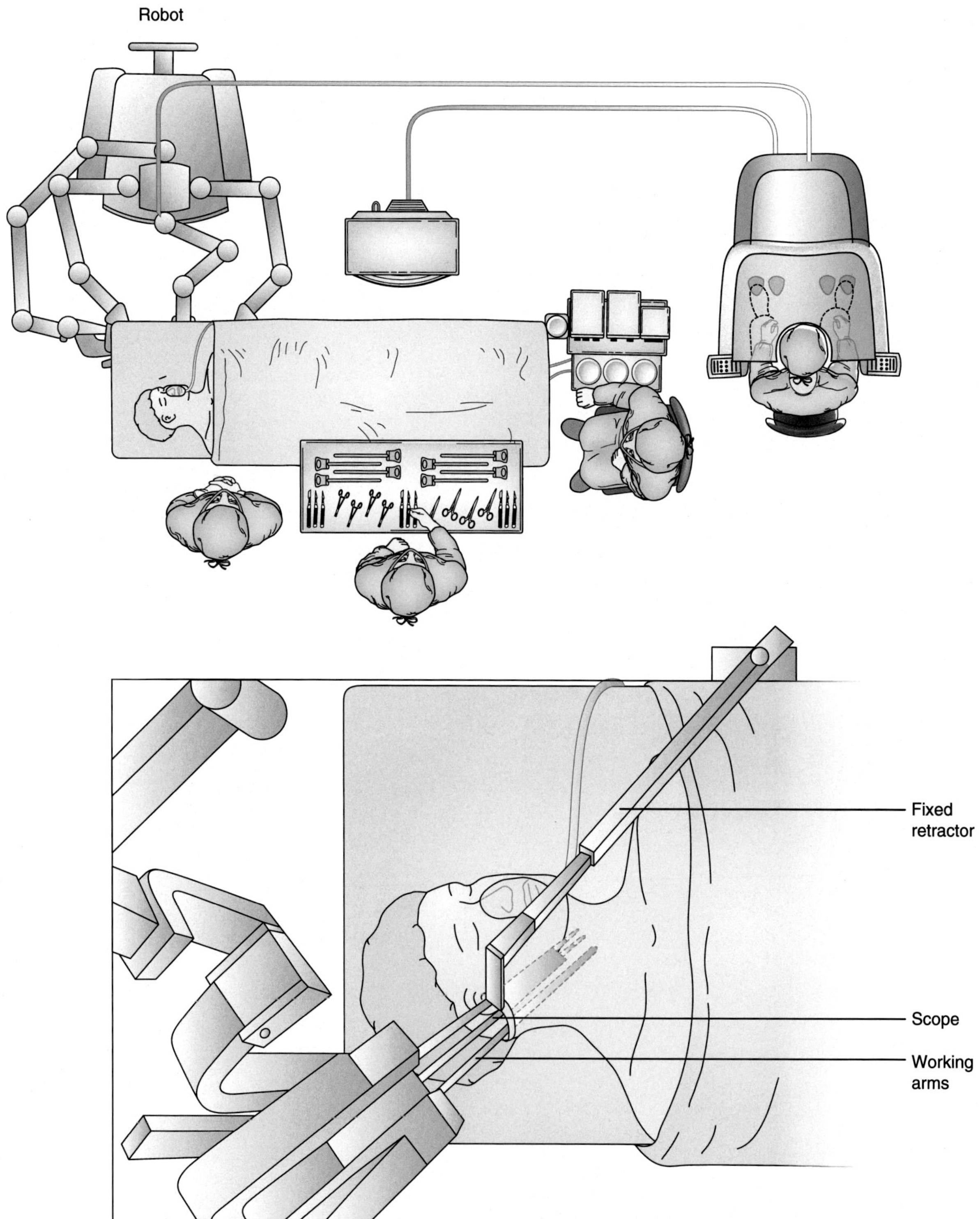

Fig. 42.7 The robotic cart in position. A Harmonic device is placed in the dominant arm (Arm 1), and a Maryland forceps is placed in the nondominant arm (Arm 2) (*Redrawn with permission from* White et al. [11])

Superior Pole Division

Sequential identification and dissection of a number of landmarks facilitate safe and effective robotic dissection of the thyroid gland. The first of these structures is the superior vascular pedicle (Fig. 42.9). It is isolated and then transected using the Harmonic device.

The superior pole is then retracted inferiorly and ventrally, exposing the inferior constrictor muscle (Fig. 42.10). This muscle is followed until its lower border is identified. The SLN travels along the surface of this muscle, and care should be taken to preserve it. The superior parathyroid gland is identified along the posterior aspect of the thyroid. It is reflected posteriorly and superiorly.

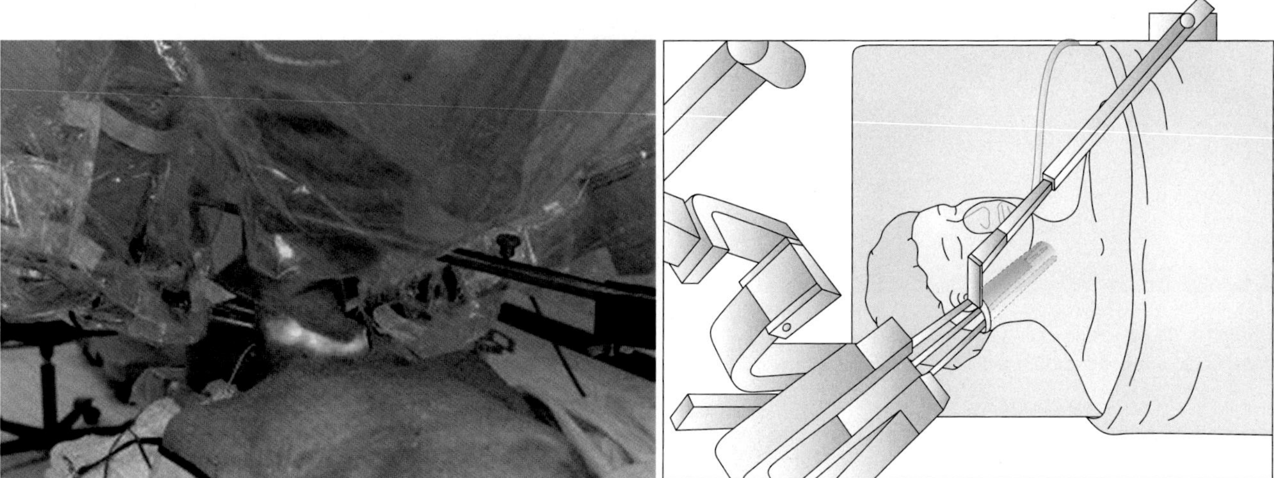

Fig. 42.8 The robotic cart in position. A Harmonic device is placed in the dominant arm (Arm 1), and a Maryland forceps is placed in the non-dominant arm (Arm 2). A second vantage point (*Reprinted with permission from* Singer et al. [2])

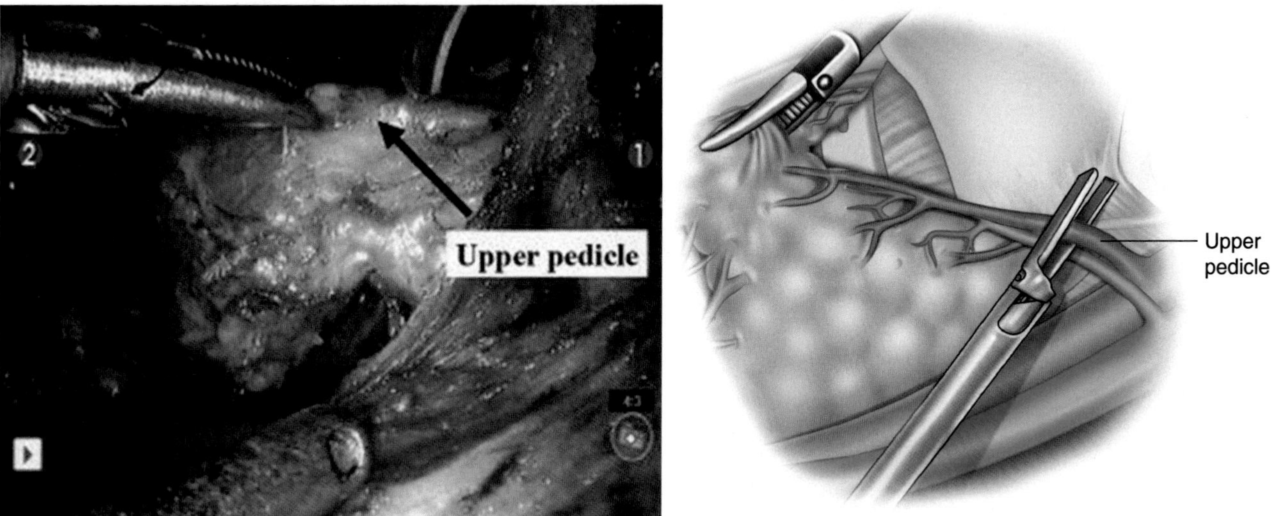

Fig. 42.9 Upper pedicle is identified (*Reprinted with permission from* Terris et al. [1])

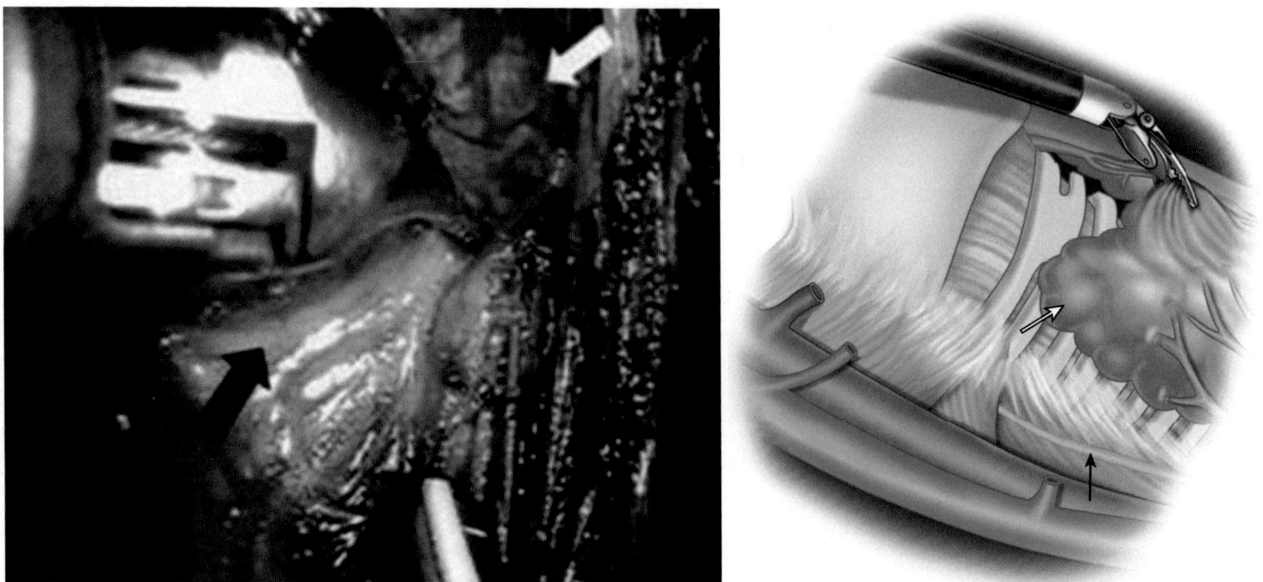

Fig. 42.10 The thyroid (*white arrow*) is retracted ventrally, and the recurrent laryngeal nerve (*black arrow*) is identified just inferior to the lower border of the inferior constrictor muscle (*Reprinted with permission from* Duke et al. [12])

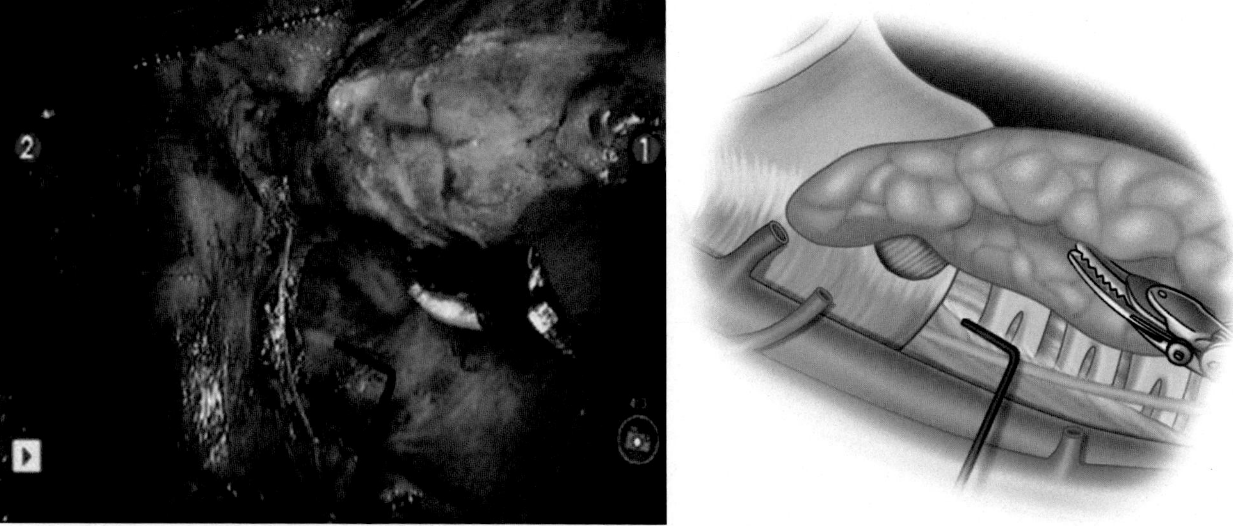

Fig. 42.11 The recurrent laryngeal nerve is identified and stimulated (*black probe*) (*Reprinted with permission from* Terris et al. [1])

The Recurrent Laryngeal Nerve Is Identified

The RLN is identified laterally as it courses under the inferior constrictor muscle (Fig. 42.11). The nerve is followed inferiorly, exposing the ligament of Berry. While visualizing the RLN, the ligament of Berry can safely be divided with the Harmonic device. The isthmus is transected. The middle thyroid vein is identified and divided using the Harmonic device.

The inferior parathyroid gland is identified and dissected inferiorly away from the thyroid. The inferior vascular pedicle can then be isolated and divided using the Harmonic device. The thyroid is then dissected free of any remaining attachments, and the specimen is removed.

Hemostasis is assured, and the robot is removed. The surgical site is irrigated, and Surgicel (Ethicon, Somerville, NJ) is placed in the thyroid bed. The skin edges are approximated with buried interrupted deep dermal sutures using a braided absorbable suture. The skin edges are sealed using a tissue adhesive, and quarter-inch Steri-Strips (3 M, St Paul, MN) are placed horizontally along the incision.

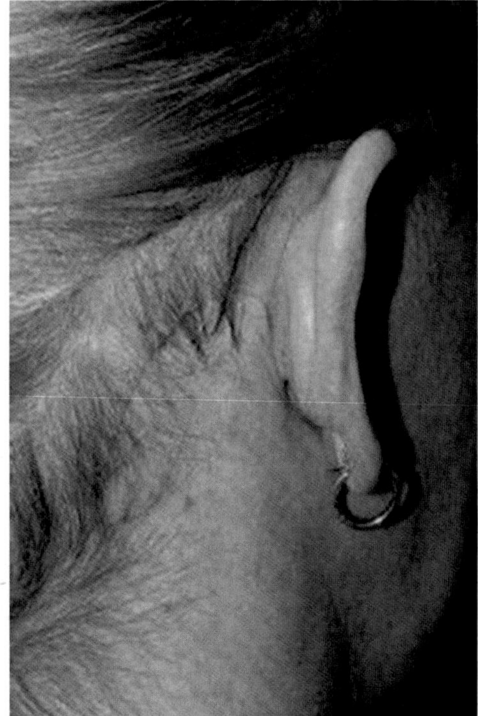
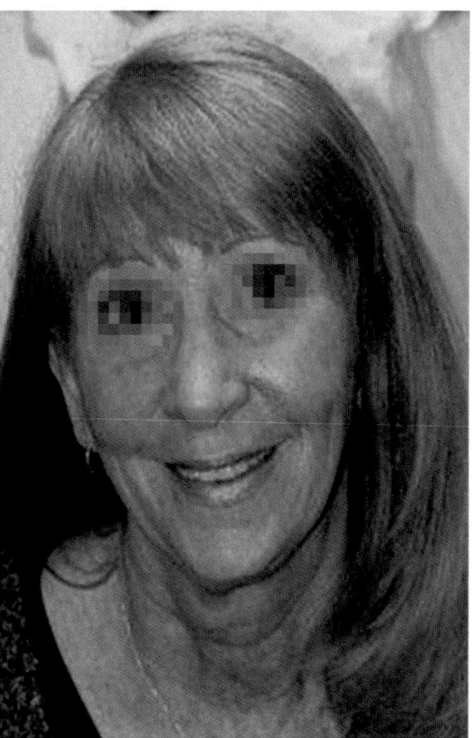

Fig. 42.12 Postoperative photographs showing no anterior cervical scar and concealed postauricular scar (*Reprinted with permission from* Terris et al. [1])

Postoperative Management

Patients are extubated while still deep under anesthesia to decrease the likelihood of bucking and coughing and subsequent hematoma formation. They are then transported to the postanesthesia care unit and discharged from the hospital 1 or 2 h later. Patients return to the office 4–6 weeks after surgery for evaluation of healing (Fig. 42.12).

Complications and Their Management

Potential complications such as hypoparathyroidism and injury to the RLN or SLN are inherent in any thyroid surgery. They are mainly prevented by meticulous dissection and identification and preservation of the nerves and parathyroid glands. An additional complication that is specific to RFT is auricular hypoesthesia. Patients should be counseled to expect up to a year of decreased auricular sensation.

Patient expectations should be appropriately tempered preoperatively, making sure to emphasize that RFT is not minimally invasive surgery. Although postoperative pain and swelling are not unique to robotic surgery, the larger extent of dissection does lead to the potential for increased pain and swelling when compared to minimally invasive approaches. This increased dissection also leads to potential seroma formation. Unless the seroma is symptomatic, we recommend conservative management to decrease the risk of introducing bacteria and precipitating a postoperative infection.

References

1. Terris DJ, Singer MC, Seybt MW. Robot facelift thyroidectomy: II. Clinical feasibility and safety. Laryngoscope. 2011;121:1636–41.
2. Singer MC, Seybt MW, Terris DJ. Robot facelift thyroidectomy: I. Preclinical simulation and morphometric assessment. Laryngoscope. 2011;121:1631–5.
3. Miccoli P, Berti P, Conte M, Bendinelli C, Marcocci C. Minimally invasive surgery for thyroid small nodules: preliminary report. J Endocrinol Investig. 1999;22:849–51.
4. McCurdy J. Considerations in Asian cosmetic surgery. Facial Plast Surg Clin North Am. 2007;15:387–97.
5. Choe JH, Kim SW, Chung KW, Park KS, Han W, Noh DY, et al. Endoscopic thyroidectomy using a new bilateral axillo-breast approach. World J Surg. 2007;31:601–6.

6. Ikeda Y, Takami H, Niimi M, Kan S, Sasaki Y, Takayama J. Endoscopic thyroidectomy by the axillary approach. Surg Endosc. 2001;15:1362–4.
7. Ohgami M, Ishii S, Arisawa Y, Ohmori T, Noga K, Furukawa T, Kitajima M. Scarless endoscopic thyroidectomy: breast approach for better cosmesis. Surg Laparosc Endosc Percutan Tech. 2000;10:1–4.
8. Shimazu K, Shiba E, Tamaki Y, Takiguchi S, Taniguchi E, Ohashi S, Noguchi S. Endoscopic thyroid surgery through the axillo-bilateral-breast approach. Surg Laparosc Endosc Percutan Tech. 2003;13:196–201.
9. Singer MC, Heffernan A, Terris DJ. Defining anatomical landmarks for robotic facelift thyroidectomy. World J Surg. 2014;38:92–5.
10. Terris D, Singer MC, Seybt MW. Robotic facelift thyroidectomy: patient selection and technical considerations. Surg Laparosc Endosc Percutan Tech. 2011;21:237–42.
11. White LC, Terris DJ. Robotic facelift thyroidectomy. Oper Techn Otolaryngol. 2013;24:120–5.
12. Duke WS, Terris DJ. Robotic thyroidectomy: facelift approach. Curr Surg Rep. 2014;2:36.
13. Duke WS, Terris DJ. Robotic thyroidectomy: facelift approach. Int J Endocr Oncol. 2014;1:217–23.

Transaxillary Robotic Modified Radical Neck Dissection

43

Eun Jeong Ban and Woong Youn Chung

Conventional neck dissection requires a long anterior neck incision and leaves a prominent scar on the neck that can be of great concern to patients (particularly young women) with early thyroid cancer and limited metastasis to one or two lateral neck lymph nodes. Remote-access endoscopic surgery of the thyroid gland has offered the opportunity to reduce the patients' burden from these surgical scars on the neck [1–3]. In 2007, we successfully performed the first robotic thyroidectomy using a gasless transaxillary approach [4]. The shift toward robotic thyroid surgery has reformed the surgical approach for thyroid disease [5–7]. With the improved ergonomics and shortened learning curve for the new robotic thyroid surgery technique, the field of head and neck surgery has witnessed a revolution in the surgical management of thyroid cancer beyond conventional transaxillary endoscopic thyroid surgery [8, 9]. Moreover, robotic neck dissection has been reported to be a safe and meticulous technique in low-risk patients who have well-differentiated thyroid cancer with lateral neck metastasis and could be an alternative operative method. The transaxillary approach for neck dissection uses a route from the axilla to the anterior neck region; thus, slightly wider flap dissection during robotic thyroid surgery offers a comprehensive operative view and working space for node dissection [10–12]. This chapter describes the latest overview in transaxillary robotic modified radical neck dissection (MRND) techniques for thyroid cancer with limited lateral neck lymph node metastasis.

Robotic surgery is designed to overcome the drawbacks of conventional open and endoscopic thyroid surgery techniques. For patients, robotic thyroid surgery offers potentially significant quality-of-life benefits, including excellent cosmetic outcomes, reductions in pain and discomfort, improvements in sensory changes, and decreases in postoperative voice changes and swallowing discomfort [13, 14]. For surgeons, the robotic technique provides a shorter operation time and a shorter learning curve than conventional endoscopic thyroidectomy and also causes less musculoskeletal discomfort than open or endoscopic thyroidectomy [15, 16]. These advantages of robotic surgery may be due to superior vision, a stable camera platform, flexible instruments, and fine coordination of robotic hands, resulting in excellent manipulations. Although robotic thyroid surgery has excellent cosmetic benefits and several other benefits, it remains a widely invasive technique compared with the conventional open procedure, but in terms of neck dissection (ND), although conventional open ND is the safest and most efficient technique, extensive surgical dissection and a long incision scar on the anterior neck are inevitable, so the application of robotic techniques to ND has been facilitated. Recent studies have shown that, compared with the conventional open technique, robotic ND is similarly safe, oncologically effective, and completely capable of compartment-oriented dissection [10–12]. This chapter describes the details of transaxillary robotic MRND techniques for thyroid cancer with involvement of lateral neck lymph nodes (LNs).

Preoperative Workup for Robotic Neck Dissection

Preoperative Diagnosis

Patients with clinically lateral neck nodes with a suspicious ultrasound appearance by preoperative staging ultrasonography should undergo fine-needle aspiration (FNA) biopsy. The presence of lateral neck LN metastasis was predicted preoperatively based on histologic examinations of ultrasonography-guided FNA biopsy or on thyroglobulin (Tg) levels of FNA biopsy washout fluid (FNA-Tg >10 ng/mL, > mean + 2 SD of FNA-Tg measured in node-negative patients, or >serum-Tg) from lateral neck LNs [17].

E. J. Ban, MD · W. Y. Chung, MD, PhD (✉)
Department of Surgery, Yonsei University College of Medicine, Seoul, South Korea
e-mail: woungyounc@yuhs.ac

Y. Fong et al. (eds.), *The SAGES Atlas of Robotic Surgery*, https://doi.org/10.1007/978-3-319-91045-1_43

Extent of Neck Dissection

At our institution, we follow general approaches to lateral neck node dissection for thyroid cancer (MRND type III, sparing the sternocleidomastoid muscle [SCM], spinal accessory nerve [SAN], and internal jugular vein [IJV]). In terms of dissection extent, the submental, submandibular, parotid, and retroauricular nodes are rarely dissected in papillary thyroid cancer [18], and level II-B and V-A LNs are not routinely dissected [19, 20]. However, if an enlarged or suspicious node is encountered by palpation or on preoperative ultrasonography at level I or II-B, or among V-A LNs, these compartments are included in the en bloc dissection. Thus, the extents of surgical dissection for ND in well-differentiated thyroid cancer with lateral neck LN metastasis are levels II-A, III, IV, V-B, and VI, conditions that also apply to robotic and open ND procedures (Fig. 43.1).

Surgical Indications

Eligibility for robotic ND requires that the patient meet the three criteria:

- Well-differentiated thyroid carcinoma with clinical lateral neck LN metastasis (cases with one or two minimal metastatic LNs on the lateral neck).
- Primary tumor size no larger than 4 cm.
- Minimal invasion to the anterior thyroid capsule and strap muscle by the primary cancer.

Several exclusion criteria also should be applied:

- Definite tumor invasion to an adjacent organ (vagus nerve, recurrent laryngeal nerve, esophagus, IJV, common carotid artery, or trachea).
- Multiple LN metastases in multiple levels of the lateral neck or conglomerated metastatic LN.
- LN metastasis on the substernal area or area below the clavicle.
- Perinodal infiltration at a metastatic LN.

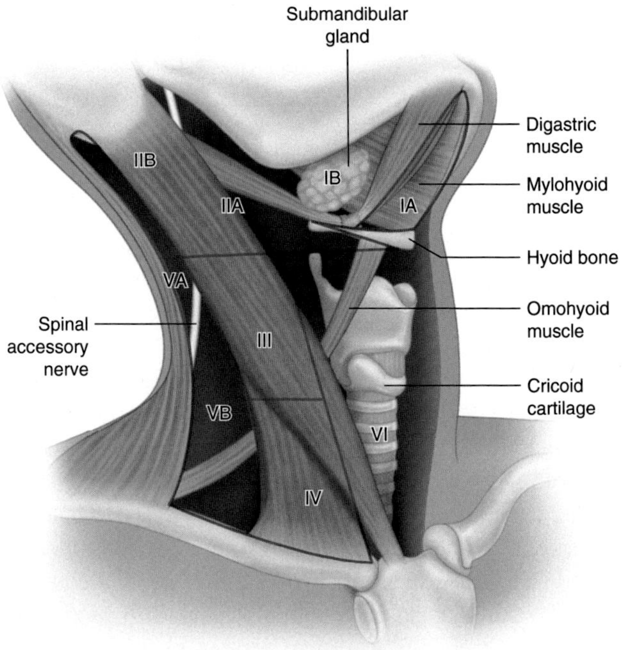

Fig. 43.1 Anatomic landmarks used to divide the lateral and central lymph node (LN) compartments among levels I through VI; the area with a deviant crease line is where LN dissection is performed during modified radical neck dissection (MRND)

Robotic Neck Dissection Procedure

Patient Position

The patient is administered general anesthesia and placed in the supine position, with mild extension of the neck with a soft pillow, and the face turned away from the lesion. The arm on the lesion side is then stretched laterally and abducted by about 80° from the body, to optimally expose the axilla and lateral neck (Fig. 43.2). The landmarks for dissection are the connecting line of the sternal notch and SCM bifurcation medially, the anterior border of the trapezius muscle laterally, and the submandibular gland superiorly.

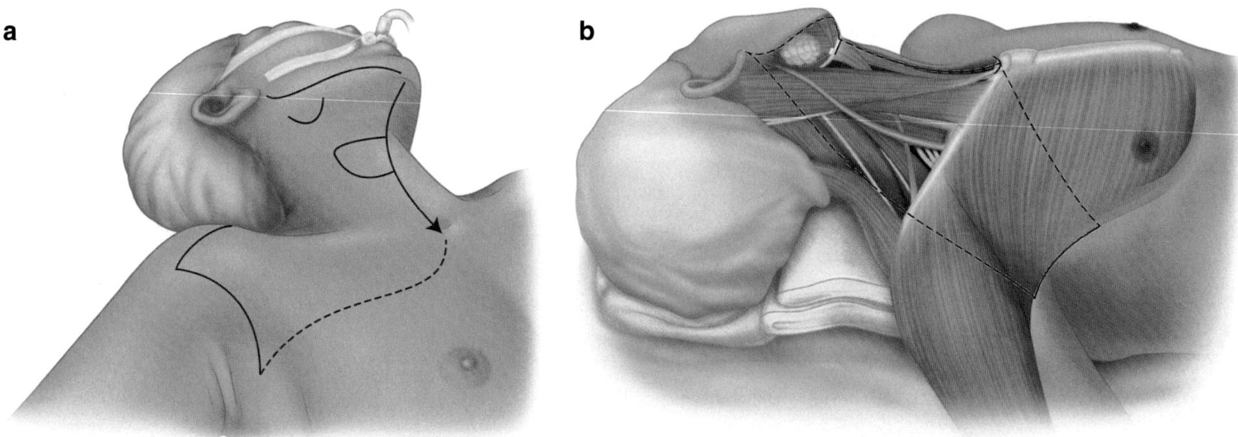

Fig. 43.2 Patient position (**a**) and superficial landmarks for flap dissection (**b**)

Development of Working Space

A 7- to 8-cm vertical incision is then made in the anterior axillary fold along the lateral border of the pectoralis major muscle, and a subcutaneous skin flap from the axilla to the anterior border of the SCM is dissected over the anterior surface of the pectoralis major muscle and clavicle by electrical cautery under direct vision. After exposing the clavicle, subplatysmal flap dissection proceeds to the upper point where the external jugular vein and great auricular nerve cross the lateral border of the SCM superiorly. The proximal external jugular vein is then clipped and divided at the crossing point of the SCM lateral border. Laterally, the flap dissection is dissected upward along its anterior border of the trapezius muscle. The SAN is then identified about 1 cm above Erb's point and exposed carefully along its course until it passes on the undersurface of the SCM muscle. To expose the level II area, the dissection is progressed along the posterior surface of the SCM until the submandibular gland and the posterior belly of the digastric muscle are exposed superiorly. Medially, the flap dissection is approached beneath the clavicular head of the SCM muscle. The clavicular head of the SCM can be transected to less than one third at the level of the clavicle-attached point, to achieve complete exposure of the junction area between the IJV and subclavian vein. Next, soft tissue and LN detachment from the posterior surface of the SCM is continued lateral to medial until the IJV and common carotid artery are exposed. The superior belly of the omohyoid muscle is divided at the level of the thyroid cartilage, the dissection is approached through the avascular space between the carotid sheath and strap muscles, and the thyroid gland is then exposed and detached from the strap muscle until the contralateral lobe is fully exposed.

The patient's face must be returned to the neutral position for bilateral total thyroidectomy after flap dissection. Afterwards, the face is once again turned away from the lesion for neck dissection. An external retractor (Chung's retractor, wide type) is used to create a working space. (The retractor's blade has suction holes that can be used to remove smoke and fumes.) The external retractor is then inserted through the axillary skin incision and located between the anterior surface of the thyroid and the strap muscles. The retractor is then used to raise and tent the skin flap at the anterior chest wall, the two heads of the SCM muscle, and the strap muscles, to create a working space (Fig. 43.3).

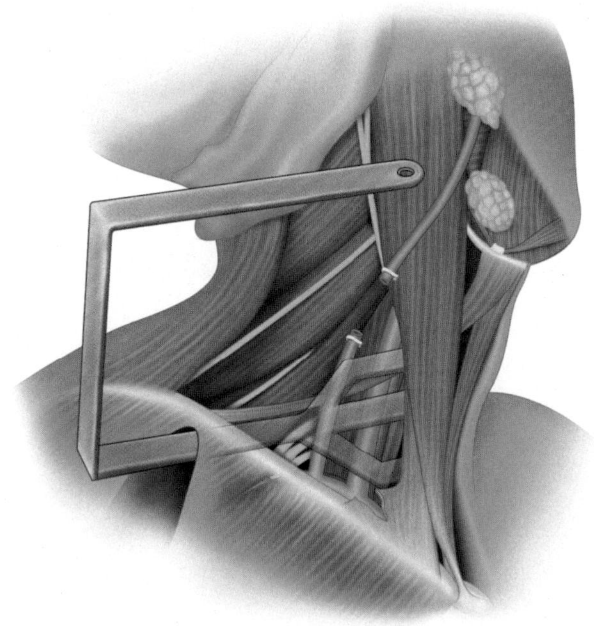

Fig. 43.3 Initial position of the external retractor for levels III, IV, and V-B dissection

Docking and Instrumentation

The robotic column is placed on the side of the patient contralateral to the main lesion, and the operative table is positioned slightly obliquely with respect to the direction of the robotic column, to allow direct alignment between the axis of the robotic camera arm and the operative approach (from the axilla to the anterior neck, which is usually also the direction of retractor blade insertion). Previously, we described a robotic ND technique that required two skin incisions—an axillary incision for access by the camera and the first and second robotic arm and an anterior chest wall incision for the third robotic arm [10, 11]. During the single-incision approach, however, the location and use of the ProGrasp™ forceps are important. The key point of the single-incision technique is that the surgeon should make proper use of the EndoWrist® of the ProGrasp™ forceps (Intuitive Surgical, Sunnyvale, CA) and minimize the movement of its external third joint to prevent collisions of the robotic arms. Four robotic arms are inserted through the axillary incision: a 30° dual-channel endoscope (Intuitive Surgical) is placed on the central camera arm through a 12-mm trocar; for the right side approach, a Harmonic® curved shears (Intuitive Surgical) is placed on the right arm of the scope through a 5-mm trocar, and a 5-mm Maryland dissector (Intuitive Surgical) is placed on the left side arm of the scope. An 8-mm trocar for the ProGrasp™ forceps is then positioned at the right of the camera, parallel to the suction tube of the retractor blade. At this point, the tip of the ProGrasp™ forceps should be positioned beneath the anterior part of the skin incision, parallel to the retractor blade. Proper introduction angles are important to prevent collisions between the robotic arms. In particular, the camera arm should be placed in the center of the axillary skin incision. This arm is inserted to face upward. (The external third joint should be placed in the lowest portion [floor] of the incision entrance, and the camera tip should be directed upward.) The Harmonic® curved shears (ultrasonic coagulator shears) and the 5-mm Maryland dissector arms should be inserted in the opposite manner to the camera arm (to face downward). Finally, the external three joints of the robotic arms should form an inverted triangle.

Robotic Modified Radical Neck Dissection Procedure

After total thyroidectomy with central compartment ND, lateral ND is initiated from the level III and IV areas around the IJV. The IJV is pulled medially using the ProGrasp™ forceps, and soft tissues and LNs are pulled laterally using a Maryland dissector and detached from the anterior surface of the IJV to the posterior aspect of the IJV until the common carotid artery and vagus nerve are identified (Fig. 43.4). The dissection is performed using a Harmonic® curved shears to allow vascular structures to be differentiated from the specimen tissues. The dissection of the IJV is progressed upward from level IV to the upper level III area.

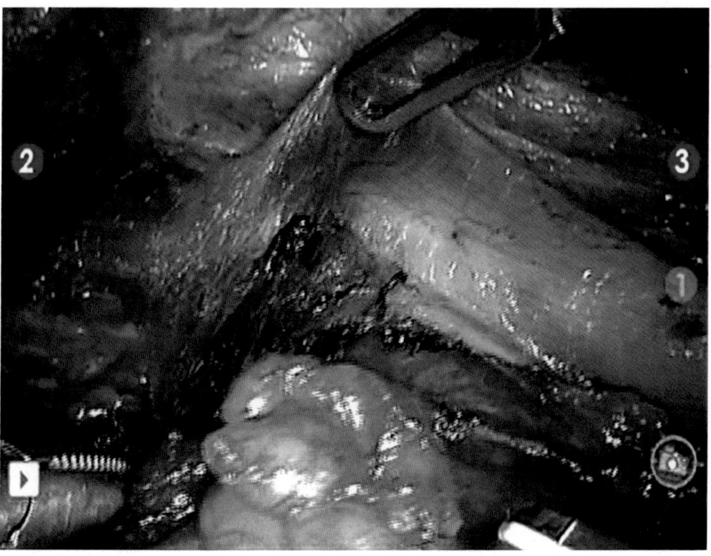

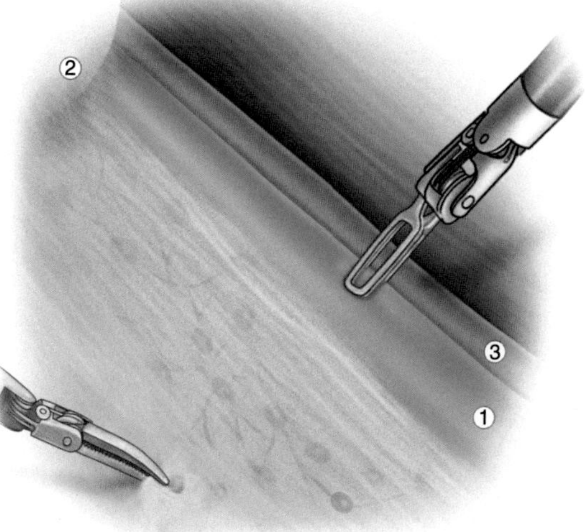

Fig. 43.4 Detachment of the soft tissues and LNs from the internal jugular vein (IJV)

At level IV, packets of LNs are then drawn superiorly using the ProGrasp™ forceps, and the LNs are meticulously detached from the junction of the IJV and the subclavian vein (Fig. 43.5). Reaching this point with a nonarticulated Harmonic® curved shears is difficult because of the clavicle. When facing such obstacles, increasing the height of the external third joint of the robotic arm while increasing its introduction angle will most likely resolve these problems. Additionally, the thoracic duct or lymphatic duct is carefully identified and divided with the Harmonic® curved shears. Further dissection is followed along the subclavian vein laterally (Fig. 43.6). The distal external jugular vein

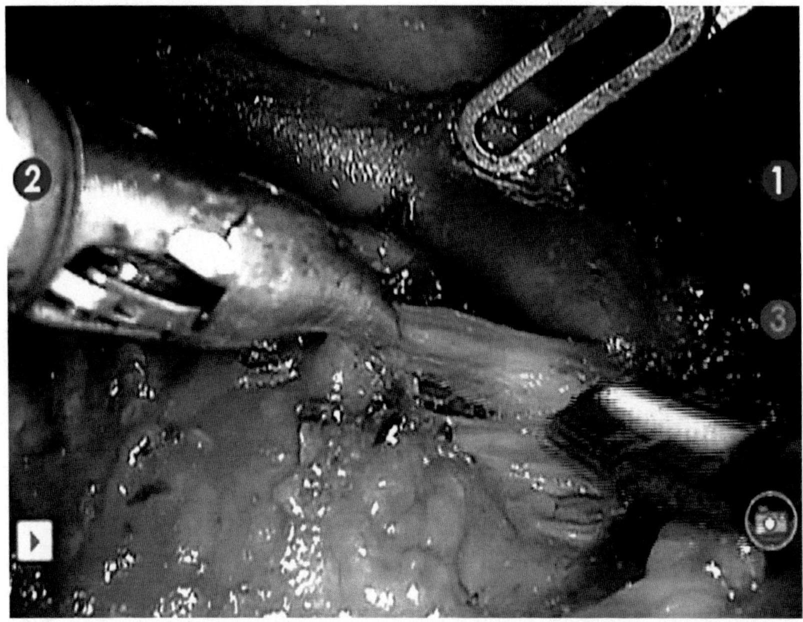

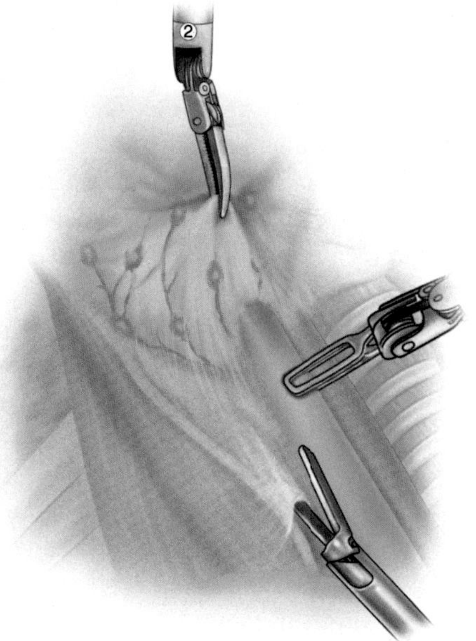

Fig. 43.5 Level IV dissection from the junction of the IJV and subclavian vein

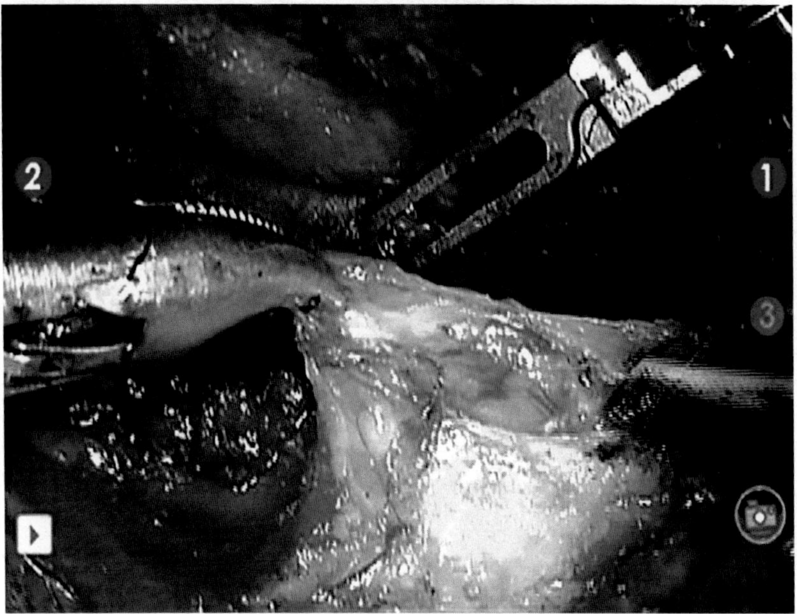

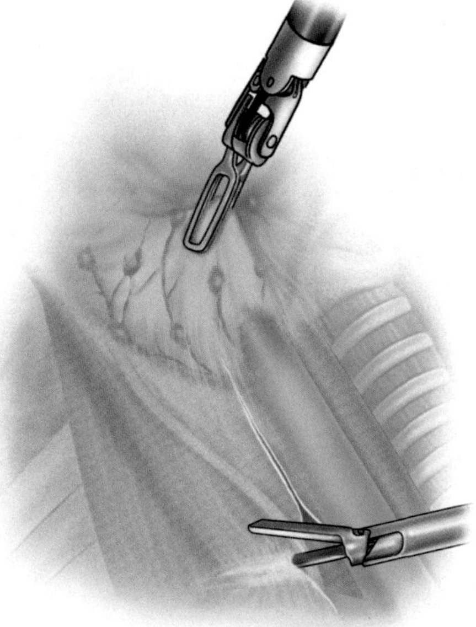

Fig. 43.6 Level IV dissection along the subclavian vein laterally on the right side

(which can join the IJV or subclavian vein) is then clipped and divided at its connection with the subclavian vein (Fig. 43.7). The inferior belly of the omohyoid muscle is cut where it meets the trapezius muscle (Fig. 43.8). In general, the transverse cervical artery (a branch of the thyrocervical trunk) courses laterally across the anterior scalene

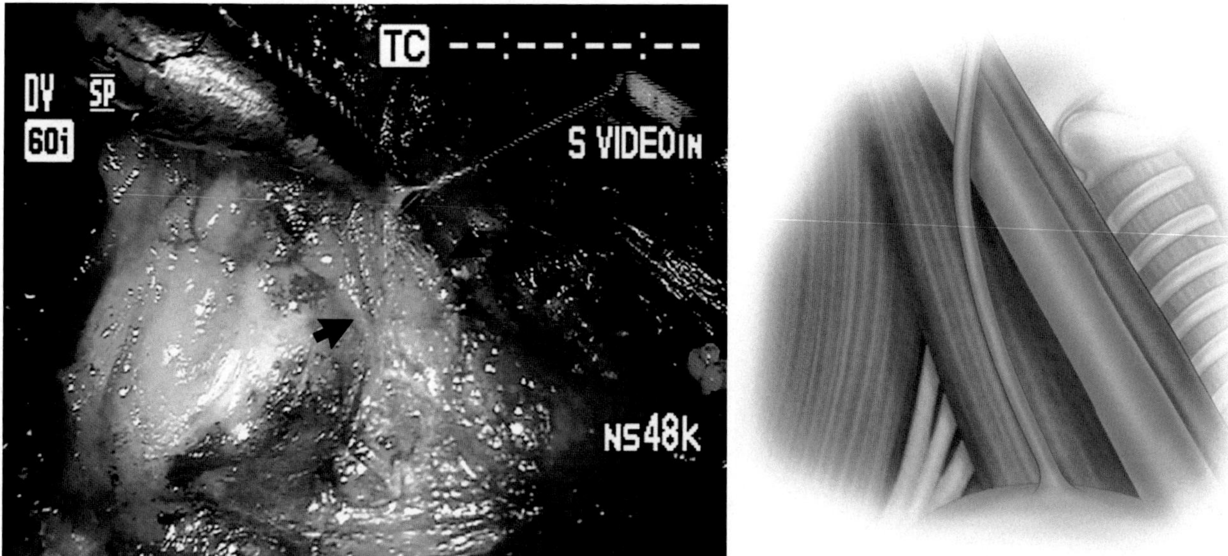

Fig. 43.7 The distal external jugular vein (*arrow*) is clipped and divided at its connection with the subclavian vein on the right side

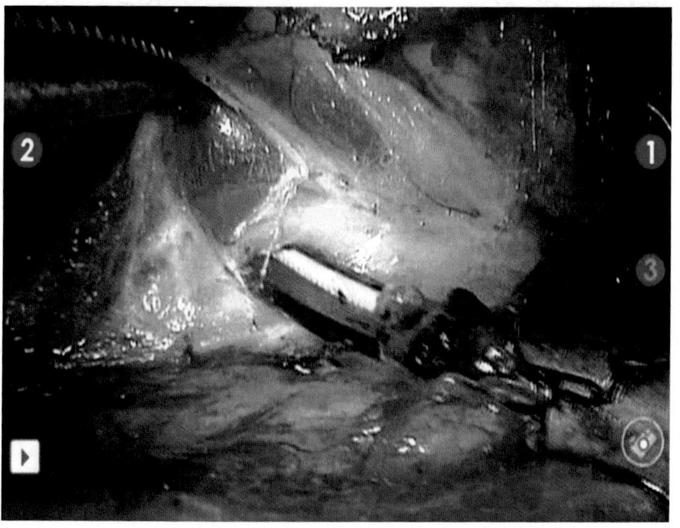

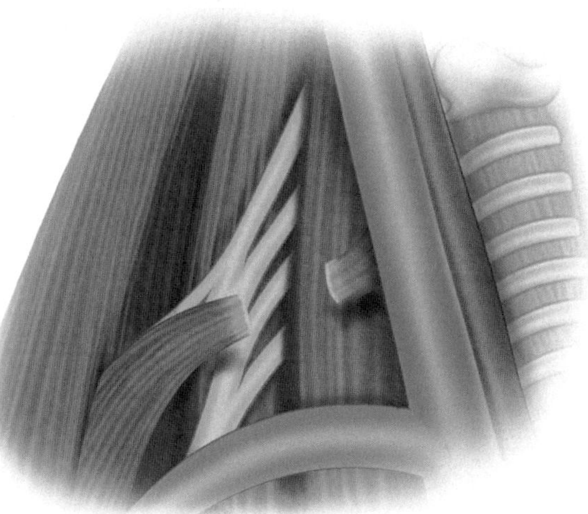

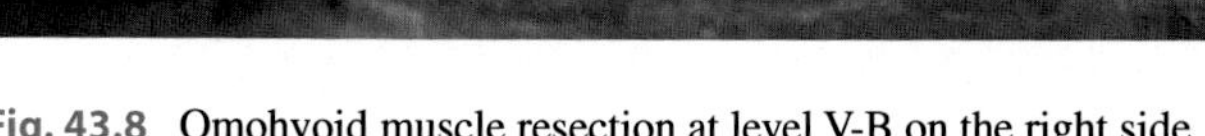

Fig. 43.8 Omohyoid muscle resection at level V-B on the right side

muscle, anterior to the phrenic nerve. Drawing the specimen tissue superiorly at level IV, these anatomic landmarks are easily exposed, and the phrenic nerve and transverse cervical artery can be preserved without injury or ligation (Fig. 43.9). Level V-B dissection in the posterior neck carefully proceeds along the anterior border of the trapezius muscle, preserving the SAN, previously identified during skin flap elevation (Fig. 43.10), and is followed by level IV dissection, while preserving the brachial nerve plexus. The individual nerves of the cervical plexus are sensory nerves, and when they are encountered during dissection, they are sacrificed to ensure complete node dissection; the phrenic nerve, ansa cervicalis, and the great auricular nerve are preserved (Fig. 43.11).

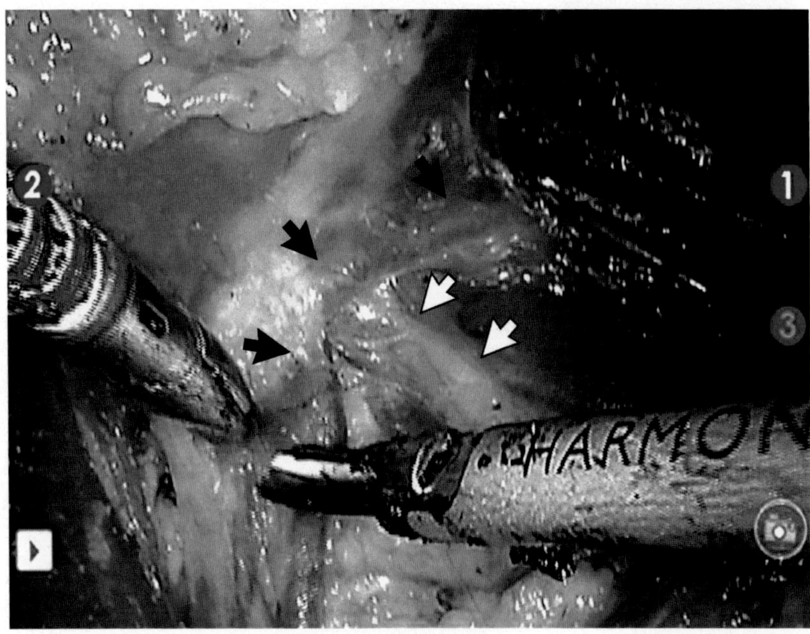

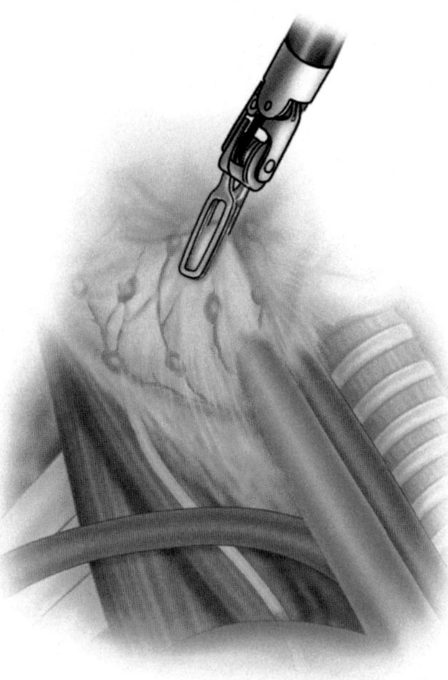

Fig. 43.9 Transverse cervical artery (*black arrow*) is exposed, and the phrenic nerve (*white arrow*) is seen beneath the fascial carpet on the right side

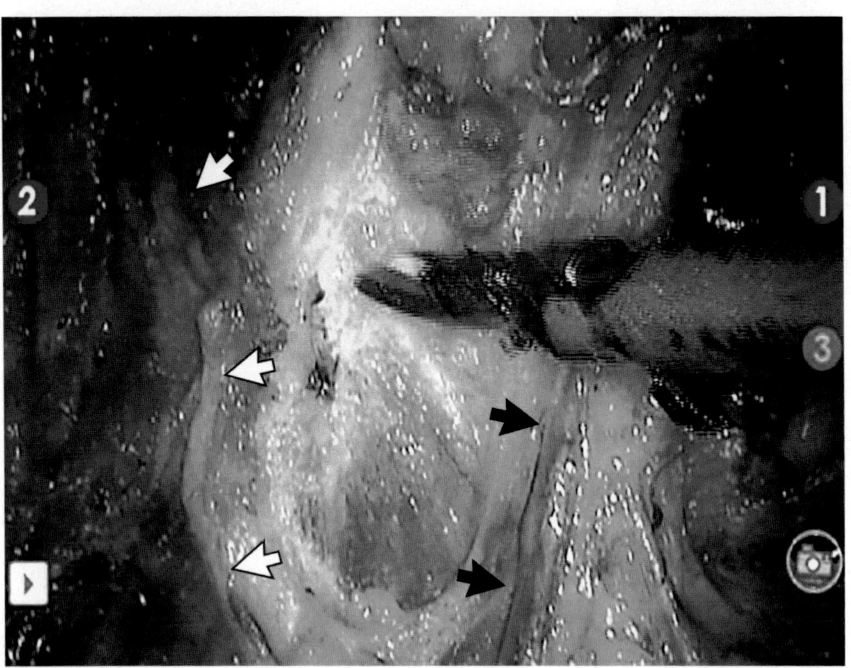

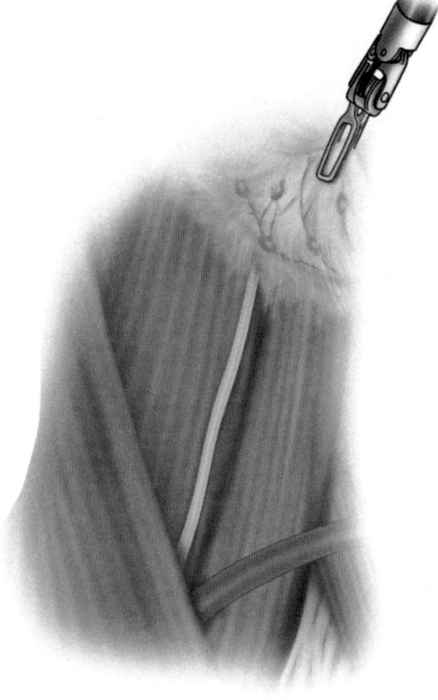

Fig. 43.10 Level V-B dissection along the anterior border of the trapezius muscle, preserving the spinal accessory nerve (*white arrow*) and the phrenic nerve (*black arrow*) on the right side

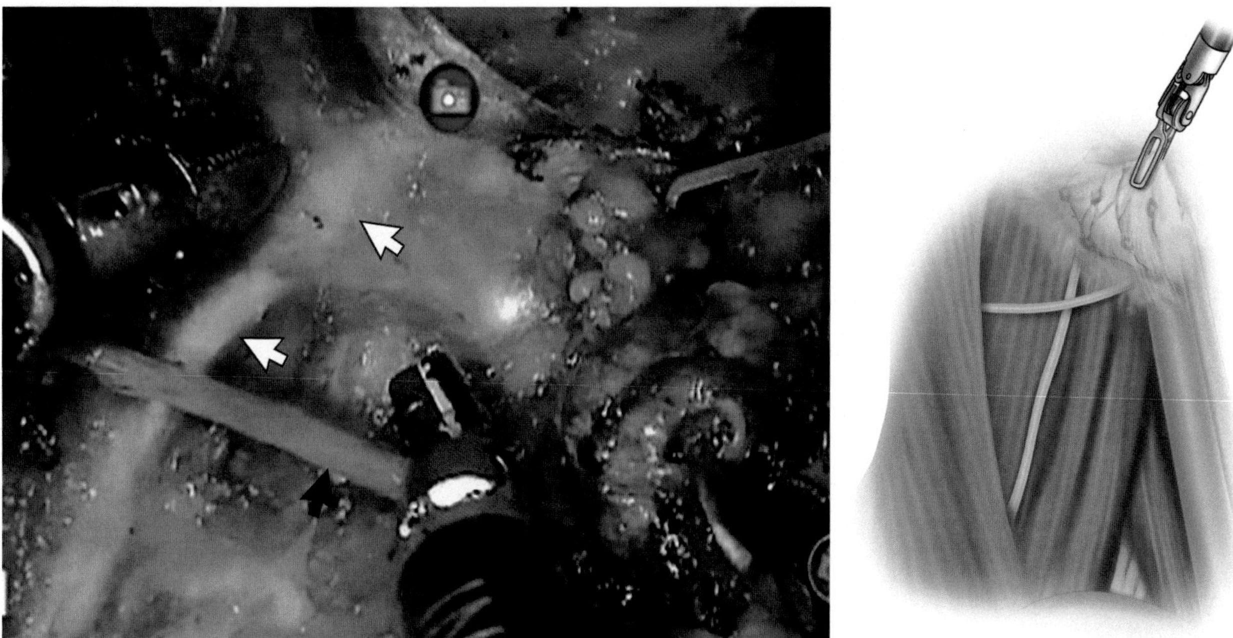

Fig. 43.11 Greater auricular nerve (*black arrow*) and spinal accessory nerve (*white arrow*) near Erb's point on the right side

After dissection of the level III, IV, and V-B nodes, the external retractor and robotic axis are repositioned to allow better exposure of the level II area. The external retractor (Chung's retractor, long type) is then reinserted through the axillary incision and directed toward the submandibular gland (Fig. 43.12). The second docking procedure is performed in the same manner as the first docking procedure; thus, the operating table should also be repositioned more obliquely with respect to the direction of the robotic column, to allow for the same alignment between the axis of the robotic camera arm and the direction of retractor blade insertion. The dissection is progressed until the posterior belly of the digastric muscle and the submandibular gland are exposed superiorly. Drawing the specimen tissue inferolaterally, soft tissues and LNs are detached from the lateral border of the sternohyoid muscle, submandibular gland, and anterior surfaces of the carotid artery and the IJV (Fig. 43.13). The dissection continues posteriorly, and the hypoglossal nerve is identified and preserved (Fig. 43.14). The upper end of the IJV and SAN is exposed under the posterior belly of the digastric muscle.

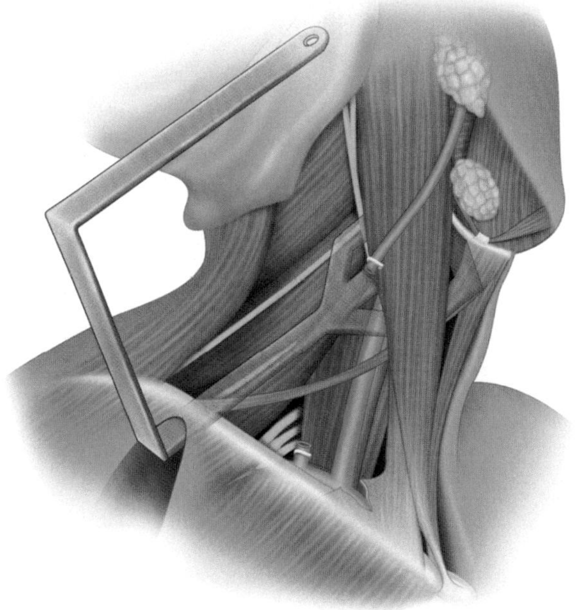

Fig. 43.12 Repositioning of the external retractor for level II dissection

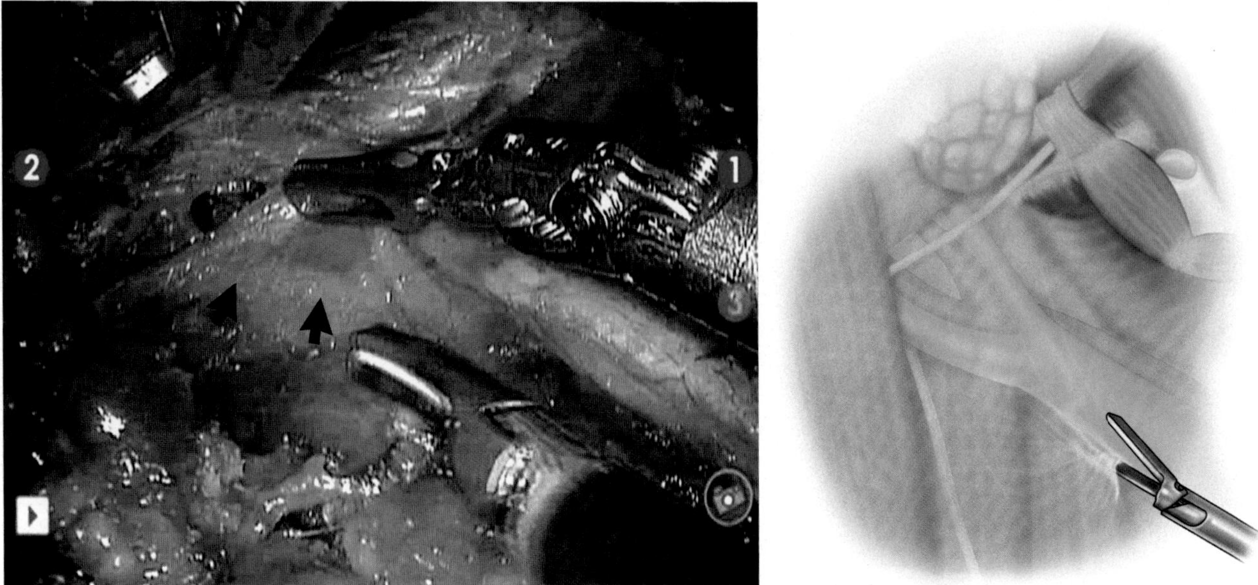

Fig. 43.13 Level II dissection from the lateral border of the IJV (*black arrow*) on the right side

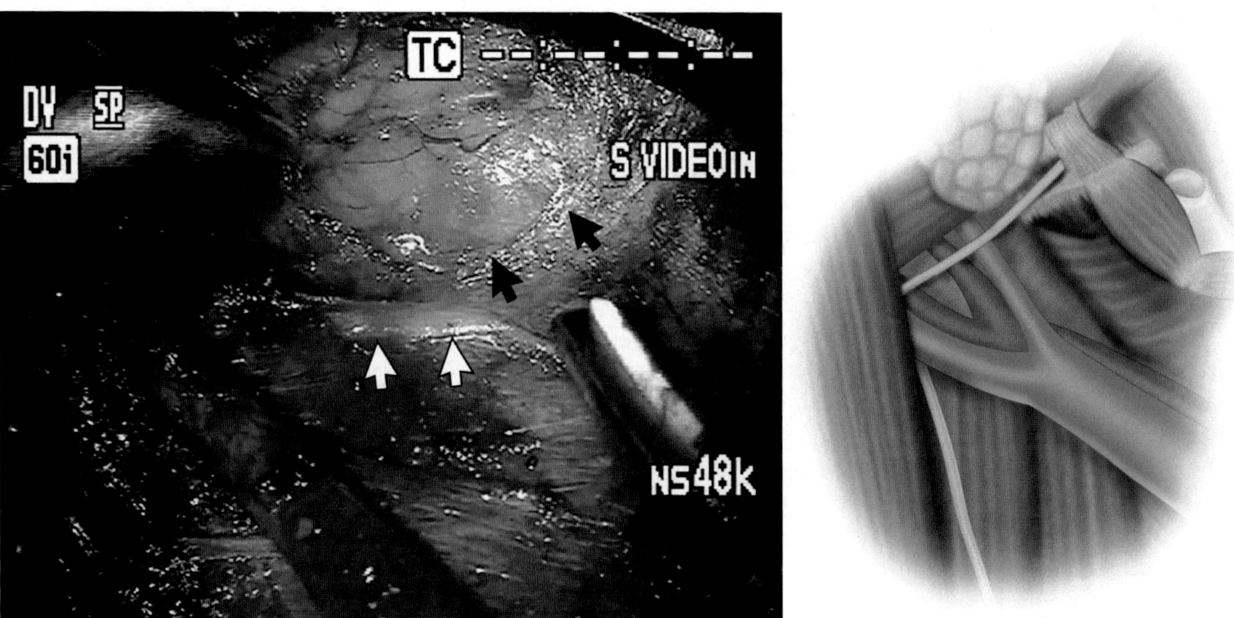

Fig. 43.14 After dissection of the level II area on the right side, the submandibular gland (*black arrow*) and hypoglossal nerve (*white arrow*) are noted

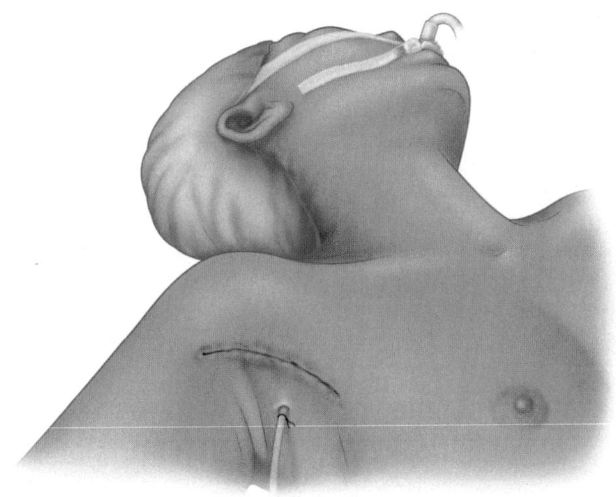

Fig. 43.15 Postoperative wound after drain insertion and skin closure

After the specimen is removed, fibrin glue is sprayed around the area of the thoracic duct and minor lymphatics, and a 3-mm closed-suction drain is inserted just under the axillary skin incision. Wounds are closed cosmetically (Fig. 43.15). The incision scar in the axilla is completely covered when the arm is in its neutral position.

The Robotic Thyroid Surgery Learning Curve and Limitations

The current robotic surgical system has several limitations, such as the lack of tactile feedback and limited instrumentation. The console surgeon and patient-side assistant must learn to use visual clues. However, experienced surgeons have reported that the current technique can be easily learned and that the loss of tactile feedback is no longer a limitation. In addition, collisions between the robotic arms during complicated surgeries occur frequently, owing to their bulky nature [21]. To lessen their complexity, future robotic systems will need to be much smaller. Another current limitation of robotic surgery is the need to train teams, including attending surgeons, surgical assistants, and nurses, to become proficient in this technique. To minimize collisions between the robotic arms, the operation team must understand the spatial relationships of the instruments outside the operative field of vision.

Robotic procedures include three stages—creating a working space, a docking stage, and a console stage (the actual operation). If the time required to create a working space and the docking stage is disregarded, the times required for robotic and conventional procedures are similar, and the operation time for patients undergoing robotic thyroidectomy with neck dissection will likely decrease as surgeons become more familiar with the robotic methods [15].

Conclusion

The recently developed advanced robotic technique in thyroid surgery has been shown to be both safe and feasible in selected patients. Moreover, this technique can expedite radical neck dissection for thyroid cancer with lateral neck node metastasis. With adequate experience, transaxillary robotic modified radical neck dissection can be performed safely, can be oncologically effective, and can become an excellent alternative to conventional open surgery for selected patients.

Acknowledgment The authors are grateful to Dong-Su Jang, (Medical Illustrator, Medical Research Support Section, Yonsei University College of Medicine, Seoul, Republic of Korea) for his help with the figures.

References

1. Ikeda Y, Takami H, Sasaki Y, Takayama J, Niimi M, Kan S. Clinical benefits in endoscopic thyroidectomy by the axillary approach. J Am Coll Surg. 2003;196:189–95.
2. Ikeda Y, Takami H, Sasaki Y, Takayama J, Kurihara H. Are there significant benefits of minimally invasive endoscopic thyroidectomy? World J Surg. 2004;28:1075–8.
3. Miccoli P, Berti P, Raffaelli M, Conte M, Materazzi G, Galleri D. Minimally invasive video-assisted thyroidectomy. Am J Surg. 2001;181:567–70.
4. Kang SW, Jeong JJ, Yun JS, Sung TY, Lee SC, Lee YS, et al. Robot-assisted endoscopic surgery for thyroid cancer: experience with the first 100 patients. Surg Endosc. 2009;23:2399–406.
5. Lee J, Chung WY. Current status of robotic thyroidectomy and neck dissection using a gasless transaxillary approach. Curr Opin Oncol. 2012;24:7–15.
6. Lee J, Chung WY. Robotic thyroidectomy and neck dissection: past, present, and future. Cancer J. 2013;19:151–61.
7. Lee J, Chung WY. Robotic surgery for thyroid disease. Eur Thyroid J. 2013;2:93–101.
8. Lee J, Yun JH, Choi UJ, Kang SW, Jeong JJ, Chung WY. Robotic versus endoscopic thyroidectomy for thyroid cancers: a multi-institutional analysis of early postoperative outcomes and surgical learning curves. J Oncol. 2012;2012:734541.

9. Lee J, Kang SW, Jung JJ, Choi UJ, Yun JH, Nam KH, et al. Multicenter study of robotic thyroidectomy: short-term postoperative outcomes and surgeon ergonomic considerations. Ann Surg Oncol. 2011;18:2538–47.
10. Kang SW, Lee SH, Ryu HR, Lee KY, Jeong JJ, Nam KH, et al. Initial experience with robot-assisted modified radical neck dissection for the management of thyroid carcinoma with lateral neck node metastasis. Surgery. 2010;148:1214–21.
11. Kang SW, Lee SH, Park JH, Jeong JS, Park S, Lee CR, et al. A comparative study of the surgical outcomes of robotic and conventional open modified radical neck dissection for papillary thyroid carcinoma with lateral neck node metastasis. Surg Endosc. 2012;26:3251–7.
12. Lee J, Kwon IS, Bae EH, Chung WY. Comparative analysis of oncological outcomes and quality of life after robotic versus conventional open thyroidectomy with modified radical neck dissection in patients with papillary thyroid carcinoma and lateral neck node metastases. J Clin Endocrinol Metab. 2013;98:2701–8.
13. Lee J, Nah KY, Kim RM, Ahn YH, Soh EY, Chung WY. Differences in postoperative outcomes, function, and cosmesis: open versus robotic thyroidectomy. Surg Endosc. 2010;24:3186–94.
14. Lee J, Na KY, Kim RM, Oh Y, Lee JH, Lee J, et al. Postoperative functional voice changes after conventional open or robotic thyroidectomy: a prospective trial. Ann Surg Oncol. 2012;19: 2963–70.
15. Lee J, Yun JH, Nam KH, Soh EY, Chung WY. The learning curve for robotic thyroidectomy: a multicenter study. Ann Surg Oncol. 2011;18:226–32.
16. Lee J, Lee JH, Nah KY, Soh EY, Chung WY. Comparison of endoscopic and robotic thyroidectomy. Ann Surg Oncol. 2011;18:1439–46.
17. Kim MJ, Kim EK, Kim BM, Kwak JY, Lee EJ, Park CS, et al. Thyroglobulin measurement in fine-needle aspirate washouts: the criteria for neck node dissection for patients with thyroid cancer. Clin Endocrinol. 2009;70:145–51.
18. Caron NR, Clark OH. Papillary thyroid cancer: surgical management of lymph node metastases. Curr Treat Options in Oncol. 2005;6:311–22.
19. Lee J, Sung TY, Nam KH, Chung WY, Soh EY, Park CS. Is level IIb lymph node dissection always necessary in N1b papillary thyroid carcinoma patients? World J Surg. 2008;32:716–21.
20. Caron NR, Tan YY, Ogilvie JB, Triponez F, Reiff ES, Kebebew E, et al. Selective modified radical neck dissection for papillary thyroid cancer--is level I, II and V dissection always necessary? World J Surg. 2006;30:833–40.
21. Liss MA, McDougall EM. Robotic surgical simulation. Cancer J. 2013;19:124–9.

Index

A
Achalasia
  barium esophagram, 397
  bronchiectasis, 397
  diagnosis, 397
  endoscopic therapy, 399
  esophageal manometry, 397, 398
  esophagogastroduodenoscopy, 397, 398
  etiology, 397
  incidence, 397
  lung abscess, 397
  medical therapy, 399
  pneumonia, 397
  subtypes, 398
  surgical management (*see* Heller myotomy)
  symptoms, 397
  treatment, 397
  vagal cholinergic motor function, 397
Acrobot® system, 8
Adhesiolysis, hernia reduction, 454
Adrenalectomy
  adrenal dissection, 129, 130
  da Vinci® robotic system, 127
  dice-5 port placement, 128
  key surgical landmarks, 129
  patient positioning, 127
  patient selection and preparation, 127
  reflection of colon, 129
  room setup, 127
  specimen extraction, 130
Advanced teleoperation laboratory, 6
Alexis wound retractor, 141, 143, 146
Anesthesia issues
  cardiopulmonary risks, 72
  communications and patient access, 78
  complications with robotic surgery, 71, 72
  position for da Vinci Si system, 72, 77
  position for pelvic procedures, 73–74
  position for upper abdominal robotic surgery, 76
  prolonged CO_2 insufflation risk, 72
  for robotic gynecological surgery, 74
  for robotic nephrectomy/pulmonary resections, 74
  from robotic positioning, 72
  during various procedures, 71
Antegrade nerve sparing, 119
Anterior longitudinal ligament (ALL), 193, 203, 204
Anterior mediastinal surgery
  bronchogenic/pericardial, 435
  ectopic parathyroid adenomas, 435
  lymphoma, 435
  patient positioning, 436
  substernal goiter, 435
  trocar placement, 438
Anterior superior pancreaticoduodenal vein (ASPDV), 224
Anthropomorphic industrial robot, 5
ARTAS system, 12
ARTEMIS surgical robot, 8
Arterial blood gas (ABG), 353
Arthrobot, 8
Automated Endoscopic System for Optimal Positioning (AESOP®), 53

B
Belgrade hand, 7
Bilateral salpingo-oophorectomy
  infundibulopelvic ligament (IP) tension, 174
  ovary and fallopian tube isolation, 175
  peritoneum dissection, 176
Bilateral vocal cord paralysis, 420
Biliary reconstruction, 318
Billroth-I reconstruction, 90
Bladder neck dissection
  anterior dissection, 117
  Foley balloon, 117
  preoperative imaging, 116
  30-degree down lens, 116
  visual cues and tissue feedback, 117
Blue Cross Blue Shield Association, 45
Brochure of Vicarm, 5
Bronchial sleeve resections, 425, 433
Bubble test, 278

C
Cadiere forceps, 186
Canadian Agency for Drugs and Technologies in Health (CADTH) database, 45
Carter-Thomason device, 164, 173
Cervical stromal dye injection, 183
Classic achalasia, 398
Cloquet's node, 134
Colectomy
  indications, 249
  outcomes, 260–261
  postoperative course, 260
  preoperative operation, 250
  robotic left colectomy and sigmoidectomy
    colorectal anastomosis, 260
    descending Colon Anastomosis, 260
    distal resection and extraction, 259
    double-docking method, 256, 257
    inferior mesenteric artery isolation and ligation, 258
    lateral-to-medial mobilization, 259
    medial-to-lateral mobilization, 259
    patient and robot positioning, 256
    single-docking method, 256, 257

Y. Fong et al. (eds.), *The SAGES Atlas of Robotic Surgery*, https://doi.org/10.1007/978-3-319-91045-1

Colectomy (*cont.*)
splenic flexure mobilization, 259
standard port setup, 256, 257
robotic right colectomy
alternative port placement, 251, 252
da Vinci Xi® robotic system, 251, 252
docking setup, 250
extracorporeal anastomosis, 254
hepatic flexure, 253
ileocolic pedicle, 252
intracorporeal anastomosis, 255
monopolar instrument, 252
patient position, 250
right colon resection, 253
standard port placement, 251
Colorectal anastomosis, 260, 278
Computer motion, 53
Computer numerically controlled (CNC) machine, 4
Coordinate system, 13
CyberKnife, 12

D
Degree of autonomy, 12
Degree of freedom (dof), 12
Denonvilliers' fascia, 132, 145
Descending colon anastomosis, 260
Direct Hassan cutdown technique, 413
Distal esophagus, 215
Distal pancreatectomy
advantages, 295
disadvantages, 295
pancreatic dissection and mobilization, 307
pancreatic exposure, 299, 300
pancreatic mobilization
with splenectomy, 302, 304, 305
without splenectomy, 306, 307
pancreatic transection methods, 308
robotic instruments, 298, 299
robotic setup, 295–297
specimen extraction, 308
splenic artery dissection, 303
Distal pancreatosplenectomy (DPS), *see* Distal pancreatectomy
Double-docking method, 256, 257
Duodenojejunal reconstruction, 318
Duodenojejunostomy, 331

E
Endo-GIA stapler, 151
Endoscopic retrograde cholangiopancreatography (ERCP), 320
EndoWrist® instrument, 129–130, 181, 186, 220, 238, 263, 292, 295, 298, 311, 314, 319, 449, 493
Enhanced recovery after surgery (ERAS), 250, 320
Esophageal cancer
incidence, 409
Ivor Lewis approach, 409
MIE, 409
surgical resection, 409
Esophageal myotomy, 399
Esophagojejunostomy, 213, 215, 216
Extended lymph node dissection (ELND), 159–161, 164
Extracervical endoscopic thyroidectomies, 465
Extracorporeal anastomosis, 254–255
Extracorporeal urinary diversion
ileal conduit
Alexis wound retractor placement, 141
ileal harvest, 141–142
robotic preparation, 141
stoma creation, 142–143
uretero-enteric anastomoses, 142
Indiana pouch formation
catheterizable limb formation, 147
ileocolonic harvest, 146–147
postoperative care, 149
pouch formation, 148
robotic/laparoscopic preparation, 146
stoma creation, 148
suprapubic catheter placement, 148
uretero-enteric anastomoses, 148
studer orthotopic ileal neobladder
ileal harvest and neobladder formation, 143–145
posterior plate reconstruction, 145
postoperative care, 146
robotic preparation, 143
uretero-enteric anastomoses, 145
urethra-neovesical anastomosis, 145, 146

F
Fascial defect, 455
Fenestrated bipolar forceps, 186
Financial considerations
cost distribution, 49
cost offset, 45
depreciation and service contracts, 49
operating costs, 49
operational concerns
governance and oversight, 47
operating room space, 46
surgeon factors and training, 46
operational expense analysis, 48
robotic program acquisition cost, 48
robotic strategy, 49
robot-specific expenses, 48
Firefly™ fluorescence imaging, 183, 187, 295, 306
Fluorescence imaging, 28, 30, 55–57, 60, 68, 110, 183, 409, 415
Force control, 13
Force refleCT(X)ion (ALF-X) robot, 12
Fossa of Marseille, 134

G
Gamma Knife system, 12
Gasless transaxillary approach, 489
Gastric cancer
radical subtotal distal gastrectomy, with D2 lymphadenectomy
complications, 231
da Vinci® surgical Systems (Si and Xi), 219
EndoWrist®, 220
gastric decompression, 222
instruments, 221
left gastric artery dissection, 227
left-sided greater curvature dissection, 223–224
limitation, 220
lymph node dissection, 222
operating room setup, 220
patient setup, 221
postoperative management, 231
proximal lesser curvature dissection, 228
proximal resection, 228
right-sided greater curvature dissection, 224

robotic surgical platform, 220
side-to-side, completely stapled loop gastrojejunostomy, 229
splenic artery dissection, 227
suprapancreatic and celiac axis dissection, 226–227
trocar placement, 221
Gastric decompression, 222
Gastroesophageal reflux disease (GERD)
antireflux medications, 379
esophageal manometry, 380
generic proton pump inhibitors, 379
laparoscopic techniques, 379
LINX® magnetic esophageal sphincter augmentation system, 379
medical treatment, 379
minimally invasive techniques, 379
pH probe/pH monitoring, 380
robot-assisted operations, 379
antireflux procedure, 380
barium upper gastrointestinal study, 380
collis gastroplasty, 389–391
diaphragmatic closure, 381, 384
hiatal hernia repair, 393
hiatus closure, 383, 389
large paraesophageal hiatus hernia, 386
Nissen fundoplication, 380, 382, 383, 385, 391
paraesophageal hernia sac, 386, 387
partial fundoplication, 388
preoperative evaluation, 380
recurrent hiatal hernia, 392, 393
recurrent GERD and, 392, 394
3D visualization, 379
Toupet and Dor fundoplication procedures, 388
side effects, 379
surgical interventions, 379
GelPOINT path, 282, 284, 285, 288
Gelport, 91, 93–95
Glove-port technique, 284

H
Hand-on compliant control, 13
Head and neck robotic emergency, 69
Heineke-Mikulicz fashion, 144, 147, 148
Heller myotomy
advantages, 399
anterior longitudinal myotomy, 403
barium esophagram, 398
blunt dissection, 402
clinical symptoms, 401
decreased esophageal perforation rates, 400
diaphragmatic hiatus, 403
dor fundoplication, 404
dysphagia, 405
esophageal myotomy, 403
esophageal perforation, 405
gastroesophageal reflux, 405
hemostasis, 404
intraoperative esophagogastroduodenoscopy, 404
with partial fundoplication, 399
patient positioning, 401
patient preparation, 401
peritoneal cavity access, 402
pneumothorax (capnothorax), 405
port placement, 402
posterior cruroplasty, 404
postoperative care, 405
postoperative hemorrhage, 405
primary outcome measures, 399
secondary outcomes, 399
Hepatectomies, 335
Hepatic duct transection, 328
Hepatic flexure mobilization, 253
Hepaticojejunostomy, 329
Hepatobiliary surgery, 96
Hepatopancreaticobiliary (HPB) surgery, 319
History of robotics, 3–7
Human papillomavirus (HPV), 445, 446, 451
Hybrid laparoscopic-robotic approach, 279
Hybrid robot-assisted surgery
ablative techniques, 97, 98
in colon surgery, 96
gynecologic malignancies, 97
hand-assisted surgery, 95
hepatobiliary surgery, 96
intestinal resections, 89, 90
laparoscopy plus robotic surgery, 95
mini-laparotomy
colectomy/proctectomy, 94
complex gastrointestinal reconstructions, 93
cystectomy, 94
gastrectomy with lymphadenectomy, 94
Gelport, 91, 93, 94
hepatectomy, 94
hysterectomy, 94
indications, 93
intra-corporeal reconstruction, 93
liver surgery, 95
neobladder construction, 93
pancreatectomy, 94
tactile sensation, 93
vascular reconstruction, 94
minimally invasive approaches, 91, 92
NOTES, 97
radical cystectomies, 89, 91
robotic pancreaticoduodenectomy, 96
selection factors, 91
total abdominal proctocolectomy, 96
total mesorectal excision, 96
Hysterectomy with bilateral salpingo-oophorectomy
docking robot, 173
patient setup, 170
port placement
camera port, 171
fascia closure, 173
low body mass index, 172
non-camera robot ports, 171
Palmer's point, 172
trocars, 173
uterine manipulators, 170
vaginal occluder, 170

I
Industrial robot, 4
Inferior mesenteric artery (IMA), 269, 270, 276
Inferior mesenteric vein (IMV), 267, 276
Inferior vena cava (IVC), 163
Inguinal hernia (IH) repair
abdominal computed tomography, 463
adhesion-resistant coated mesh, 458
analgesic use, 463
anterior dissection, 461

Inguinal hernia (IH) repair (*cont.*)
  with applied flat mesh, 462
  bowel obstruction, 458
  cigarette smoking, 457
  circumferential hernia dissection, 461
  concomitant herniorrhaphy, 463
  da Vinci Surgical System robot, 458
  extraperitoneal approach, 459
  extraperitoneal laparoscopic radical prostatectomy, 458
  healthcare resources, 458
  incidence rate, 457
  intraperitoneal inguinal hernia repair, 458
  lateral dissection, 460
  mesh infection, 458
  midline incision, 457
  operative variables and complications, 463
  peritoneal integrity, 458
  preoperative physical examination, 463
  prosthetic mesh, 458
  radical prostatectomy, 457
  randomized-controlled trials, 458, 463
  recurrence rates, 463
  reperitonealization, 458
  risk factors, 457
  robotic-assisted radical prostatectomy, 458, 459
  scarring, preperitoneal space, 458
  smoking history, 457
  systematic detection, 463
  transversalis fascia, 458
  urine sterilization, 458
Intracorporeal anastomosis, 255
Intracorporeal urinary diversion
  bowel isolation
    Endo-GIA stapler, 151
    final staple load, 151
    staple load, 150
    stay sutures, 150
    umbilical tape, 149
  ileal conduit, 152
  instrumentation, 149
  patient positioning, 149
  port placement, 149
  specimen removal, 153
  stoma maturation, 153
  studer orthotopic neobladder
    pouch creation, 154–155
    urethral anastomosis, 153–154
    Wiklund neobladder, 155, 156
    Y-pouch neobladder, 156
Intuitive Surgical da Vinci® Sp system, 54, 55
Ivor Lewis approach to MIE, *see* Robot-assisted minimally invasive esophagectomy (RAMIE)

J

Joint Commission on Accreditation of Hospitals (JCAH) standards, 39

L

Laparoscopic Roux-en-Y gastric bypass (LRYGB)
  bariatric surgery volume, 355
  intracorporeal suturing, 355
  learning curve, 355
  physiological tremor, 355
  port site trauma, 355
  vs. robot-assisted RYGB, 361
  tissue dissection, 355
Laparoscopic stapler, 132, 135–137
Large needle driver, 220
Left gastric artery (LGA) dissection, 227
Left lower lobectomy, 432
Left upper lobectomy, 430
Lesser curvature dissection, 225–226
Ligament of Treitz, 212, 215, 267, 276, 324, 330, 360, 371
LigaSure bipolar cautery, 138
Limited lymph node dissection (LLND), 160, 161
Lingulectomy, 433
Liver parenchymal transection, 335
Liver resection
  anesthesia and postoperative care, 335
  mortality rate, 335
  surgeon's dexterity, 335
Liver retraction, 222
Low anterior resection (LAR)
  complications, 279, 280
  limitations, 279–280
  operative technique
    colorectal anastomosis, 278
    distal rectum, 278
    drain placement, 279
    hybrid laparoscopic-robotic approach, 279
    mobilization, 276–277
    operating room configuration, 274
    ostomy construction, 279
    patient position, 274
    port placement, 275
    preparation, 274
    robot docking, 275
    robotic stapler, 278
    specimen extraction, 278
    total mesorectal excision, 276–278
    transanal approach, 279
  outcomes, 280
  postoperative management, 279
  preoperative planning, 273–274
  with total mesorectal excision, 273
Lower lobe superior segmentectomies, 433
Lymph node dissection (LND)
  completed extended pelvic lymph node dissection, 120, 121
  dorsal venous complex control, 122
  European Association of Urology guidelines, 120
  pelvic LND, 120
  peritoneal incision, 120
  proximal extent of dissection, 120
  staple control, 122
  suture control, 123
Lymphadenectomy, 215

M

MacDonald trial, 209
MAGIC trial, 209
Maryland Bipolar Forceps, 186
Mauna Kea's Cellvizio® microendoscope, 58
Mazor Robotics, 12
Mechanical Turk, 3
Medial-to-lateral mobilization, 277
Mediastinal masses, 435
Mediastinum
  anatomy, 435
  median sternotomy/thoracotomy, 435
  postoperativec care, 442

right phrenic nerve, 441
thymectomies, 435
thymic veins, 441
video-assisted thoracic surgery and robotics, 435
Mega™ Suture Needle Driver, 220
Middle colic vein (MCV), 224, 301
Middle colic vessels, 265, 266
Minimally invasive esophagectomy (MIE), 409
Minimally invasive surgery (MIS) technique, 209
Minimally invasive total abdominal colectomy, 263
MIRO surgical system, 10
Modified radical neck dissection (MRND) techniques, *see* Transaxillary robotic modified radical neck dissection neck
Monopolar cautery, 134
Monopolar curved scissors, 186
Multidisciplinary program, 50
Multiport cholecystectomy
Calot's triangle, 238, 239
cosmetic benefit, 233
cystic duct and artery, 238, 239
cystic plate, 240
da Vinci Single-Site® port and cannulae, 234
docking, 237–238
efficacy and feasibility, 233
gallbladder, initial exposure, 238
learning curve, 247
ligation, 238
monopolar instruments, 238
near-infrared fluorescence cholangiography, 238, 240
patient preparation, 236
port placement, 236–237
preoperative considerations, 235
retraction and dissection, 238
room setup, 235
suction/irrigation, 238
Myasthenia Gravis (MG) without thymoma, 435, 436

N
Narrowband imaging (NBI), 58
Natural orifice transluminal endoscopic surgery (NOTES), 97
Neck dissection, *see* Transaxillary robotic modified radical neck dissection neck
Nephron-sparing surgery (NSS), 103
Nerve-sparing neurovascular bundle dissection, 136
NeuroMate system, 10
NeuroSAFE technique, 119
Neurovascular bundle preservation, 118, 119

O
Olympus Endoeye® Flex 3D, 54, 55
Omentectomy, 213
Operating room (OR)
additional space, 22
bed position, 68
cabling, 22
case workflow checklist, 67
circulation space, 16, 19, 20
critical dimensions and clearances, 16
cords, tubes, and cables securing and positioning, 68
departure of patient, 22
disruption of independent tasks, 22, 26
emergency conversion tray, 68
initial preparations, 67
instrumentation, 68, 69
lighting design, 22
operator space, 16
optimal spacing, 68
optional position of robot, 22, 25
patient positioning, 67
physical footprint, 16
remote console space, 22
restricted environment, 16
restrictive requirements for circulation, 22
robot setup, 16
robotic video images, 28
room setup, 67
room size, 16
staffing, 68
staff support spaces, 22
stereo imaging, 28
sterile field size, 22
support and repair spaces, 21
surgical suite, 16
3-D visualization, 28
training spaces, 21
video system development, 28
workflow and traffic, 22, 27
Optical endoscopy
acquisition of image mosaics, 58, 59
camera and optics in tip, 54
camera elements outside the body, 53, 54
fluorescence imaging, 55–57
incoherent fiber optic bundles, 53
intuitive Surgical da Vinci® Sp system, 54, 55
narrowband imaging, 58
NBI, 58
Olympus Endoeye® Flex 3D, 54, 55
stereo endoscopes, 54
sterile drape interface, 54
tissue scattering and absorption, 58
white balance and left-right eye alignment, 54
Ostomy, 279

P
Palatopharyngoplasty, 450
Pancreaticogastrostomy, anterior approach, 317
Pancreaticojejunostomy, 316, 330
Pancreatic transection, 326
Pancreatoduodenectomy (PD)
anastomosis, 316
anterograde cholecystectomy, 313
biliary reconstruction, 311
cephalic peripancreatic lymph node stations, 313
common bile duct, 313
distal bile duct transection, 313
duodenojejunal flexure, 313
gastrocolic ligament, 312, 313
gastroduodenal artery, 313
gastrointestinal anastomosis, 311
hepatoduodenal ligament, 313
jejunal loop transition, 313
Kocher maneuver, 312
liver hilum exploration and arterial control, 313
mortality rate, 311
nononcological resections, 311
oncological results, 311
pancreatic anastomosis, 311
pancreatic fistula rate, 311
pancreatic neck transection, 314

Pancreatoduodenectomy (PD) (*cont.*)
  patient positioning, 311
  patient selection, 311
  port setting, 312
  right colonic flexure mobilization, 312
  right gastroepiploic and gastric arteries, 313
  specimen extraction and closure, 318
  superior mesenteric vein dissection, 314
  trocar positioning and docking, 311, 312
  uncinate process dissection, 314, 315
  vascular and lymphatic connections, 313
  vascular isolation, 311
Pancreatojejunostomy, 316
Parenchymal transection, 344, 349, 352, 353
Parks transanal excision for rectal neoplasms, 292
Partial hepatectomy, 352
  aggressive dieresis, 353
  aggressive fluid resuscitation, 353
  bariatric robotic port, 353
  blood urea nitrogen, 353
  central venous pressure, 344, 353
  coagulation studies, 353
  complete blood count, 353
  complete metabolic panel, 353
  contraindications, 343, 344
  da Vinci Si system, 346
  formal anatomic lobectomy, 352
  indications, 343
  liver assessment, 348
  parenchymal transection, 349, 352
  patient positioning, 345, 346
  perioperative stage, 344
  peripheral hepatic lesions, 343
  phosphorous and magnesium levels, 353
  port placement, 347, 348, 352
  postoperative monitoring, 353
  preoperative studies, 344
  radiologic staging, 344
  reverse Trendelenburg position, 345
  robotic/handheld staplers, 351
  Si port placement, 347
  specimen extraction site, 353
  staple articulation, 352
  stapler positioning, 352
  supine patient positioning, 345
  ultrasound staging, 348
  venous thromboembolic prophylaxis, 353
Partial nephrectomy
  hilar exposure, 106
  intraoperative ultrasound imaging, 106
  near infrared fluorescence imaging, 109, 110
  patient selection, 103
  planning site of excision, 106, 107
  port placement and instruments, 104, 105
  reflection of colon, 105
  renorrhaphy, 109
  room setup and patient positioning, 103, 104
  specimen extraction, 110
  treatment outcomes, 111
  tumor excision, 107–109
  upper pole dissection of hepatorenal ligaments, 106
PathFinder, 10
Pedicle ligation, 352
Pelvic lymph node dissection (PLND), prostate cancer
  patient selection, 159
  technique and steps, 160–161
Pelvic organ prolapse (POP), 193
Perivesical fat space dissection, 118
Piver-Rutledge-Smith system, 182
Pneumo-occluder, 190, 191
Pneumoperitoneum, 213
Position/kinematic control, 13
Posterior mediastinal surgery, 436
  patient positioning, 437
  trocar placement, 439
Presacral space, 193, 194, 197, 202, 203
PROBOT system, 8, 53
ProGrasp™ forceps, 176, 186, 199, 299, 466, 472, 473, 493
Prostate cancer, RPLND
  patient selection, 159
  technique and steps, 160
Proximal duodenum, 214
Proximal lesser curvature dissection, 228
Pulmonary artery injuries, 427
Pulmonary resection
  bipolar dissecting instruments, 427
  hilar dissection, 427
  lateral decubitus position, 426
  lower lobe bronchus, 432
  lower lobe vein, 430
  lymph node removal, 427
  mediastinal lymph node dissection, 427
  nonanatomic wedge resections, 425
  passive retraction, 427
  port placement, 427
  Si robot, 427
PUMA 200 robot, 53
Puma 500 robotic arm, 6
Pyloroplasty, 415
Pylorus-preserving pancreatoduodenectomy, 313

Q

Querleu-Morrow system, 182

R

Radical cystoprostatectomy
  extracorporeal urinary diversion (*see* Extracorporeal urinary diversion)
  female patient
    anterior exenteration completion, 140
    bladder mobilization, 139
    bowel mobilization, 137
    lymph node dissection, 138
    ureteral dissection, 138
    uterine-sparing cystectomy, 140
    vaginal closure, 140
    vascular pedicles division, 138–139
  intracorporeal urinary diversion (*see* Intracorporeal urinary diversion)
  male patient
    bladder mobilization, 136
    bowel mobilization, 132
    extended pelvic lymph node dissection, 134–135
    nerve-sparing neurovascular bundle dissection, 136–137
    seminal vesicle/posterior dissection, 132
    ureteral dissection, 133–134
    vascular pedicles ligation, 135
  patient positioning, 131
  patient selection, 131
  port placement, 131, 132
  preoperative preparation, 131
Radical hysterectomy
  for cervical cancer, 181–182
  cost-effectiveness, 183

docking, 185
instrument selection, 186
operative steps
colpotomy, 190
infundibulopelvic ligament, 186
knot-tying, 190
parametria dissection, 188
rectovaginal space, 188, 189
uterine artery, 188
uterosacral ligament transection, 188, 189
vaginal closure, 190, 191
vesicouterine space, 187
patient positioning, 183
sentinel lymph node, 182
SLN dye injection, 183
trocar placement, 184
uterine manipulator, 184
Radical prostatectomy
hernia repair, 457
prostate cancer, 457
with lymph node dissection, 457
Radical subtotal distal gastrectomy
with D2 lymphadenectomy
da Vinci® surgical systems (Si and Xi), 219
complications, 231
EndoWrist®, 220
instruments, 221
left gastric artery dissection, 227
left-sided greater curvature dissection, 223–224
lesser curvature dissection, 225–226
limitation, 220
liver retraction, 222
lymph node dissection, 222
operating room setup, 220
patient setup, 221
postoperative management, 231
proximal lesser curvature dissection, 228
proximal resection, 228
right-sided greater curvature dissection, 224
robotic surgical platform, 220
side-to-side, completely stapled loop gastrojejunostomy, 229
splenic artery dissection, 227
trocar placement, 221
Raven II surgical robot, 11
Rectal cancer
surgical management, 273
treatment, 273
Remote center technology, 355
Remote-access endoscopic surgery of the thyroid gland, 489
Renal cell and upper tract urothelial carcinoma, 164
RPLND
patient positioning, 164
patient selection, 164
port placement, 164
technique and steps, 164
Renorrhaphy, 109
Retrograde nerve sparing, 120
Retroperitoneal lymph node dissection (RPLND)
renal cell carcinoma and upper tract urothelial carcinoma
patient positioning, 164
patient selection, 164
port placement, 164
technique and steps, 164
testicular cancer
management, 159
patient positioning, 162
patient selection, 162
port placement, 162
room setup, 162
technique and steps, 163–164
Right gastroepiploic vein (RGEV), 224
Right lower lobectomies, 430
Right middle lobectomy, 432, 433
Right upper lobe apical segmentectomy, 433
Right upper lobectomy using a fissure-last technique, 428, 429
Right-sided greater curvature dissection, 223–225
Right-sided lobectomy, 426
RIO Robotic Arm Interactive Orthopedic system, 12
ROBODOC system, 8, 12, 53, 62
Robot-assisted laparoscopic hysterectomy
bladder mobilization away from the uterus/cervix, 176
cardinal ligaments isolation and transection, 177
colpotomy incision, 177–178
morbid obesity, 179
pelvic organs vizualization, 179
uterine morcellation, 179
uterine vessels isolation, 177
vaginal cuff closure, 178
vs. abdominal approach, 176
Robot assisted microsurgery workstation
(RAMS) system, 9, 53
Robot-assisted minimally invasive esophagectomy (RAMIE)
abdominal phase
celiac and retrogastric lymphadenectomy, 414
gastric conduit formation, 416
gastric mobilization, 415
gastric tubularization, 416
gastroepiploic arcade, 415
hiatal dissection, 414
pyloroplasty, 415, 416
retrogastric dissection, 414
anastomotic leaks, 420
antibiotics and prophylactic subcutaneous heparin, 410
anvil insertion, 418
circular-S stapled anastomosis
stapler anvil, 418
stapler insertion and firing, 419
clinical staging, 410
conduit formation, 416
en bloc esophageal mobilization
conduit advancement and deep mediastinal dissection, 418
pericardial and hiatal dissection, 417
subcarinal dissection, 417, 418
superior mediastinal and para-aortic dissection, 418
gastric mobilization, 415
healthcare system, 410
induction chemotherapy and radiation, 410
intraoperative airway injury, 420
intraoperative setup, 411
intrapleural position. CO_2 insufflation, 413
intrathoracic anastomoses, 420
intrathoracic robotic approaches, 420
operative approach, 410
patient positioning, 410
port placement, 411
postoperative care, 419
postoperative complications, 422
robotic arm collisions, 413
robotic cart and console placement, 411
stapler preparation and anastomosis, 419
subcarinal dissection, 417, 420
thoracic phase, 417–419
thoracoscopic-assisted approach, 420
tissue diagnosis, esophageal cancer, 410
transhiatal approach, 420
Trendelenburg positioning, 413

Robot-assisted minimally invasive telesurgery, 8
Robot-assisted radical prostatectomy (RARP)
  antegrade nerve sparing, 119
  bladder neck dissection
    anterior dissection, 117
    Foley balloon, 117
    preoperative imaging, 116
    30-degree down lens, 116
    visual cues and tissue feedback, 117
  Denonvilliers fascia incision, 116
  dissection behind prostate, 116
  laparoscopic closure device, 124
  LND (*see* Lymph node dissection (LND))
  neurovascular bundle preservation, 118, 119
  patient selection, 113
  perivesical fat space dissection, 118
  port placement
    extraperitoneal approach, 114, 115
    transperitoneal approach, 114, 115
  retrograde nerve sparing, 120
  Retzius space development, 116
  room setup and positioning, 113
  specimen extraction, 124
  transperitoneal approach, 113
  treatment outcomes, 113
  vas deferens and seminal vesicles dissection, 115–117
  vesicourethral anastomosis, 123, 124
Robot-assisted RYGB (RRYGB), 361, 362
Robot-assisted stereotaxic brain surgery, 8
Robot cart, 274
Robot docking, 274, 275
  multiport cholecystectomy, 237–238
  robotic total colectomy, 264, 265
  single-site cholecystectomy, 243
Robotic-assisted herniorrhaphy, 453
Robotic-assisted sacrocolpopexy (RASC)
  anesthesia, 194
  endoscopic instrumentation, 199
  indications for surgery, 194
  patient cart positioning, 198
  patient positioning
    Trendelenburg positioning, 194
    with hysterectomy, 195, 196
    without hysterectomy, 197
  postoperative care, 206
  trocar placement, 197
  with hysterectomy steps, 199–201
    vaginal cuff, 199, 200
  without hysterectomy steps
    peritoneal closure, 204, 205
    sacral mesh attachment, 204, 205
    sacral promontory dissection, 202–203
    vaginal dissection, 201–202
    vaginal mesh attachment, 203
Robotic cholecystectomy
  cost, 246
  multiport
    Calot's triangle, 238, 239
    cosmetic benefit, 233
    cystic duct and artery, 238, 239
    cystic plate, 240
    da Vinci Single-Site® port and cannulae, 234
    docking, 237–238
    gallbladder, initial exposure, 238
    learning curve, 247
    ligation, 238
    monopolar instruments, 238
    near-infrared fluorescence cholangiography, 238, 240
    patient preparation, 236
    port placement, 236–237
    preoperative considerations, 235
    retraction and dissection, 238
    room setup, 235
    suction/irrigation, 238
  postoperative care, 246
  procedure-specific complications, 246
  single-site
    cosmetic benefit, 233
    da Vinci Single-Site® system, 245
    docking, 243
    instruments, 244
    operative steps, 244–246
    patient preparation, 241
    preoperative considerations, 235
    room setup, 241
    single-Site® silicone port, 241, 242
  training, 247
Robotic credentialing, 48
Robotic facelift thyroidectomy (RFT)
  anterior cervical incision, 480
  anterior cervical scar, 487
  axillary techniques, 479
  cervical anatomy, 479, 480
  complications, 487
  conservative management, 487
  cosmetic outcomes, 479, 480
  hypoparathyroidism, 487
  indications, 480
  inferior constrictor muscle, 480
  laryngeal nerve, 486
  muscle flap, 481, 482
  muscular triangle, 482
  occipital hairline, 479
  open dissection, 481
  operative pocket with retractors, 483
  patient expectations, 487
  patient marking, 480
  patient positioning, 481
  postauricular scar, 487
  postoperative management, 487
  recurrent laryngeal nerve, 486
  remote access techniques, 479
  retractor system, 483
  RLN/SLN injury, 487
  robotic cart in position, 484, 485
  robotic console, 483, 484
  robotic deployment, 481
  robotic dissection, 481
  selection criteria, 480
  soft-tissue flap, 479
  strap muscles, 483
  superior pole division, 485
  thyroid gland, superior pole, 483
Robotic first assistants (RFAs), 46
Robotic left colectomy and sigmoidectomy
  colorectal anastomosis, 260
  descending colon anastomosis, 260
  distal resection and extraction, 259
  double-docking method, 256, 257
  inferior mesenteric artery isolation and ligation, 258
  lateral-to-medial mobilization, 259
  medial-to-lateral mobilization, 259

patient and robot positioning, 256
single-docking method, 256, 257
splenic flexure mobilization, 259
standard port setup, 256, 257
Robotic pancreaticoduodenectomy, 96
Robotic pylorusic-preserving pancreaticoduodenectomy
AirSeal® Access Port incision, 332
contraindications, 320
da Vinci Xi® system, 319
dusky duodenum, 326
ERAS protocol, 320
gastrocolic omentum, 326
hand-assisted and hybrid laparoscopic-robotic techniques, 319
indications, 320
intraoperative fluid administration, 333
Kocher maneuver, 324
operating room setup, 321
for pancreatic ductal adenocarcinoma, 319
pancreatic exposure, 325
pancreatic parenchyma, 326, 327
patient placement, 320
perioperative goal-directed fluid therapy principles, 333
perioperative outcomes, 319
port placement, 321
Porta hepatis dissection, 322–324
postoperative complications, 333
preparation and operative strategy, 320
reconstruction techniques, 319, 329
relative infancy, 319
specimen removal, 327, 328
surgical techniques, 319
trocar/port placement, 322
two-layer anastomosis, 330
vision system, 319
Robotic right colectomy
alternative port placement, 251
da Vinci Xi® robotic system, 251, 252
docking setup, 250
extracorporeal anastomosis, 254
hepatic flexure, 253
ileocolic pedicle, 252
intracorporeal anastomosis, 255
monopolar instrument, 252
patient position, 250
right colon resection, 253
standard port placement, 251
Robotic right hepatectomy, 341
contraindications, 335
diagnostic laparoscopy, 336
falciform ligament, 338
hemostatic agent, 341
hilum dissection, 338
indications, 335
operative room disposition, 336
parenchymal transection, 339, 340
patient positioning, 336
Pfannenstiel incision, 341
pneumoperitoneum, 336
port setting, 337
right hepatic duct and indocyanine green fluorescence assessment, 338
surgical technique, 337
vascular invasion, 335
vena cava preparation, 339
Robotic single-site platform, 234
Robotic surgery coordinator, 46
Robotic surgery platform
da Vinci units, 29
evidence-based medicine, 31, 32
FDA clearance, 29
financial considerations, 31
fluorescence imaging system, 30
number and type of annual worldwide procedures, 30
urology and gynecology, 30
Robotic surgery steering committee
on administrative side, 33
bedside assistant, 34
careful surgical planning, 34
checklist, 34
on clinical side, 33
credentialing and privileging surgeons, 33, 34
docking and undocking process, 34
marketing and community education, 35
operating surgeon, 34
troubleshooting, 34
Robotic surgical malpractice action, 37–38
Robotic thymectomy, 436, 437
general anesthesia, 436
left-sided thoracoscopic approach, 437
patient positioning
anterior mediastinal mass resections, 436
posterior mediastinal masses, 437
Robotic to open procedure conversion, 69
Robotic total colectomy
da Vinci Xi® system, 263
dual docking approach, 264
indications, 263
operative technique
ileocolic pedicle, 265, 266
inferior mesenteric artery, 269, 270
inferior mesenteric vein exposure, 267
left ureter identification, 269
lesser sac opening, 268
middle colic vessels, 265, 266
patient rotation, 265
rectal dissection, 270
rectal transection, 270
right colon lateral attachments, 267
robot docking, 265
patient position, 264
trocar placement, 265
Robotic transanal surgery (RTS), 281, 283
custom rigid port, 286
for endoluminal local excision, 282
for local excision of neoplasia, 288, 290
glove port, 283, 284, 286
transanal access device, 284, 285
Rosebud stoma, 142
Roux-en-Y gastric bypass (RYGB)
advantages, 355
alimentary limb, 374
anastomosis, 361
antecolic versus retrocolic, 356
in bariatric surgery, 365
benefits and safety, 365
biliopancreatic diversion, 377
body mass index, 355
boom-mounted arms, 377
complications, 365
da Vinci® patient cart, 358
da Vinci® robotic system, 366, 376
end-gastric-pouch to side-jejunal-loop fashion, 371

Roux-en-Y gastric bypass (RYGB) (*cont.*)
  enterotomy, 360
  gastric pouch, 359, 360, 369, 370
  gastrojejunal anastomosis, 371–373
  gastrojejunostomy, 355, 356, 361
  gastrotomy and enterotomy, 376
  harmonic scalpel, 372
  hybrid *vs.* totally robotic, 356
  indications, 365
  instrumentation, 356
  jejunal loop, 373
  jejuno-jejunal anastomosis, 373, 374
  jejunojejunostomy, 355, 360
  leak test, 375
  mesenteric defect, 374
  obesity-related comorbidities, 355, 365
  operating room setup, 357
  operative times, 365
  patient cart positioning, 357
  patient factors, 376
  patient positioning, 357, 366, 367, 369
  perigastric dissection, 359
  Petersen's defect, 361
  port position and docking, 358
  postoperative care, 375
  preoperative preparation, 365, 366
  prophylaxis for deep venous thrombosis, 361
  revisional bariatric procedures, 355
  robotic *vs.* laparoscopic approaches, 365
  single docking *vs.* double docking, 356
  staple line reinforcements/oversewing, 356
  trocar placement, 368
  trocars placement, 368
  Xi system, 376, 377
Roux-en-Y jejunojejunostomy, 215
RUMI II uterine manipulator device, 170

S
SAGES-MIRA Robotic Surgery Consensus Group, 355
Segmentectomy, 433
Selective Compliant Articulated Robot for Assembly (SCARA), 6
Sensor-equipped robots, 5
SENTICOL study, 182
Sentinel lymph node (SLN), 182–183
Sigmoid colon, 132, 135, 137, 156
Single-docking method, 256, 257
Single Port Orifice Robotic Technology (SPORT), 12
Single-site cholecystectomy
  cosmetic benefit, 233
  da Vinci Single-Site® system, 245
  docking, 241–244
  instruments, 244
  operative steps, 244–246
  patient preparation, 241
  preoperative considerations, 235
  room setup, 241
  single-Site® silicone port, 241, 242
Spacemaker™, 105, 128
Spastic achalasia, 398
SPIDER (Single-Port Instrument Delivery Extended Research) device, 247
Spleen-preserving distal pancreatectomy, 300
Splenic artery dissection, 227
Split-and-roll technique, 134, 135
Squamous cell carcinoma (SCC)
  da Vinci® Si System, 445
  patient selection, 446
  physical examination, 446
  preoperative history, 446
  single-modality surgical management, 445
  staging workup, 446
  tobacco/alcohol use, 445
  transoral exposure, 446
  transoral robot use, 445
  upper aerodigestive tract, 445
Stanford arm, 4
Stereo endoscopes, 54
Stereoscopic camera-based implementations, 53
Suprapancreatic and celiac axis dissection, 226–227
Surgenius surgical robot, 11
Surgeon's Operating Force-feedback Interface Eindhoven (SOFIE) robotic system, 11
Surgical case diversification, 49
Surgical robot litigation
  collateral estoppel, 41, 42
  corporate negligence, 39
  credentialing protocols, 39
  delineation of privilege, 39
  informed consent, 38, 39
  learned intermediary doctrine, 41
  medical training and certification, 39
  proximate cause, 38
  robot malfunction, 40, 41
  standard operating practices for proctors, 40
  strict product liability, 40
SurgiQuest AirSeal insufflation system, 104, 128
Surveillance, Epidemiology, and End Results Program (SEER) database, 409

T
T1 adenocarcinomas, 281
Telerobotic surgery, 435
Testicular cancer, RPLND
  patient positioning, 162
  patient selection, 162
  port placement, 162
  room setup, 162
  technique and steps, 163
Thoracoscopic lobectomy, 425
Thoracoscopic surgical resection, robotically assisted resections, 436
Three-hole esophagectomy with robotic assistance, 420
Three Laws of Robotics, 3
3 M™ Bair Hugger™, 104
Thymectomy technique, 435, 436, 440–442
Tomographic imaging
  accuracy and speed, 60
  PUMA 200 robot, 53
  surgical workflow, 60
    mapping of coordinate frames, 61
    registration of preoperative CT images, 62
    ROBODOC® registration, 62
    segmentation, 63
    semiautomated registration techniques, 61
    visualization, 64
Total abdominal proctocolectomy, 96
Total gastrectomy
  operative steps
    conversion to open, 213
    distal esophagus division, 215
    greater curvature dissection, 214

lymphadenectomy, 215
omentectomy, 213–214
procedural setup, 213
proximal duodenum division, 214
Roux-en-Y jejunojejunostomy, 215–217
specimen retrieval, 215
patient positioning, 210–212
patient selection, 209–210
postoperative care and complications, 217
postoperative outcomes, 217
Total mesorectal excision (TME), 273
Transanal endoscopic microsurgery (TEM), 281
Transanal endoscopic operation (TEO), 281, 287
indications, 281
RTS approach, 292
Transanal excision (TAE) technique
colon and rectal cancer screening and prevention, 282
early-stage malignancy, 282
indications for RTS, 281
local excision and clinical surveillance, 281
mechanical bowel preparation, 282
over-the-colonoscope suturing device, 291
prone-jackknife split-leg position, 282
robotic suturing, surgical defect, 290
S and Xi Surgical Systems, 282
transanal access port, 284
Transanal minimally invasive surgery (TAMIS) technique, 281
Transanal repair of complex rectourethral fistulae, 281
Transanal total mesorectal excision (taTME), 281
Transaxillary approach for neck dissection, 489
Transaxillary robotic modified radical neck dissection
lateral neck lymph nodes
auricular nerve, 497
brachial nerve plexus, 496
distal external jugular vein, 494
docking and instrumentation, 493
docking procedure, 497
exclusion criteria, 490
external retractor and robotic axis, 492, 497
flap dissection, 492
Harmonic® curved shears, 493
hypoglossal nerve, 498
metastasis, 489
nonarticulated Harmonic® curved shears, 494
omohyoid muscle resection, 495
patient positioning, 491
phrenic nerve and transverse cervical artery, 496
postoperative wound, 499
preoperative ultrasonography, 489, 490
ProGrasp™ forceps, 493
skin flap elevation, 496
soft tissue and LN detachment, 492, 493
spinal accessory nerve, 497
stages, 499
subclavian vein, 494
submandibular gland, 498
surgical indications, 490
tactile feedback and limited instrumentation, 499
thoracic/lymphatic duct, 494
transverse cervical artery, 495
open and endoscopic thyroid surgery techniques, 489
surgical management, 489
thyroid cancer, lateral neck metastasis, 489
Transaxillary robotic thyroidectomy
breast lighted retractor, 467
central compartment neck dissection, 473–475
clinical practice, 465
complications, 476
contralateral superior thyroidal vessels, 475
contralateral upper pole dissection, 476
conventional open method, 465
curvilinear skin incision, 470
docking and instrumentation, 472, 473
enlarged thyroid, 466
equipments, 466
external retractor system, 468, 470, 471
follicular neoplasm, 466
Harmonic® curved shears, 473
instruments, 466
ipsilateral recurrent laryngeal nerve (RLN) identification, 474
limitations, 476
mechanical technology, 476
minimally invasive approaches, 465
nerve integrity monitor, 476
omohyoid muscle, 470
patient positioning, 469
postoperative pain, 476
postoperative wound, 475
recurrent laryngeal nerve, 465
remote site incisions, 465
robotic instrument placement, 473
skin incision, 465
sternocleidomastoid muscle, 470
subcutaneous skin flap, 470
superior parathyroid gland, 474
superior thyroidal vessels, 473
surgical indications, 465
tracheoesophageal groove, 466
transaxillary approach, 471
Western medicine, 465
Transient ipsilateral arm paralysis, 476
Transoral anvil, 215, 216
Transoral robotic radical tonsillectomy, 449, 450
Transoral robotic surgery (TORS)
da Vinci® system patient cart, 448
disease control, 451
HPV-positive oropharyngeal cancer, 451
ICU on intravenous steroids, 451
mandibulotomy, 451
nonrobotic surgical tools, 448
patient positioning, 447
postoperative management, 451
primary chemoradiation, 451
single-port system, 451
surgical instruments, 449
tongue retractors, 448
upper aerodigestive tract, 445
Transperitoneal laparoscopic adrenalectomy, 127
Trauma Pod, 10
Tri-Staple™, 150, 151

U

Unimation robot, 4
Ureteral dissection, 133
Ureteral stents, 274
Uretero-enteric anastomosis, 142
Urgent and emergent conversions
contingency plan
during hemorrhage, 85
emergency conversion time-out, 85
instruments, 85

Urgent and emergent conversions (*cont.*)
lost needle, instrument, or sponge, 86
robotic emergency time-out, 85
senior surgeon tricks, 86
simulations, 86
conversion to open operation causes, 80
foreign objects removal, 80
personnel roles, risk of bleeding, 85
planning rescue strategies, 79
preoperative planning and communications, 80–85
undocking causes, 80

V
Vascular pedicles ligation, 135
Ventral hernia repair
abdominal wall reconstructions, 455
adhesions, 454
benefits, 453
extensive adhesiolysis, 456
general anesthesia, 453
indications, 453
intra-abdominal pressure, 456
intracorporeal closure, 453, 455
mesh fixation, 455
myofascial advancement flaps, 455
myofascial release and complex repairs, 453
postoperative pain control, 456
preoperative systemic antibiotic for wound infection prophylaxis, 453
recurrence rates, 453
tackers and transabdominal sutures, 453
Veress technique, 336
Vesicourethral anastomosis, 123, 124
Video game-based simulation, 48
Virtual fixture, 12
Virtual reality simulators, 13
Volumetric imaging, 53

W
WABOT-1, 7
Warshaw's technique, 306
Whipple technique, 316
Wiklund neobladder, 155, 156

X
Xi Robotic system, 77, 83, 84, 104, 114, 115, 131, 162, 171, 173, 181, 183, 235, 426, 456

Y
Y-pouch neobladder, 156

Z
Zeus surgical robotic system, 8, 10